The Complete Book of
Symptoms and Treatments

THE COMPLETE BOOK OF

Symptoms & Treatments

Your Comprehensive Guide
to the Safety and Effectiveness of
Alternative and Complementary
Medicine for
Common Ailments

Roland Bettschart
Gerd Glaeske
Kurt Langbein
Reinhard Saller
Christian Skalnik

Edited by Edzard Ernst

ELEMENT

Shaftesbury, Dorset • Boston, Massachusetts
Melbourne, Victoria

First published in Germany as *Bittere Naturmedizin, Wirkung und Bewertung der alternativen Behandlungsmethoden, Diagnoseverfahren und Arneimittel*
© Verlag Kiepenheuer & Witsch, Köln 1995

© Element Books Limited 1998
Translation © D Wood 1998

This edition first published in the USA in 1998 by
Element Books, Inc.
160 North Washington Street, Boston, MA 02114

Published in the UK in 1998 by
Element Books Limited
Shaftesbury, Dorset SP7 8BP

Published in Australia in 1998 by
Element Books and distributed
by Penguin Books Australia Limited
487 Maroondah Highway, Ringwood,
Victoria 3134

Cover design by Slatter-Anderson
Typeset by Bournemouth Colour Press
Printed and bound in the USA by
Courier Westford
British Library Cataloguing in Publication
data available

Library of Congress Cataloging-in-Publication data
Bittere Naturmedizin. English.
The book of symptoms & treatments: a comprehensive guide to the
safety and effectiveness of alternative and complementary medical
treatments for common ailments / Roland Bettschard ... [et al.];
edited by Edzrd Ernst & translated by David Wood
p.   cm.
Includes bibliographical references and index.
ISBN 1–86204–424–7 (hb: alk. paper)
1. Alternative medicine. 2. Symptomatology. 3. Medicine.
Popular. 4. Self-care. Health. I. Bettschard. Roland. II. Ernst.
E. (Edzard) III. Title.
R733.B5713 1998
615.5—dc21
98–3697
CIP

ISBN 1 86204 424 4

Acknowledgments

The Editor is grateful to Jo Barnes, B Pharm (Hons), for a revision of the chapters on herbal treatments and to David Wood for translating from the German.

Contents

Introduction   xiii
The boom in complementary medicine and its implications   xiii
How to use this book   xvi
   The approach   xvi
   The main scientific principles of *The Complete Book of Symptoms and Treatments*   xvii
   The rating system used in *The Complete Book of Symptoms and Treatments*   xviii
You the consumer   xx
   "Alternative" or "complementary" medicine   xx
   Placebo   xxi
   Risk versus benefit   xxii
   Treatment plan and limited period trial   xxiii
   Finding the right therapist   xxiv

Prevention   1
Diet   2
   Changing poor eating habits   2
   What is healthy eating?   2
   Fat in various meats   4
   Organic diets   4
   Obesity and crash diets   6
Sports and exercise   8
Immune system modulation   10
   Orthodox treatment   10
   Complementary therapies   11

Part 1 Symptoms and disorders

Pain   23
Headaches and migraines   23
Neuralgia   36
Toothaches   47

Psyche and nervous system   57
Addiction to illicit and prescription drugs   57
Alcohol and nicotine withdrawal   66
Alzheimer's disease   75
Anxiety and worry   84
Bedwetting (enuresis)   93
Depression   100
Insomnia (sleeplessness)   109
Multiple sclerosis   120
Myalgic encephalomyelitis (ME) and chronic fatigue   130
Neuropathy   140
Parkinson's disease   149
Psychotic disorders   157

Muscles, bones, and joints   167
Back pain   167
Gout   180
Muscle soreness   187
Osteoporosis (brittle bone disease)   195
Rheumatism   202
Sprains and strains   216
Tendons and ligaments   222

Respiratory ailments   229
Asthma   229
Colds   239
Hoarseness and laryngitis   261
Mouth ulcers   267
Pneumonia   277
Sinusitis   286
Sore throat   297

Allergies   304

Skin   314
Acne   314

Herpes   322
Itching   331
Lice and mites   338
Neurodermatitis   341
Warts   350

Eyes   359
Conjunctivitis   359

Ears   363
Middle ear infection and earache   363
Tinnitus   372

Urinary system   380
Kidney and urinary tract disease   380
Prostate enlargement   391
Prostatitis   400

Heart and circulation   409
Angina pectoris   409
Atherosclerosis   420
High blood pressure (hypertension)   431
Low blood pressure (hypotension)   443
Cardiac arrhythmia   454
Heart attack   464
Heart failure (cardiac insufficiency)   474
Stroke   488
Varicose veins, phlebitis, and chronic venous insufficiency   499

Stomach, intestine, digestive system   512
Constipation   512
Diarrhea   525
Gall bladder disease   536
Gastritis, heartburn, gastric ulcers and duodenal ulcers   548
Hemorrhoids   564
Irritable bowel syndrome   574
Lack of appetite   583
Liver disease   598
Vomiting   608
Wind (meteorism and flatulence)   613
Worms   624

Metabolic disorders   627
Diabetes   627

High cholesterol   635
Thyroid disorders (goiter, hyperthyroidism and
hypothyroidism)   641

Sexual organs and secondary sexual characteristics   648
Breast disorders (mastopathy and mastodynia)   648
Fertility problems   656
Infections of the sexual organs, discharge   664
Menopause   672
Premenstrual syndrome (PMS)   682
Sexual problems   692

Cancer   701

AIDS   715

Ailments of the elderly   726

Children's ailments   742

Part 2 The therapies used in complementary medicine

Acupressure and shiatsu   769
Acupuncture   772
Anthroposophical medicine (AM)   781
Aromatherapy   786
Ayurveda   789
Bioresonance therapy (BRT)   794
Cell therapy   796
Chelation therapy   800
Electroacupuncture according to Voll (EAV)   802
Electroneural therapy according to Croon (ENT)   806
Eliminative methods   809
   Bloodletting   810
   Cantharidal poultices   812
   Cupping, bloody   815
   Cupping, unbloody   817
   Enemas   819
   Leeches   822
Enzyme therapy   824

Flower remedies 828
Homeopathy 831
Hypnosis and self-hypnosis 837
Magnetic field therapy 841
Manual therapies (chiropractic, osteopathy) 844
Massage 847
   Classical massage 847
   Lymphatic drainage 850
Medical herbalism (phytotherapy) 853
Nutritional therapies 858
   Hay's diet 858
   Macrobiotics 861
   Therapeutic fasting 864
Physical therapies 867
   Exercise therapy 868
   Hydrotherapy and hydrothermal therapy 871
Probiotics 878
Reflex therapies 881
   Reflexology 883
   Transcutaneous electrical nerve stimulation (TENS) 886
Relaxation techniques 888
   Autogenic training (basic level) 888
   Biofeedback 891
   Muscle relaxation according to Jacobson 893
Traditional Chinese medicine 895
Vitamins 900

Part 3 The diagnostic techniques used in complementary medicine

Applied kinesiology (AK) 907
Bioelectronics according to Vincent 909
Dowsing 910
Electroacupuncture according to Voll (EAV) 912
Electroneural diagnosis according to Croon 914
Hair mineral analysis 915
Iridology 917
Kirlian photography 918

Optical blood testing   920
Pendulum diagnosis   921
Thermoregulation diagnosis (TRD)   923
Tongue diagnosis   925

Glossary   927

Useful addresses   930

Authors and advisers   938

Index   941

Introduction

The boom in complementary medicine and its implications

This book is intended to be a reference to complementary medicine. The authors aim to guide you toward using both mainstream and complementary medicine in the best possible way, maximizing the benefits and minimizing the risks. Complementary healthcare has made a quantum leap over the last two decades, evolving from a fascinating side branch of medicine to a full-blown industry. With more and more being spent on nonorthodox therapies, it is reported from some countries that as much as a third of total expenditure on diagnosis and treatment falls to the nonorthodox sector. Surveys conducted in Europe and the USA have revealed a growing public awareness of, and interest in, the "gentle" and "holistic" types of medicine. Patients are increasingly seeking complementary treatments—either in addition to a conventional regime or as an alternative to it. This is perhaps because of a general, often deeply felt, disillusionment with mainstream medicine, perhaps out of mere curiosity, or perhaps out of a desire to assume responsibility for one's own health and well-being. Who does not have a friend or relative who has, at one time or another, resorted to a "natural" remedy to treat cold or flu symptoms? How many people would not themselves be prepared to give complementary medicine a try if all other attempts at treating a chronic or recurrent complaint have failed?

In the media there is no stopping the steady, trend reinforcing coverage given to complementary healthcare practices. There is likewise no apparent shortage of high-profile claims by celebrities to have been cured by this or that treatment. In some countries there are practitioners (and even doctors) who, in the press and on TV talk shows, promise what is tantamount to a complete cure. In glossy health magazines manufacturers and practitioners sponsor articles that promote their own natural products and treatments; the promises they make are sometimes honored—but are also often expensive.

Moreover, how natural is "natural"? Some procedures are based on high-tech wizardry, and the fact that the "person" is not necessarily their main focus is borne out by therapists' overflowing waiting rooms, the conveyor-belt processing of patients in some practice centers, and the fact that a not inconsiderable number of treatment providers seem to arrive monotonously at the same "diagnosis" and recommend the same therapy to their patients. In other words, the situation in some complementary centers is often very similar to that in orthodox medical practices. These are, it seems, drawbacks that exist in both worlds—medicine does not always come up to scratch, regardless of whether it is complementary or mainstream. This book will therefore expose some of the darker sides of complementary medicine. This is not intended to be alarmist, just to guide you safely to those practices which may do you more good than harm.

The boom in complementary medicine, the burgeoning number of therapies available and the ever more extravagant diagnostic procedures cannot gloss over the fact that discerning patients requiring reliable evidence that promises are being kept are often disappointed; there is indeed sometimes very little hard and fast proof to substantiate alternative practitioners' claims. The efficacy and mode of action of most complementary healthcare practices are more often than not only sparsely documented. Controlled clinical studies (*see* page xix), the backbone of orthodox medical science, are the exception in the complementary field. Little general credibility can be given to the typically euphoric outcome reports of some alternative practitioners or to the testimonials of over-enthused patients. Persons persuaded by promises made by complementary therapists are often walking on thin ice. Having said that, it must be recognized that while there may be no direct proof of the efficacy of some remedies, anecdotal evidence may indicate that they do work for many people. So absence of scientific evidence does not necessarily indicate that a remedy is ineffective.

One reason for the general lack of documentation relating to the presumed strengths and weaknesses of complementary medicine is the fact that, while as recently as two decades ago, the number of nonorthodox practitioners was too low to warrant serious scientific research, today many proponents of modern complementary medicine are not interested in supporting rigorous scientific research into the services they provide. On the one hand, to fare badly in an investigation would play into the hands of their opponents. On the other, there is currently no shortage of patients, so most practitioners seem to be happy with the status quo. Some providers of complementary medicine also maintain that their therapies defy the methodologies used for testing mainstream medicines. This is clearly not true. These methodologies may require a degree of adaptation, but there are no good reasons why they cannot also be used for testing complementary therapies.

The waters are also muddied by the fact that the debate between orthodoxy and nonorthodoxy is typically conducted in the form of a religious war, with "bunglers and charlatans" locked in battle with "proponents of cold, high-tech medicine." Information available to patients seeking advice almost always comes either from biased proponents of orthodox medicine or from the apologists of alternative medicine who promise a cure almost as the inevitable outcome of treatment. In practice the distinction between these two standpoints is being whittled away. While orthodox medical academia remains sceptical, at times downright dismissive, toward complementary medicine, there is now a new breed of mainstream doctors who are also prepared to reap the financial rewards of providing complementary healthcare or who take a more holistic approach to healthcare.

All this only serves to blur the picture and does little to help the patient separate the wheat from the chaff. Unfortunately it is the consumer who suffers. It may well be, however, that lack of sound information is preventing patients from enjoying the benefit of an appropriate complementary treatment. From another perspective, a scarcity of proper information may mean that certain procedures receive too much positive emphasis, while their risks are underestimated; or that rash promises by complementary practitioners are depriving the patient of sound orthodox diagnosis and/or therapy. In the latter case, even complementary medicine can metamorphose from a gentle healing technique into a risk factor. This book, we hope, will enable you to avoid the risks and fully enjoy the benefits of complementary medicine.

How to use this book

The philosophy behind this book is a desire to make available the best that mainstream and complementary medicine can offer.

The approach

The Complete Book of Symptoms and Treatments is divided into three parts. Part One addresses the most common ailments and symptoms, arranging them, where possible, according to type of complaint or organ affected. Each chapter opens with a brief description of the ailment or symptom, followed by a brief summary of the orthodox medical approach to its treatment, and then by a résumé of complementary therapies, with cautions where appropriate. A system of cross-references will guide you to other relevant sections. There follows an alphabetical table of the most commonly used complementary treatments, which gives a benefit rating and details of possible risks. The therapies listed are those that are used frequently for the respective condition; procedures that find only scant use or that are practiced by the "fringe element" are not included. Each chapter closes with a list of the most popular herbal remedies (phytotherapeutics) that may be employed to alleviate that ailment or its associated symptoms, again with a rating of potential benefit and warnings of potential risks.

Part Two is an A–Z review of the most popular complementary therapies available. It starts by presenting the rationale of each therapy, followed by an explanation of how it works and a rating of the potential benefit to the patient. The yardstick used to rate each therapy is the total body of scientific knowledge available today. Criteria for choosing a reputable practitioner are provided, with useful addresses (e.g. of professional organizations).

Part Three describes the main principles of the diagnostic techniques commonly used in complementary medicine and examines the rationale of each method followed by a rating of practitioners' own claims as to how it works and its diagnostic precision. The current body of scientific knowledge is again taken as the yardstick for rating each therapy.

The main scientific principles of *The Complete Book of Symptoms and Treatments*

The Complete Book of Symptoms and Treatments certainly is not aimed against alternative or complementary medicine, nor does it promote this field of healthcare. Its aim is, in fact, to provide a critical appraisal of individual complementary healthcare practices and realistically assess individual techniques used to treat the commonest ailments and symptoms. It might be seen as an aid to maintaining your bearings in the jungle of complementary medical practices, and will help you, the patient, view complementary remedies responsibly and as objectively as possible. The ratings were compiled by a panel of scientific experts. They are based on

- available published data on the efficacy of individual complementary practices
- available published data on the possible risks of individual complementary therapies
- available published data on how individual complementary therapies work
- particularly in the absence of "hard data," the panel's subjective appraisal of the potential efficacy of, and risks inherent in, individual complementary therapies when used for that ailment or set of symptoms; special weighting was given to these subjective appraisals in any case where there was a lack of empirical data

Information sources included:

- the Medline, Embase, Current Contents, and other medical databases

- British, American, German, and French journals of complementary medicine
- complementary medicine textbooks and other standard works published within the last 50 years

The Complete Book of Symptoms and Treatments is *not* an exhaustive medical reference text and is in no way intended as a replacement for the diagnosis and care provided by a physician. Anyone with unexplained symptoms *must* consult a qualified doctor.

The rating system used in *The Complete Book of Symptoms and Treatments*

All ratings assigned to the complementary diagnostic and therapeutic techniques, and the potential benefit that can be expected to be derived from them in the treatment or alleviation of individual ailments and symptoms, are based on the appraisals of our panel of scientific advisers and on the current body of scientific knowledge. The ratings themselves, like the reasons for defining them thus, are subjective assessments that are based on state of the art scientific research and on detailed analyses of the medical literature; they can be justified scientifically.

As in any branch of medicine, all statements made regarding the efficacy of, or the risk/benefit evaluation assigned to, a given therapy are founded on statistical probability, so the rating "efficacious" does not necessarily imply efficacy in every single patient.

- **Useful** means that, in the view of our panel of experts, the efficacy of a complementary procedure or of the active principle(s) of a herbal remedy in dealing with a given ailment or set of symptoms is supported by a favorable body of evidence and that, used competently, the anticipated benefit to the patient outweighs the inherent risks.
- **Only useful** implies that, in the view of our panel of experts, the efficacy of a complementary procedure or of the active principle(s) of a herbal remedy in dealing with one or more symptoms of an ailment is only supported by a favorable body of evidence for a circumscribed set of conditions but that, with competent use, the anticipated benefit to the

patient outweighs the inherent risks. In the case of a herbal remedy "only useful" may also imply a limitation in terms of the way in which it is administered.

- **May be of some use** signifies that, in the view of our panel of experts, there is some good evidence to suggest that the complementary procedure or the active principle(s) of a remedy might be effective in dealing with specific ailments, complaints or symptoms, but that there is insufficient evidence to permit a definitive judgment.
- **Of little use** means that, in the view of our panel of experts, the efficacy of a complementary procedure or of the active principle(s) of a remedy in dealing with one or more symptoms of an ailment is only supported by weak evidence but that, with competent use, the inherent risk is considered to be small.
- **Inappropriate** means that, in the view of our panel of experts, a complementary procedure is not suitable for treating a primary disease (e.g. AIDS, multiple sclerosis, etc.). Whether and to what degree it can address secondary symptoms is rated separately.
- **Not advised** means that, in the view of our panel of experts, there is no or only insufficient evidence to prove the efficacy of a complementary procedure or the active principle(s) of a remedy, either alone or in combination, but that there is evidence of potential risks.

The rating is followed by a statement of the nature of that body of evidence on which it was based.

- **Controlled clinical studies**. These are employed to enable the efficacy of a procedure to be seen divorced from other possibly beneficial factors, such as the special doctor/patient relationship. Ideally, treatment allocation is "randomized," which means that chance alone decides which patients receive the experimental treatment and which the control or sham treatment. This method ensures the two groups are comparable. Clinical studies are often carried out "double blind," which means that neither the patient nor the therapist knows whether the treatment being studied is the real one or the sham (*see* Placebo, page xxi). Randomized double-blind studies are the mainstay of orthodox drug testing. When conducted against a placebo control, they show whether and to what extent the drug is superior to a placebo.

- **Post-marketing surveillance studies**. These are documents detailing the history of treatments administered to a patient and on which the clinical outcome, positive or negative, must be recorded. In practice they are often tantamount to an accumulation of case reports, but with more detail. They provide little useful information regarding the efficacy of the treatment, as there is no comparison (unlike in controlled clinical studies) and no allowance is made for possible placebo effects (*see* page xxi). They can, however, be valuable for assessing risks.

- **Case reports**. These are used by practitioners simply to document the fact that a treatment was carried out, and what the outcome was. As with post-marketing studies, it is impossible to deduce conclusively to what extent the outcome, or the patient's condition after treatment, was due to the treatment given. Often, not all treatments are recorded—only those with a positive outcome. Case reports thus give no indication of success rates. What is more, most of the positive outcome reports tend to be anecdotal and passed on by word of mouth.

- **Case studies**. Case studies consist of series of case reports, usually from one and the same practitioner. Unlike controlled clinical trials, they are not comparative and therefore do not account for possible placebo effects (*see* page xxi). Positive selection by the investigator can produce misleading results.

- **Testimonials**. Testimonials are anecdotal accounts by patients about the benefits they claim to have derived personally from a treatment. Testimonials are, almost by nature, of a positive character and are normally seen published in the form of newspaper advertisements. As evidence they have little to offer.

You the consumer

"Alternative" or "complementary" medicine?

"Alternative medicine" used to be a catchall phrase denoting any healing practice that failed to meet the approval of the orthodox medical world. The label "alternative," in a political sense, also typified the stance taken by certain groups or individuals who were vehemently opposed to what they saw as the choking principles of orthodoxy and proposed their own practices as a counterpoint to those of the medical establishment. In the meantime, the term "complementary medicine" has come to be the more accepted term. Reputable proponents of complementary medicine do not see their relationship with mainstream medicine in terms of "either/or" but rather as supportive and collaborative. Their aim, in particular, is to open to patients a broader range of therapies and make available the best that mainstream *and* complementary medicine jointly have to offer; this is also the philosophy behind *The Complete Book of Symptoms and Treatments*.

Placebo

Placebo is the Latin for "I shall please." In clinical research, a placebo is a dummy drug, identical in taste and appearance to the real thing, but containing no active constituents. What is remarkable is that, through a suggestive effect, a placebo can elicit a positive response to treatment and, indeed, actually cure patients who strongly believe that they have taken a real drug. Believing in a drug or therapy is an extremely powerful force in medicine. Clinical researchers use placebos to try and isolate the effect of the active agent contained in a drug from the suggestive effect of treatment: for instance, from that produced by the special doctor/patient relationship. Randomized double-blind trials are studies in which patients are split up randomly into subgroups and assigned to a doctor, with neither the doctor nor the patient knowing whether the treatment is the real one or the control treatment; both the doctor and patient are "blind."

Investigations of this type are designed to show whether and by what margin the drug is more efficacious than the placebo. Placebos have also been known to have adverse effects.

Mind–health connections such as the placebo effect have for some time now been the object of heightened scientific research. The relatively new discipline of psychoneuroimmunology (PNI) is trying to make sense of the long suspected and frequently observed links between emotions and the immune system, and to put them into a scientific framework. Though the links themselves have not yet been fully elucidated, PNI researchers have managed time and again to demonstrate the effects of emotional phenomena such as stress, bereavement, hope, and euphoria on the numbers of certain types of immune cells circulating in the blood.

Treatment with a placebo can certainly not be equated with a treatment that simply does not work. What is more, a placebo effect may be patient-specific. This means in practice that, even with complementary therapies, no treatment that has not been the subject of controlled clinical study may be substituted willy-nilly for another in the same patient without there being some difference in effect. Little is known at present about the finer aspects of these links. This makes it all the more difficult to judge what is a placebo response and what is the specific effect of treatment.

Whether treatment with a placebo is effective or not depends on a number of factors, which include the doctor/patient relationship, the patient's aspirations and expectations, and his/her emotional and mental state; and also on certain suggestive, symbolic, and cultural elements (in cultures where people believe in it, for example, voodoo is actually capable of killing).

There are no grounds for concluding, just because a placebo effect is presumed in a patient, that the condition is psychosomatic or even imagined. Pain researchers can confirm, for instance, that placebo reactions seem to be more powerful, and to occur more frequently, in patients with truly physical pain than in those presenting with pain of psychosomatic origin.

Complex connections such as these have made it incredibly difficult to evaluate complementary healthcare practices definitively. There is no doubt, though, that all branches of medicine would profit from being able to study the results of long overdue controlled clinical trials into the placebo effect.

Risk versus benefit

Wherever controlled clinical studies have been conducted into the efficacy of a therapy, the results do enable a risk/benefit evaluation to be made. However, it is important to remember that a medical prediction is based simply on probabilities, so that no definitive predictions are possible for an individual patient.

Whether the patient belongs to that group in which, statistically, the expected benefit *is* seen, or in which adverse effects *are* to be expected, cannot be said with certainty before treatment. This problem is compounded by the fact that there have been few controlled clinical studies in complementary medicine. Given this situation, it is easy to appreciate the difficulties involved in predicting not only how an individual patient will react but, indeed, in a larger group, even how the majority will react.

In all branches of medicine, any treatment is, by nature, an experiment. Controlled clinical studies do play a significant part, therefore, in optimizing the experimental preconditions, in maximizing the chance of benefit to the patient and minimizing the possible risk.

Any therapeutic decision, taken responsibly, will take account of what might be achieved with other therapies. For example, a patient with severe cancer pains may well be relieved by judicious use of a complementary procedure. The main question to ask, of course, is whether the patient might not be better served by an appropriate dose of morphine.

Considerations such as these make it necessary to draw up a treatment plan that has a defined goal, as a yardstick by which the efficacy of treatment in a given patient and his/her quality of life may be measured.

Treatment plan and limited-period trial

In the complementary health sector treatments may become very protracted for want of a precise diagnosis. A claim made by a practitioner that the patient has a buildup of waste products, or that his/her body contains disease-causing foci (*see* page 928) or toxins (*see* page 929), or that there is an energy imbalance (*see* page 927) or a precancerous condition, or that his/her immunological age is too high, generally defies rational investigation to the same extent that it is impossible to verify the efficacy or otherwise of the treatment subsequently given.

Such "universal diagnoses" are part of the standard repertoire of some complementary practitioners. It is therefore essential that the practitioner draws up a treatment plan setting out a clear and appropriate time frame and defining the aim to be achieved by the therapy, with due consideration being given to quality of life. Whether the particular therapy is working or not should then be monitored in a limited term course of treatment. Decision-making may be aided of course by previous experience.

If the treatment is not coming up to expectation, it should be discontinued. Even useful therapies become pointless, not to mention expensive, when used for too long without being monitored for a successful outcome. Insisting on a written treatment plan or contract will put you in a position where you can assert your rights if you have recourse to the law.

Finding the right therapist

Most complementary therapies may be carried out by doctors or healthcare practitioners without special training and qualification. In some countries qualified doctors specifically describe themselves as naturopaths, acupuncturists, or homeopaths. These titles generally reveal little about the individual's knowledge and skills. Many professional organizations certify their members as having received proper training in their particular complementary discipline. Most patients, however, have difficulty in judging the genuineness of these organizations; some, for instance, are closely allied to manufacturers of products or equipment, some see themselves as lobby groups. For this reason, you should not view the professional organizations listed in this book as being specifically endorsed by us; they are rather to be seen as organizations and associations from which you can obtain information. While, in most cases, the fact that a practitioner is a member of a reputable professional association does give some assurance as to the type and quality of training he/she has received and of the standards of treatment that can be expected, it does not provide any guarantee as to the appropriateness of that treatment.

A good therapist will generally not offer treatment until the patient's condition has been conventionally diagnosed; he/she will involve the patient in formulating a treatment goal, then draw up a treatment plan (*see* page xxiii), initially for limited term treatment, to enable the patient's progress to be monitored. No credence should be given to practitioners promising a complete or instantaneous cure.

Practitioner checklist

A good therapist

- will talk to you at length to find out about any conventional diagnoses already made and any treatments you are already receiving, and will examine aspects of your life, work, diet, and exercise
- will carry out a thorough examination and explain the basis on which the diagnosis is founded
- will talk to you about what the examination has revealed and what treatment he/she proposes
- will formulate a proper plan for limited term treatment, explain why he/she thinks this treatment will help, and give details of other (possibly conventional) treatments that may help
- will discuss with you any changes to the treatment plan
- will discuss with you how earlier or existing treatments or prescribed medications can be made to fit into the treatment plan
- will willingly provide information about credentials, training, qualifications, and indemnity
- will discuss the cost of treatment with you and help you claim for the treatment through your health insurance, if you have it

A bad therapist

- will claim to be able to cure your ailment completely or instantaneously
- will suggest that he/she knows exactly what is wrong with you
- will shun conventional medicine and even other alternative therapies
- will advise you to start treatment immediately, even for non-acute conditions, to prevent awful repercussions
- will omit to tell you about the possible side effects of the treatment, or assure you there is not the slightest risk
- will decline to discuss treatment with you in advance
- will insist you throw out all other treatments and medications
- will dissuade you from obtaining a second opinion from an

independent doctor or therapist, or even try to prevent you from speaking to anyone before carrying out the treatment
- will sometimes ask for cash up front for more protracted treatments
- will often have dubious degrees or diplomas, usually from an untraceable source

Prevention

Health, in the definition of the World Health Organization (WHO), is the state of complete physical, mental, and social well-being and not simply the absence of disease and infirmity. The rather optimistic attempt to juxtapose the fairly mechanistic approach to health by the orthodox medical world—which does, hand on heart, sometimes reduce its view of health to the absence of physical disease—with what is otherwise a fairly "holistic" ideal is beset with problems. Is there anyone who does permanently enjoy a state of physical, mental, and social well-being?

To bridge the gap between reality and the WHO's almost impossible ideal is the aim of a loud army of health gurus, nutritional experts, fitness freaks, and the like, warning of impending doom and giving conflicting advice which it is often impossible to follow. Anyone who does not heed their advice—preferably immediately—is faced with the hideous prospect of lifelong obesity and poor health.

There is no disputing that one's lifestyle is shaped through one's education and life experiences and through environmental influences. A lifestyle is a very difficult thing to change, which is why health damaging habits are better modified a step at a time, to give the successes achieved a chance to be absorbed. (Only scientific research can help define what habits are actually detrimental to health.) Consequently, the resolve to lead a healthier lifestyle should be integrated gradually into one's everyday life. The way to improved physical well-being may have less to do with self-denial and strict discipline than with pleasure and *joie de vivre*. Social factors play a significant role, of course, since stress, job dissatisfaction, and lack of personal fulfillment can all make you ill.

Diet

In many parts of Europe people consume, statistically speaking, 50 percent more calories than they actually require. Overeating is the cause of many of the classic ills of civilization. Obesity and high blood cholesterol levels may bring on atherosclerosis, (*see* page 564), heart disease, and circulatory problems (*see* pages 409). Obesity is also a contributory factor in diabetes (*see* page 622) and even arthritis. Eating too much meat results in too high an intake not only of fat and cholesterol but also of protein; excessive protein consumption overloads the kidneys and is known to be one of the causes of gout. Eating less meat lessens the risk of cancer and heart disease. Too much sugar can cause obesity and tooth decay.

Changing poor eating habits

In many people eating and drinking are processes that are not controlled rationally, being driven instead by emotions and force of habit. The first step toward correcting poor eating habits might be an attempt to discover their causes:

- When and why do I eat too much?
- Do I eat too hastily, consuming more than is good for me?
- Do I often skip a meal, only to binge later?
- What would I like to weigh, and why?
- Why am I overweight or underweight?

Nutritional experts often advise people to keep a precise log of all they eat and drink over a period of several days. Did I eat simply to satisfy my appetite or were there other factors: boredom, stress, frustration, or a specific set of circumstances such as watching TV? Once the causes have been analyzed, a way can be sought to limit the craving for calories. Speaking to a professional dietician may help. *See also* pages 858–67.

What is healthy eating?

There are enough books, magazines, and TV programs offering advice as to what constitutes "healthy eating." Many have one thing in common: they advocate, sometimes quite vociferously, a specific type of diet, ranging from a vegetarian diet on the one hand to a so-called "Eskimo diet," which is anything but vegetarian, on the other. While vegans and believers in macrobiotics consider dairy products to be unhealthy, modern research ascribes to fermented dairy products and lactic acid bacteria a whole raft of beneficial effects. For some dietary faddists even moderate consumption of alcohol is anathema; the latest wisdom is, however, that a glass or two of wine will possibly ward off heart and circulatory disease.

So what is the right path to health? There is general consensus among nutritional experts that modern eating habits are an unhealthy development. Since the mid-1940s we have as a society reduced our intake of roughage in the form of cereals and vegetables, but at the same time increased our consumption of meat. One effect of eating animal fat, it is now felt, is that it increases the flow of bile, which is suspected of causing bowel cancer. Dietary fiber is thought to absorb bile acids and so ensure that they are eliminated as quickly as possible from the body. Another point to remember is that fats contain more than twice as many calories as proteins and carbohydrates; high consumption of fatty meat is thus a principal cause of obesity. One further point: meat contains purines, and the breakdown products of these organic substances are known to cause gout.

The great meat-eating debates of years gone by were usually won by the proponents of a vegetarian lifestyle. Various long-term studies showed that people who consume little or no meat tend, on balance, to be in better health and live longer; and also to be more likely to have an ideal weight (*see* pages 6–8), lower blood pressure, lower uric acid and blood lipid levels, and better kidney function. They are also deemed to be exempt from the risk factors that lie at the root of nearly all modern lifestyle diseases.

However, such arguments are deceptive and should not be used to advocate a diet that shuns meat entirely. Other research has shown that strict vegans (that is to say those who refuse any animal product, including honey) are in poorer health than moderate meat eaters. The latest investigations have shown that it is advisable to maintain a relatively low level of meat consumption and to opt more for low-fat varieties such as chicken and turkey. However, even pork or beef, given the right cuts, can be eaten as part of a reasonably low-fat diet.

Fat in various meats

The fat contents of selected cuts of pork and beef are as follows (weight of fat in grams per 4 ounces of uncooked meat):

- escalope of pork 1.9g/4oz
- pork tenderloin 2.0g/4oz
- beef tenderloin 4.0g/4oz
- lean roast beef 4.5g/4oz
- pork chop 5.2g/4oz
- roast joint of beef 8.1g/4oz
- boiled fillet of beef 9.3g/4oz
- knuckle of pork 12.2g/4oz
- belly of pork 29.0g/4oz

Some agencies recommend that our diet should consist of 55 percent carbohydrates and that our energy intake should consist of no more than 30 percent fats. For the man in the street, however, these recommendations are hard to follow as, to provide all the required nutritional elements, it takes numerous complex calculations just for one day's meal plan. Pragmatic nutritionists therefore recommend a simpler approach that is based on the assignment of foods to groups. The most important groups are made up of foods of plant origin—namely cereals, cereal products, and potatoes; vegetables and pulses; and fruit. Other groups are: fluids (beverages); milk and dairy products; meat, fish, and eggs; and fats and oils. Each day's meals should include foods from every group, with the emphasis always being on the plant groups. The diet will then automatically be varied and well balanced and prevent deficiencies.

Organic diets

An organic diet is one that not only complies with physiological, nutritional, and toxicological aspects but also takes account of ecological and social factors. Foods are expected to be produced locally, where possible, by organic farmers and market gardeners (to reduce the environmental impact of transporting them to market), and to be packaged in an environmentally friendly way.

Organic foods make appetizing meals. The chief organic foods are wholegrain products, vegetables and fruit, potatoes, pulses, and milk and dairy produce, which may be combined with small amounts of meat, fish, or eggs. Roughly half of a person's food intake should be made up of fresh, uncooked food. Meals should be prepared gently, with as little fat as possible.

An organic diet can guard to a degree against such problems as obesity, diabetes, gout, kidney stones, arteriosclerosis, cardiovascular disease, high blood pressure, digestive disorders, and tooth decay. Researchers have discovered a lower incidence of breast and bowel cancer, for instance, in people who eat a low-fat diet, and of bowel cancer in people who eat a high-fiber diet. Fiber, or roughage, is the coarse bulky component of foods, mostly plant, that is relatively indigestible for humans. There is a high proportion of fiber in fruit and vegetables, fresh salads, and wholegrain cereals. Fiber is effective in lowering blood glucose and cholesterol levels and reducing the toxicity of environmental pollutants, as well as in promoting normal bowel function. In recent years there have been indications that an adequate supply (not yet quantified) of selenium, beta-carotene, and the vitamins C and E may influence certain phenomena implicated in the development of cancer (*see* Vitamins, page 900).

A relatively new area of research is now actively looking into the curative effects of certain phytochemicals, bioactive substances, and other secondary components that occur widely in fruit, vegetables, and cereals. Plants synthesize these active principles, of which there are thought to be some 5,000–10,000, in secondary metabolic processes. As they are "non-essential," the human body does not need them to survive. It was assumed for a long time that they are produced by plants as a protection against pests, as growth regulators, or as color, smell, and taste defining substances. However, tests on animals and *in vitro* are showing more and more that some phytochemicals might be effective against modern lifestyle diseases such as cancer and cardiovascular disease, and new buzzwords are making the rounds: "dietary pharmacology" and "chemoprevention." It is thought that these secondary principles in plants are able, *inter alia*, to slow down the development of certain types of cancer or even prevent them altogether, to regulate blood pressure and blood glucose levels, to reduce blood fats, to kill bacterial and fungal infections, to inhibit inflammation, and to stimulate the immune system. The implications of this research for the human organism as yet remain unclear, however. *See also* pages 858–67.

Obesity and crash diets

One formula used in the past to define a person's ideal weight went as follows: men should weigh, in kilograms, as much as their height in centimetres less a hundred, while for women the figure should be the same less a further 10 percent. Health was deemed to be at risk whenever a person was more than 10 percent over his/her normal weight.

Today there is much controversy surrounding these figures, and uncertainty prevails. Likewise, the premise that an ideal weight, such as that proposed at one time by some US insurance companies, leads to the highest life expectancy turned out to be flawed. A person's ideal weight may well be that at which he or she feels most at ease. The "ideal" can turn out to be a millstone if attempts to attain it become obsessive.

Judging by the number of television features and the wealth of books and magazine articles, losing weight is a topic that rarely fails to attract an audience. There is no shortage of neatly packaged promises. Hardly a year goes by in which a new diet is not added to the already long list of classical crash diets. However, the promises and the associated "wand-waving" sometimes verge on quackery. Quick fix diets promising maximum weight loss are usually ineffective in the medium term—and often even harmful.

- When a person is on a high-protein crash diet, the body is unable to eliminate the excess waste products formed. Crash diets may lead to a situation in which uric acid builds up in the blood and crystals of urea form in the joints, possibly leading to gout. Excessive protein consumption produces nitrogenous waste with which the kidneys can no longer cope. Persons with a kidney problem should therefore steer clear of such diets.
- High-fat dieting programs are known to damage health. Anyone overindulging in this type of program runs the risk

of increased blood fat and uric acid values, and the likelihood of gout or cardiovascular disease. There is increasing reason to suspect that excessive fat intake may also favor bowel cancer.

- After just a couple of days without carbohydrates there is a change in kidney function, leading to significant losses of water and electrolytes. This may set in train a very risk-laden process: the person's blood pressure falls, in the elderly possibly leading to stroke (*see* page 488). Losing calcium also irritates the heart and may lead to cardiac arrhythmia (*see* page 454).

Any hopes of converting the initial weight loss achieved in high-fat and high-protein diets into longer-term success are generally dashed; 70 percent of the lost pounds are accounted for by loss of fluids, and only 30 percent through an actual reduction in body fat. In low-fat diets the desired effects generally take longer to achieve but, by contrast, with a comparable calorie intake the body will lose about 80 percent body fat and 20 percent water.

Though some people might indeed lose weight through a high-fat, high-protein diet, only a minuscule number manage to keep the pounds off in the long term. Nutritional experts have an explanation for this—and for why you might end up even fatter than before. Because it is unable to tell the difference between a natural famine and a dieting program, the body initiates its own survival strategies. First, leaving its fat reserves (for the time being) untouched, it turns its attention to its energy reserves, which it uses to overcome food shortage in the short term. The energy reserves are located chiefly in the liver and muscle tissues and consist of sugars and glycogen. Every ounce of these, however, is combined with about 4 ounces of water. The relatively high weight loss seen at the start of a dieting program is thus due primarily to water loss which, unfortunately, cannot be sustained indefinitely.

It is only after about the fifth day of a weight-loss program that the body actually starts to draw on its fat reserves. Again, it adopts various defensive strategies. When deprived of calories it releases and produces the hormones and enzymes responsible for storing fat in the cells: for example, the enzyme lipoprotein lipase (LPL). This enzyme, which is probably already present in excess in persons with a hereditary predisposition to obesity, is then also produced by persons of normal weight. After several days of dieting, the body's so-called basal metabolic rate is lowered. This is a measure of the number of calories that can be ingested without a person gaining weight. In dieting programs of this type the body soon becomes used to managing with fewer calories. At the end of the program, if the dieter gives way to his or her voracious appetite, any calories that are eaten over and above the readjusted baseline requirement are converted into fat at an even greater rate than before. LPL remains fully functional beyond the end of the diet and, with the body now accustomed to a lower metabolic turnover, continues to replenish depleted fat cells at a significant rate. The infamous yo-yo effect is preprogrammed, and the person's hopes of acquiring a slim figure disappear over the horizon.

Modern nutritionists would suggest that the most appropriate diet is one that involves only a slightly reduced calorie intake leading to slow breakdown of fatty tissues. Indeed, the daily intake should be between 500 and 1,000 calories, with the diet leading to a long-term change in eating habits. A modest level of exercise will certainly be a beneficial adjunct to this type of diet, as it builds up the muscles. Compared to fat, muscle tissue has a high rate of metabolism and also has the advantage of using up calories. *See also* pages 858–67.

Sports and exercise

Stamina, strength, agility, and good coordination are important for health. Sport can heighten the feeling of well-being, give you a "buzz," and guard against a number of ailments. When properly done, endurance training can slow down the pulse by strengthening the heart muscle, so the body's oxygen requirement can be covered with fewer heart contractions. Anyone who can reduce their pulse from 85 to 65 beats per minute will spare their heart 864,000 beats per month, meaning that it "wears out" less quickly.

Endurance exercise can down-regulate the autonomic nervous system and reduce the total amount of stress hormones released. This again serves to slow down the pulse and lengthen the recovery phase between two heartbeats. Blood circulation is improved and oxygen transport becomes more efficient. The heart itself needs less oxygen and the risk of infarction decreases.

Such exercise can also slow down the ageing process. Fit muscles and ligaments are much less likely to be damaged in the event that they have to take a sudden strain. Glandular functions improve. The sense organs remain functional for longer and the risk of osteoporosis (*see* page 195) can be reduced. Some experts would even claim that, with proper exercise, life expectancy can be prolonged by as much as 25 percent.

Regular exercise and sports can also positively influence existing ailments. In diabetes mellitus (*see* page 627) it can lower blood glucose readings and reduce levels of fat in the blood (*see* page 7). Stretching, swimming, and cycling can help people with rheumatism (*see* page 202) to overcome the dreaded morning stiffness and bent finger syndrome. Regular exercise will also ease arthritis and help persons with depressive moods cope better.

On the down side, however, a highly competitive mentality, the stress associated with important events, and the injuries occasionally sustained can add a significant element of risk to sports. What one should do, perhaps, is think less competitively and have the courage to slow down. According to one classical definition, fitness should enable you to achieve physical and mental well-being to help you deal with the rigors of everyday life.

An important point to remember when you are training is that all exercise should remain aerobic; in other words, you should not work the muscles beyond the point at which they are still just able to meet their oxygen needs with oxygen carried in the blood. Overworking muscles, on the other hand, produces anaerobic conditions and the muscle must then find its own supply of oxygen, which it achieves through metabolic changes that do more harm than good.

Adults intending to take up sports, for the first time or again, are urgently advised to ask their doctor to give them a thorough medical checkup, or at least to test the function of their lungs, muscles, and heart. It is advisable to start with a coordinated program of circulation and muscle exercises under trained supervision. Limbering up properly will reduce the risk of torn muscles and ligaments. For those over 50, gentle stamina building exercises are advised; newcomers should avoid explosive or "all-out" disciplines such as weightlifting or sprinting.

It does not really take too much effort to become, and remain, fit: exercising for 30 minutes three times a week is probably adequate. Swimming, walking, rowing, and jogging, in moderation, are deemed particularly beneficial as they are dynamic and concentrate on building up stamina. So you see, even noncompetitive sports will help you improve your general fitness.

Stop and rest frequently. Children, when playing, do this frequently after a short burst of activity. They run, stop, then carry on—automatically.

Immune system modulation

The immune system is highly complex and linked to virtually all of the body's physical functions and mental processes. This means it has a key role in almost any disease a person may develop, but often its mechanisms and effects are rather unclear.

Immunotherapies are now used in the treatment of various diseases, including some forms of cancer. They are based on the latest research findings and liable to change as new information emerges. Most of the treatments offered cannot be neatly categorized as "immunostimulation" or "immunosuppression" and tend to modulate rather than simply stimulate or suppress in isolation. Attempts at achieving immunomodulation are currently being made in experimental cancer therapy, with various substances being used in an attempt to elicit reactions within the body, in the hope that these will slow the progression of the disease or eliminate it altogether.

There has been very little research, for most diseases, into the efficacy of, and the balance of risk versus benefit achieved with, this type of immunological approach.

Orthodox treatment

Orthodox treatment of immunological disorders is at the clinical study stage and has only been routinely used so far in a very limited number of clinical situations, for example, during organ transplantation. Immunosuppression has been tried experimentally in certain diseases such as severe forms of rheumatism. Benefit and risk cannot be directly deduced from experimental research or from theoretical considerations. Benefit can only be confirmed through reproducible clinical results and controlled clinical studies. Some complementary treatments and remedies may have an immunomodulating effect, though the clinical significance of these findings is yet to be established.

Complementary therapies

Some complementary treatments focus on immunomodulation. However, for most diseases, in particular the more severe ones, there have been few if any clinical studies, so no risk/benefit assessments can be given. Many such approaches to the immune system fail to take account of the body of scientific knowledge and of the problems associated with administering this type of treatment to the patient.

Treatment plan and limited trial

Before administering a complementary treatment, every therapist should draw up a treatment plan (*see* page xxiii) that sets out a clear time-frame and defines the goal that the treatment is designed to achieve. Treatment should then be tried for a limited term to test the patient's response.

Warning

In those diseases or other conditions where immunological therapy is an accepted practice, present findings indicate that complementary treatments are no substitute for orthodox immunotherapy.

Complementary treatments to modulate the immune system

Treatment	Rating	Point of delivery/risks
Acupressure This treatment (*see* page 769), otherwise known as pressure-point massage, is claimed to activate the immune system when the appropriate pressure points are stimulated.	**Of little use** Acceptable as a short-term treatment attempt. Case reports and field studies claim efficacy; however, success is probably seen in only a small proportion of patients (*see* Placebo, page xxi).	**Suitable for DIY** Qualified guidance is recommended. **Risks:** Unlikely provided treatment is carried out competently.
Acupuncture Acupuncture in its various forms (*see* page 772) aims to encourage the flow of energy (*see* page 927) or to act directly on the immune system. The acupuncture points chosen can vary from one practitioner to another.	**Of little use** Acceptable as a short-term treatment attempt. Case reports and field studies claim efficacy; however, success is probably seen in only a proportion of patients (*see* Placebo, page xxi).	**Requires a qualified practitioner** Practitioners should be properly qualified and should propose a treatment plan. **Risks:** Probably rare provided treatment is carried out competently.
Anthroposophical medicine AM (*see* page 781) holds mistletoe extract in great regard as an immuno-modulating agent, particularly in the treatment of cancer. It is claimed to build up the body's defences and improve general well-being. Some therapists even take the view that mistletoe preparations are able to arrest tumor growth.	**May be of some use** as a supportive treatment attempt for cancer. Some studies claim efficacy; however, success is probably seen in only a proportion of patients (*see* Placebo, page xxi). There have not been any controlled clinical trials to substantiate claims that mistletoe preparations are able to inhibit growth of tumors.	**Requires a qualified practitioner** Practitioners should be properly qualified and should propose a treatment plan. **Risks:** Allergies, toxic reactions, or intolerance are possible.

Treatment	Rating	Point of delivery/risks
Aromatherapy Essential oils (*see* page 786) are used to soothe and relax, or to invigorate, thereby stimulating the immune system. The essences may be taken orally, used externally as massage oils or bathing emulsions, or inhaled as vapors.	**Of little use** Acceptable as a short-term treatment attempt aimed at improvement of mood or well-being. Some case reports claim efficacy in terms of modulation of the immune system; however, success is probably seen in only a proportion of patients (*see* Placebo, page xxi).	**Suitable for DIY** Qualified guidance is recommended. The effects of individual essential oils differ widely. **Risks:** Allergies or intolerance are possible. Some oils are carcinogenic in test systems and possibly in humans.
Bioresonance therapy Bioresonance therapists use electrical devices in an attempt to discover the causes of illness and claim to be able to regulate pathogenic energies and disease related vibrations (*see* page 794).	**Of little use** Possibly acceptable as a short-term, supportive treatment attempt for chronic and persistent complaints when simpler, more established methods have been unsuccessful. Some case reports claim efficacy; however, success is probably seen, if at all, in only a small proportion of patients (*see* Placebo, page xxi).	**Requires a qualified practitioner** Practitioners should be properly qualified and should propose a treatment plan. **Risks:** Fairly unlikely.
Cell therapy Injecting or ingesting products extracted from the tissues of newborn animals or animal fetuses is said to have a rejuvenating and revitalizing effect and to enhance the healing of human tissues and organs (*see* page 796).	Based on present knowledge, thymus treatment and cell therapy are **of little use**. The efficacy and mode of action of these costly and relatively risky procedures remain unproven.	**Requires a qualified practitioner** Practitioners should be properly qualified and should propose a treatment plan. **Risks:** Injecting foreign proteins into the body can provoke (possibly fatal) allergic reactions. Also, pathogens such as those that cause bovine spongiform encephalopathy (BSE) or other serious infections may be introduced.

Treatment	Rating	Point of delivery/risks
Electroacupuncture according to Voll By taking readings of the electrical conductivity of the skin (*see* page 802), therapists claim to be able to derive an insight into diseased areas of the body, pathogenic foci (*see* page 928), and stress factors (*see* Toxins, page 929).	**Of little use** Possibly acceptable as a short-term, supportive treatment attempt for chronic and persistent complaints when simpler, more established methods have been unsuccessful. Some case reports claim efficacy; however, success is probably seen, if at all, in only a small proportion of patients (*see* Placebo, page xxi).	**Requires a qualified practitioner** Practitioners should be properly qualified and should propose a treatment plan. No credence should be given to anyone promising immediate or total success. **Risks:** A second opinion must always be obtained from a qualified physician before any attempt is made to "eliminate foci" (e.g. by surgery).
Electroneural therapy according to Croon According to the theory, readings taken at various reactive sites on the skin highlight diseased areas within the body. Based on these readings, targeted neurotherapeutic measures can be undertaken to build up the body's defences (*see* page 806).	**Of little use** Possibly acceptable as a short-term, supportive treatment attempt for chronic and persistent complaints when simpler, more established methods have been unsuccessful. Some case reports claim efficacy; however, success is probably seen, if at all, in only a small proportion of patients (*see* Placebo, page xxi).	**Requires a qualified practitioner** Practitioners should be properly qualified and should propose a treatment plan. **Risks:** Proponents themselves warn that treatment should not be given in acute inflammatory conditions.
Eliminative methods, bloody Bloody cupping (*see* page 815) is said to detoxify the body and stimulate the immune system.	Bloody cupping is **of little use**. Some case reports claim efficacy; however, success is probably seen in only a proportion of patients (*see* Placebo, page xxi).	**Requires a qualified practitioner** Practitioners should be properly qualified and should propose a treatment plan. **Risks:** Bloody cupping can cause infection and scarring and, if the immune system is weakened, may be associated with poor wound healing.

Treatment	Rating	Point of delivery/risks
Eliminative methods, unbloody Sweating (*see* page 877), unbloody cupping (*see* page 817), and cantharide poultices (*see* page 812) are supposed to eliminate accumulated waste products, detoxify the body, and stimulate the immune system.	Sweating **may be of some use** in treating common colds. **Of little use**, on the other hand, are cantharide poultices and unbloody cupping, these being acceptable at most as short-term treatment attempts aimed at dealing with persistent complaints. Case reports claim efficacy; however, success is probably seen in only a proportion of patients (*see* Placebo, page xxi).	**Suitable for DIY** Unbloody cupping is best carried out under the guidance of a qualified practitioner. Treatment with cantharide poultices requires a qualified practitioner. **Risks:** Unlikely provided treatment is carried out competently. Cantharide poultices can cause second-degree burns.
Enzyme therapy The enzymes that are used reportedly stimulate the immune system, as well as dispelling and destroying "immune complexes" that course in the blood and are responsible, for instance, for sustaining inflammatory processes (*see* page 824).	**Of little use** Some case reports and studies claim efficacy for this little researched therapy; however, success is probably seen in only a small proportion of patients (*see* Placebo, page xxi).	**Requires a qualified practitioner** Practitioners should propose a treatment plan. Non-prescription formulations are suitable for do-it-yourself. **Risks:** Allergies or intolerance are possible.
Flower remedies Flower remedies (*see* page 828) are said to restore emotional balance, assist in psychic healing, and stimulate the immune system.	**Of little use** Acceptable as a short-term, supportive, treatment attempt aimed at sootheing and relaxing. Case reports claim efficacy in terms of modulation of the immune system; however, success is probably seen in only a proportion of patients (*see* Placebo, page xxi).	**Suitable for DIY** Qualified guidance is recommended. Practitioners should propose a treatment plan. **Risks:** Possible intolerance.

Treatment	Rating	Point of delivery/risks
Homeopathy Highly diluted (potentized) solutions are believed able to redress vital energy imbalances and strengthen the body's defences. Organo- and functiotropic (*see* page 833) homeopathy is claimed to be effective for dealing with individual diseases on a symptomatic basis (*see* pages 831–6).	**Of little use** Acceptable as a short-term, supportive therapeutic attempt at dealing with chronic and persistent infections. Some case reports claim success for homeopathic treatments; however, success is probably seen in only a proportion of patients (*see* Placebo, page xxi).	**Requires a qualified practitioner** Homeopaths should be properly qualified and should propose a treatment plan. Ready-formulated preparations are suitable for do-it-yourself. **Risks:** Allergies and intolerance are possible.
Manual therapies Chiropractors and osteopaths use a series of manipulations to realign allegedly displaced vertebrae that, it is believed, have a negative influence on the immune system (*see* page 844).	**Of little use** Possibly acceptable as a short-term therapeutic attempt at addressing chronic and persistent complaints when less risky, more established methods have been unsuccessful. Case reports claim efficacy; however, success is probably seen, if at all, in only a small proportion of patients (*see* Placebo, page xxi).	**Requires a qualified practitioner** Practitioners should be properly qualified and should propose a treatment plan. **Risks:** Spinal manipulations can cause serious injury. Osteoporosis is one of several risk factors.
Massage Lymphatic drainage (*see* page 850) is thought to boost the body's defences.	**Of little use** Acceptable as a treatment attempt at soothing and relaxing the patient. Whether lymphatic drainage does boost the body's defences is unclear. Some case reports claim efficacy; however, success is probably seen in only a proportion of patients (*see* Placebo, page xxi).	**Requires a qualified practitioner** Practitioners should be properly qualified. **Risks:** Some people are sensitive to manual stimuli; others find it hard to tolerate close physical contact.

Treatment	*Rating*	*Point of delivery/risks*
Nutritional therapies An organic diet (*see* page 4) provides the body with essential nutrients that are believed to exercise a multitude of positive effects and to be capable, *inter alia*, of strengthening the immune system. Other dietary approaches may achieve similar objectives (*see* pages 2–8).	**Useful** as a preventive measure. Various studies suggest that dietary therapies are successful to a certain extent in building up the body's defence system.	**Suitable for DIY** Qualified guidance is recommended. **Risks:** Avoid imbalanced or intolerable diets. They can cause deficiencies with serious consequences. Children are at particular risk.
Physical therapies Exercise therapy (*see* page 868), various hydrotherapeutic techniques (*see* pages 871–8) and Kneipp treatments (*see* page 871) are said to stimulate the immune system. Saunas (see page 876) are supposed to eliminate accumulated waste products, detoxify the body, and stimulate the immune system.	**May be of some use** as a short-term treatment attempt. Case studies, case reports, and field studies claim efficacy; however, success is probably seen in only a proportion of patients (*see* Placebo, page xxi).	**Suitable for DIY** Qualified guidance is recommended though not essential. Practitioners should propose a treatment plan. **Risks:** Skin damage may be caused to persons with diminished temperature sensation when extreme temperatures are applied. Exercise should not be overdone.
Probiotics The introduction of certain bacteria into the gut is claimed to bring the intestinal flora back into balance and to have a beneficial effect on the immune system (*see* page 878).	**Of little use** for generally stimulating the immune system. **May be of some use** as a short-term treatment attempt for persistent complaints. Case reports and studies claim efficacy; however, success is probably seen in only a proportion of patients (*see* Placebo, page xxi).	**Requires a qualified practitioner** Practitioners should be properly qualified and should propose a treatment plan. Non-prescription preparations are suitable for do-it-yourself. **Risks:** Fairly unlikely provided treatment is carried out competently.

Treatment	*Rating*	*Point of delivery/risks*
Reflex therapies Connective tissue massage and reflexology (*see* page 883) are thought to be good for strengthening the body and stimulating the immune system.	**Of little use** Acceptable as a short-term, supportive treatment attempt. Some case reports claim efficacy; however, success is probably seen in only a proportion of patients (*see* Placebo, page xxi).	**Requires a qualified practitioner** Practitioners should be properly qualified and should propose a treatment plan. **Risks:** Some people are sensitive to manual stimuli; others find it hard to tolerate close physical contact.
Relaxation techniques Autogenic training (*see* page 888), muscle relaxation according to Jacobson (*see* page 893), and various biofeedback techniques (*see* page 891) are said to relieve muscle tension and inner unrest, and might be effective in alleviating stress and its potential negative effect on the immune system.	**May be of some use** as a therapeutic attempt at addressing stress and its consequences. Case reports and field studies claim efficacy; however, success is probably seen in only a proportion of patients (*see* Placebo, page xxi).	**Suitable for DIY** Once a sound understanding of the technique has been acquired from a trainer, patients can perform exercises themselves. Therapists should be properly qualified. **Risks:** Fairly unlikely.
Vitamins and trace elements Beta-carotene, vitamins A, B12, C, E, folic acid, and selenium are thought to bring a number of benefits by addressing the problem of free radical formation and supplementing the body's own antioxidative defence systems (*see* page 900).	**May be of some use** as a supportive measure. No endorsements can be given based on present knowledge. Recommended dosages vary widely but are probably set to rise.	**Suitable for DIY** Qualified guidance is recommended though not essential. **Risks:** Intolerance and overdosage are possible. Recent findings imply that beta-carotene and vitamin A might increase the risk of cancer.

Herbal remedies to strengthen the immune system

Active ingredient/preparation	Rating
Boneset (*Eupatorium perfoliatum*)	**May be of some use** for generally increasing resistance to infection. **Dosage:** As instructed by the manufacturer/prescriber. **Risks:** Boneset, like coltsfoot, which is similarly used supportively to strengthen the body's defences against influenza, contains, according to some but not all sources, pyrrolizidines; these substances are potentially carcinogenic and cause liver damage, particularly when used in sustained high dosages.
Preparations containing **Echinacea** (*Echinacea angustifolia* root and coneflower, *Echinacea purpurea* root)	**Of little use**. Whether *Echinacea angustifolia* root and coneflower and *Echinacea purpurea* root are efficacious is debatable; there is little evidence to support claims that they are effective immune system stimulants. **Dosage:** As instructed by the manufacturer/prescriber. **Risks:** These preparations should be used with caution in systemic diseases such as tuberculosis, leukosis, collagenosis, multiple sclerosis, myelitis, and others, as they may exacerbate the causative factors.
Preparations containing **Echinacea** (*Echinacea pallida* root, *Echinacea purpurea* coneflower)	Preparations containing extracts of *Echinacea pallida* root or *Echinacea purpurea* coneflower **may be of some use** as an attempt to reduce susceptibility to infection, also in children. **Dosage:** As instructed by the manufacturer/prescriber. **Risks:** Do not use in progressive systemic diseases. Do not use for more than eight weeks consecutively. Take when no infection is present or at the very start of an infection. These preparations must not be injected, as they can provoke allergic reactions including shock, swelling of the pharynx, and breathing difficulty. There have also been isolated reports of allergy following oral administration.

Active ingredient/preparation	*Rating*
Combination preparations containing **Echinacea**	**Of little use**. It is doubtful whether combination preparations can increase resistance to infection. **Dosage:** As instructed by the manufacturer/prescriber.
Mistletoe for injection	**May be of some use** in stimulative and immunemodulation therapy, in the treatment of precancerous conditions, and as an adjunct to other treatments. **Dosage:** As instructed by the manufacturer/prescriber. Standardized mistletoe preparations enable an accurately controlled dose to be administered and are thus the preparations of choice. **Risks:** Shivering attacks, a raised temperature (a slight rise is desirable for interferon induction), headaches, angina pectoris, circulatory disorders, allergic reactions. Do not use in protein allergy, chronic infection, or acute, highly febrile, inflammatory disease. Caution: The berries must not be used.
Thuja (*Thuja occidentalis*)	**May be of some use** as a supportive treatment attempt for malignant tumor, acute and chronic respiratory infections, colds, and influenza. **Parts used:** dried young shoots. **Dosage:** As instructed by the manufacturer/prescriber. **Risks:** Cramps, visual disturbance, cardiac arrhythmia, also symptoms of kidney and liver damage. Thuja extract contains thujone, which is toxic; it is vital, therefore, not to exceed the recommended dosage. **Caution:** Not to be used during pregnancy.

PART 1

Symptoms and disorders

Pain

Headaches and migraines

Causes and symptoms

With a third of the population of Western industrialized countries suffering from the occasional tension headache and one in ten people affected at least twice a week, headaches are one of the classic diseases of civilization. Between 8 and 12 percent of the population is thought to suffer from migraines.

Headaches may vary in intensity from slight pressure in the head to a full migraine attack with visual disturbances, slurred speech, sensitivity to light, and vomiting. Headaches can be triggered by various factors, such as climatic changes, colds, eye strain, abuse of alcohol or nicotine, excessive noise, air pollution, or too much sun. There is also a phenomenon known as a coffee-withdrawal headache, when a person who is addicted to caffeine (more than eight to ten cups of coffee a day) suddenly goes "cold turkey." Headaches are also very often the first sign of a number of physical ailments, including high or low blood pressure and a brain tumor. Anyone experiencing recurrent or persistent headaches *must* consult a doctor.

Headaches may have a variety of psychological, as well as physical, causes: strained relationships at home or at work, emotional stress, nervous tension, or suppressed aggression. Research into the psychosomatic causes of illness has shown that approximately 60 percent of all migraine sufferers are unable to cope with stressful situations.

Headaches that are due to, or triggered by, emotional factors can be treated by psychological counselling or psychotherapy, or through participation in a self-awareness group. What these therapies do is help patients cope better with their emotional problems and conflicts.

Orthodox treatment

Painkillers

One person in ten regularly takes painkillers. In Europe the number of painkilling tablets sold per year is in the billions if not trillions. But taking painkillers to relieve headaches may lead to other serious problems, first because they suppress what is essentially a warning signal (of what might be a potentially serious disease) and secondly because they only alleviate symptoms temporarily instead of removing the underlying cause. Also, persons taking analgesic preparations that contain caffeine or codeine risk becoming physically or psychologically addicted. Experts consider that half of all chronic pain sufferers have a drug problem.

There are also problems with combination medicines that contain several active ingredients. Rather than making the medicine more effective, such combinations often just increase the risk of side effects.

Prolonged use of painkillers may start a vicious circle of events:

- As pain suppression diminishes, the painkillers may actually induce headaches. Patients need to take increasing numbers of tablets to remain pain-free.
- Regular use of painkillers over a number of years can damage the kidneys and even cause kidney failure. Their excessive use is said to be responsible for the kidney damage suffered by as many as a third of all renal dialysis and kidney transplant patients.

Medicines containing acetylsalicylic acid (aspirin), ibuprofen or paracetamol, used briefly, are effective and relatively safe. If any of these, in proper doses, fails to provide relief from pain, a combination preparation containing a mild opiate such as codeine may be taken for a limited period.

Coffee

Taking a painkiller with a cup of coffee may bring temporary relief from a headache. Also, if the stomach can take it, coffee with lemon juice is a useful cure.

Complementary therapies

Natural remedies can be used to relieve headaches and migraines; they either act directly or by inducing a state of general relaxation.

Treatment plan and limited trial

The effect a therapy has on a particular person should be evaluated in a short-term trial, full details of which should be discussed between the patient and the doctor or therapist. Even therapies that are wholly appropriate may become problematic if used in the long term without any checks as to their continuing efficacy.

Cautions

Before receiving treatment for chronic or persistent headaches, every patient must be examined by an orthodox doctor to rule out possible physical causes such as a systemic illness, pathological processes in the head or neck region, vascular disease, or a brain tumor. Most complementary treatments are better suited to a supportive, rather than an exclusive, style of use.

Complementary treatments for headaches and migraines

Treatment	Rating	Point of delivery/risks
Acupressure This treatment (*see* page 769), otherwise known as pressure-point massage, is claimed to alleviate pain and relieve tension when the appropriate pressure points are stimulated.	**May be of some use** as a short-term treatment attempt. Various case reports and field studies claim efficacy; however, success is probably seen in only a small proportion of patients (*see* Placebo, page xxi).	**Suitable for DIY** Qualified guidance is recommended. Therapists should be properly qualified. **Risks:** Unlikely provided treatment is carried out competently.
Acupuncture Acupuncture in its various forms (*see* page 772) aims to encourage the flow of energy (*see* page 927) or to directly alleviate pain and relieve tension. The acupuncture points chosen can vary from one practitioner to another.	**May be of some use** as a short-term treatment attempt for chronic headaches and migraines, as a preventive measure, and as a means of reducing the quantities of painkillers consumed. Investigations have shown that success is probably seen in only a proportion of patients treated (*see* Placebo, page xxi). There are numerous positive observational studies relating to the use of acupuncture in acute pain. The efficacy claimed in some studies was perhaps seen in only a proportion of patients treated (*see* Placebo, page xxi).	**Requires a qualified practitioner** Practitioners should be properly qualified and should propose a treatment plan. **Risks:** Probably rare provided treatment is carried out competently.

Treatment	Rating	Point of delivery/risks
Anthroposophical medicine Biographical work, dialog, art therapy, and the constitutional remedy Kephalodoron (with iron, quartz, and sulphur) are said to regulate the activity of the body's four constituent elements, to contribute to a change of behavior and well-being, and so ease headaches and migraines (*see* page 781).	**May be of some use** as a treatment attempt for chronic headaches and migraines, as a preventive measure, and as a means of reducing the quantities of painkillers consumed, providing that the patient has given his/her approval. Some case reports claim efficacy; however, success is probably seen in only a proportion of patients (*see* Placebo, page xxi).	**Requires a qualified practitioner** Practitioners should be properly qualified and should propose a treatment plan. **Risks:** Hypersensitivity to Kephalodoron or gastric intolerance are possible.
Aromatherapy Essential oils (*see* page 786) are used to soothe and relax, and may alleviate headaches. The essences may be taken orally, used externally as massage oils or bathing emulsions, or inhaled as vapors.	**May be of some use** as a supportive attempt at soothing and relaxing the patient. Some case reports and studies claim efficacy in the treatment of headaches and migraines; however, success is probably seen in only a proportion of patients (*see* Placebo, page xxi).	**Suitable for DIY** Qualified guidance is recommended. The effects of individual essential oils differ widely. **Risks:** Allergies or intolerance are possible. Some oils are carcinogenic in test systems and possibly in humans.
Bioresonance therapy Bioresonance therapists use electrical devices in an attempt to discover the causes of illness and claim to be able to regulate pathogenic energies and disease related vibrations (*see* page 794).	**Of little use** for treating headaches. Possibly acceptable as a short-term, supportive treatment attempt aimed at improving general well-being when simpler, more established methods have been unsuccessful. Some case reports claim efficacy against headaches; however, success is probably seen, if at all, in only a small proportion of patients (*see* Placebo, page xxi).	**Requires a qualified practitioner** Practitioners should be properly qualified and should propose a treatment plan. No credence should be given to anyone promising immediate or total success. **Risks:** Fairly unlikely.

Treatment	Rating	Point of delivery/risks
Cell therapy Injecting or ingesting products extracted from the tissues of newborn animals or animal fetuses is said to have a rejuvenating and revitalizing effect and to enhance the healing of human tissues and organs (*see* page 796).	**Not advised** Based on present knowledge, there is no satisfactory evidence of the efficacy and mode of action of these costly and relatively risky procedures.	**Risks:** Injecting foreign proteins into the body can provoke (possibly fatal) allergic reactions. Also, pathogens such as those that cause bovine spongiform encephalopathy (BSE) or other serious infections may be introduced.
Electroacupuncture according to Voll By taking readings of the electrical conductivity of the skin (*see* page 802), therapists claim to be able to derive an insight into diseased areas of the body, pathogenic foci (*see* page 928), and stress factors (*see* Toxins, page 929).	**Of little use** Possibly acceptable as a short-term treatment attempt for chronic and persistent headache when simpler, more established methods of pain relief have been unsuccessful. Some case reports claim efficacy; however, success is probably seen, if at all, in only a small proportion of patients (*see* Placebo, page xxi).	**Requires a qualified practitioner** Practitioners should be properly qualified and should propose a treatment plan. No credence should be given to anyone promising immediate or total success. **Risks:** A second opinion must always be obtained from a qualified physician before any attempt is made to "eliminate foci" (e.g. by surgery).
Electroneural therapy according to Croon According to the theory, readings taken at various reactive sites on the skin highlight diseased areas within the body (*see* page 860). Based on these readings, targeted neurotherapeutic measures can be undertaken.	**Of little use** Possibly acceptable as a short-term treatment attempt for chronic and persistent headaches when simpler, more established methods of pain relief have been unsuccessful. Some case reports claim efficacy; however, success is probably seen, if at all, in only a small proportion of patients (*see* Placebo, page xxi).	**Requires a qualified practitioner** Practitioners should be properly qualified and should propose a treatment plan. No credence should be given to anyone promising immediate or total success. **Risks:** Proponents themselves warn that treatment should not be given in acute inflammatory conditions.

Treatment	Rating	Point of delivery/risks
Eliminative methods, bloody Bloody cupping (*see* page 815) is said to ease headaches and migraines. The technique is often used as part of a holistic approach (*see* page 928) rather than directly against the headache.	**Of little use** Possibly acceptable as a short-term treatment attempt for chronic or persistent conditions when less invasive, more established methods have been unsuccessful. Some case reports claim efficacy; however, success is probably seen in only a small proportion of patients (*see* Placebo, page xxi).	**Requires a qualified practitioner** Practitioners should be properly qualified and should propose a treatment plan. **Risks:** Bloody cupping can cause infections and scarring. Furthermore, it should not be practiced in patients with bleeding disorders.
Eliminative methods, unbloody Enemas (*see* page 819) and unbloody cupping (*see* page 817) are frequently applied to treat headaches. These techniques are often used as part of a holistic approach (*see* page 928) rather than directly against the headache.	**Of little use** Possibly acceptable as a short-term treatment attempt when more established methods have been unsuccessful. Some case reports claim efficacy; however, success is probably seen in only a proportion of patients (*see* Placebo, page xxi).	**Suitable for DIY** Professional guidance is recommended. **Risks:** Unlikely provided treatment is carried out competently.
Flower remedies Flower remedies (*see* page 828) are said to restore emotional balance and well-being.	**May be of some use** as a short-term, supportive treatment attempt aimed at soothing, relaxing, and bringing peace of mind. Some case reports claim efficacy against headaches; however, success is probably seen in only a small proportion of patients (*see* Placebo, page xxi).	**Suitable for DIY** Qualified guidance is recommended. Practitioners should propose a treatment plan. **Risks:** Possible intolerance.

Treatment	Rating	Point of delivery/risks
Homeopathy Highly diluted (potentized) solutions (*see* page 831) are believed to be able to redress vital energy imbalances. Organo- and functiotropic (*see* page 833) homeopathy is claimed to be effective in dealing with headaches and migraines.	**May be of some use** as a short-term treatment attempt for chronic headaches, as a preventive measure, and as a means of reducing the quantities of painkillers consumed. Some case reports and field studies claim success for homeopathic treatments; however, success is probably seen in only a proportion of patients (*see* Placebo, page xxi).	**Requires a qualified practitioner** Homeopaths should be properly qualified and should propose a treatment plan. Ready-formulated preparations are suitable for do-it-yourself. **Risks:** Allergies and intolerance are possible.
Hypnosis and self-hypnosis In the relaxed and generally altered state of awareness that is induced in hypnosis or self-hypnosis (*see* page 837), physical conditions can be addressed and headaches relieved, or at least made less intense. Hypnosis is often used in combination with other psycho- and behavioral therapies.	**May be of some use** as a short-term treatment attempt for chronic and persistent headaches when simpler, more established methods of pain relief have been unsuccessful. Some case reports and field studies claim efficacy; however, success is probably seen in only a proportion of patients treated (*see* Placebo, page xxi).	**Requires a qualified practitioner** Hypnotherapists should be properly qualified and should propose a treatment plan. No credence should be given to anyone promising immediate or total success. **Risks:** Unlikely provided treatment is carried out competently.
Manual therapies Chiropractors and osteopaths (*see* page 844) use a series of manipulations to realign allegedly displaced vertebrae that, it is believed, irritate the nerves to cause headaches.	**May be of some use** as a short-term treatment attempt for chronic and persistent headaches when less risky, more established methods have been unsuccessful. Studies suggest that some 50–60 percent of patients find at least passing relief from headaches.	**Requires a qualified practitioner** Practitioners should be properly qualified and should propose a treatment plan. **Risks:** Spinal manipulations of the neck can cause serious injury. Osteoporosis is one of several risk factors.

Treatment	Rating	Point of delivery/risks
Massage Classical massage (*see* page 847) can ease muscular and emotional tension; some techniques aim to induce counterirritation to obscure pain at least temporarily. Ice massage is said to exert a beneficial influence via reflex channels.	**May be of some use** in headaches. Massage is generally experienced as being agreeable and relaxing. Some studies claim efficacy in the treatment of headaches; however, success is probably seen, if at all, in only a proportion of patients (*see* Placebo, page xxi).	**Suitable for DIY** Qualified guidance is recommended. Masseurs/masseuses should propose a treatment plan. **Risks:** Some people are sensitive to cold, manual stimuli; others find it hard to tolerate close physical contact.
Nutritional therapies An organic diet (*see* page 4) provides the body with essential and secondary nutrients that are believed to exercise a multitude of positive effects and to be capable, *inter alia*, of fending off some of the mechanisms that lead to headaches.	**Useful** as an individually directed supportive measure. Elimination and rotation diets may be of some assistance in identifying the cause of chronic food allergy induced headaches.	**Suitable for DIY** Qualified guidance is recommended. See your doctor before starting an elimination or rotation diet. **Risks:** Avoid imbalanced or intolerable diets. They can cause deficiencies with serious consequences. Children are particularly at risk.
Physical therapies Hydro- and hydrothermic therapy, and electrotherapy (*see* page 871) can provide stimuli to induce relaxation, improve the circulation, and reduce pain.	**Of little use** in headaches. Possibly acceptable as a supportive measure aimed at providing an improved feeling of well-being. Some case reports and field studies claim efficacy in the treatment of headaches; however, success is probably seen in only a proportion of patients (*see* Placebo, page xxi).	**Suitable for DIY** Qualified guidance is recommended. Practitioners should be appropriately qualified and propose a treatment plan. **Risks:** Skin damage may be caused to persons with diminished temperature sensation when extreme temperatures are applied.

Treatment	Rating	Point of delivery/risks
Probiotics The introduction of certain bacteria into the gut is claimed to bring the intestinal flora back into balance and to have a beneficial effect in persons with headaches caused by gastric or intestinal disorders (*see* page 878).	**Only useful** as a short-term treatment attempt for digestion related headaches. Some case reports claim efficacy in the treatment of this type of headache; however, success is probably seen in only a small proportion of patients (*see* Placebo, page xxi).	**Suitable for DIY** Qualified guidance is essential. Therapists should propose a treatment plan. **Risks:** Unlikely provided treatment is carried out competently.
Reflex therapies Reflex zone massage, cold sprays, and TENS (*see* page 886) are said to exert a beneficial influence via reflex channels (*see* page 881).	**May be of some use** as a short-term treatment attempt. Some field studies and case reports claim efficacy; however, success is probably seen in only a proportion of patients (*see* Placebo, page xxi). When compared, the various techniques seem to be equally effective, though the benefits they provide vary greatly from person to person.	**Suitable for DIY** Qualified guidance is essential. Therapists should be properly qualified and should propose a treatment plan. **Risks:** Some people are sensitive to cold, electrical, or manual stimuli, rubber electrodes, etc. others find it hard to tolerate close physical contact.
Relaxation techniques Autogenic training (*see* page 888), muscle relaxation according to Jacobson (*see* page 893), and various biofeedback techniques (*see* page 891) are said to relieve muscle tension and inner unrest. These techniques are frequently used in combination with other psycho- and behavioral therapies.	**Useful** as a medium-term treatment attempt for chronic headaches and acute migraines, as a preventive measure, and as a means of reducing the intake of painkillers. Case reports and studies reveal these techniques as being effective in a number of patients.	**Suitable for DIY** Once a sound understanding of the technique has been acquired from a trainer, patients can perform exercises themselves. Therapists should be properly qualified. **Risks:** Fairly unlikely.

Treatment	Rating	Point of delivery/risks
Vapor inhalation Vapor inhalations (of infusions of elderflowers, camomile, peppermint, or limeflowers) are primarily aimed at headaches associated with colds (*see* page 239).	**Only useful** for headaches associated with colds. Some controlled trials claim efficacy.	**Suitable for DIY Risks:** Scalding or nausea if proper care is not taken.

Herbal remedies for headaches

Active ingredient/preparation	Rating
Caffeine from coffee beans or leaf tea	Caffeine **may be of some use** as a treatment attempt for headaches. **Daily dose:** 600mg (six to eight cups of coffee); individual dose: 80–100mg to a cup of hot water. **Risks:** More than 200mg of caffeine can cause users to overestimate their own abilities. Habitual intake of more than 600mg daily can lead to withdrawal headaches if consumption is stopped abruptly, e.g. at weekends if you regularly drink lots of coffee at work.
Cajeput oil (*Melaleuca leucadendron*)	Cajeput oil, massaged into the temples, **may be of some use** as a supportive treatment attempt during acupressure. To apply, lightly massage in the oil for five to ten minutes in a circular motion. **Dosage:** Use externally as a 5 percent alcoholic solution. **Risks:** Be careful not to get the oil into the eyes, as it will cause them to sting painfully. Do not apply to the face and nostrils of infants. Not to be used on sensitive persons. Inhalation may lead to inflammation of the respiratory system. Extensive external use may lead to kidney problems and disorders of the central nervous system. Cajeput oil can irritate the mucous membranes and cause skin allergies.

Active ingredient/preparation	Rating

Fir needle oil
(*Abies sibirica*)

Fir needle oil, massaged into the temples, **may be of some use** as a supportive treatment attempt during acupressure. To apply, lightly massage in the oil for five to ten minutes in a circular motion.
Dosage: Apply a few drops before massaging; otherwise use as instructed by the manufacturer/prescriber.
Risks: Be careful not to get the oil into the eyes, as it will cause them to sting painfully. This oil may irritate the mucous membranes if incorrectly used; because of this irritant effect, it must not be used by persons with asthma or whooping cough.

Mint oil
(essential oil of *Mentha arvensis*)

Mint oil, massaged into the temples, **may be of some use** as a supportive treatment attempt during acupressure. To apply, lightly massage in the oil for five to ten minutes in a circular motion.
Dosage: Apply a few drops before massaging; otherwise use as instructed by the manufacturer/prescriber.
Risks: Be careful not to get the oil into the eyes, as it will cause them to sting painfully. Do not apply to the face and nostrils of infants. This oil may irritate the mucous membranes if incorrectly used and can cause skin allergies.

Peppermint oil
(*Mentha piperita*)

Peppermint oil, massaged into the temples, is **useful** as a supportive treatment attempt during acupressure. To apply, lightly massage in the oil for five to ten minutes in a circular motion.
Dosage: Apply a few drops before massaging; otherwise use as instructed by the manufacturer/prescriber.
Risks: Be careful not to get the oil into the eyes, as it will cause them to sting painfully. Peppermint oil can cause allergic reactions. Do not apply to the nose and face of infants and young children.

Active ingredient/preparation	Rating

Pine needle oil
(*Pinus pinaster*)

Pine needle oil, massaged into the temples, **may be of some use** as a supportive treatment attempt during acupressure. To apply, lightly massage in the oil for five to ten minutes in a circular motion.
Dosage: Apply a few drops before massaging; otherwise use as instructed by the manufacturer/prescriber.
Risks: Be careful not to get the oil into the eyes, as it will cause them to sting painfully. Do not apply to the face and nostrils of infants. Not to be used on sensitive persons. Inhalation may lead to inflammation of the respiratory system. Extensive external use may lead to kidney problems and disorders of the central nervous system. Pine needle oil can cause skin allergies.

Turpentine oil
(*Terebinthina laricina*)

Turpentine oil, massaged into the temples, **may be of some use** as a supportive treatment attempt during acupressure. To apply, lightly massage in the oil for five to ten minutes in a circular motion.
Dosage: Apply a few drops before massaging; otherwise use as instructed by the manufacturer/prescriber.
Risks: Be careful not to get the oil into the eyes, as it will cause them to sting painfully. Oil should be used fresh. Do not apply to the face and nostrils of infants. Hypersensitivity and allergies are possible; inhalation may cause acute inflammation of the respiratory tract.

Willow bark extract
(*Salix fragilis*)

Willow bark extract, taken orally, **may be of some use** as a treatment attempt for muscular pain. Willow bark is a febrifuge, analgesic, and anti-inflammatory agent. Aspirin was originally derived from it.
Individual dose: 2.0g willow bark contains approximately 20mg salicin. Use ready-formulated preparations as instructed by the manufacturer/prescriber.
Daily dose: 60–120mg total salicin.
Risks: Skin allergies, asthmatic symptoms (bronchospasm), and gastrointestinal complaints may occur in persons sensitive to aspirin or other salicylates.

Neuralgia

Causes and symptoms

Neuralgia is pain arising through irritation of a nerve, hence its name. Trigeminal neuralgia, for instance, is a pain affecting the trigeminal nerve in the face; intercostal neuralgia affects the nerves in the region between the ribs. Neuralgia can be caused by poor circulation or by a virus such as *Herpes zoster* (the shingles virus). Other possible causes are vitamin B deficiency as a result of poor eating, alcoholism, diabetic neuropathy (*see* Neuropathy, page 140), or triggers such as inflammation, scars, trapped nerves, or pressure. Psychological factors and central nervous disorders can also play a key role.

Nerve irritation is felt as a severe shooting pain that normally lasts for only a few seconds but may occur dozens of times a day. Pain may be brought on by certain movements or even by slight pressure on trigger points (*see* page 929). Often actions as mundane as chewing, swallowing, speaking, shaving, or brushing teeth are enough to bring on a painful attack. In exceptional cases the condition may be so severe that sufferers hardly dare to speak, eat, or brush their teeth and, as they try to avoid such normal function, their quality of life deteriorates.

Orthodox treatment

Simple analgesic drugs containing only acetylsalicylic acid (aspirin), paracetamol, or ibuprofen are generally unable to alleviate neuralgic pain. Severe neuralgia often calls for more potent painkillers (*see* page 24) or even for a preparation containing carbamazepine. If pain is persistent and excruciating, a neurosurgeon will sometimes operate to remove an offending nerve. A specialist in psychosomatic disorders or a psychotherapist can sometimes detect the origin of neuralgia that does not have an obvious physical cause.

Complementary therapies

Certain complementary therapists claim to be successful in directly alleviating neuralgic pain, though the procedures they propose are usually no substitute for conventional treatments.

Treatment plan and limited trial

Before administering a complementary treatment, every therapist should draw up a treatment plan (see page xxiii) that sets out a clear time-frame and defines the goal that the treatment is designed to achieve. Treatment should then be tried for a limited term to test the patient's response.

Cautions

Before receiving complementary treatment for recurrent neuralgia, patients must be examined by an orthodox doctor.

Most nonconventional treatments are more suitable as a supportive measure than as the sole treatment.

Complementary treatments for neuralgia

Treatment	Rating	Point of delivery/risks
Acupressure This treatment (*see* page 769), otherwise known as pressure-point massage, is claimed to alleviate pain and relieve tension when the appropriate pressure points are stimulated. The points chosen can vary from one practitioner to another.	**May be of some use** as a short-term attempt at pain relief. Outcome studies claim efficacy; however, success is probably seen in only a proportion of patients (*see* Placebo, page xxi).	**Suitable for DIY** Qualified guidance is essential. Therapists should be properly qualified and should propose a treatment plan. **Risks:** Unlikely provided treatment is carried out competently.

Treatment	Rating	Point of delivery/risks
Acupuncture Acupuncture in its various forms (*see* page 772) aims to alleviate neuralgic pain and relieve tension. The acupuncture points chosen can vary from one practitioner to another.	**May be of some use** as a short-term attempt to bring relief from pain. There are several studies and case reports that claim that some patients achieved relief from pain and that the incidence of pain declined (*see* Placebo, page xxi).	**Requires a qualified practitioner** Acupuncturists should be properly qualified and should propose a treatment plan. **Risks:** Probably rare provided treatment is carried out competently.
Anthroposophical medicine Aconite can be massaged in as an oil or swallowed as a potentized (*see* page 831) preparation. It is claimed to act preventively as well as to bring relief from acute pain, thus allowing the numbers of painkillers that are consumed to be reduced (*see* page 781).	**May be of some use** as a short-term attempt to bring relief from pain. Some case reports claim efficacy; however, success is probably seen in only a proportion of patients (*see* Placebo, page xxi).	**Requires a qualified practitioner** Practitioners should be properly qualified and should propose a treatment plan. **Risks:** Allergies and intolerance are possible.
Aromatherapy Essential oils (*see* page 786) are used to soothe and relax, and may thus also alleviate neuralgic pain. The essences may be taken orally, used externally as massage oils or bathing emulsions, or inhaled as vapors.	**Of little use** Acceptable as a short-term treatment attempt aimed at soothing and relaxing. Some case reports claim efficacy; however, success is probably seen in only a small proportion of patients (*see* Placebo, page xxi).	**Suitable for DIY** Qualified guidance is recommended. Aromatherapists should be properly qualified and should propose a treatment plan. **Risks:** Allergies or intolerance are possible. Some oils are carcinogenic in test systems and possibly in humans.

Treatment	Rating	Point of delivery/risks
Bioresonance therapy Bioresonance therapists use electrical devices in an attempt to discover the causes of illness and claim to be able to regulate pathogenic energies and disease related vibrations (*see* page 794).	**Of little use** Possibly acceptable as a short-term treatment attempt when simpler, more established methods have been unsuccessful. Some case reports claim efficacy; however, success might well be seen in only a proportion of patients (*see* Placebo, page xxi).	**Requires a qualified practitioner** Practitioners should be properly qualified and should propose a treatment plan. No credence should be given to anyone promising immediate or total success. **Risks:** Fairly unlikely.
Cell therapy Injecting or ingesting products extracted from animal tissues or organs is said to have an immune system modulating effect (*see* page 10) and to enhance the healing of human tissues and organs (*see* page 796). It is also said to be instrumental in combating neuralgia.	Cell therapy is **not advised**. Organ extracts are **of little use** and are, at most, acceptable as a limited treatment attempt when better established methods of pain relief have been unsuccessful. Descriptions in field studies and other documents (of the efficacy of such extracts in pain reduction and reversal of inflammation) probably apply to only a minority of patients receiving treatment (*see* Placebo, page xxi).	**Administration of organ extracts requires a qualified practitioner.** Practitioners should be properly qualified and should propose a treatment plan. No credence should be given to anyone promising immediate or total success. **Risks:** Injecting foreign proteins into the body can provoke (possibly fatal) allergic reactions. Also, pathogens such as those that cause bovine spongiform encephalopathy (BSE) or other serious infections may be introduced.

Treatment	Rating	Point of delivery/risks
Electroacupuncture according to Voll By taking readings of the electrical conductivity of the skin (*see* page 802), therapists claim to be able to derive an insight into diseased areas of the body, pathogenic foci (*see* page 928), and stress factors (*see* Toxins, page 929).	**Of little use** Possibly acceptable as a short-term treatment attempt in persistent cases when simpler, more established methods have been unsuccessful. Some case reports claim efficacy; however, success is probably seen, if at all, in only a small proportion of patients (*see* Placebo, page xxi).	**Requires a qualified practitioner** Practitioners should be properly qualified and should propose a treatment plan. No credence should be given to anyone promising immediate or total success. **Risks:** A second opinion must always be obtained from a qualified physician before any attempt is made to "eliminate foci" (e.g. by surgery).
Electroneural therapy according to Croon According to the theory, readings taken at various reactive sites on the skin highlight diseased areas within the body. Based on these readings, targeted neurotherapeutic measures can be undertaken to build up the body's defences (*see* page 806).	**Of little use** Possibly acceptable as a short-term, supportive treatment attempt in persistent cases when simpler, more established methods have been unsuccessful. Some case reports claim efficacy; however, success is probably seen, if at all, in only a small proportion of patients (*see* Placebo, page xxi).	**Requires a qualified practitioner** Practitioners should be properly qualified and should propose a treatment plan. No credence should be given to anyone promising immediate or total success. **Risks:** Proponents themselves warn that treatment should not be given in acute inflammatory conditions.
Eliminative methods, unbloody Enemas (*see* page 819) and unbloody cupping (*see* page 817) are said to offer some relief from neuralgic pain.	**Of little use** Acceptable as a short-term treatment attempt. Some case reports claim efficacy; however, success is probably seen in only a proportion of patients (*see* Placebo, page xxi).	**Suitable for DIY** Professional guidance is recommended. **Risks:** Unlikely provided treatment is carried out competently.

Treatment	Rating	Point of delivery/risks
Enzyme therapy The enzymes used are said to dispel and destroy "immune complexes" (*see* page 824) that course in the blood and that are responsible, for instance, for sustaining inflammatory processes.	**Of little use** Some case reports claim this little researched therapy works against neuralgia; however, success is probably seen in only a small proportion of patients (*see* Placebo, page xxi).	**Requires a qualified practitioner** Practitioners should propose a treatment plan. Nonprescription preparations are suitable for do-it-yourself. **Risks:** Allergies or intolerance are possible.
Flower remedies Flower remedies (*see* page 828) are said to restore emotional balance and bring peace of mind. Bach Rescue Remedy is often used for acute attacks.	**Of little use** Acceptable as a short-term, supportive treatment attempt aimed at relaxing the patient and improving the body's own regulatory systems. Some case reports claim efficacy; however, success is probably seen in only a proportion of patients (*see* Placebo, page xxi).	**Suitable for DIY** Qualified guidance is recommended. Practitioners should be properly qualified and propose a treatment plan. **Risks:** Possible intolerance.
Homeopathy Highly diluted (potentized) solutions are believed to be able to redress vital energy imbalances and strengthen the body's defences. Organo- and functiotropic (*see* page 833) homeopathy is claimed to be effective for symptomatic treatment of neuralgic pain.	**May be of some use** as a short-term treatment attempt. Some case reports and field studies claim success for homeopathic treatments; however, success is probably seen in only a proportion of patients (*see* Placebo, page xxi).	**Requires a qualified practitioner** Homeopaths should be properly qualified and should propose a treatment plan. Ready-formulated preparations are suitable for do-it-yourself. **Risks:** Possible intolerance.

Treatment	Rating	Point of delivery/risks
Hypnosis and self-hypnosis In the relaxed and generally altered state of awareness that is induced in hypnosis or self-hypnosis (*see* page 837), physical conditions can be addressed and pain relieved.	**May be of some use** as a short-term, supportive treatment attempt. There is a lack of reliable information. Some case reports claim efficacy; however, success is probably seen in only a proportion of patients treated (*see* Placebo, page xxi).	**Requires a qualified practitioner** Hypnotherapists should be properly qualified and should propose a treatment plan. **Risks:** Unlikely provided treatment is carried out competently.
Magnetic field therapy The use of magnetic field generators, magnetic strips, bracelets, and other objects (*see* page 841) allegedly encourages cell metabolism and so relieves pain.	**Inappropriate** Based on present knowledge, there is inadequate evidence of the efficacy and mode of action of magnetic field therapy in neuralgia.	Operation of magnetic field equipment **requires a qualified practitioner**. **Risks:** Magnetic field equipment can cause implanted cardiac pacemakers to malfunction.
Manual therapies Chiropractors and osteopaths use a series of manipulations to realign allegedly displaced vertebrae and joints that, it is believed, might be co-responsible for neuralgia (*see* page 844).	**May be of some use** as a short-term treatment attempt when less risky, more established methods have been unsuccessful. Some case reports and field studies claim efficacy; however, success is probably seen in only a proportion of patients (*see* Placebo, page xxi).	**Requires a qualified practitioner** Practitioners should be properly qualified and should propose a treatment plan. **Risks:** Spinal manipulations can cause serious injury. Osteoporosis is one of several risk factors.
Massage Classical massage (*see* page 847) can ease muscular and perhaps also emotional tension and thus may be instrumental in relieving neuralgic pain; some hard techniques aim to induce counterirritation to obscure pain at least temporarily. Ice massage is said to ease pain and relax the patient.	**Useful** as a supportive treatment attempt aimed at bringing relaxation and increasing general well-being. Some case reports claim efficacy in the treatment of pain; however, success is probably seen in only a proportion of patients (*see* Placebo, page xxi).	**Suitable for DIY** Qualified guidance is recommended. Masseurs/masseuses should propose a treatment plan. **Risks:** Some people are sensitive to cold or manual stimuli; others find it hard to tolerate close physical contact.

Treatment	Rating	Point of delivery/risks
Nutritional therapies An organic diet (*see* page 4) provides the body with essential and secondary nutrients that are believed to exercise a multitude of positive effects.	**May be of some use** as an individually directed supportive measure. Numerous studies offer general support for the claim that organic diets are beneficial.	**Suitable for DIY** Qualified guidance is recommended, though not essential. **Risks:** Avoid imbalanced or intolerable diets. They can cause deficiencies with serious consequences, particularly in children.
Physical therapies Cold sprays, cold compresses, and electrostimulative techniques are said to relieve pain (*see* page 871).	**May be of some use** as a short-term attempt to treat pain. Field studies and case reports claim efficacy; however, success is probably seen in only a proportion of patients (*see* Placebo, page xxi).	**Suitable for DIY** Qualified guidance is recommended, but not essential. Therapists should be properly qualified and should propose a treatment plan. **Risks:** Severe skin damage may be caused to persons with diminished temperature sensation when extreme temperatures are applied.
Probiotics The introduction of certain bacteria into the gut is claimed to bring the intestinal flora back into balance and to have a beneficial effect in persons with neuralgia (*see* page 878).	**Of little use** Possibly acceptable as a short-term treatment attempt when more established techniques have been unsuccessful. Some case reports claim efficacy in the treatment of this condition; however, success is probably seen in only a small proportion of patients (*see* Placebo, page xxi).	**Suitable for DIY** Qualified guidance is essential. Therapists should propose a treatment plan. **Risks:** Unlikely provided treatment is carried out competently.

Treatment	Rating	Point of delivery/risks
Reflex therapies Reflex zone massage, cold sprays, reflexology (*see* page 883), and TENS (*see* page 886) are said to ease pain and relax the patient via reflex channels (*see* page 881).	**May be of some use** as a short-term treatment attempt aimed at alleviating acute neuralgic pain. When compared, the various techniques seem to be equally effective, though the benefits they provide vary greatly from person to person. Field studies and case reports claim efficacy; however, success is probably seen in only a proportion of patients (*see* Placebo, page xxi).	**Suitable for DIY** Qualified guidance is essential. Therapists should be properly qualified and should propose a treatment plan. **Risks:** Some people are sensitive to cold, electrical, or manual stimuli, etc.; others find it hard to tolerate close physical contact.
Relaxation techniques Autogenic training (*see* page 888), muscle relaxation according to Jacobson (*see* page 893), and various biofeedback techniques (*see* page 891) are said to relieve muscle tension and inner unrest, and could thus be instrumental in alleviating neuralgic pain as well as being a possibly effective preventive measure.	**May be of some use** as a supportive attempt to bring relaxation and to help the patient come to terms with his/her condition and so reduce the consumption of painkillers. Some studies have reported a reduction in the need for painkillers in some patients. The efficacy that some case reports describe as having been achieved in pain prevention and relief might be seen in only a proportion of patients receiving treatment (*see* Placebo, page xxi).	**Suitable for DIY** Once a sound understanding of the technique has been acquired from a trainer in group sessions or through individual tuition, patients can perform exercises themselves. Therapists should be properly qualified. **Risks:** Fairly unlikely.

Treatment	Rating	Point of delivery/risks
Vitamins and trace elements The painkilling properties of vitamin B6 are thought to contribute to pain relief. The antioxidative properties of vitamin E and selenium are, it is supposed, instrumental in the suppression of inflammation and in combating neuralgia (*see* page 900).	**Of little use** Acceptable as a supportive measure when a patient cannot tolerate the full dose of a painkiller or when vitamin deficiency is suspected. Field studies ascribe a degree of success to vitamin B in the treatment of pain.	**Suitable for DIY** Medical supervision is recommended though not essential. **Risks:** Intolerance and overdosage are possible. Vitamin B6 in high doses can cause serious side effects.

Herbal remedies for neuralgia

Active ingredient/preparation	Rating
Cajeput oil (*Melaleuca leucadendron*)	Used externally, cajeput oil **may be of some use** as a treatment attempt for painful muscles and joints. It contains the rubefacient and skin-warming ingredient cineol. To apply, massage a few drops several times daily into the painful area. **Dosage:** Use externally as a 5 percent alcoholic solution. **Risks:** Be careful not to get the oil into the eyes, as it will cause them to sting painfully. Do not apply to the face and nostrils of infants. Not to be used on sensitive persons. Inhalation may lead to inflammation of the respiratory system. Extensive external use may lead to kidney problems and disorders of the central nervous system. Cajeput oil can irritate the mucous membranes and cause skin allergies.

Active ingredient/preparation	*Rating*
Fir needle oil (*Abies sibirica*)	**Only useful** as an external treatment attempt for neuralgia. Fir needle oil improves the circulation and has a gentle warming effect. **Dosage:** Use externally in a 10–50 percent concentration. To apply, massage a few drops several times daily into the area giving pain. Use ready-formulated preparations as instructed by the manufacturer/prescriber. **Risks:** Be careful not to get the oil into the eyes, as it will cause them to sting painfully. This oil may irritate the mucous membranes if incorrectly used; because of this irritant effect, it must not be used by persons with asthma or whooping cough.
Mint oil (essential oil of *Mentha arvensis*)	**Only useful** as an external treatment attempt for muscle pain and neuralgia. Mint oil has a cooling effect. **Dosage:** Use as a 5–20 percent alcoholic preparation. When using it as a massage oil, apply and work in a few drops several times daily. Use ready-formulated preparations according to the manufacturer's instructions. **Risks:** Be careful not to get the oil into the eyes, as it will cause them to sting painfully. Do not apply to the face and nostrils of infants. This oil may irritate the mucous membranes if incorrectly used and can cause skin allergies.
Pine needle oil (*Pinus pinaster*)	**Only useful** as an external treatment attempt for neuralgia. Pine needle oil improves the circulation and has a gentle warming effect. **Dosage:** Use externally in a 10–50 percent concentration. To apply, massage a few drops several times daily into the area giving pain. Use ready-formulated preparations as instructed by the manufacturer/prescriber. **Risks:** Be careful not to get the oil into the eyes, as it will cause them to sting painfully. Do not apply to the face and nostrils of infants. Not to be used on sensitive persons. Inhalation may lead to inflammation of the respiratory system. Extensive external use may lead to kidney problems and disorders of the central nervous system. Pine needle oil can cause skin allergies.

Active ingredient/preparation	Rating
Turpentine oil (*Terebinthina laricina*)	**Only useful** as an external treatment attempt for painful conditions of the nerves and musculature, for rheumatic pains, and for neuralgia. Turpentine oil improves the circulation and has a gentle warming effect. **Dosage:** In liquid and semisolid formulations 10–20 percent (e.g. mixed with isopropyl alcohol). When using it as a massage oil, apply and work in a few drops several times daily. Use ready-formulated preparations according to the manufacturer's instructions. **Risks:** Be careful not to get the oil into the eyes, as it will cause them to sting painfully. Oil should be used fresh. Do not apply to the face and nostrils of infants. Hypersensitivity and allergies are possible; inhalation may cause acute inflammation of the respiratory tract.

Toothaches

Causes and symptoms

Some nine persons out of every ten have tooth decay or periodontosis. More than two-thirds of all six-year-olds have dental problems, due largely to poor oral hygiene and to diets containing too much sugar and white flour.

Much of the pain, suffering, and needless extra expenditure on dental treatment is the result of a poor dental health policy. The way the Swiss manage dental health is a shining example of successful preventive medicine. Thanks to a series of awareness and prevention campaigns, to the regular brushing of teeth in most schools, and to the establishment of pediatric dentistry as a separate academic discipline, by the age of 12 only one Swiss child in ten will have had a filling, let alone a tooth extracted.

In most cases toothaches are preventable. The most effective prevention is regular cleaning, two or three times a day, with a toothbrush and dental floss, plus additional cleaning after sugary foods and drinks. This is the only sure way of removing plaque from the dental enamel (plaque is the bacterial film that continually forms on teeth, causing decay and periodontosis). Test tablets can be used to show whether the teeth have been cleaned properly or whether plaque has been allowed to build up.

Contrary to what the advertisements would have us believe, toothpaste consists almost entirely of a mild abrasive plus a glidant. It has the disadvantage of creating a false sense of freshness and cleanliness. Research has shown brushing with water alone to be just as effective as brushing with toothpaste.

Toothaches are nearly always an acute warning that something is wrong and in need of treatment. Self-treatment is out of the question, so the most effective cure for a toothache is a visit to the dentist.

Toothaches may arise through:

- tooth decay (caries) which has eaten through the enamel and reached the dentin
- inflammation of the tooth pulp or root (abscesses, granuloma, fistules, or cysts) resulting from untreated caries
- destruction of supporting structures, e.g. periodontosis and periodontitis, as a result of untreated gum inflammation
- sensitivity in the neck of the tooth when the gums have receded through periodontosis
- misalignment and faulty occlusion as a result of grinding and applying undue pressure to the teeth
- dental treatments such as drilling and polishing, both of which generate heat; unlined metal fillings, which conduct heat and cold; poorly positioned fillings, crowns, and bridges; chemical irritation from fillings
- trigeminal neuralgia (*see* page 36)
- trigger points (*see* page 929) in the jaw region that, when irritated, cause referred pain to appear in other parts of the body

Amalgam fillings leak mercury, which affects the teeth and surrounding tissue. It is absorbed by the mucous membranes and may be carried by the bloodstream to affect virtually any organ or functional system.

Orthodox treatment

The fact that toothaches sometimes disappears by themselves does not mean that the cause has disappeared. Only a dentist can identify and eradicate the cause. Patients who are in pain can expect priority dental treatment.

To relieve intense pain, a simple analgesic preparation containing paracetamol, ibuprofen, or acetylsalicylic acid (aspirin) (*see* page 24) can be taken for a short period. It should be noted, however, that aspirin is also an anticoagulant (i.e. it makes any bleeding more profuse) and might cause problems if a tooth has been, or is likely to be, extracted.

A doctor can prescribe a weak opiate such as codeine if the painkillers listed above do not work.

Complementary therapies

Not only are bad teeth a source of pain, but as disease-causing foci (*see* page 928) they are also believed to cause and perpetuate many conditions. No complementary therapy is able to cure pain caused by tooth decay or gum disease. The most complementary treatments will do is occasionally improve a patient's subjective well-being temporarily by soothing and making him/her feel more relaxed. Some therapies will also perhaps alleviate pain following dental surgery, as well as referred pain.

Various nutritional therapies (*see* page 858), especially organic diets, have been shown to be good at preventing tooth decay.

Treatment plan and limited trial

Any therapy should be tried initially for a limited period (*see* page xxiii) to test patient response. Full details of the therapy should be discussed between the patient and the doctor or therapist. Even useful treatments may become problematic if used in the long term without checks for a positive patient response.

Cautions

No complementary treatment is suitable as a substitute for proper dental treatment. An alternative treatment should at most be used in support of treatment by a conventional dentist.

Failure to obtain an orthodox dental diagnosis may result in the patient receiving inappropriate treatment for a serious dental problem.

Complementary treatments for toothaches

Treatment	Rating	Point of delivery/risks
Acupressure This treatment (*see* page 769), otherwise known as pressure-point massage, is claimed to alleviate pain and relieve tension when the appropriate pressure points are stimulated.	**Inappropriate** as the sole form of treatment for dental problems. **May be of some use** as a short-term, supportive treatment attempt aimed at the elimination of pain before and after dental surgery. Investigations have shown a beneficial effect to have been achieved in some patients (*see* Placebo, page xxi).	**Suitable for DIY** Qualified guidance is recommended. Practitioners should be properly qualified and should propose a treatment plan. **Risks:** Unlikely provided treatment is carried out competently.
Acupuncture Acupuncture in its various forms (*see* page 772) aims to encourage the flow of energy (*see* page 927) or to directly alleviate a toothache, relieve discomfort in the jaw, or act preventively against treatment pain.	**Inappropriate** as the sole form of treatment for dental problems. **May be of some use** as a short-term, supportive treatment attempt aimed at eliminating pain before and after dental surgery. Investigations have shown a beneficial effect to have been achieved in some patients (*see* Placebo, page xxi).	**Requires a qualified practitioner** Practitioners should be properly qualified and should propose a treatment plan. **Risks:** Probably rare provided treatment is carried out competently.
Anthroposophical medicine The "compositions" (*see* page 783) Arnica Phytolacca and Lachesis are said to reduce inflammation, arrest bleeding, and reverse swelling in patients with pain associated with dental treatment, swelling after tooth extraction, and children's dental problems.	**Inappropriate** as the sole form of treatment for dental problems. Acceptable as a treatment attempt for pain associated with dental treatment, swelling after tooth extraction, or dental problems in children. Field studies claim efficacy; however, success is probably seen in only a small proportion of patients (*see* Placebo, page xxi).	**Requires a qualified practitioner** Practitioners should be properly qualified and should propose a treatment plan. **Risks:** Allergies, toxic reactions, or intolerance are possible.

Treatment	Rating	Point of delivery/risks
Aromatherapy Essential oils (*see* page 786) are used to soothe and relax, or to invigorate, thereby helping to ease a toothache. The essences may be taken orally, used externally as massage oils or bathing emulsions, or inhaled as vapors.	**Inappropriate** as the sole form of treatment for dental problems. Acceptable as a supportive treatment attempt when the patient perceives it to be calming and relaxing. Some case reports claim efficacy; however, success is probably seen in only a proportion of patients (*see* Placebo, page xxi).	**Suitable for DIY** Qualified guidance is recommended. Aromatherapists should be properly qualified and should propose a treatment plan. **Risks:** Allergies or intolerance are possible. Some oils are carcinogenic in test systems and possibly in humans.
Bioresonance therapy Bioresonance therapists use electrical devices in an attempt to discover the causes of illness and claim to be able to regulate pathogenic energies and disease related vibrations (*see* page 794).	**Inappropriate** as the sole form of treatment for dental problems. Possibly acceptable as a short-term, supportive treatment attempt for chronic and persistent toothaches when simpler, more established methods of pain relief have been unsuccessful. Some case reports claim efficacy; however, success is probably seen, if at all, in only a small proportion of patients (*see* Placebo, page xxi).	**Requires a qualified practitioner** Practitioners should be properly qualified and should propose a treatment plan. **Risks:** Fairly unlikely.
Electroacupuncture according to Voll By taking readings of the electrical conductivity of the skin (*see* page 802), therapists claim to be able to derive an insight into diseased areas of the body, pathogenic foci (*see* page 928), and stress factors (*see* Toxins, page 929).	**Inappropriate** as the sole form of treatment for dental problems. Possibly acceptable as an additional, supportive attempt to locate foci when orthodox dental techniques have been unsuccessful. Some case reports claim efficacy; however, success is probably seen, if at all, in only a small proportion of patients (*see* Placebo, page xxi).	**Requires a qualified practitioner** Practitioners should be properly qualified and should propose a treatment plan. No credence should be given to anyone promising immediate or total success. **Risks:** A second opinion must always be obtained from a qualified physician before any attempt is made to "eliminate foci" (e.g. by surgery).

Treatment	Rating	Point of delivery/risks
Electroneural therapy according to Croon According to the theory, readings taken at various reactive sites on the skin highlight diseased areas within the body. Based on these readings, targeted neurotherapeutic measures can be undertaken to combat toothaches (*see* page 806).	**Inappropriate** as the sole form of treatment for dental problems. Possibly acceptable as a short-term, supportive treatment attempt for nagging toothaches when simpler, more established methods have been unsuccessful. Some case reports claim efficacy; however, success is probably seen, if at all, in only a small proportion of patients (*see* Placebo, page xxi).	**Requires a qualified practitioner** Practitioners should be properly qualified and should propose a treatment plan. No credence should be given to anyone promising immediate or total success. **Risks:** Proponents themselves warn that treatment should not be given in acute inflammatory conditions.
Flower remedies To the flower therapist a toothache can be an expression of psychological problems. Flower remedies (*see* page 828), especially Bach Rescue Remedy in the case of a toothache, are said to restore emotional balance and bring peace of mind.	**Inappropriate** as the sole form of treatment for dental problems. Acceptable as a supportive treatment attempt aimed at soothing and relaxing, or for acting preventively against worries about receiving dental treatment. Some case reports claim efficacy; however, success is probably seen in only a proportion of patients (*see* Placebo, page xxi).	**Suitable for DIY** Qualified guidance is recommended. Bach flower therapists should be properly qualified and should propose a treatment plan. **Risks:** Possible intolerance.

Treatment	Rating	Point of delivery/risks
Homeopathy Highly diluted (potentized) solutions (*see* page 831) are believed to be able to redress vital energy imbalances. Organo- and functiotropic (*see* page 833) homeopathy is claimed to be effective in dealing symptomatically with toothaches.	**Inappropriate** as the sole form of treatment for dental problems. Acceptable as a supportive treatment attempt (e.g. for chronic inflammation) when orthodox dental treatment has been unsuccessful. Some case reports claim success for homeopathic treatments; however, success is probably seen in only a small proportion of patients (*see* Placebo, page xxi).	**Requires a qualified practitioner** Homeopaths should be properly qualified and should propose a treatment plan. **Risks:** Possible intolerance.
Hypnosis and self-hypnosis In the relaxed and generally altered state of awareness that is induced in hypnosis or self-hypnosis (*see* page 837), physical conditions can be addressed and toothaches associated with disorders of the musculoskeletal system (e.g. in the jaw) may be lessened. Some professionally organized courses in self-hypnosis are now available.	**Inappropriate** as the sole form of treatment for dental problems. Acceptable as a short-term treatment attempt when simpler, more established methods of pain relief have been unsuccessful. Some case reports claim efficacy; however, success is probably seen in only a proportion of patients treated (*see* Placebo, page xxi).	**Requires a qualified practitioner** Hypnotherapists should be properly qualified and should propose a treatment plan. **Risks:** Unlikely provided treatment is carried out competently.

Treatment	*Rating*	*Point of delivery/risks*
Manual therapies Chiropractors and osteopaths use a series of manipulations to realign the jaw and any vertebrae that may be displaced. This is said to reduce the irritation of trigger points (*see* page 929) thought to be responsible for generating referred toothaches (*see* page 844).	**Inappropriate** as the sole form of treatment for dental problems. Acceptable as a short-term treatment attempt for persistent referred toothaches when less risky, more established methods have been unsuccessful. Some case reports claim efficacy; however, success is probably seen in only a proportion of patients (*see* Placebo, page xxi).	**Requires a qualified practitioner** Practitioners should be properly qualified and should propose a treatment plan. **Risks:** Manipulations carried out on the head and neck can cause serious arterial damage, dislocations, and even bone fractures. Osteoporosis is a prevalent risk factor.
Nutritional therapies An organic diet (*see* page 4) provides the body with essential and secondary plant nutrients that are believed to exercise a multitude of positive effects and to be capable, *inter alia*, of preventing tooth decay.	**Inappropriate** as the sole form of treatment for dental problems. **Useful** as a preventive measure. Various controlled studies suggest that dietary therapies afford effective caries prophylaxis.	**Suitable for DIY** Qualified guidance is recommended, though not essential. **Risks:** Avoid imbalanced or intolerable diets. They can cause deficiencies with serious consequences, particularly in children.
Physical therapies Exercise therapy (*see* page 868), various hydrotherapeutic techniques (*see* pages 871–8), and Kneipp treatments (*see* page 871) are said to stimulate the immune system.	**Inappropriate** as the sole form of treatment for dental problems. Acceptable as a short-term therapeutic attempt in cases where other methods of pain relief are not available. Some case studies claim efficacy; however, success is probably seen in only a proportion of patients (*see* Placebo, page xxi).	**Suitable for DIY** Qualified guidance is recommended though not essential. Practitioners should propose a treatment plan. **Risks:** Skin damage may be caused to persons with diminished temperature sensation when extreme temperatures are applied.

Treatment	Rating	Point of delivery/risks
Reflex therapies This technique (*see* page 881) is founded on the belief that, through the reflex channels (*see* page 882), certain parts of the body can exert an influence on other, sometimes distant, parts where pain is actually experienced.	**Inappropriate** as the sole form of treatment for dental problems. **Useful** as a treatment attempt for referred pain. There are few reliable reports of a definite beneficial effect. When compared, the various techniques all seem to offer the same degree of effectiveness, though the individual benefits they provide vary greatly from person to person.	**Suitable for DIY** Qualified guidance is essential. **Risks:** Some people are sensitive to cold or electrical stimuli; others find rubber electrodes hard to tolerate.
Relaxation techniques Autogenic training (*see* page 888), muscle relaxation according to Jacobson (*see* page 893), and various biofeedback techniques (*see* page 891) may reduce toothaches associated with disorders of the musculoskeletal system (e.g. in the jaw), and may be of benefit in relaxing tense muscles and easing inner unrest.	**Inappropriate** as the sole form of treatment for dental problems. **May be of some use** as a supportive attempt to provide relaxation for an acute toothache and to cut down on the intake of painkillers. Some case studies indicate that relaxation techniques are successful in temporarily reducing the severity of toothaches. Various controlled clinical studies report success in reducing the amounts of painkillers required by some patients.	**Suitable for DIY** Once a sound understanding of the technique has been acquired from a trainer in group sessions or through individual tuition, patients can perform exercises themselves. Therapists should be properly qualified. **Risks:** Fairly unlikely.

Treatment	Rating	Point of delivery/risks
TENS The use of low frequency electrical currents on the surface of the skin is said to act through so-called reflex channels (*see* page 882) to reduce toothaches (see page 886).	**Inappropriate** as the sole form of treatment for dental problems. **Useful** as a treatment attempt for referred pain. Controlled clinical studies and field studies confirm the efficacy of TENS in some patients suffering from toothaches associated with disorders of the musculoskeletal system (e.g. in the jaw).	**Requires a qualified practitioner** Practitioners should be properly qualified and should propose a treatment plan. **Risks:** Some people react sensitively to electrical stimuli or rubber electrodes.

Herbal remedy for toothaches

Active ingredient/preparation	Rating
Clove oil (essential oil of cloves *Caryophylli atheroleum*)	Clove oil **may be of some use** as a treatment attempt for inflammation of the oral and pharyngeal mucosa, and for fast analgesia through the local anasthetic effect of its active principle, eugenol. To apply, soak a cotton swab or piece of cotton wool and apply to the painful tooth as required. **Risks:** Can have an irritant or numbing effect on the surrounding gum.

Psyche and nervous system

Addiction to illicit and prescription drugs

Causes and symptoms

With hashish, marijuana, and cocaine the overriding problem is that of psychological addiction. Fast onset physiological dependence has only been noted so far for crack and opiates such as heroin. The serious health and sociological consequences of taking "hard drugs" result less from the drug itself than from the lifestyle the addict is forced to adopt through criminalization of the drug. The problems are: health damage through living in a subculture, indebtedness, and criminality as a way of financing a drug habit; the risk of contracting diseases such as AIDS (*see* page 715), hepatitis B, and other infections by using nonsterile needles; and the risk to life itself through a fatal overdose or through "cut" and impure illicit drugs.

In Western, industrialized countries addiction to prescription drugs is second only to alcohol addiction. In the UK the number of people addicted to tranquilizers and sleeping tablets can be put in the hundreds of thousands, if not millions. Substances having the greatest potential for misuse and causing habituation are: potent painkillers, virtually all types of sleeping tablets and other soporific preparations, central nervous stimulants, appetite suppressants, and laxatives. Cough mixtures containing codeine or other opiates are also sometimes abused.

Psychological addiction comes from a powerful craving in people to re-experience an earlier "high" they attained with the drug, to alleviate anxiety or pain, or to obliterate their worries for a while.

With physiological dependence the person usually, but not always, becomes increasingly hooked on the drug so that ever higher doses have to be taken to achieve the same effect. Abrupt discontinuance of the drug may induce severe withdrawal reactions, especially with hypnotics and sedatives of the benzodiazepine type. Misuse of prescription drugs, depending on the substance taken, can have a variety of consequences: personality changes, perception disorders, poor general health, malnutrition, and protein and vitamin deficiency. It can also produce serious physical damage (for example, kidney failure through taking painkillers over a number of years).

Orthodox treatment

Withdrawal begins with a detoxification phase, usually with supportive medication. Methadone is often prescribed as a heroin substitute or for support during withdrawal. However, this morphinelike substance can itself lead to habituation. Detoxification is usually followed by medium- or long-term psychotherapy to resocialize the patient.

Complementary therapies

Some complementary therapies claim to alleviate withdrawal symptoms and help the person overcome the addiction.

Treatment plan and limited trial

The therapist should start by defining a treatment goal and setting a time-frame (*see* page xxiii). At the end of this initial treatment period the success, or otherwise, of the therapy should be critically appraised.

Caution

No complementary procedure is by itself able to overcome severe withdrawal reactions.

Complementary treatments for addiction to illicit and prescription drugs

Treatment	Rating	Point of delivery/risks
Acupressure This treatment (*see* page 769), otherwise known as pressure-point massage, is used to reduce nausea and vomiting during withdrawal and to improve general well-being. The pressure points chosen may differ from one practitioner to another.	**May be of some use** as a short-term treatment attempt aimed at alleviating nausea and vomiting. Case reports claim efficacy; however, success is probably seen in only a proportion of patients (*see* Placebo, page xxi).	**Suitable for DIY** Qualified guidance is recommended. Practitioners should be properly qualified and should propose a treatment plan. **Risks:** Unlikely provided treatment is carried out competently.
Acupuncture Acupuncture in its various forms (*see* page 772) aims to alleviate withdrawal pain, reduce addiction, and ease tension. The acupuncture points chosen can vary from one practitioner to another. Semi-permanent ear implants are sometimes used (*see* page 776).	**May be of some use** as a short-term, supportive treatment attempt aimed at alleviating withdrawal symptoms and reducing addiction. Trials and field studies indicate that this technique has a degree of efficacy in a proportion of patients. Semi-permanent implants have a similar effect.	**Requires a qualified practitioner** Acupuncturists should be properly qualified and should propose a treatment plan. **Risks:** Probably rare provided treatment is carried out competently.
Anthroposophical medicine Anthroposophically oriented psychotherapy (*see* page 784) is said to strengthen the ego as part of an all-round treatment plan and so make withdrawal easier.	**May be of some use** as a treatment attempt when the patient accepts this type of approach. Case reports claim efficacy; however, success is probably seen in only a proportion of patients (*see* Placebo, page xxi).	**Requires a qualified practitioner** Practitioners should be properly qualified and should propose a treatment plan. **Risks:** Unlikely provided treatment is carried out competently.

Treatment	Rating	Point of delivery/risks
Aromatherapy Essential oils (*see* page 786) are used to soothe and relax, thereby easing withdrawal symptoms. The essences may be taken orally, used externally as massage oils or bathing emulsions, or inhaled as vapors.	**May be of some use** as a supportive attempt at mood improvement and relaxation. Some case reports claim efficacy; however, success is probably seen in only a proportion of patients (*see* Placebo, page xxi).	**Suitable for DIY** Qualified guidance is recommended. The effects of individual essential oils differ widely. **Risks:** Allergies or intolerance are possible. Some oils are carcinogenic in test systems and possibly in humans.
Bioresonance therapy Bioresonance therapists (*see* page 794) use electrical devices allegedly to weaken or turn around pathogenic energies and vibrations and so reduce the craving for drugs.	**Of little use** Possibly acceptable as a short-term, supportive treatment attempt when simpler, more established methods have been unsuccessful. The efficacy in withdrawal crises described in some case reports is probably seen, if at all, in only a small proportion of patients (*see* Placebo, page xxi).	**Requires a qualified practitioner** Practitioners should be properly qualified and should propose a treatment plan. No credence should be given to anyone promising immediate or total success. **Risks:** Fairly unlikely.
Cell therapy Injecting or ingesting products extracted from calf thymus is said to have a rejuvenating and revitalizing effect and to stimulate human tissues and organs (*see* page 796).	Based on present knowledge, thymus treatment is **of little use**. The efficacy and mode of action of this costly and relatively risky procedure remain unproven. Fresh cell therapy is **not advised**.	**Requires a qualified practitioner** Practitioners should be properly qualified and should propose a treatment plan. **Risks:** Injecting foreign proteins into the body can provoke (possibly fatal) allergic reactions. Also, pathogens such as those that cause bovine spongiform encephalopathy (BSE) or other serious infections may be introduced. Using needles in former addicts may make it more difficult for them to kick the habit.

Treatment	*Rating*	*Point of delivery/risks*
Electroacupuncture according to Voll By taking readings of the electrical conductivity of the skin, therapists claim to be able to derive an insight into diseased areas of the body, intoxications, and pathogenic foci (*see* page 928) said to be conducive to addiction. Afterwards the cause of addiction can be eliminated and the body "detoxified" (*see* page 802).	**Of little use** Possibly acceptable as a short-term, supportive treatment attempt for chronic and persistent complaints when simpler, more established methods have been unsuccessful. Some case reports claim efficacy; however, success is probably seen, if at all, in only a small proportion of patients (*see* Placebo, page xxi).	**Requires a qualified practitioner** Practitioners should be properly qualified and should propose a treatment plan. No credence should be given to anyone promising immediate or total success. **Risks:** A second opinion must always be obtained from a qualified physician before any attempt is made to "eliminate foci" (e.g. by surgery).
Electroneural therapy according to Croon According to the theory, readings taken at various reactive sites on the skin highlight diseased areas of the body, pathogenic foci (*see* page 928), and stress factors (*see* Toxins, page 929). Afterwards the addiction can be addressed using electrostimulative therapy (*see* page 806).	**Of little use** Possibly acceptable as a short-term, supportive treatment attempt when simpler, more established methods have been unsuccessful. Some case reports claim efficacy; however, success is probably seen, if at all, in only a small proportion of patients (*see* Placebo, page xxi).	**Requires a qualified practitioner** Practitioners should be properly qualified and should propose a treatment plan. No credence should be given to anyone promising immediate or total success. **Risks:** Proponents themselves warn that treatment should not be given in acute inflammatory conditions.
Eliminative methods, unbloody Sweating (*see* page 877) is supposed to ease withdrawal symptoms, encourage metabolism, accelerate the elimination of drug residues, and improve the body's own regulatory systems.	**May be of some use** as a supportive treatment attempt when the patient perceives sweating as pleasant. The easing of symptoms described in some case reports and field studies is probably seen in only a proportion of patients (*see* Placebo, page xxi).	**Suitable for DIY** Qualified guidance is recommended. **Risks:** Intense sweating can be a cause of physical stress. The motor unrest present in acute alcohol withdrawal precludes the use of sweating.

Treatment	*Rating*	*Point of delivery/risks*
Enzyme therapy The enzymes that are used reportedly prevent and destroy "immune complexes" that course in the blood and are responsible, for instance, for sustaining inflammatory processes (*see* page 824).	**Of little use** Some case reports claim this little researched therapy works; however, success is probably seen in only a small proportion of patients (*see* Placebo, page xxi).	**Requires a qualified practitioner** Practitioners should propose a treatment plan. Non-prescription formulations are suitable for do-it-yourself. **Risks:** Allergies or intolerance are possible.
Flower remedies Flower remedies (*see* page 828) are said to restore emotional balance and assist the body's psychic ability to heal itself. Bach Rescue Remedy is often used to counter withdrawal symptoms.	**Of little use** Acceptable as a short-term, supportive treatment attempt aimed at soothing and relaxing. The efficacy in withdrawal crises described in some case reports is probably seen in only a proportion of patients (*see* Placebo, page xxi).	**Suitable for DIY** Qualified guidance is recommended. Practitioners should propose a treatment plan. **Risks:** Possible intolerance.
Homeopathy Highly diluted (potentized) solutions (*see* page 831), the use of which may be either symptom or personality oriented, are believed to be able to redress vital energy imbalances. Organo- and functiotropic (*see* page 833) homeopathy is claimed to be an effective way of tackling drug addiction.	**Of little use** Acceptable as a short-term, supportive treatment attempt for withdrawal symptoms. The success of organotropic homeopathic remedies described in case reports and field studies is probably seen in only a proportion of patients (*see* Placebo, page xxi).	**Suitable for DIY** Qualified guidance is recommended. Homeopaths should be properly qualified and should propose a treatment plan. **Risks:** Possible intolerance.

Treatment	Rating	Point of delivery/risks
Hypnosis and self-hypnosis In the relaxed and generally altered state of awareness that is induced in hypnosis or self-hypnosis (*see* page 837), the patient's mental state can be positively influenced, pain can be alleviated, and addictive behavior modified. Hypnosis is frequently used in association with other psycho- and behavioral therapies.	**May be of some use** as a short-term, supportive treatment attempt aimed at relaxing the patient and modifying his/her addictive behavior. Case reports and field studies claim efficacy; however, success is probably seen in only a proportion of patients (*see* Placebo, page xxi).	**Requires a qualified practitioner** Hypnotherapists should be properly qualified and should propose a treatment plan. No credence should be given to anyone promising immediate or total success. **Risks:** Unlikely provided treatment is carried out competently.
Manual therapies Chiropractors and osteopaths use a series of manipulations to realign allegedly displaced vertebrae and joints that, it is believed, may be co-responsible for pain (*see* page 844).	**Of little use** Acceptable as a short-term, supportive treatment attempt during withdrawal. The efficacy of this relatively risky procedure described in some case reports is probably seen, if at all, in only a proportion of patients (*see* Placebo, page xxi).	**Requires a qualified practitioner** Practitioners should be properly qualified and should propose a treatment plan. **Risks:** Spinal manipulations can cause serious injury. Osteoporosis is one of several risk factors.
Massage Classical massage (*see* page 847) can improve general well-being, as well as ease muscular and perhaps also emotional tension; certain techniques can be used to induce counterirritation to obscure withdrawal pain. Ice massage is said to generate counterstimuli to mask acute withdrawal pain at least temporarily.	**May be of some use** as a supportive treatment attempt aimed at increasing general well-being. The easing of withdrawal pain described in case reports and field studies is probably seen in only a proportion of patients (*see* Placebo, page xxi).	**Suitable for DIY** Qualified guidance is recommended. Masseurs/masseuses should propose a treatment plan. **Risks:** Some people are sensitive to manual stimuli; others find it hard to tolerate close physical contact.

Treatment	Rating	Point of delivery/risks
Nutritional therapies An organic diet (*see* page 4), through its high content of dietary fiber, vitamins (*see* page 900), and secondary plant constituents, exercises a multitude of positive effects within the body.	**Useful** for general support during withdrawal. Case reports and field studies claim efficacy; however, success is probably seen in only a proportion of patients (*see* Placebo, page xxi).	**Suitable for DIY** Qualified guidance is recommended though not essential. **Risks:** Avoid imbalanced or intolerable diets. They can cause deficiencies with serious consequences, particularly in children.
Physical therapies Cold sprays or cold compresses are said to generate counterstimuli to mask acute withdrawal pain at least temporarily. Baths, warm compresses, and exercise, it is believed, help the patient relax and give an increased feeling of well-being. (*see* page 867). Saunas are supposed to ease withdrawal symptoms, encourage metabolism, accelerate the elimination of drug residues, and improve the body's own regulatory systems.	**Useful** as a short-term, supportive attempt aimed at alleviating pain and increasing general well-being. Case reports and field studies claim efficacy; however, success is probably seen in only a proportion of patients (*see* Placebo, page xxi). Saunas **may be of some use** as a supportive treatment.	**Suitable for DIY** Qualified guidance is recommended, but not essential. Therapists should be properly qualified and should propose a treatment plan. **Risks:** Severe skin damage may be caused to persons with diminished temperature sensation when extreme temperatures are applied. The motor unrest present in acute alcohol withdrawal precludes the use of saunas.
Probiotics The introduction of certain bacteria into the gut is claimed to bring the intestinal flora back into balance and to have a beneficial effect on other parts of the immune system (*see* page 878).	**Of little use** Possibly acceptable as a short-term, supportive treatment attempt aimed at improving poor digestion. The efficacy of this little researched technique, as described in some case reports, is probably seen in only a proportion of patients (*see* Placebo, page xxi).	**Requires a qualified practitioner** Practitioners should be properly qualified and should propose a treatment plan. Non-prescription formulations are **suitable for do-it-yourself**. **Risks:** Fairly unlikely provided treatment is carried out competently.

Treatment	*Rating*	*Point of delivery/risks*
Reflex therapies Various techniques such as reflex zone massage (*see* page 883) or TENS (*see* page 886) are said to free blocked energy and lessen pain via reflex channels (*see* page 881). These techniques, it is claimed, can also relax the patient and ease withdrawal symptoms.	**Useful** as a short-term, supportive treatment attempt during withdrawal. Case reports and (in the case of TENS) initial controlled studies claim efficacy; however, success is probably seen in only a proportion of patients (*see* Placebo, page xxi).	**Suitable for DIY** Qualified guidance is essential. **Risks:** Some people find it hard to tolerate the pressure applied during massage; others cannot stand close physical contact, electrical stimuli, or rubber electrodes.
Relaxation techniques Autogenic training (*see* page 888), muscle relaxation according to Jacobson (*see* page 893), and various biofeedback techniques (*see* page 891) are said to relieve muscle tension and inner unrest, to ease symptoms, and to prevent renewed cravings. These techniques are frequently combined with other psycho- or behavioral therapies.	**Useful** as a supportive treatment attempt aimed at relaxing the patient, easing symptoms, and preventing strong cravings. Case reports and field studies claim efficacy; however, success is probably seen in only a proportion of patients (*see* Placebo, page xxi).	**Suitable for DIY** Once a sound understanding of the technique has been acquired from a trainer, patients can perform exercises themselves. Therapists should be properly qualified. **Risks:** Fairly unlikely.
Vitamins and trace elements The painkilling properties of vitamin B6 are thought to contribute to pain relief. The anti-oxidative properties of vitamins C and E and of selenium are, it is supposed, instrumental in the suppression of inflammation (*see* page 900).	**Useful** in vitamin deficiency as a result of drug abuse. Based on present knowledge it is not possible to make any definitive recommendations regarding the dosage of antioxidative vitamins and trace elements.	**Suitable for DIY** Medical guidance is recommended though not essential. **Risks:** Intolerance and overdosage are possible. Vitamin B6 in high doses can cause serious side effects.

Herbal remedies for withdrawal of illicit and prescription drugs

There are no recommended herbal remedies for use in this indication. However, herbal remedies for anxiety (*see* page 91) and depression (*see* page 109) may be used supportively during withdrawal.

Alcohol and nicotine withdrawal

Causes and symptoms

Alcohol dependence is a major social and health issue. Regular heavy drinking can damage not only the liver (*see* page 598) but also the stomach, heart, vascular system, mucous membranes, nervous system, and skin, as well as affecting the person's libido and sexual performance. Regular or excessive drinking by expectant mothers can seriously damage their unborn children. Too much alcohol also considerably increases the risk of a person developing certain types of cancer, such as cancer of the mouth, pharynx, bowels, or liver, and can lead to psychological and emotional changes, with all their social, professional, and economic repercussions.

Every pack of cigarettes nowadays carries a health warning. Tobacco smoke, as well as containing nicotine and tar, harbors some 4,500 other chemical substances such as carbon monoxide, oxides of nitrogen, traces of radioactive plutonium, arsenic, prussic acid, and various free radical forming agents (*see* page 902). Smoking will cause arteriosclerosis, cardiovascular disease (*see* pages 409–511), smoker's leg, stomach ulcers (*see* page 548), cancer (*see* page 701), possibly spinal damage (*see* page 167), and even male impotence. It may also exacerbate osteoporosis (*see* page 195). Eighty-five percent of all lung cancer sufferers are, or have been, smokers.

Smoking by expectant mothers induces alimentary disease in the embryo; the children of smoking mothers are born smaller and lighter than the children of mothers who did not smoke during their pregnancy. Smoking also leads to premature ageing and wrinkling of the skin.

Orthodox treatment

Medically supervised alcohol withdrawal generally begins with the person being admitted to a hospital or private clinic. During the initial detoxification phase, medical staff monitor the patient for withdrawal symptoms and any disease that might have been brought on through the addiction. The patient subsequently undergoes social and behavioral therapy to help him/her stay dry.

Kicking the nicotine habit may be supported by the use of nicotine gum, sprays, inhalators or patches, all of which do, indeed, increase the success rate in persons trying to give up smoking. Numerous controlled studies have confirmed the superiority of these products over a dummy treatment (*see* Placebo, page xxi). Psychotherapy may be required to underpin a change in behavior.

Complementary therapies

Some complementary therapies claim to alleviate withdrawal symptoms and help the person overcome the addiction.

Treatment plan and limited trial

The therapist should start by defining a treatment goal and setting a time frame (*see* page xxiii). At the end of this initial treatment period the success, or otherwise, of the therapy should be critically appraised.

Caution

No complementary procedure is in itself an adequate means of overcoming severe alcohol or other addiction.

Complementary treatments for alcohol and nicotine withdrawal

Treatment	Rating	Point of delivery/risks
Acupressure This treatment (*see* page 769), otherwise known as pressure-point massage, is used to reduce withdrawal pains and ease tension. Special bracelets can be worn to stimulate points associated with addiction and withdrawal problems.	**May be of some use** as a short-term treatment attempt aimed at alleviating withdrawal pains. The easing of symptoms and long periods without relapse described in case reports and field studies are probably seen in only a proportion of patients (*see* Placebo, page xxi).	**Suitable for DIY** Qualified guidance is recommended. Practitioners should be properly qualified and should propose a treatment plan. **Risks:** Unlikely provided treatment is carried out competently.
Acupuncture Acupuncture in its various forms (*see* page 772) aims to alleviate withdrawal pain, reduce addiction, and ease tension. The acupuncture points chosen can vary from one practitioner to another. Semi-permanent ear implants are sometimes used (*see* page 776).	**May be of some use** as a treatment attempt aimed at alleviating withdrawal pain and reducing addiction. The efficacy during withdrawal described in field studies and—for nicotine addiction—in various studies is probably seen in only a proportion of patients (*see* Placebo, page xxi).	**Requires a qualified practitioner** Acupuncturists should be properly qualified and should propose a treatment plan. **Risks:** Probably rare provided treatment is carried out competently.
Anthroposophical medicine Anthroposophically oriented psychotherapy (*see* page 784) is said to strengthen the ego as part of an all-round treatment plan and so make withdrawal easier.	**May be of some use** as a treatment attempt when the patient accepts this sometimes elaborate procedure. Case reports claim efficacy; however, success is probably seen in only a proportion of patients (*see* Placebo, page xxi).	**Requires a qualified practitioner** Practitioners should be properly qualified and should propose a treatment plan. **Risks:** Unlikely provided treatment is carried out competently.

Treatment	Rating	Point of delivery/risks
Aromatherapy Essential oils (*see* page 786) are used to soothe and relax, thereby easing the pain of withdrawal. The essences may be taken orally, used externally as massage oils or bathing emulsions, or inhaled as vapors.	**May be of some use** as a supportive attempt at mood improvement and relaxation. The efficacy during withdrawal described in some case reports is probably seen in only a proportion of patients (*see* Placebo, page xxi).	**Suitable for DIY** Qualified guidance is recommended. The effects of individual essential oils differ widely. **Risks:** Allergies or intolerance are possible. Some oils are carcinogenic in test systems and possibly in humans.
Bioresonance therapy Bioresonance therapists (*see* page 794) use electrical devices allegedly to weaken or turn around pathogenic energies and vibrations and so reduce the craving for alcohol or nicotine.	**Of little use** If it is at all acceptable, then only as a short-term, supportive treatment attempt when simpler, more established methods have been unsuccessful. The efficacy during withdrawal described in some case reports is probably seen, if at all, in only a proportion of patients (*see* Placebo, page xxi).	**Requires a qualified practitioner** Practitioners should be properly qualified and should propose a treatment plan. No credence should be given to anyone promising immediate or total success. **Risks:** Fairly unlikely.
Electroacupuncture according to Voll By taking readings of the electrical conductivity of the skin (*see* page 802), therapists claim to be able to derive an insight into diseased areas of the body, intoxications, and pathogenic foci (*see* page 928) said to be conducive to addiction. Afterwards the cause of addiction can be eliminated and the body "detoxified."	**Of little use** Possibly acceptable as a short-term, supportive treatment attempt when more established methods have been unsuccessful. Some case reports claim efficacy; however, success is probably seen, if at all, in only a small proportion of patients (*see* Placebo, page xxi).	**Requires a qualified practitioner** Practitioners should be properly qualified and should propose a treatment plan. No credence should be given to anyone promising immediate or total success. **Risks:** A second opinion must always be obtained from a qualified physician before any attempt is made to "eliminate foci" (e.g. by surgery).

Treatment	Rating	Point of delivery/risks
Electroneural therapy according to Croon According to the theory, readings taken at various reactive sites on the skin highlight diseased areas of the body and pathogenic foci (*see* page 928) said to be conducive to alcohol or nicotine addiction. Afterwards the cause of addiction can be eliminated by electrostimulative therapy (*see* page 806).	**Of little use** Possibly acceptable as a short-term, supportive treatment attempt when simpler, more established methods have been unsuccessful. Some case reports claim efficacy; however, success is probably seen, if at all, in only a small proportion of patients (*see* Placebo, page xxi).	**Requires a qualified practitioner** Practitioners should be properly qualified and should propose a treatment plan. No credence should be given to anyone promising immediate or total success. **Risks:** Proponents themselves warn that treatment should not be given in acute inflammatory conditions.
Eliminative methods, unbloody Sweating (*see* page 877) is supposed to ease withdrawal symptoms, encourage metabolism, accelerate the elimination of alcohol and nicotine residues, and improve the body's own regulatory systems.	**May be of some use** as a supportive treatment attempt when the patient perceives sweating as pleasant. The easing of symptoms described in case reports and field studies is probably seen in only a proportion of patients (*see* Placebo, page xxi).	**Suitable for DIY** Qualified guidance is recommended though not essential. **Risks:** Intense sweating can be a cause of physical stress. The motor unrest present in acute alcohol withdrawal precludes the use of sweating.
Flower remedies Flower remedies (*see* page 828) are said to restore emotional balance and assist the body's psychic ability to heal itself. Bach Rescue Remedy is often used to counter withdrawal symptoms.	**Of little use** Acceptable as a short-term, supportive treatment attempt aimed at soothing and relaxing. The efficacy during withdrawal crises described in some case reports is probably seen in only a proportion of patients (*see* Placebo, page xxi).	**Suitable for DIY** Qualified guidance is recommended. Practitioners should propose a treatment plan. **Risks:** Possible intolerance.

Treatment	Rating	Point of delivery/risks
Homeopathy Highly diluted (potentized) solutions (*see* page 831), the use of which may be either symptom or personality oriented, are believed to be able to redress vital energy imbalances and thus remove the cause of addiction.	**Of little use** Acceptable as a short-term, supportive treatment attempt. The success of symptom oriented homeopathy in the alleviation of symptoms, as described in case reports and field studies, is probably seen in only a proportion of patients (*see* Placebo, page xxi).	**Requires a qualified practitioner** Homeopaths should be properly qualified and should propose a treatment plan. **Risks:** Possible intolerance.
Hypnosis and self-hypnosis In the relaxed and generally altered state of awareness that is induced in hypnosis or self-hypnosis (*see* page 837), pain and other symptoms can be alleviated. Hypnosis is frequently used in association with other psycho- and behavioral therapies.	**May be of some use** as a short-term, supportive treatment attempt. The easing of symptoms described in case reports is probably seen in only a proportion of patients (*see* Placebo, page xxi).	**Requires a qualified practitioner** Hypnotherapists should be properly qualified and should propose a treatment plan. **Risks:** Unlikely provided treatment is carried out competently.
Manual therapies Chiropractors and osteopaths use a series of manipulations to realign displaced vertebrae and joints that, it is believed, are the cause of a number of pathological conditions (*see* page 844).	**Of little use** Possibly acceptable as a short-term, supportive therapeutic attempt at alleviating pain. The efficacy of this relatively risky procedure described in some case reports is probably seen in only a proportion of patients (*see* Placebo, page xxi).	**Requires a qualified practitioner** Practitioners should be properly qualified and should propose a treatment plan. **Risks:** Spinal manipulations can cause serious injury. Osteoporosis is one of several risk factors.

Treatment	Rating	Point of delivery/risks
Massage Classical massage (*see* page 847) can improve general well-being, as well as ease muscular and perhaps also emotional tension; certain techniques can be used to induce counterirritation to obscure withdrawal pain. Ice massage is said to generate counterstimuli to mask acute withdrawal pain at least temporarily.	**May be of some use** as a supportive treatment attempt aimed at increasing general well-being. The easing of withdrawal pain described in case reports is probably seen in only a proportion of patients (*see* Placebo, page xxi).	**Suitable for DIY** Qualified guidance is recommended. **Risks:** Some people are sensitive to manual stimuli; others find it hard to tolerate close physical contact.
Nutritional therapies An organic diet (*see* page 4), through its high content of dietary fiber, vitamins (*see* page 900), and secondary plant constituents, exercises a multitude of positive effects within the body.	**Useful** for general support during withdrawal. Case reports and field studies claim efficacy; however, success is probably seen in only a proportion of patients (*see* Placebo, page xxi).	**Suitable for DIY** Qualified guidance is recommended though not essential. **Risks:** Avoid imbalanced or intolerable diets. They can cause deficiencies with serious consequences, particularly in children.

Treatment	Rating	Point of delivery/risks
Physical therapies Cold sprays and cold compresses are said to generate counterstimuli to mask acute withdrawal pain at least temporarily. Warm compresses, it is believed, improve circulation, and help the patient relax. Kneipp treatments are claimed to stimulate the body and give an increased feeling of well-being. Saunas are supposed to ease withdrawal symptoms, encourage metabolism, accelerate the elimination of alcohol and nicotine residues, and improve the body's own regulatory systems (*see* pages 867–78).	**May be of some use** as a short-term, supportive attempt aimed at alleviating pain and increasing general well-being. Case reports and field studies claim efficacy; however, success is probably seen in only a proportion of patients (*see* Placebo, page xxi).	**Suitable for DIY** Qualified guidance is recommended, but not essential. Therapists should be properly qualified and should propose a treatment plan. **Risks:** Severe skin damage may be caused to persons with diminished temperature sensation when extreme temperatures are applied. Excessive sessions in a sauna can be a cause of physical stress. The motor unrest present in acute alcohol withdrawal precludes the use of saunas.
Probiotics The introduction of certain bacteria into the gut is claimed to bring the intestinal flora back into balance and to have a beneficial effect on other parts of the immune system (*see* page 878).	**Of little use** Possibly acceptable as a short-term, supportive treatment attempt aimed at improving poor digestion. Some case reports claim efficacy; however, success is probably seen in only a small proportion of patients (*see* Placebo, page xxi).	**Requires a qualified practitioner** Practitioners should be properly qualified and should propose a treatment plan. Non-prescription formulations are suitable for do-it-yourself. **Risks:** Fairly unlikely provided treatment is carried out competently.

Treatment	Rating	Point of delivery/risks
Reflex therapies Various techniques such as reflex zone massage (*see* page 883) or TENS (*see* page 886) are said to free blocked energy and lessen pain via reflex channels (*see* page 881). These techniques, it is claimed, can also improve the body's own regulatory systems.	**May be of some use** as a short-term treatment attempt aimed at alleviating pain and improving general well-being. The easing of symptoms described in case reports and field studies is probably seen in only a proportion of patients (*see* Placebo, page xxi).	**Suitable for DIY** Qualified guidance is essential. Therapists should be properly qualified and should propose a treatment plan. **Risks:** Some people find it hard to tolerate the pressure applied during massage; others cannot stand close physical contact, electrical stimuli, or rubber electrodes.
Relaxation techniques Autogenic training (*see* page 888), muscle relaxation according to Jacobson (*see* page 893), and various biofeedback techniques (*see* page 891) are said to relieve muscle tension and inner unrest, to ease symptoms, and to prevent renewed cravings. These techniques are frequently combined with other psycho- or behavioral therapies.	**Useful** as a supportive treatment attempt aimed at relaxing the patient, easing symptoms, and preventing strong cravings. Case reports and field studies claim efficacy; however, success is probably seen in only a proportion of patients (*see* Placebo, page xxi).	**Suitable for DIY** Once a sound understanding of the technique has been acquired from a trainer, patients can perform exercises themselves. Therapists should be properly qualified. **Risks:** Fairly unlikely.
Vitamins and trace elements The painkilling properties of vitamin B6 are thought to contribute to pain relief. The anti-oxidative properties of vitamins C and E and of selenium are, it is supposed, instrumental in the suppression of inflammation (*see* page 900).	**Of little use** Acceptable in vitamin deficiency resulting from alcohol or nicotine abuse. **May be of some use** for pain relief. The efficacy ascribed to vitamin B6 in some field studies is probably seen in only a proportion of patients (*see* Placebo, page xxi).	**Suitable for DIY** Medical guidance is recommended though not essential. **Risks:** Intolerance and overdosage are possible. High doses of vitamin B6 can cause serious side effects.

Herbal remedies for alcohol and nicotine withdrawal

There are no recommended herbal remedies for use in this indication. However, herbal remedies for anxiety (*see* page 91) and depression (*see* page 109) may be used supportively during withdrawal.

Alzheimer's disease

Causes and symptoms

Alzheimer's disease is one of several forms of dementia. Its cause is not known. A dementia is a degenerative brain condition leading to progressive and/or permanent loss of mental function.

Alzheimer's disease occurs when certain brain as cells die and the brain shrinks. Sufferers become disoriented and withdrawn, and sometimes revert to an earlier period in their life. Their personality gradually degenerates. In the early stages of the illness, symptoms may vary widely, often presenting as depressive moods (*see* Depression, page 100) anxiety (*see* page 84), or paranoia, though there may be other mental signs.

Orthodox treatment

As the illness progresses, comprehensive nursing care will usually be required; orthodox medicine is unable to propose any treatment other than tender loving care. There are suggestions that certain drugs may be able to slow the inevitable progression of the disease.

Complementary therapies

No complementary therapy has been shown to be effective for curing Alzheimer's disease. There may be merit in some therapies, however, as part of an appropriate program of care or in terms of delaying the rapidity of mental decline.

Treatment plan and limited trial

Before administering a complementary treatment, every therapist should propose a treatment plan (*see* page xxiii) that sets out a clear time frame and defines the goal that the treatment is designed to achieve. Treatment should then be tried for a limited term to test the patient's response.

Caution

Any complementary treatment attempted must take account of the patient's overall condition.

Complementary treatments for Alzheimer's disease

Treatment	Rating	Point of delivery/risks
Acupressure This treatment (*see* page 769), otherwise known as pressure-point massage, is claimed to invigorate, energize, and stimulate the patient and relieve symptoms. The pressure points chosen can vary from one practitioner to another.	**Inappropriate** as a treatment for Alzheimer's disease. **May be of some use** in the initial stages of the disease as a short-term, supportive attempt to address symptoms and stimulate the patient, assuming he/she tolerates the treatment. Case reports claim efficacy; however, success is probably seen in only a small proportion of patients (*see* Placebo, page xxi).	**Suitable for DIY** Qualified guidance is recommended. Practitioners should be properly qualified and should propose a treatment plan. **Risks:** unlikely provided treatment is carried out competently.

Treatment	Rating	Point of delivery/risks
Acupuncture Acupuncture in its various forms (*see* page 772) aims to encourage the flow of energy (*see* page 927) or to address symptoms directly. The acupuncture points chosen can vary from one practitioner to another.	**Inappropriate** as a treatment for Alzheimer's disease. **May be of some use** in the initial stages of the disease as a short-term, supportive attempt to address symptoms and stimulate the patient, assuming he/she tolerates the treatment. Case reports claim efficacy; however, success is probably seen in only a proportion of patients (*see* Placebo, page xxi).	**Requires a qualified practitioner** Acupuncturists should be properly qualified and should propose a treatment plan. **Risks:** Probably rare provided treatment is carried out competently.
Anthroposophical medicine Anthroposophically oriented doctors (*see* page 781) see early signs of sclerosis as an expression of imbalance and overloading of the nerve–sense system. Potentized lead and silver preparations are used (e.g. Scleron).	**Inappropriate** as a treatment for Alzheimer's disease. **May be of some use** in the early stages of the disease as a supportive attempt to address symptoms. Some studies claim efficacy; however, success is probably seen in only a proportion of patients (*see* Placebo, page xxi).	**Requires a qualified practitioner** Practitioners should be properly qualified and should propose a treatment plan. **Risks:** Allergies or intolerance are possible.
Aromatherapy Essential oils (*see* page 786) are used to soothe and relax, or to invigorate, thereby alleviating symptoms. The essences may be taken orally, used externally as massage oils or bathing emulsions, or inhaled as vapors.	**Inappropriate** as a treatment for Alzheimer's disease. **May be of some use** as a supportive treatment attempt aimed at soothing and relaxing the patient. Some case reports claim efficacy; however, success is probably seen in only a small proportion of patients (*see* Placebo, page xxi).	**Suitable for DIY** Qualified guidance is recommended. The effects of individual essential oils differ widely. **Risks:** Allergies or intolerance are possible. Some oils are carcinogenic in test systems and possibly in humans.

Treatment	Rating	Point of delivery/risks
Bioresonance therapy Bioresonance therapists use electrical devices in an attempt to discover the causes of illness and claim to be able to weaken or turn around pathogenic energies and disease related vibrations (*see* page 794).	**Inappropriate** as a treatment for Alzheimer's disease. Possibly acceptable in the early stages of the disease as a short-term, supportive treatment attempt when simpler, more established methods have been unsuccessful. Some case reports claim efficacy; however, success is probably seen, if at all, in only a small proportion of patients (*see* Placebo, page xxi).	**Requires a qualified practitioner** Practitioners should be properly qualified and should propose a treatment plan. No credence should be given to anyone promising immediate or total success. **Risks:** Fairly unlikely.
Cell therapy Injecting or ingesting products extracted from the tissues of newborn animals or animal fetuses is said to have a rejuvenating and revitalizing effect and to enhance the healing of human tissues and organs (*see* page 796).	**Not advised** Based on present knowledge, there is a lack of satisfactory evidence regarding the efficacy and mode of action of these costly and relatively risky procedures.	**Risks:** Injecting foreign proteins into the body can provoke (possibly fatal) allergic reactions. Also, pathogens such as those that cause bovine spongiform encephalopathy (BSE) or other serious infections may be introduced.
Chelation therapy The chelating agent EDTA (*see* page 800) is able, it is claimed, to bind calcareous deposits and heavy metals in the blood vessels. These are subsequently eliminated from the body, so that arteriosclerotic disease can, according to the theory, be reversed.	**Not advised** Evidence of the therapeutic usefulness of this risky procedure is lacking.	**Risks:** EDTA can cause a deficit of calcium and essential heavy metals and, in extreme cases, can lead to cardiac arrhythmia, respiratory failure, cramps, and death.

Treatment	Rating	Point of delivery/risks
Electroacupuncture according to Voll By taking readings of the electrical conductivity of the skin (*see* page 802), therapists claim to be able to derive an insight into diseased areas of the body, pathogenic foci (*see* page 928), and stress factors (*see* Toxins, page 929). Then measures can be taken to address the causative factors.	**Inappropriate** as a treatment for Alzheimer's disease. Possibly acceptable in the initial stages of the disease as a short-term, supportive treatment attempt when simpler, more established methods have been unsuccessful and assuming the patient actually tolerates the treatment. Some case reports claim efficacy; however, success is probably seen, if at all, in only a small proportion of patients (*see* Placebo, page xxi).	**Requires a qualified practitioner** Practitioners should be properly qualified and should propose a treatment plan. No credence should be given to anyone promising immediate or total success. **Risks:** A second opinion must always be obtained from a qualified physician before any attempt is made to "eliminate foci" (e.g. by surgery).
Electroneural therapy according to Croon According to the theory, readings taken at various reactive sites on the skin highlight diseased areas within the body. Based on these readings, targeted neurotherapeutic measures can be undertaken to address the cause of symptoms (*see* page 806).	**Inappropriate** as a treatment for Alzheimer's disease. Possibly acceptable in the early stages of the disease as a short-term, supportive treatment attempt when more established methods have been unsuccessful and assuming the patient actually tolerates the treatment. Some case reports claim efficacy; however, success is probably seen, if at all, in only a small proportion of patients (*see* Placebo, page xxi).	**Requires a qualified practitioner** Practitioners should be properly qualified and should propose a treatment plan. No credence should be given to anyone promising immediate or total success. **Risks:** Proponents themselves warn that treatment should not be given in acute inflammatory conditions.
Eliminative methods, bloody Bloody cupping (*see* page 815) is said to improve the body's own regulatory systems and alleviate symptoms.	**Not advised** Evidence for the efficacy and mode of action of this invasive and sometimes risky procedure is lacking.	**Risks:** Bloody cupping should not be practiced in patients with bleeding disorders.

Treatment	Rating	Point of delivery/risks
Eliminative methods, unbloody Unbloody cupping (*see* page 817) is said to improve the body's own regulatory systems and alleviate symptoms.	**Inappropriate** as a treatment for Alzheimer's disease. **May be of some use** in the early stages of the disease as a short-term, supportive treatment attempt aimed at relieving pain, provided the patient tolerates the treatment. Some case reports claim efficacy; however, success is probably seen in only a proportion of patients (*see* Placebo, page xxi).	**Requires a qualified practitioner** Practitioners should be properly qualified and should propose a treatment plan. **Risks:** Unlikely provided treatment is carried out competently. Patients often show motor unrest.
Enzyme therapy The enzymes that are used reportedly dispel and destroy "immune complexes" that course in the blood and are responsible, for instance, for sustaining inflammatory and degenerative processes (*see* page 824).	**Of little use** Some case reports claim this little researched therapy works; however, success is probably seen in only a small proportion of patients (*see* Placebo, page xxi).	**Requires a qualified practitioner** Practitioners should propose a treatment plan. Non-prescription preparations are suitable for do-it-yourself. **Risks:** Possible intolerance.
Flower remedies Flower remedies (*see* page 828) are said to restore emotional balance and assist the body's psychic ability to heal itself.	**Inappropriate** as a treatment for Alzheimer's disease. **May be of some use** in the initial stages of the disease as a short-term, supportive treatment attempt aimed at soothing and relaxing the patient. Some case reports claim efficacy; however, success is probably seen in only a small proportion of patients (*see* Placebo, page xxi).	**Suitable for DIY** Qualified guidance is recommended. The patient must be able to participate actively in his/her treatment. **Risks:** Possible intolerance.

Treatment	Rating	Point of delivery/risks
Homeopathy Highly diluted (potentized) solutions (*see* page 831) are believed to be able to redress vital energy imbalances and strengthen the body's defences. Organo- and functiotropic (*see* page 833) homeopathy is claimed to be effective for dealing with individual diseases on a symptomatic basis.	**Inappropriate** as a treatment for Alzheimer's disease. **May be of some use** in the initial stages of the disease as a supportive therapeutic attempt aimed at addressing symptoms. Some case reports claim success for homeopathic treatments; however, success is probably seen in only a proportion of patients (*see* Placebo, page xxi).	**Requires a qualified practitioner** Homeopaths should be properly qualified and should propose a treatment plan. Ready-formulated preparations are suitable for do-it-yourself. **Risks:** Possible intolerance.
Manual therapies Chiropractors and osteopaths use a series of manipulations to realign allegedly displaced vertebrae. This, it is claimed, alleviates symptoms and has a beneficial effect on the patient's condition (*see* page 844).	**Not advised** Based on present knowledge, evidence of the mode of action and efficacy of these relatively risky procedures is lacking.	**Risks:** Spinal manipulations can cause serious injury. Osteoporosis is a prevalent risk factor.
Massage Classical massage (*see* page 847) can invigorate the patient, as well as ease muscular and perhaps also emotional tension.	**Inappropriate** as a treatment for Alzheimer's disease. **Useful** as a supportive treatment attempt aimed at relaxing the patient and improving his/her general well-being assuming he/she actually tolerates the treatment. Some case reports claim efficacy; however, success is probably seen in only a proportion of patients (*see* Placebo, page xxi).	**Requires a qualified practitioner** Masseurs/masseuses should be properly qualified and should propose a treatment plan. **Risks:** Some people are sensitive to manual stimuli; others find it hard to tolerate close physical contact.

Treatment	Rating	Point of delivery/risks
Physical therapies Warm bathing and rinsings are said to soothe and relax and improve general well-being (*see* page 871).	**Inappropriate** as a treatment for Alzheimer's disease. **May be of some use** as a supportive measure provided that the patient perceives the treatment as soothing and relaxing. Case reports claim efficacy; however, success is probably seen in only a proportion of patients (*see* Placebo, page xxi).	**Suitable for DIY** Qualified guidance is recommended though not essential. Practitioners should propose a treatment plan. **Risks:** Skin damage may be caused to persons with diminished temperature sensation when extreme temperatures are applied.
Probiotics The introduction of certain bacteria into the gut is claimed to bring the intestinal flora back into balance and to have a beneficial effect on the immune system and change the course of the disease for the better (*see* page 878).	**Inappropriate** as a treatment for Alzheimer's disease. Possibly acceptable as a short-term treatment attempt aimed at addressing inflammatory processes when more established methods have been unsuccessful. Some case reports claim efficacy; however, success is probably seen in only a proportion of patients (*see* Placebo, page xxi).	**Requires a qualified practitioner** Practitioners should be properly qualified and should propose a treatment plan. Non-prescription formulations are suitable for do-it-yourself. **Risks:** Fairly unlikely provided treatment is carried out competently.
Reflex therapies Reflex zone massage (*see* page 883) can invigorate the patient, as well as ease muscular and perhaps emotional tension.	**Inappropriate** as a treatment for Alzheimer's disease. **Useful** as a supportive treatment attempt aimed at relaxing the patient and improving his/her general well-being, assuming he/she actually tolerates the treatment. Some case reports claim efficacy; however, success is probably seen in only a proportion of patients (*see* Placebo, page xxi).	**Requires a qualified practitioner** Practitioners should be properly qualified and should propose a treatment plan. **Risks:** Some people are sensitive to manual stimuli; others find it hard to tolerate close physical contact.

Treatment	Rating	Point of delivery/risks
Relaxation techniques Autogenic training (*see* page 888), muscle relaxation according to Jacobson (*see* page 893), and various biofeedback techniques (*see* page 891) are said to relieve muscle tension and inner unrest, and might help the patient become more aware of his/her physical and emotional states.	**Inappropriate** as a treatment for Alzheimer's disease. Acceptable in the initial stages of the disease as a short-term supportive treatment attempt, assuming the patient actually tolerates the treatment. Some case reports claim efficacy; however, success is probably seen, if at all, in only a small proportion of patients (*see* Placebo, page xxi).	**Suitable for DIY** Once a sound understanding of the technique has been acquired from a trainer in group sessions or through individual tuition, patients can perform exercises themselves. Therapists should be properly qualified. **Risks:** Fairly unlikely.
TENS The use of low frequency electrical currents on the surface of the skin is said to energize the patient, reduce pain, and change the course of the disease for the better (*see* page 886).	**Inappropriate** as a treatment for Alzheimer's disease. Suggestions that TENS might work have not been adequately substantiated.	**Requires a qualified practitioner** Practitioners should be properly qualified and should propose a treatment plan. **Risks:** Some people react sensitively to electrical stimuli or rubber electrodes.
Vitamins and trace elements The antioxidative properties of beta-carotene, vitamins C and E, and selenium are, it is supposed, instrumental in tackling free radical formation, in boosting the body's antioxidative defence systems and in exercising a number of beneficial effects in the body (*see* page 900).	**Inappropriate** as a treatment for Alzheimer's disease. **Useful** in vitamin deficiency. Based on present knowledge, taking slightly raised doses of antioxidants would appear to be expedient; no definitive statements can be made, however, regarding dosage and efficacy.	**Suitable for DIY** Qualified guidance is recommended though not essential. **Risks:** Intolerance and overdosage are possible. Recent findings imply that beta-carotene might increase the risk of cancer.

Herbal remedies for Alzheimer's disease

Recent, well-conducted clinical trials have convincingly demonstrated that regular medication with Ginkgo leaves (*Ginkgo biloba*) can be helpful. This does not cure Alzheimer's but it delays the decline in mental function that is the hallmark of this disease. No serious side effects of Gingko leaves are known. The dose should be as recommended on the package.

Anxiety and worry

Causes and symptoms

Anxiety and worry have a number of causes: the stresses of everyday life, personal problems, events in life with which the sufferer has not come to terms, psychosocial conflicts, and the effects or ramifications of a physical disease.

Anxiety and worry vary in intensity from person to person—from slight irritability to severe anxiousness and panic attacks.

Orthodox treatment

Anxiety can mostly be treated with anxiolytic drugs, usually of the benzodiazepine type. These should only be taken for a short time, as they are addictive. Counselling is sometimes proposed to help long-term sufferers.

Complementary therapies

In complementary medicine, anxiety is frequently seen as the outward manifestation of a chronic intoxication or of adverse environmental influences. It is sometimes considered to be constitutional in origin or due to the patient's life force (*see* page 928) being out of balance.

There have been field studies and controlled clinical trials showing certain complementary treatments to be effective in alleviating the symptoms of slight to moderate anxiety and worry.

Treatment plan and limited trial

Before administering a complementary treatment, every therapist should propose a treatment plan (*see* page xxiii) that sets out a clear time-frame and defines the goal that the treatment is designed to achieve. Treatment should then be tried for a limited term to test the patient's response.

Caution

No complementary treatment, on its own, can adequately deal with severe anxiety and worry.

Complementary treatments for anxiety and worry

Treatment	Rating	Point of delivery/risks
Acupressure This treatment (*see* page 769), otherwise known as pressure-point massage, is used to ease anxiety and worry, relieve tension, and improve general well-being. Acupressure is also used as a method of imparting vital energy (*see* Life force, page 928).	**May be of some use** as an acute treatment or short-term treatment attempt. Case reports and field studies claim efficacy; however, success is probably seen in only a proportion of patients (*see* Placebo, page xxi).	**Suitable for DIY** Qualified guidance is recommended. Practitioners should be properly qualified. **Risks:** Unlikely provided treatment is carried out competently.
Acupuncture Acupuncture in its various forms (*see* page 772) aims to encourage the flow of energy (*see* page 927) or to alleviate anxiety and worry directly. The acupuncture points chosen can vary from one practitioner to another.	**May be of some use** as a short-term treatment attempt for recurrent symptoms. Case reports and field studies claim efficacy; however, success is probably seen in only a proportion of patients (*see* Placebo, page xxi).	**Requires a qualified practitioner** Practitioners should be properly qualified and should propose a treatment plan. **Risks:** Probably rare provided treatment is carried out competently.
Anthroposophical medicine Biographical work is said to help in identifying the causes of anxiety and worry, which are then subsequently tackled by carrying out a constitutional treatment (*see* page 781).	**May be of some use** as a short-term treatment attempt when the patient accepts this form of treatment. Some case reports claim efficacy; however, success is probably seen in only a proportion of patients (*see* Placebo, page xxi).	**Requires a qualified practitioner** Practitioners should be properly qualified and should propose a treatment plan. **Risks:** Allergies, toxic reactions, or intolerance are possible.

Treatment	Rating	Point of delivery/risks
Aromatherapy Essential oils (*see* page 786) are used to soothe and relax, or to invigorate, and so might play a part in alleviating anxiety, unrest, and tension. The essences may be taken orally, used externally as massage oils or bathing emulsions, or inhaled as vapors.	**May be of some use** as a short-term treatment attempt aimed at calming and relaxing the patient. Case reports claim efficacy; however, success is probably seen in only a proportion of patients (*see* Placebo, page xxi).	**Suitable for DIY** Qualified guidance is recommended. The effects of individual essential oils differ widely. **Risks:** Allergies or intolerance are possible. Some oils are carcinogenic in test systems and possibly in humans.
Bioresonance therapy Bioresonance therapists use electrical devices in an attempt to discover the causes of illness and claim to be able to weaken or turn around pathogenic energies and disease related vibrations (*see* page 794).	**Of little use** Possibly acceptable as a short-term, supportive treatment attempt for pronounced symptoms when simpler, more established methods have been unsuccessful. Some case reports claim efficacy; however, success is probably seen, if at all, in only a small proportion of patients (*see* Placebo, page xxi).	**Requires a qualified practitioner** Practitioners should be properly qualified and should propose a treatment plan. No credence should be given to anyone promising immediate or total success. **Risks:** Fairly unlikely.
Cell therapy Injecting or ingesting products extracted from the tissues of newborn animals or animal fetuses is said to have a rejuvenating and revitalizing effect and to enhance the healing of human tissues and organs (*see* page 796).	**Not advised** Based on present knowledge, there is little evidence of the efficacy and mode of action of these costly and relatively risky procedures.	**Risks:** Injecting foreign proteins into the body can provoke (possibly fatal) allergic reactions. Also, pathogens such as those that cause bovine spongiform encephalopathy (BSE) or other serious infections may be introduced.

Treatment	Rating	Point of delivery/risks
Electroacupuncture according to Voll By taking readings of the electrical conductivity of the skin (*see* page 802), therapists claim to be able to derive an insight into diseased areas of the body, pathogenic foci (*see* page 928), and stress factors (*see* Toxins, page 929). The causes of anxiety and unrest can then be addressed.	**Of little use** Possibly acceptable as a short-term, supportive treatment attempt for pronounced symptoms when simpler, more established methods have been unsuccessful. Some case reports claim efficacy; however, success is probably seen, if at all, in only a small proportion of patients (*see* Placebo, page xxi).	**Requires a qualified practitioner** Practitioners should be properly qualified and should propose a treatment plan. No credence should be given to anyone promising immediate or total success. **Risks:** A second opinion must always be obtained from a qualified physician before any attempt is made to "eliminate foci" (e.g. by surgery).
Electroneural therapy according to Croon According to the theory, readings taken at various reactive sites on the skin highlight diseased areas within the body. Based on these readings, targeted neurotherapeutic measures can be undertaken to combat anxiety and worry (*see* page 806).	**Of little use** Possibly acceptable as a short-term treatment attempt for pronounced anxiety and worry when simpler, more established methods have been unsuccessful. Some case reports claim efficacy; however, success is probably seen, if at all, in only a small proportion of patients (*see* Placebo, page xxi).	**Requires a qualified practitioner** Practitioners should be properly qualified and should propose a treatment plan. No credence should be given to anyone promising immediate or total success. **Risks:** Proponents themselves warn that treatment should not be given in acute inflammatory conditions.
Eliminative methods, bloody Bloody cupping (*see* page 815) is said to improve the body's own regulatory systems in patients with anxiety or worry.	**Not advised** There is insufficient evidence regarding the efficacy and mode of action of this little researched, invasive procedure.	**Risks:** Bloody cupping must not be practiced in patients with bleeding disorders.

Treatment	Rating	Point of delivery/risks
Eliminative methods, unbloody Sweating (*see* page 822), colonic irrigation, or unbloody cupping (*see* page 817) are said to improve the body's own regulatory systems and relieve anxiety and tension.	**May be of some use** as a short-term, supportive treatment attempt. Case reports claim efficacy; however, success is probably seen in only a proportion of patients (*see* Placebo, page xxi).	**Suitable for DIY** by a friend or relative. Unbloody cupping is best carried out with the guidance of a qualified practitioner. **Risks:** Unlikely provided treatment is carried out competently.
Flower remedies Flower remedies (*see* page 828) are said to restore emotional balance and assist the body's psychic ability to heal itself.	**May be of some use** as a short-term treatment attempt. Some case reports claim efficacy; however, success is probably seen in only a proportion of patients (*see* Placebo, page xxi).	**Suitable for DIY** Qualified guidance is recommended. Practitioners should propose a treatment plan. **Risks:** Possible intolerance.
Homeopathy Highly diluted (potentized) solutions (*see* page 831) are believed to be able to encourage the body to regulate its disturbed vital energy. Organo- and functiotropic (*see* page 833) homeopathy is claimed to be effective for dealing with anxiety or worry.	**May be of some use** as a short-term treatment attempt for pronounced states of anxiety and worry. Case reports claim efficacy; however, success is probably seen in only a proportion of patients (*see* Placebo, page xxi).	**Requires a qualified practitioner** Homeopaths should be properly qualified and should propose a treatment plan. Ready-formulated preparations are suitable for do-it-yourself. **Risks:** Possible intolerance.

Treatment	Rating	Point of delivery/risks
Hypnosis and self-hypnosis In the relaxed and generally altered state of awareness that is induced in hypnosis or self-hypnosis (*see* page 837), physical and mental conditions can be addressed. Some professionally organized courses in self-hypnosis are now available. Hypnosis is often used in combination with other psycho- and behavioral therapies to effect a change in lifestyle.	**Useful** as a short-term treatment attempt for frequent and pronounced symptoms, for inducing relaxation, and for effecting a change in lifestyle when simpler, more established methods have been unsuccessful. Case reports and field studies claim efficacy; however, success is probably seen in only a proportion of patients (*see* Placebo, page xxi).	**Requires a qualified practitioner** Hypnotherapists should be properly qualified and should propose a treatment plan. No credence should be given to anyone promising immediate or total success. **Risks:** Unlikely provided treatment is carried out competently.
Manual therapies Chiropractors and osteopaths use a series of manipulations to realign displaced vertebrae. This, it is claimed, is instrumental in freeing energy blockage (*see* page 927), thus removing the basis for anxiety and worry (*see* page 844).	**Of little use** Possibly acceptable as a short-term treatment attempt for frequent and pronounced symptoms when less risky, more established methods have been unsuccessful. Some case reports claim efficacy; however, success is probably seen, if at all, in only a small proportion of patients (*see* Placebo, page xxi).	**Requires a qualified practitioner** Practitioners should be properly qualified and should propose a treatment plan. **Risks:** Spinal manipulations can cause serious injury. Osteoporosis is one of several risk factors.
Massage Classical massage (*see* page 847) can soothe and relax the patient, as well as ease muscular and perhaps also emotional tension.	**Useful** as a short-term treatment attempt for frequent and pronounced states of anxiety and worry. Case reports and field studies claim efficacy; however, success is probably seen in only a proportion of patients (*see* Placebo, page xxi).	**Requires a qualified practitioner** Masseurs/masseuses should be properly qualified and should propose a treatment plan. **Risks:** Some people are sensitive to manual stimuli; others find it hard to tolerate close physical contact.

Treatment	Rating	Point of delivery/risks
Nutritional therapies An organic diet (*see* page 4) provides the body with essential and secondary plant nutrients that are believed to exercise a multitude of positive effects and to be capable, *inter alia*, of taking some of the load off the digestive system (*see* pages 858–67).	**Useful** as a supportive measure for addressing frequent and pronounced states of anxiety and worry associated with food intolerance or, in the elderly, with vitamin deficiency. Case reports claim efficacy; however, success is probably seen in only a proportion of patients (*see* Placebo, page xxi).	**Suitable for DIY** Qualified guidance is recommended though not essential. **Risks:** Avoid imbalanced or intolerable diets. They can cause deficiencies with serious consequences, particularly in children.
Physical therapies Exercise therapy (*see* page 868), the application of heat, various hydrotherapeutic techniques (*see* pages 871–8), and Kneipp treatments (*see* page 871) are said to have a calming and relaxing, or else an invigorating, effect. Saunas are said to improve the body's own regulatory systems.	**Useful** as a short-term treatment attempt for frequent or pronounced symptoms. Controlled studies of exercise demonstrate efficacy. Saunas **may be of some use** as a short-term, supportive treatment attempt; however, success is probably seen in only a small proportion of patients.	**Suitable for DIY** A specific treatment plan should be defined together with the treating physician. **Risks:** Severe skin damage may be caused to persons with diminished temperature sensation when extreme temperatures are applied.
Probiotics The introduction of certain bacteria into the gut is claimed to bring the intestinal flora back into balance and to have a beneficial effect in patients with anxiety and worry (*see* page 878).	**Of little use** Acceptable as a short-term attempt at addressing pronounced symptoms associated with disturbance and impairment of the gastrointestinal tract. Some case reports claim efficacy; however, success is probably seen in only a proportion of patients (*see* Placebo, page xxi).	**Requires a qualified practitioner** Practitioners should be properly qualified and should propose a treatment plan. Non-prescription formulations are suitable for do-it-yourself. **Risks:** Fairly unlikely provided treatment is carried out competently.

Treatment	Rating	Point of delivery/risks
Reflex therapies The application of reflex zone massage (*see* page 883), reflexology (*see* page 883), and TENS (*see* page 886) are said to relax the patient through reflex channels (*see* page 881) and exercise a beneficial effect on a number of physical functions.	**May be of some use** as a short-term treatment attempt for pronounced symptoms. Case reports claim efficacy; however, success is probably seen in only a proportion of patients (*see* Placebo, page xxi).	**Suitable for DIY** Qualified guidance is required. Practitioners should be properly qualified and should propose a treatment plan. **Risks:** Some people find it hard to tolerate the pressure applied during massage; others cannot stand electrical stimuli or rubber electrodes.
Relaxation techniques Autogenic training (*see* page 888), muscle relaxation according to Jacobson (*see* page 893), and various biofeedback techniques (*see* page 891) are said to relieve muscle tension and inner unrest, and might help the patient become more aware of his/her physical and emotional states.	**Useful** as a treatment attempt for frequent and pronounced anxiety and worry. Some case reports and field studies claim efficacy; however, success is probably seen in only a proportion of patients (*see* Placebo, page xxi).	**Suitable for DIY** Once a sound understanding of the technique has been acquired from a trainer, patients can perform exercises themselves. Therapists should be properly qualified. **Risks:** Fairly unlikely.

Herbal remedies for anxiety and worry

Active ingredient/preparation	Rating
Hops (*Humulus lupulus*)	Taken orally, hops are **useful** as a treatment attempt for conditions such as restlessness, anxiety, and insomnia. **Individual dose:** Infuse 0.5g dried flowers with 1 cup of hot water. Use ready-formulated preparations as instructed by the manufacturer/prescriber. A hop pillow **may be of some use** for inducing restfulness and sleep. Fill a small linen bag with hop strobiles and place it near the headboard. The sedative agent, lupulin, is emitted. Renew after three to four weeks. Suitable for long-term use. **Risks:** Hops are not thought to carry any significant risks, but should not be used by persons with marked depression.

Active ingredient/preparation	Rating

Kava root
(*Piper methysticum*)

Taken orally, kava is **useful** as a treatment attempt for nervousness, tension, and anxiety.
Daily dose: 1.5–2g drug. **Individual dose:** Infuse 0.5g drug with 1 cup of hot water. Use ready-formulated preparations as instructed by the manufacturer/prescriber.
Risks: Not to be taken during pregnancy or lactation. Not to be taken in depression. The action of kava may be potentiated when it is taken with alcohol, barbiturates, or psychotropic drugs.
Not to be taken for longer than three months except on a doctor's advice. Even in recommended dosages, kava affects vision and the ability to drive and operate machinery. Prolonged use may result in yellowing of the skin, allergic skin reactions, difficulty in focusing the eyes and pupil dilation. Use of kava root extracts is not advised for children under 12 years.

Lavender flowers
(*Lavandula angustifolia*)

Used internally or externally, lavender flowers **may be of some use** as a treatment attempt for worry and sleeplessness or, when used as a bath additive, as a treatment attempt for functional circulation problems.
Daily dose: 3–5g dried herb. Pour 1 cup of boiling water over 1–2 teaspoons (1–2g) of dried herb, infuse for five minutes, and drink. Alternatively, use 1–4 drops of oil (20–80mg); for use externally as a relaxing bath, add 1–4oz dried herb to 5 gallons of bath water. Use ready-formulated preparations as instructed by the manufacturer/prescriber.
Risks: Lavender flowers are not known to have any serious side effects.

Active ingredient/preparation	Rating
Lemon balm leaves (*Melissa officinalis*)	Used internally, lemon balm **may be of some use** as a treatment attempt for anxiety states and sleeplessness. **Daily dose:** 8–10g dried herb. **Individual dose:** Pour 5oz of hot water over 1.5–2g of dried herb and infuse for five to ten minutes.
Passionflower (*Passiflora incarnata*)	Used internally, passionflower **may be of some use** as a treatment attempt for restlessness and anxiety. **Daily dose:** As an infusion: 4–8g dried herb. **Individual dose:** Pour a cup of hot water over about 2g of dried herb and infuse. Use ready-formulated preparations as instructed by the manufacturer/prescriber. **Risks:** There are not thought to be any significant risks.
Valerian root (*Valeriana officinalis*)	Taken orally, valerian is **useful** as an attempt to promote natural sleep and relieve worry. **Dosage:** As an infusion: infuse 2–3g dried root with boiling water. Tincture: 15–20 drops one to three times daily. Full bath: 4oz dried root. **Risks:** Ready-formulated preparations frequently contain 3–5 percent so-called valepotriates, which reportedly cause cell damage, especially in the liver. Headaches, restlessness, and cardiac effects are possible. Only *Valeriana officinalis* should be taken.

Bedwetting (enuresis)

Causes and symptoms

There is no hard and fast rule for the age from which a child should be dry. In Europe bedwetting is only recognized as a medical condition when a child of five years or more wets the bed frequently and no urinary infection can be found. Causes of bedwetting tend to be emotional rather than physical in nature.

Orthodox treatment

Apart from counselling, a mild antidepressant or hormone treatment might be helpful. The long-term success of such approaches to the disorder is disputed. Placing a rubber sheet over a mattress and using a buzzer to wake the child if dampness is detected is said to have roughly a 70 percent success rate.

Complementary therapies

Some complementary treatments claim to act directly on the bladder through energy links (*see* page 928). Foci (*see* page 928) and energy imbalances (*see* page 927) are often blamed for a child's bedwetting.

Treatment plan and limited trial

Before administering a complementary treatment, every therapist should propose a treatment plan (see page xxiii) that sets out a clear time-frame and defines the goal that the treatment is designed to achieve. Treatment should then be tried for a limited term to test the child's response.

Cautions

Many complementary treatments ignore possible psychological causes of bedwetting. Therapies such as needling may cause the child undue pain and even be dangerous.

Complementary treatments for bedwetting

Treatment	Rating	Point of delivery/risks
Acupressure This treatment (*see* page 769), otherwise known as pressure-point massage, is used to calm and relax, and also to activate points associated with the bladder.	**Of little use** Acceptable as a short-term treatment attempt. Some case reports claim efficacy; however, success is probably seen in only a proportion of patients (*see* Placebo, page xxi).	**Suitable for DIY** Qualified guidance is recommended. **Risks:** Unlikely provided treatment is carried out competently.
Acupuncture Acupuncture in its various forms (*see* page 772) aims to encourage the flow of energy (*see* page 927) or to act directly (symptomatically) to reduce bedwetting. The acupuncture points chosen can vary from one practitioner to another.	**Of little use** Possibly acceptable as a short-term treatment attempt when less painful procedures have been unsuccessful. Some case reports and field studies claim efficacy; however, success is probably seen in only a proportion of patients (*see* Placebo, page xxi).	**Requires a qualified practitioner** Acupuncturists should be properly qualified and should propose a treatment plan. **Risks:** Probably rare provided treatment is carried out competently.
Anthroposophical medicine In AM (*see* page 781), bedwetting in older children is seen as a constitutional, physical, and emotional problem that can be addressed, it is claimed, by seeking the psychological causes and treating them with anthroposophically oriented psychotheraphy and various medicines referred to as "compositions."	**May be of some use** as a short-term treatment attempt. Some studies claim efficacy; however, success is probably seen in only a small proportion of patients (*see* Placebo, page xxi).	**Requires a qualified practitioner** Practitioners should be properly qualified and should propose a treatment plan. **Risks:** Allergies or intolerance are possible.

Treatment	Rating	Point of delivery/risks
Aromatherapy Essential oils (*see* page 786) are used to soothe and relax, thereby leading to a reduction, it is claimed, in bedwetting. The essences may be taken orally, used externally as massage oils or bathing emulsions, or inhaled as vapors.	**Of little use** Acceptable as a short-term, supportive treatment attempt aimed at soothing and relaxing. Some case reports claim efficacy; however, success is probably seen in only a small proportion of patients (*see* Placebo, page xxi).	**Suitable for DIY** Qualified guidance is recommended. The effects of individual essential oils differ widely. **Risks:** Allergies or intolerance are possible. Some oils are carcinogenic in test systems and possibly in humans.
Bioresonance therapy Bioresonance therapists use electrical devices in an attempt to discover the causes of illness and claim to be able to weaken or turn around pathogenic energies and disease related vibrations (*see* page 794).	**Of little use** Possibly acceptable as a short-term treatment attempt when simpler, more established methods have been unsuccessful. Some case reports claim efficacy; however, success is probably seen, if at all, in only a small proportion of patients (*see* Placebo, page xxi).	**Requires a qualified practitioner** Practitioners should be properly qualified and should propose a treatment plan. No credence should be given to anyone promising immediate or total success. **Risks:** Fairly unlikely.
Electroacupuncture according to Voll By taking readings of the electrical conductivity of the skin (*see* page 802), therapists claim to be able to derive an insight into diseased areas of the body, pathogenic foci (*see* page 928), and stress factors (*see* Toxins, page 929). The causative factors for bedwetting can then be addressed.	**Of little use** Possibly acceptable as a short-term treatment attempt when simpler, more established methods have been unsuccessful. Some case reports claim efficacy; however, success is probably seen, if at all, in only a small proportion of patients (*see* Placebo, page xxi).	**Requires a qualified practitioner** Practitioners should be properly qualified and should propose a treatment plan. No credence should be given to anyone promising immediate or total success. **Risks:** A second opinion must always be obtained from a qualified physician before any attempt is made to "eliminate foci" (e.g. by surgery).

Treatment	Rating	Point of delivery/risks
Electroneural therapy according to Croon According to the theory, readings taken at various reactive sites on the skin highlight diseased areas within the body. Based on these readings, targeted electrostimulative measures can be undertaken to address the causative factors of bedwetting (*see* page 806).	**Of little use** Possibly acceptable as a short-term, supportive treatment attempt when more established methods have been unsuccessful. Some case reports claim efficacy; however, success is probably seen, if at all, in only a small proportion of patients (*see* Placebo, page xxi).	**Requires a qualified practitioner** Practitioners should be properly qualified and should propose a treatment plan. No credence should be given to anyone promising immediate or total success. **Risks:** Proponents themselves warn that treatment should not be given in acute inflammatory conditions.
Eliminative methods, unbloody Unbloody cupping (*see* page 817) is sometimes used in bedwetting to improve the body's own regulatory systems, or as a reflex therapy (*see* page 881) aimed at strengthening the bladder.	**Of little use** Possibly acceptable as a short-term treatment attempt when simpler, more established methods have been unsuccessful. Case reports claim efficacy; however, success is probably seen, if at all, in only a proportion of patients (*see* Placebo, page xxi).	**Suitable for DIY** Unbloody cupping is best carried out under the guidance of a qualified practitioner. **Risks:** Unlikely provided treatment is carried out competently.
Flower remedies Flower remedies (*see* page 828) are said to restore emotional balance and assist the body's psychic ability to heal itself.	**Of little use** Acceptable as a short-term, supportive attempt aimed at soothing and relaxing. Case reports claim efficacy; however, success is probably seen in only a proportion of patients (*see* Placebo, page xxi).	**Suitable for DIY** Qualified guidance is recommended. Practitioners should propose a treatment plan. **Risks:** Possible intolerance.

Treatment	Rating	Point of delivery/risks
Homeopathy Highly diluted (potentized) solutions (*see* page 831) are believed to be able to encourage the body to regulate its disturbed vital energy. Organo- and functiotropic (*see* page 833) homeopathy is claimed to be effective for dealing with bedwetting.	**Of little use** Acceptable as a short-term treatment attempt when the treatment shows signs of working. Case reports claim efficacy; however, success is probably seen in only a proportion of patients (*see* Placebo, page xxi).	**Requires a qualified practitioner** Homeopaths should be properly qualified and should propose a treatment plan. Ready-formulated preparations are suitable for do-it-yourself. **Risks:** Possible intolerance.
Hypnosis and self-hypnosis In the relaxed and generally altered state of awareness that is induced in hypnosis or—in older children—in self-hypnosis (*see* page 837), the patient's physical and mental state can be positively influenced. Hypnosis is frequently used in association with other psycho- and behavioral therapies.	**May be of some use** as a short-term treatment attempt aimed when simpler, more established methods have been unsuccessful. Case reports claim efficacy; however, success is probably seen in only a proportion of patients (*see* Placebo, page xxi).	**Requires a qualified practitioner** Hypnotherapists should be properly qualified and should propose a treatment plan. **Risks:** Unlikely provided treatment is carried out competently.
Massage Classical massage (*see* page 847) can invigorate the patient, as well as ease muscular and perhaps also emotional tension.	**Of little use** Acceptable as a short-term treatment attempt aimed at soothing and relaxing. Case reports claim efficacy; however, success is probably seen in only a proportion of patients (*see* Placebo, page xxi).	**Suitable for DIY** Qualified guidance is recommended. Masseurs/masseuses should propose a treatment plan. **Risks:** Some people are sensitive to manual stimuli; others find it hard to tolerate close physical contact.

Treatment	Rating	Point of delivery/risks
Physical therapies Rising temperature foot baths, warm sitz baths (*see* page 874), cold washing, and other forms of Kneipp treatment (*see* page 871) are said to be effective in preventing bedwetting.	**Of little use** Acceptable as a short-term supportive treatment attempt. Case reports and field studies claim efficacy; however, success is probably seen in only a proportion of patients (*see* Placebo, page xxi).	**Suitable for DIY** Qualified guidance is recommended though not essential. **Risks:** Skin damage may be caused to persons with diminished temperature sensation when extreme temperatures are applied.
Reflex therapies Certain techniques (*see* Connective tissue massage and Reflexology, page 883) are said to be an effective means of affecting bladder function.	**Of little use** Acceptable as a short-term, supportive treatment attempt. Some case reports claim efficacy; however, success is probably seen in only a proportion of patients (*see* Placebo, page xxi).	**Requires a qualified practitioner** With qualified guidance, also suitable for DIY. Practitioners should be properly qualified. **Risks:** Unlikely provided treatment is carried out competently.
Relaxation techniques Autogenic training (*see* page 888), muscle relaxation according to Jacobson (*see* page 893), and various biofeedback techniques (*see* page 891) are said to relieve muscle tension and inner unrest, and might help the patient become more aware of his/her physical and emotional states.	**May be of some use** as a short-term treatment attempt. Case reports and field studies claim efficacy; however, success is probably seen in only a proportion of patients (*see* Placebo, page xxi).	**Suitable for DIY** Once a sound understanding of the technique has been acquired from a trainer in group sessions or through individual tuition, patients can perform exercises themselves **Risks:** Fairly unlikely provided treatment is carried out competently.

Treatment	Rating	Point of delivery/risks
TENS The application of low frequency electrical current to the surface of the skin serves as a reflex therapy (see page 886) in bedwetting to influence bladder function.	**Of little use** Acceptable as a short-term treatment attempt. Case reports and field studies claim efficacy; however, success is probably seen in only a proportion of patients (*see* Placebo, page xxi).	**Requires a qualified practitioner** Practitioners should be properly qualified and should propose a treatment plan. **Risks:** Some people react sensitively to electrical stimuli or rubber electrodes.

Herbal remedy for bedwetting

Active ingredient/preparation	Rating
St. John's wort (*Hypericum perforatum*)	Taken orally, St. John's wort **may be of some use** as a treatment attempt for bedwetting, though its claimed beneficial effect has not been fully substantiated. **Daily dose:** 2–4g dried herb. **Individual dose:** Infuse 1–2g of dried herb with 1 cup of hot water. **Risks:** Photosensitization (persons with a light complexion should avoid bright sunlight after taking St. John's wort, or they may suffer allergic skin irritation).

Depression

Causes and symptoms

Depression is a mood disorder. It may be of short or long duration and of varying severity ranging from a slightly pessimistic view of life to a feeling of total despair and worthlessness. Sufferers often show suicidal tendencies. Classic physical symptoms of depression are headaches and muscular aches, chronic tiredness, and sleep disorders. Depression may sometimes be brought on by a physical disease or by taking certain medications.

Orthodox treatment

Apart from counselling and psychotherapy, the main orthodox approach is to prescribe antidepressants.

Complementary therapies

Much of complementary medicine sees depression either through the eyes of mainstream doctors or as a sign of a weakened vital force, as an energy imbalance (*see* page 927), or as a result of exposure to toxins. There have been numerous controlled clinical trials that ascribe a beneficial effect to herbalism (*see* page 853).

Treatment plan and limited trial

Before administering a complementary treatment, every therapist should propose a treatment plan (*see* page xxiii) that sets out a clear time frame and defines the goal that the treatment is designed to achieve. Treatment should then be tried for a limited term to test the patient's response.

Caution

Complementary treatments alone usually do not constitute an adequate means of dealing with severe depression. Some therapies may be useful, however, in a supportive role. Failure to obtain an orthodox diagnosis may result in the patient receiving inappropriate treatment for what is a serious medical condition.

Complementary treatments for depression

Treatment	Rating	Point of delivery/risks
Acupressure This treatment (*see* page 769), otherwise known as pressure-point massage, is used to reduce pain, ease tension, and improve general well-being. Acupressure is also used to impart vital energy (*see* Life force, page 928).	**May be of some use** as a short-term, supportive treatment attempt for depression or for symptoms such as pain or nausea. Some case and field studies claim efficacy; however, success is probably seen in only a small proportion of patients (*see* Placebo, page xxi).	**Suitable for DIY** Qualified guidance is recommended. Therapists should propose a treatment plan. **Risks:** Unlikely provided treatment is carried out competently. Some people find it hard to tolerate pressure or close physical contact.
Acupuncture Acupuncture in its various forms (*see* page 772) aims to encourage the flow of energy (*see* page 927) or to treat the symptoms of depression. The acupuncture points chosen can vary from one practitioner to another.	**May be of some use** as a short-term treatment attempt for slight to moderate depression. Some case reports and field studies claim efficacy; however, success is probably seen in only a proportion of patients (*see* Placebo, page xxi).	**Requires a qualified practitioner** Practitioners should be properly qualified and should propose a treatment plan. **Risks:** Probably rare provided treatment is carried out competently.
Anthroposophical medicine Anthroposophically oriented doctors (*see* page 781) see depression or a lack of drive as being associated with the liver. Liver therapy, art therapy and, occasionally, anthroposophical dialog therapy will usually be the mainstays of treatment.	**May be of some use** as a short-term, supportive treatment attempt for slight to moderate depression when the patient accepts this form of treatment. Some case reports and field studies claim efficacy; however, success is probably seen in only a proportion of patients (*see* Placebo, page xxi).	**Requires a qualified practitioner** Practitioners should be properly qualified and should propose a treatment plan. **Risks:** Allergies or intolerance are possible.

Treatment	*Rating*	*Point of delivery/risks*
Aromatherapy Essential oils (*see* page 786) are used to soothe and relax, or to invigorate, thereby helping to alleviate depression. The essences may be taken orally, used externally as massage oils or bathing emulsions, or inhaled as vapors.	**Of little use** Acceptable as a short-term, supportive treatment attempt aimed at soothing and relaxing or, alternatively, at invigorating the patient. Some case reports claim efficacy; however, success is probably seen in only a proportion of patients (*see* Placebo, page xxi).	**Suitable for DIY** Qualified guidance is recommended. The effects of individual essential oils differ widely. **Risks:** Allergies or intolerance are possible. Some oils are carcinogenic in test systems and possibly in humans.
Bioresonance therapy Bioresonance therapists use electrical devices in an attempt to discover the causes of illness and claim to be able to weaken or turn around pathogenic energies and disease related vibrations (*see* page 794).	**Of little use** Possibly acceptable as a short-term, supportive treatment attempt when simpler, more established methods have been unsuccessful. Some case reports claim efficacy; however, success is probably seen, if at all, in only a small proportion of patients (*see* Placebo, page xxi).	**Requires a qualified practitioner** Practitioners should be properly qualified and should propose a treatment plan. No credence should be given to anyone promising immediate or total success. **Risks:** Fairly unlikely.
Cell therapy Injecting or ingesting products extracted from the tissues of newborn animals or animal fetuses is said to have a rejuvenating and revitalizing effect and to enhance the healing of human tissues and organs (*see* page 796).	**Not advised** Based on present knowledge, there is little evidence of the efficacy and mode of action of these costly and relatively risky procedures.	**Risks:** Injecting foreign proteins into the body can provoke (possibly fatal) allergic reactions. Also, pathogens such as those that cause bovine spongiform encephalopathy (BSE) or other serious infections may be introduced.

Treatment	Rating	Point of delivery/risks
Electroacupuncture according to Voll By taking readings of the electrical conductivity of the skin (*see* page 802), therapists claim to be able to derive an insight into diseased areas of the body, pathogenic foci (*see* page 928), and stress factors (*see* Toxins, page 929). The factors that may be causing depression can then be addressed.	**Of little use** Possibly acceptable as a short-term, supportive treatment attempt when simpler, more established methods have been unsuccessful. Case reports claim efficacy; however, success is probably seen, if at all, in only a small proportion of patients (*see* Placebo, page xxi).	**Requires a qualified practitioner** Practitioners should be properly qualified and should propose a treatment plan. No credence should be given to anyone promising immediate or total success. **Risks:** A second opinion must always be obtained from a qualified physician before any attempt is made to "eliminate foci" (e.g. by surgery).
Electroneural therapy according to Croon According to the theory, readings taken at various reactive sites on the skin highlight diseased areas within the body. Based on these readings, targeted neurotherapeutic measures can be undertaken to combat depression (*see* page 806).	**Of little use** Possibly acceptable as a short-term, supportive treatment attempt when simpler, more established methods have been unsuccessful. Some case reports claim efficacy against concomitant symptoms such as pain; however, success is probably seen, if at all, in only a small proportion of patients (*see* Placebo, page xxi).	**Requires a qualified practitioner** Practitioners should be properly qualified and should propose a treatment plan. No credence should be given to anyone promising immediate or total success. **Risks:** Proponents themselves warn that treatment should not be given in acute inflammatory conditions.
Eliminative methods, bloody Bloody cupping (*see* page 815) is said to improve the body's own regulatory systems and so alleviate depression.	**Not advised** Evidence for the efficacy of this invasive and relatively risky procedure is lacking.	**Requires a qualified practitioner** Practitioners should be properly qualified and should propose a treatment plan. **Risks:** Bloody cupping must not be practiced in patients with bleeding disorders.

Treatment	*Rating*	*Point of delivery/risks*
Eliminative methods, unbloody Unbloody cupping (*see* page 817) is supposed to bring about changes in the body's own regulatory systems and energize the patient (*see* page 927), alleviating depression.	**Of little use** Possibly acceptable as a treatment attempt for mild depression. Some case reports claim efficacy; however, success is probably seen in only a small proportion of patients (*see* Placebo, page xxi).	**Suitable for DIY** Unbloody cupping is best carried out under the guidance of a qualified practitioner. **Risks:** Unlikely provided treatment is carried out competently.
Flower remedies To the flower therapist depression might be an expression of an emotional imbalance. Flower remedies (*see* page 828) are supposed to restore emotional balance and assist the body's psychic ability to heal itself.	**Of little use** Acceptable as a short-term, supportive treatment attempt aimed at soothing and relaxing persons with mild depression. Some case reports claim efficacy; however, success is probably seen in only a proportion of patients (*see* Placebo, page xxi).	**Suitable for DIY** Qualified guidance is recommended. Practitioners should be properly qualified and should propose a treatment plan. **Risks:** Possible intolerance.
Homeopathy Highly diluted (potentized) solutions (*see* page 831) are believed to be able to encourage the body to regulate its disturbed vital energy. Organo- and functiotropic (*see* page 833) homeopathy is claimed to be effective for dealing symptomatically with depression.	**Of little use** Possibly acceptable as a short-term treatment attempt for depression. Case reports claim efficacy; however, success is probably seen in only a proportion of patients (*see* Placebo, page xxi).	**Requires a qualified practitioner** Homeopaths should be properly qualified and should propose a treatment plan. Ready-formulated preparations are suitable for do-it-yourself. **Risks:** Possible intolerance.

Treatment	Rating	Point of delivery/risks
Hypnosis and self-hypnosis In the relaxed and generally altered state of awareness that is induced in hypnosis or self-hypnosis (*see* page 837), the patient's physical and mental state can be positively influenced. Hypnosis is frequently used in association with other psycho- and behavioral therapies to bring about a positive change in lifestyle or to help the patient come to terms better with his/her condition.	**Of little use** Possibly acceptable in chronic depression as a short-term measure forming part of an overall psychotherapeutic program. Some case reports claim efficacy; however, success is probably seen in only a proportion of patients (*see* Placebo, page xxi).	**Requires a qualified practitioner** Hypnotherapists should be properly qualified and should propose a treatment plan. No credence should be given to anyone promising immediate or total success. **Risks:** Unlikely provided treatment is carried out competently.
Manual therapies Chiropractors and osteopaths use a series of manipulations to realign allegedly displaced vertebrae that, it is believed, may be responsible for causing depression and energy blockage (*see* page 844).	**Of little use** Possibly acceptable in chronic depression when an initial treatment attempt has shown positive results. Some case reports claim efficacy for these relatively risky procedures; however, success is probably seen, if at all, in only a proportion of patients (*see* Placebo, page xxi).	**Requires a qualified practitioner** Practitioners should be properly qualified and should propose a treatment plan. **Risks:** Spinal manipulations can cause serious injury. Osteoporosis is a prevalent risk factor.
Massage Classical massage (*see* page 847) can invigorate the patient, as well as ease muscular and perhaps also emotional tension.	**Useful** as a short-term, supportive treatment attempt aimed at relaxing the patient. Case reports claim efficacy; however, success is probably seen in only a proportion of patients (*see* Placebo, page xxi).	**Suitable for DIY** Qualified guidance is recommended. **Risks:** Some people are sensitive to manual stimuli; others find it hard to tolerate close physical contact.

Treatment	Rating	Point of delivery/risks
Nutritional therapies An organic diet (*see* page 4) provides the body with essential and secondary plant nutrients that are believed to exercise a multitude of positive effects.	**May be of some use** as a supportive measure and as a treatment attempt when elimination or rotation diets are used to identify the cause of a food intolerance that is perhaps to blame for affecting the psyche.	**Suitable for DIY** Qualified guidance is recommended. See your doctor before starting an elimination or rotation diet. **Risks:** Avoid imbalanced or intolerable diets. They can cause deficiencies with serious consequences, particularly in children.
Physical therapies Exercise therapy (*see* page 868) and other forms of physical activity can influence the production of endorphins, which in turn may ease depression. Kneipp treatments (*see* page 871) are also said to have a stimulating effect and to give the patient an improved feeling of well-being. Saunas are supposed to bring about changes in the body's own regulatory systems and energize the patient.	**Useful** as a short-term treatment attempt. Controlled studies of exercise demonstrate efficacy. Saunas are of **little use**, but possibly acceptable as a treatment for mild depression. Success is probably seen in only a small proportion of patients (*see* Placebo, page xxi).	**Suitable for DIY** Qualified guidance is recommended though not essential. **Risks:** Possible physical injuries. However, unlikely if saunas are used, provided treatment is carried out competently.
Probiotics The introduction of certain bacteria into the gut is claimed to bring the intestinal flora back into balance and occasionally to have a beneficial effect on the body's own regulatory systems (*see* page 878).	**Of little use** Possibly acceptable as a short-term treatment attempt in persistent cases. Some case reports claim efficacy; however, success is probably seen in only a proportion of patients (*see* Placebo, page xxi).	**Requires a qualified practitioner** Practitioners should be properly qualified and should propose a treatment plan. Non-prescription preparations are suitable for do-it-yourself. **Risks:** Fairly unlikely provided treatment is carried out competently.

Treatment	Rating	Point of delivery/risks
Reflex therapies Certain techniques (*see* Reflex zone massage, page 883; TENS, page 886) are said to release blocked energy and ease muscular tension, as well as, it is claimed, improve the body's own regulatory systems.	**Of little use** Possibly acceptable as a short-term, supportive treatment attempt in patients suffering pain, dizziness, or nausea. Some case reports claim efficacy; however, success is probably seen in only a proportion of patients (*see* Placebo, page xxi).	**Suitable for DIY** Qualified guidance is required. **Risks:** Some people are sensitive to electrical stimuli or rubber electrodes; some may perceive physical contact as menacing.
Relaxation techniques Autogenic training (*see* page 888), muscle relaxation according to Jacobson (*see* page 893), and various biofeedback techniques (*see* page 891) are said to relieve muscle tension and inner unrest, and might help the patient become more aware of his/her physical and emotional states. These techniques are frequently combined with other psycho- or behavioral therapies.	**May be of some use** as a treatment attempt for depression when the technique is part of an overall psychotherapeutic program. Case reports claim efficacy; however, success is probably seen in only a proportion of patients (*see* Placebo, page xxi).	**Suitable for DIY** Once a sound understanding of the technique has been acquired from a trainer in group sessions or through individual tuition, patients can perform exercises themselves. Therapists should be properly qualified. **Risks:** Fairly unlikely.
Vitamins and trace elements The antioxidative properties of beta-carotene, vitamins C and E, and selenium are thought to give a boost to the body's defence against free radical formation and consequently to exercise a number of beneficial effects (*see* page 900).	**Of little use** as the sole measure. Possibly acceptable as a short-term, supportive treatment attempt or when used in patients with a massive fear of environmental poisons. Case reports and studies claim efficacy; however, success is probably seen in only a proportion of patients (*see* Placebo, page xxi).	**Suitable for DIY** Qualified guidance is recommended though not essential. **Risks:** Intolerance and overdosage are possible. Recent findings imply that beta-carotene might increase the risk of cancer.

Herbal remedies for depression

Active ingredient/preparation	Rating
St. John's wort (*Hypericum perforatum*)	Taken orally, St. John's wort is **useful** as a treatment for mild to moderate depression and anxiety. **Daily dose:** As an infusion 2–4g dried herb. **Individual dose:** Infuse 1–2g of dried herb with 1 cup of hot water; otherwise 0.2 –1.0mg total hypericin. Use ready-formulated preparations as instructed by the manufacturer/prescriber. **Risks:** Photosensitization (persons with a light complexion should avoid bright sunlight after taking St. John's wort, or they may suffer allergic skin irritation).
St. John's wort in combination with kava-kava	**Of little use** for treating depression. The other herbal extracts contained in this type of preparation usually have a sedative effect. Possibly acceptable when anxiety accompanies depression. **Dosage:** As instructed by the manufacturer/prescriber.
St. John's wort in combination with rauwolfia	**Not advised**. Preparations containing St. John's wort alone should be used in preference. **Risks:** At high dosages, extracts of rauwolfia root may exacerbate, or even induce, extreme mental depression.

Insomnia (sleeplessness)

Causes and symptoms

It is thought that in the UK as many as 10 million people may suffer from some form of sleep disorder, usually involving difficulty in getting to sleep, waking during sleep, or feeling generally exhausted during the day. Sufferers never feel refreshed by sleep, often take a long time to get going in the morning, and find it difficult to concentrate. Women are twice as likely as men to suffer from a sleep disorder.

Of course, there is no rule book for effective sleeping. Sleeping and waking cycles are affected by climate and cultural influences. It is also accepted that a "night owl's" sleep requirement differs fundamentally from an "early bird's."

Sleep disturbance has many causes. For example, too much alcohol can affect the most important phase of sleep, REM sleep, while jetlag and nightshifts can turn the body's biological clock on its head; extraneous noise may upset the autonomic nervous system; there has been a tendency of late to blame poor sleep on environmental pollutants and electromagnetic radiation; stress and difficult life situations can cause difficulty in getting to sleep or mean the patient wakes frequently in the night; drugs such as appetite suppressants, analgesics, some cold cure preparations, and asthma medications may also be stimulants and thus cause sleep disorders.

Orthodox treatment

Though effective to start with, many of the sleeping tablets that doctors prescribe can cause addiction if taken for any length of time, sometimes if taken for just a couple of weeks. Withdrawal symptoms are not uncommon and many people, having once taken a sleeping preparation, will become habitual users (the figure is something like one in five).

Recurrent or persistent insomnia is appropriately treated with sleeping tablets in the short term as part of an overall course of treatment. Help may also be available from the numerous sleep research units and sleep disorder clinics that have been established, as well as from specialist counsellors.

Complementary therapies

Various natural treatments try to eliminate sleep disturbance, mostly by helping the person relax.

Treatment plan and limited trial

Before administering a complementary treatment, every therapist should propose a treatment plan (*see* page xxiii) that sets out a clear time frame and defines the goal that the treatment is designed to achieve. Treatment should then be tried for a limited term to test the patient's response.

Cautions

Accurate diagnosis by a qualified doctor is essential before any complementary treatment is attempted against recurrent or persistent sleep disturbance, to exclude all physical, neurological, or psychiatric causes. If the disturbance is associated with stress or emotional problems, counselling or behavioral therapy might be appropriate.

Complementary treatments for sleeplessness

Treatment	*Rating*	*Point of delivery/risks*
Acupressure This treatment (*see* page 769), otherwise known as pressure-point massage, is claimed to bring relief to persons with sleeping disorders when the appropriate pressure points are stimulated. The pressure points chosen may differ from one practitioner to another. Special bracelets are sometimes used.	**Useful** as a short-term treatment attempt aimed at helping patients fall asleep, sleep longer, and wake up less frequently. Case reports claim efficacy; however, success is probably seen in only a proportion of patients (*see* Placebo, page xxi).	**Suitable for DIY** Qualified guidance is recommended. **Risks:** Unlikely provided treatment is carried out competently.
Acupuncture Acupuncture in its various forms (*see* page 772) aims to encourage the flow of energy (*see* page 927) or to act directly against sleeplessness. The acupuncture points chosen can vary from one practitioner to another.	**Useful** as a short-term treatment attempt for persistent or recurrent sleep problems (or pain, if this is the cause of sleeplessness). Case reports and field studies claim efficacy; however, success is probably seen in only a proportion of patients (*see* Placebo, page xxi).	**Requires a qualified practitioner** Practitioners should be properly qualified and should propose a treatment plan. **Risks:** Probably rare provided treatment is carried out competently.

Treatment	Rating	Point of delivery/risks
Anthroposophical medicine Constitutional therapy (*see* page 781) and anthroposophically oriented psychotherapy are said to remove the physical, mental, and emotional causes of sleeplessness. The "composition" Avena Sativa Compositum is frequently prescribed as a sedative.	**May be of some use** as a short-term treatment attempt when the patient accepts this form of treatment. Some studies claim efficacy; however, success is probably seen in only a small proportion of patients (*see* Placebo, page xxi).	**Requires a qualified practitioner** Practitioners should be properly qualified and should propose a treatment plan. **Risks:** Allergies and intolerance are possible.
Aromatherapy Essential oils (*see* page 786) are used to soothe and relax, and so can possibly overcome sleeplessness. The essences may be taken orally, used externally as massage oils or bathing emulsions, or inhaled as vapors.	**May be of some use** as a short-term treatment attempt aimed at soothing and relaxing. Some case reports claim efficacy; however, success is probably seen in only a proportion of patients (*see* Placebo, page xxi).	**Suitable for DIY** Qualified guidance is recommended. The effects of individual essential oils differ widely. **Risks:** Allergies or intolerance are possible. Some oils are carcinogenic in test systems and possibly in humans.
Bioresonance therapy Bioresonance therapists use electrical devices in an attempt to discover the causes of illness and claim to be able to weaken or turn around pathogenic energies and disease related vibrations (*see* page 794).	**Of little use** Possibly acceptable as a short-term, supportive treatment attempt when simpler, more established methods have been unsuccessful. Some case reports claim efficacy; however, success is probably seen, if at all, in only a small proportion of patients (*see* Placebo, page xxi).	**Requires a qualified practitioner** Practitioners should be properly qualified and should propose a treatment plan. No credence should be given to anyone promising immediate or total success. **Risks:** Fairly unlikely.

Treatment	Rating	Point of delivery/risks
Cell therapy Injecting or ingesting products extracted from the tissues of newborn animals or animal fetuses is said to have a rejuvenating and revitalizing effect and to enhance the healing of human tissues and organs (*see* page 796).	**Not advised** Based on present knowledge, there is inadequate evidence of the efficacy and mode of action of these costly and relatively risky procedures.	**Risks:** Injecting foreign proteins into the body can provoke (possibly fatal) allergic reactions. Also, pathogens such as those that cause bovine spongiform encephalopathy (BSE) or other serious infections may be introduced.
Electroacupuncture according to Voll By taking readings of the electrical conductivity of the skin (*see* page 802), therapists claim to be able to derive an insight into diseased areas of the body, pathogenic foci (*see* page 928), and stress factors (*see* Toxins, page 929). The supposed causes of sleeplessness can then be addressed.	**Of little use** Possibly acceptable as a short-term, supportive treatment attempt when simpler, more established methods have been unsuccessful. Some case reports claim efficacy; however, success is probably seen, if at all, in only a small proportion of patients (*see* Placebo, page xxi).	**Requires a qualified practitioner** Practitioners should be properly qualified and should propose a treatment plan. No credence should be given to anyone promising immediate or total success. **Risks:** A second opinion must always be obtained from a qualified physician before any attempt is made to "eliminate foci" (e.g. by surgery).
Electroneural therapy according to Croon According to the theory, readings taken at various reactive sites on the skin highlight diseased areas within the body. Based on these readings, targeted electrostimulative measures can be undertaken to address the causes of sleeplessness (*see* page 806).	**Of little use** Possibly acceptable as a short-term, supportive treatment attempt when simpler, more established methods have been unsuccessful. Some case reports claim efficacy; however, success is probably seen, if at all, in only a small proportion of patients (*see* Placebo, page xxi).	**Requires a qualified practitioner** Practitioners should be properly qualified and should propose a treatment plan. No credence should be given to anyone promising immediate or total success. **Risks:** Proponents themselves warn that treatment should not be given in acute inflammatory conditions.

Treatment	Rating	Point of delivery/risks
Eliminative methods, bloody Bloody cupping (*see* page 815) and bloodletting (*see* page 810) are said to improve the body's own regulatory systems in people with sleep disorders.	Bloody cupping is **not advised**; other methods are **of little use**. Possibly acceptable as a short-term treatment attempt for persistent sleep disorders when less invasive, more established methods have been unsuccessful. Some case reports claim efficacy; however, success is probably seen in only a proportion of patients (*see* Placebo, page xxi).	**Requires a qualified practitioner** Practitioners should be properly qualified and should propose a treatment plan. No credence should be given to anyone promising immediate or total success. **Risks:** Bloody cupping can cause infection and scarring. Furthermore, these procedures should not be carried out in persons with bleeding disorders.
Eliminative methods, unbloody Colonic irrigation (see page 819) and unbloody cupping (*see* page 817) are supposed to improve the body's own regulatory systems in persons with sleep disorders and also alleviate symptoms.	**May be of some use** as a short-term, supportive treatment attempt aimed at inducing relaxation. Some case reports claim efficacy; however, success is probably seen in only a proportion of patients (*see* Placebo, page xxi).	**Suitable for DIY** by friends and relatives. Unbloody cupping is best carried out under the guidance of a qualified practitioner. **Risks:** Unlikely provided treatment is carried out competently.
Flower remedies Flower remedies (*see* page 828) are said to restore emotional balance and assist the body's psychic ability to heal itself.	**May be of some use** as a short-term treatment attempt aimed at soothing and relaxing. Some case reports claim efficacy; however, success is probably seen in only a proportion of patients (*see* Placebo, page xxi).	**Suitable for DIY** Qualified guidance is recommended. Practitioners should propose a treatment plan. **Risks:** Possible intolerance.

Treatment	Rating	Point of delivery/risks
Homeopathy Highly diluted (potentized) solutions (*see* page 831) are believed to be able to redress vital energy imbalances and strengthen the body's defences. Organo- and functiotropic (*see* page 833) homeopathy is claimed to be effective for dealing with sleeplessness.	**May be of some use** as a short-term, supportive treatment attempt and for helping the patient come to terms emotionally with his/her condition. Case reports claim success for homeopathic treatments; however, success is probably seen in only a proportion of patients (*see* Placebo, page xxi).	**Requires a qualified practitioner** Homeopaths should be properly qualified and should propose a treatment plan. Ready-formulated preparations are suitable for do-it-yourself. **Risks:** Allergies and intolerance are possible.
Hypnosis and self-hypnosis In the relaxed and generally altered state of awareness that is induced in hypnosis or self-hypnosis (*see* page 837), physical and mental conditions can be addressed. Hypnosis is often used in combination with other psycho- and behavioral therapies.	**May be of some use** as a short-term treatment attempt for chronic and persistent sleeplessness when simpler, more established methods have been unsuccessful. Case reports claim efficacy; however, success is probably seen in only a proportion of patients (*see* Placebo, page xxi).	**Requires a qualified practitioner** Hypnotherapists should be properly qualified and should propose a treatment plan. No credence should be given to anyone promising immediate or total success. **Risks:** Unlikely provided treatment is carried out competently.
Manual therapies Chiropractors and osteopaths use a series of manipulations to realign allegedly displaced vertebrae. This is said to reduce pain, release energy blockages (*see* page 927), and address factors that may be at the root of sleeplessness (*see* page 844).	**Useful** as a short-term treatment attempt aimed at pain that may be responsible for sleeplessness. Some case reports claim efficacy for these potentially risky procedures; however, success is probably seen, if at all, in only a small proportion of patients (*see* Placebo, page xxi).	**Requires a qualified practitioner** Practitioners should be properly qualified and should propose a treatment plan. **Risks:** Spinal manipulations can cause serious injury. Osteoporosis is one of several risk factors.

Treatment	Rating	Point of delivery/risks
Massage Classical massage (*see* page 847) can soothe the patient, as well as ease muscular and perhaps also emotional tension. Certain techniques can be used to induce counterirritation to obscure existing pain.	**Useful** as a short-term, supportive treatment attempt aimed at relaxing the patient. The easing of pain described in case reports and field studies is probably seen in only a proportion of patients (*see* Placebo, page xxi).	**Requires a qualified practitioner** Masseurs/masseuses should be properly qualified and should propose a treatment plan. **Risks:** Some people are sensitive to manual stimuli; others find it hard to tolerate close physical contact.
Nutritional therapies An organic diet (*see* page 4) provides the body with essential and secondary plant nutrients (dietary fiber, antioxidants) that are believed to exercise a multitude of positive effects.	**Useful** as a supportive measure when foods that are the cause of sleeplessness are eliminated from the diet.	**Suitable for DIY** Qualified guidance is recommended though not essential. **Risks:** Avoid imbalanced or intolerable diets. They can cause deficiencies with serious consequences, particularly in children.
Physical therapies Foot, arm, and full-immersion baths, walking in water, cold wraps, cold sitz baths in the evening, arm and knee douches, Kneipp treatments, and exercise therapy are said to relax or invigorate and so bring relief from sleep disorders. Saunas are supposed to improve the body's own regulatory systems in people with sleep disorders and alleviate symptoms (*see* pages 867–78).	**Useful** as a short-term treatment attempt. Case reports and field studies claim efficacy; however, success is probably seen in only a proportion of patients (*see* Placebo, page xxi). The effects of these procedures may differ from person to person. Saunas **may be of some use** as a short-term, supportive treatment attempt aimed at inducing relaxation.	**Suitable for DIY** Qualified guidance is recommended. An individual plan of treatment should be defined in association with the treating physician. **Risks:** Skin damage may be caused to persons with diminished temperature sensation when extreme temperatures are applied.

Treatment	Rating	Point of delivery/risks
Reflex therapies Reflex zone massage (*see* page 883), reflexology (*see* page 883), and TENS (*see* page 886) are claimed to act via reflex channels (*see* page 881) to ease pain that may be co-responsible for sleeplessness.	**Useful** as a short-term treatment attempt aimed at alleviating pain. Field studies, case reports, and clinical studies (for TENS) ascribe a certain efficacy to these treatments in some patients (*see* Placebo, page xxi).	**Suitable for DIY** Qualified guidance is essential. **Risks:** Some people are sensitive to electrical stimuli and rubber electrodes; others find it hard to tolerate manual stimulation or close physical contact.
Relaxation techniques Autogenic training (*see* page 888), muscle relaxation according to Jacobson (*see* page 893), and various biofeedback techniques (*see* page 891) are said to relieve muscle tension and inner unrest, and might be instrumental in addressing sleeplessness.	**Useful** as a treatment attempt for acute and chronic sleep disorders. Case reports and field studies claim efficacy; however, success is probably seen in only a proportion of patients (*see* Placebo, page xxi).	**Suitable for DIY** Once a sound understanding of the technique has been acquired from a trainer, patients can perform exercises themselves. Therapists should propose a treatment plan. **Risks:** Fairly unlikely.
Vitamins and trace elements Undiagnosed vitamin deficiencies, especially in the elderly, may be responsible for a variety of problems, including sleep disorders (*see* page 900). Administration of certain vitamins and trace elements is reported to eliminate these deficiencies.	**Useful** as a short-term treatment attempt when dietary trace element or vitamin deficiency is suspected in an elderly patient. Recommended dosages vary widely but are probably set to rise.	**Suitable for DIY** Qualified guidance is recommended. Vitamin deficiency is a diagnosis that must be made by the treating physician. **Risks:** Intolerance and overdosage are possible. Recent findings imply that beta-carotene and vitamin A might increase the risk of cancer. Vitamin B6 in high doses can cause serious side effects.

Herbal remedies for insomnia

Active ingredient/preparation	Rating
California poppy (*Eschscholzia californica*)	**Of little use** as a sedative. Its efficacy is in some doubt.
Carmelite water (spirit of melissa) (*Spiritus melissae*)	**Not advised.** Such highly alcoholic remedies as this are not helpful. They have a significant potential for misuse and should not be taken for medicinal purposes.
Holewort root (*Corydalis cava*)	**Of little use** for encouraging sleep. Its efficacy is in doubt.
Hops (*Humulus lupulus*)	Taken orally, hops are **useful** as a treatment attempt for conditions such as restlessness, anxiety, and insomnia. **Individual dose:** Infuse 0.5g dried flowers with 1 cup of hot water, to be drunk before retiring to bed. Use ready-formulated preparations as instructed by the manufacturer/prescriber. A hop pillow **may be of some use** for inducing restfulness and sleep. Fill a small linen bag with hop strobiles and place near the headboard. The sedative agent lupulin is emitted. Renew after three to four weeks. Suitable for long-term use. **Risks:** Hops are not thought to carry any significant risks, but should not be used by persons with marked depression.
Jamaica dogwood (*Piscidia erythrina*)	**Of little use** as a soporific. Its efficacy is in doubt. **Caution:** While not being as poisonous to humans as it is to cold-blooded creatures (e.g. fish), Jamaica dogwood is a remedy that must be used with great care, and only by trained practitioners.

Active ingredient/preparation	*Rating*

Lavender flowers
(*Lavandula angustifolia*)

Taken orally, lavender flowers **may be of some use** as a potential means of encouraging restfulness and sleep.
Daily dose: 6–8g dried herb. **Individual dose:** Pour 1 cup of boiling water over 1–2 teaspoons (2.5g) of dried herbs, infuse for five to ten minutes and drink. Alternatively, use 1–4 drops of oil (20–80mg); for use externally as a relaxing bath, add 20–100g dried herbs to 5 gallons of bath water. Use ready-formulated preparations as instructed by the manufacturer/prescriber.
Risks: There are not thought to be any significant risks.

Lemon balm leaves
(*Melissa officinalis*)

May be of some use as an attempted treatment for nervous sleeplessness.
Daily dose: 5–6g herb. **Individual dose:** Pour 1 cup of hot water over 1.5–2g of dried leaves and infuse.
Risks: Hypersensitivity reactions have been reported.

Oats
(*Avena sativa*)

Of little use as a sedative. Its efficacy is in some doubt.

Passionflower
(*Passiflora incarnata*)

Taken orally, passionflower **may be of some use** as an attempted treatment for nervous restlessness and to encourage sleep.
Daily dose: 2–4g dried leaves. **Individual dose:** Pour a cup of hot water over 1g of dried herbs and infuse. Use ready-formulated preparations as instructed by the manufacturer/prescriber.
Risks: Passionflower is not known to have any serious side effects.

Phytotherapeutics in combination with chemical sedatives such as diphenhydramine

Not advised. Mixing phytotherapeutics and chemical sedatives will interfere with the mild soporific effects of the pure phytotherapeutics. Combination preparations are thus not advised.

Active ingredient/preparation	Rating
Valerian root (*Valeriana officinalis*)	Taken orally, valerian is **useful** as an attempt to promote natural sleep and relieve worry. **Dosage:** Infusion: infuse 2–3g fresh or dried root with boiling water one to several times daily. Tincture: 15–20 drops one to three times daily. Full bath: 100g fresh or dried root. Use ready-formulated preparations as instructed by the manufacturer/prescriber. **Risks:** Headaches, restlessness, and cardiac effects are possible. Only *Valeriana officinalis* should be taken. Ready-formulated preparations frequently contain 3–5 percent so-called valepotriates, which reportedly cause cell damage, especially in the liver.
Valerian in combination with St. John's wort	**Of little use**, because St. John's wort's primary action is antidepressant, not soporific. Preparations containing just valerian, or valerian in combination with hops or passion flower, should be used in preference.

Multiple sclerosis

Causes and symptoms

Multiple sclerosis (MS) is one of the major diseases of the central nervous system. It may at first be episodic, progressing later to a stage in which the symptoms gradually become more pronounced.

In MS the sheath of fatty tissue (myelin) that protects the nerve fibers in the central nervous system becomes inflamed and later sclerotized. This gives rise to a wide variety of symptoms, including loss of motor coordination and muscle control, sensory problems, and paralysis. MS seriously affects the patient's mobility and makes constant care a necessity. Other problems arise, such as loss of bladder function. MS sufferers are frequently depressive.

The later stages of MS are associated with a variety of complications, such as urinary tract infection (*see* page 381), thrombosis, pressure sores, and osteoporosis (see page 195).

Progression of the disease varies from one patient to another. Sometimes it develops slowly and imperceptibly, and sometimes with remissions and sudden relapses.

Orthodox treatment

Treatment is usually just symptomatic. Through effective management and control of symptoms, however, it has been possible, over the last few decades, to raise the life expectancy of MS sufferers quite significantly. Statistically, MS patients now have a life expectancy equivalent to around 80 percent of normal. It is difficult to say with certainty what has led to this success, or to differentiate clearly between the spontaneous course of the disease and the possible effects of the treatments given.

Drugs used experimentally during treatment have ranged from anti-inflammatory agents and/or immune system modulators (*see* Immunomodulation, page 10), including certain interferons (soluble small proteins that are produced by the cells). Physio- and occupational therapies are encouraged as they can help the sufferer with everyday tasks.

Complementary therapies

Like orthodox treatments, complementary therapies will include various physical procedures.

Complementary approaches frequently concentrate on alleviating symptoms. Some therapists believe MS to be triggered by exposure to toxins (*see* page 929), by foci (*see* page 928), or by damage to the immune system. Others see it as a constitutional problem (*see* Constitution, page 927) or as a manifestation of the patient's life force (*see* page 928) being out of balance. There is at present no reliable evidence to suggest that these approaches have anything to offer in terms of patient care, though certain complementary therapies may be found to offer some relief.

Treatment plan and limited trial

Before administering a complementary treatment, every therapist should propose a treatment plan (*see* page xxiii) that sets out a clear time-frame and defines the goal that the treatment is designed to achieve. Treatment should then be tried for a limited term to test the patient's response.

Cautions

Accurate diagnosis is essential and must involve orthodox neurological examination. Complementary treatments are no substitute for proper physio- or occupational therapy.

Complementary treatments for multiple sclerosis

Treatment	Rating	Point of delivery/risks
Acupressure This treatment (*see* page 769), otherwise known as pressure-point massage, is used to reduce pain and nausea, ease tension, and improve general well-being. The procedure is also used to impart vital energy (*see* Life force, page 928).	**May be of some use** as a short-term treatment attempt for pain, muscle tension, and nausea. Some case reports claim efficacy; however, success is probably seen in only a proportion of patients (*see* Placebo, page xxi).	**Suitable for DIY** Qualified guidance is recommended. **Risks:** Unlikely provided treatment is carried out competently.
Acupuncture Acupuncture in its various forms (*see* page 772) aims to encourage the flow of energy (*see* page 927) or to act directly against pain or functional disturbance. The acupuncture points chosen can vary from one practitioner to another.	**May be of some use** as a short-term attempt to bring relief from pain or functional disorders. There is no reliable information regarding the way in which it might influence the course of the disease. Some case reports claim efficacy; however, success is probably seen in only a small proportion of patients (*see* Placebo, page xxi).	**Requires a qualified practitioner** Acupuncturists should be properly qualified and should propose a treatment plan. **Risks:** Probably rare provided treatment is carried out competently. Care should be taken when inserting needles in areas where nerves have been damaged.

Treatment	Rating	Point of delivery/risks
Aromatherapy Essential oils (*see* page 786) are used to soothe and relax, or to invigorate, thereby alleviating symptoms. The essences may be taken orally, used externally as massage oils or bathing emulsions, or inhaled as vapors.	**Of little use** Acceptable as a short-term, supportive treatment attempt aimed at soothing and relaxing the patient. Some case reports claim efficacy; however, success is probably seen in only a proportion of patients (*see* Placebo, page xxi).	**Suitable for DIY** Qualified guidance is recommended. The effects of individual essential oils differ widely. **Risks:** Allergies or intolerance are possible. Some oils are carcinogenic in test systems and possibly in humans.
Bioresonance therapy Bioresonance therapists use electrical devices in an attempt to discover the causes of illness and claim to be able to weaken or turn around pathogenic energies and disease related vibrations (*see* page 794).	**Of little use** Possibly acceptable as a short-term treatment attempt when simpler, more established methods have been unsuccessful. Some case reports claim efficacy; however, success is probably seen, if at all, in only a small proportion of patients (*see* Placebo, page xxi).	**Requires a qualified practitioner** Practitioners should be properly qualified and should propose a treatment plan. **Risks:** Fairly unlikely.
Cell therapy Injecting or ingesting products extracted from the tissues of newborn animals or animal fetuses is said to have a rejuvenating and revitalizing effect and to enhance the healing of human tissues and organs (*see* page 796).	**Not advised** Based on present knowledge, there is inadequate evidence of the efficacy and mode of action of these costly and relatively risky procedures.	**Risks:** Injecting foreign proteins into the body can provoke (possibly fatal) allergic reactions. Also, pathogens such as those that cause bovine spongiform encephalopathy (BSE) or other serious infections may be introduced.

Treatment	*Rating*	*Point of delivery/risks*
Chelation therapy The chelating agent EDTA (*see* page 800) is able, it is claimed, to bind heavy metals in the bloodstream thought to be the cause of multiple sclerosis. These are subsequently eliminated from the body.	**Not advised** Based on present knowledge, the idea that multiple sclerosis is caused by intoxication is purely speculative. Evidence of the efficacy of this risky procedure is lacking.	**Risks:** EDTA can cause a deficit of calcium and essential heavy metals and, in extreme cases, can lead to cardiac arrhythmia, respiratory failure, cramps, and death.
Electroacupuncture according to Voll By taking readings of the electrical conductivity of the skin (*see* page 802), therapists claim to be able to derive an insight into diseased areas of the body, pathogenic foci (*see* page 928), and stress factors (*see* Toxins, page 929). The factors that may be causing multiple sclerosis can then be addressed.	**Of little use** Possibly acceptable as a short-term, supportive treatment attempt when simpler, more established methods have been unsuccessful. Some case reports claim efficacy; however, success is probably seen, if at all, in only a small proportion of patients (*see* Placebo, page xxi).	**Requires a qualified practitioner** Practitioners should be properly qualified and should propose a treatment plan. No credence should be given to anyone promising immediate or total success. **Risks:** A second opinion must always be obtained from a qualified physician before any attempt is made to "eliminate foci" (e.g. by surgery).
Electroneural therapy according to Croon According to the theory, readings taken at various reactive sites on the skin highlight diseased areas within the body. Based on these readings, electrostimulative therapy can then be used to address the factors that may be causing multiple sclerosis (*see* page 806).	**Of little use** Possibly acceptable as a short-term, supportive treatment attempt when simpler, more established methods have been unsuccessful. Some case reports claim efficacy; however, success is probably seen, if at all, in only a small proportion of patients (*see* Placebo, page xxi).	**Requires a qualified practitioner** Practitioners should be properly qualified and should propose a treatment plan. No credence should be given to anyone promising immediate or total success. **Risks:** Proponents themselves warn that treatment should not be given in acute inflammatory conditions.

Treatment	*Rating*	*Point of delivery/risks*
Eliminative methods, unbloody Unbloody cupping (*see* page 817) is claimed to alleviate pain, to improve the body's own regulatory systems, to energize the patient, and to modulate the immune system (*see* page 10).	**Of little use** Acceptable as a short-term treatment attempt aimed at relieving pain. Some case reports claim efficacy; however, success is probably seen in only a small proportion of patients (*see* Placebo, page xxi).	**Suitable for DIY** Unbloody cupping is best carried out under the guidance of a qualified practitioner. **Risks:** Care must be taken when cups are applied to areas of the body where the nerves have been damaged.
Enzyme therapy The enzymes that are used reportedly prevent and destroy "immune complexes" that course in the blood and are responsible, for instance, for sustaining inflammatory processes (*see* page 824).	**Of little use** Some case reports claim this little researched therapy works; however, success is probably seen in only a small proportion of patients (*see* Placebo, page xxi).	**Requires a qualified practitioner** Practitioners should propose a treatment plan. Non-prescription formulations are suitable for do-it-yourself. **Risks:** Allergies or intolerance are possible.
Flower remedies Flower remedies (*see* page 828) are said to restore emotional balance and assist the body's psychic ability to heal itself.	**Of little use** Acceptable as a short-term, supportive treatment attempt aimed at soothing and relaxing. Some case reports claim efficacy; however, success is probably seen in only a small proportion of patients (*see* Placebo, page xxi).	**Suitable for DIY** Qualified guidance is recommended. Practitioners should propose a treatment plan. **Risks:** Possible intolerance.

Treatment	Rating	Point of delivery/risks
Homeopathy Highly diluted (potentized) solutions (*see* page 831) are believed to be able to encourage the body to regulate its disturbed vital energy. Organo- and functiotropic (*see* page 833) homeopathy is claimed to be effective for dealing symptomatically with MS.	**Of little use** Possibly acceptable as a short-term, supportive treatment attempt aimed at addressing symptoms. Some case reports claim success for homeopathic treatments; however, success is probably seen in only a small proportion of patients (*see* Placebo, page xxi).	**Requires a qualified practitioner** Homeopaths should be properly qualified and should propose a treatment plan. Ready-formulated preparations are suitable for do-it-yourself. **Risks:** Possible intolerance.
Hypnosis and self-hypnosis In the relaxed and generally altered state of awareness that is induced in hypnosis or self-hypnosis (*see* page 837), physical conditions can be addressed and pain relieved. Some professionally organized courses in self-hypnosis are now available. Hypnosis is often used in combination with other psycho- and behavioral therapies.	**May be of some use** as a short-term, supportive treatment attempt aimed at relaxing the patient and helping him/her come to terms better with his/her condition. Some case reports claim efficacy; however, success is probably seen in only a proportion of patients treated (*see* Placebo, page xxi).	**Requires a qualified practitioner** Hypnotherapists should be properly qualified and should propose a treatment plan. No credence should be given to anyone promising immediate or total success. **Risks:** Unlikely provided treatment is carried out competently.
Magnetic field therapy The use of magnetic field generators, magnetic strips, bracelets, and other objects (*see* page 841) allegedly encourages cell metabolism and so relieves pain.	**Of little use** Based on present knowledge, there is inadequate evidence of the efficacy and mode of action of magnetic field therapy in MS.	Operation of magnetic field equipment **requires a qualified practitioner**. **Risks:** Magnetic field equipment can cause implanted cardiac pacemakers to malfunction.

Treatment	*Rating*	*Point of delivery/risks*
Manual therapies Chiropractors and osteopaths use a series of manipulations to realign allegedly displaced vertebrae. This, it is believed, may ease pain and free blocked energy (*see* page 844).	**Of little use** Acceptable as a short-term treatment attempt for pain relief in the musculoskeletal system. Some case reports claim efficacy for this relatively risky procedure; however, success is probably seen, if at all, in only a small proportion of patients (*see* Placebo, page xxi).	**Requires a qualified practitioner** Practitioners should be properly qualified and should propose a treatment plan. **Risks:** Spinal manipulations can cause serious injury. Osteoporosis is a prevalent risk factor.
Massage Classical massage (*see* page 847), lymphatic drainage (*see* page 850), and reflex zone massage (*see* page 883) can invigorate the patient, as well as ease muscular and perhaps also emotional tension.	**May be of some use** as a short-term, supportive treatment attempt aimed at relaxing the patient and increasing general well-being. Case reports claim efficacy; however, success is probably seen in only a proportion of patients (*see* Placebo, page xxi).	**Requires a qualified practitioner** Practitioners should be properly qualified and should propose a treatment plan. **Risks:** Some people are sensitive to manual stimuli; others find it hard to tolerate close physical contact.
Nutritional therapies An organic diet (*see* page 4) provides the body with essential and secondary plant nutrients (dietary fiber, antioxidants), that are believed to exercise a multitude of positive effects.	**May be of some use** as an individually directed supportive measure.	**Suitable for DIY** Qualified guidance is recommended though not essential. **Risks:** Avoid imbalanced or intolerable diets. They can cause deficiencies with serious consequences, particularly in children.

Treatment	Rating	Point of delivery/risks
Physical therapies Exercise and physiotherapy (*see* page 868) may help the patient cope better with everyday living despite his/her difficulties.	**Useful** as an individually directed, supportive measure. Case reports and field studies claim efficacy; however, success is probably seen in only a proportion of patients (*see* Placebo, page xxi).	**Suitable for DIY** Qualified guidance is required. **Risks:** Fairly rare provided treatment is carried out competently.
Probiotics The introduction of certain bacteria into the gut is claimed to bring the intestinal flora back into balance and to have a beneficial effect on the immune system (*see* page 878).	**Of little use** Possibly acceptable as a short-term, supportive treatment attempt when more established methods have been unsuccessful. Some case reports claim efficacy; however, success is probably seen in only a proportion of patients (*see* Placebo, page xxi).	**Requires a qualified practitioner** Practitioners should be properly qualified and should propose a treatment plan. Non-prescription preparations are suitable for do-it-yourself. **Risks:** Fairly unlikely provided treatment is carried out competently.
Reflex therapies Reflex zone massage (*see* page 883) and TENS (*see* page 886) are said to alleviate pain and exercise a number of beneficial effects via reflex channels (*see* page 881).	**May be of some use** as a short-term attempt to address symptoms. Some case reports and one recent clinical trial claim efficacy; however, success is probably seen in only a proportion of patients (*see* Placebo, page xxi).	**Suitable for DIY** Qualified guidance is essential. **Risks:** Some people are sensitive to pressure applied during massage; others find it hard to tolerate close physical contact or rubber electrodes.

Treatment	Rating	Point of delivery/risks
Relaxation techniques Autogenic training (*see* page 888), muscle relaxation according to Jacobson (*see* page 893), and various biofeedback techniques (*see* page 891) are said to relieve muscle tension and inner unrest, and might be instrumental in helping the patient come to terms better with his/her condition.	**May be of some use** as a supportive treatment attempt aimed at relaxing the patient and helping him/her come to terms better with his/her condition. Some case reports and field studies claim efficacy; however, success is probably seen in only a proportion of patients (*see* Placebo, page xxi).	**Suitable for DIY** Once a sound understanding of the technique has been acquired from a trainer in group sessions or through individual tuition, patients can perform exercises themselves. Therapists should be properly qualified. **Risks:** Fairly unlikely provided treatment is carried out competently.
Vitamins and trace elements Vitamin B6 is said to alleviate pain. The anti-oxidative properties of beta-carotene, vitamins C and E ,and selenium are thought to be instrumental in improving the body's own defence systems (*see* page 900).	**Of little use** Possibly acceptable as a short-term, supportive treatment attempt. No definitive recommendations can be given based on present knowledge.	**Suitable for DIY** Qualified guidance is recommended though not essential. **Risks:** Intolerance and overdosage are possible. Recent findings imply that beta-carotene might increase the risk of cancer. In high doses, vitamin B6 can cause serious side effects.

Herbal remedy for multiple sclerosis

Active ingredient/preparation	Rating
Evening primrose oil (*Oenothera biennis*)	**Of little use**. Herbal remedies are not recommended for multiple sclerosis. However, as an adjunct to other treatments, certain saturated vegetable fatty acids, including evening primrose oil (which contains gamma-linolenic acid), are sometimes tentatively employed. Borage oil is another remedy that contains gamma-linolenic acid. **Dosage:** As instructed by the manufacturer/prescriber. **Risks:** To prevent epileptic attacks, patients taking potentially epileptogenic agents, e.g. certain neuroleptics (phenothiazines), should not receive simultaneous treatment with evening primrose oil. Nausea, digestive problems, headaches, abdominal pain, and skin hypersensivity may occasionally be experienced.

Myalgic encephalomyelitis (ME) and chronic fatigue

Causes and symptoms

Studies in the UK and the USA have shown that roughly a quarter of the population experiences chronic fatigue. It seems to be one of the modern ills—the result perhaps of an over-stressful lifestyle. Chronic stress drives sufferers to become lethargic and resigned in the face of situations with which they feel they cannot cope.

There are many supposed causes of chronic fatigue. Some environmentalists consider modern man to be chronically exposed to toxins, while some doctors with an immunological leaning blame deficiencies in the body's immune system. Others attribute chronic fatigue to a hectic way of life. It may, however, also be a symptom of a severe physical or mental condition.

The incidence of ME has reached almost epidemic proportions. There is still no convincing explanation, though, for the raft of symptoms which many of those affected present to their doctor. ME, sometimes also called chronic fatigue syndrome (CFS), usually differs from simple chronic fatigue in that sufferers become severely debilitated and lethargic, complaining of muscle aches and other symptoms. The condition sometimes lasts for months or even years. Some studies point to psychological and/or psychosomatic factors as possible triggers that spark off ME.

Orthodox treatment

The medical profession has long been sceptical of, at times even hostile to, people presenting with chronic fatigue. What is usually offered simply addresses the symptoms that accompany chronic fatigue (aching muscles, headaches, depressive moods) rather than its root cause. There has not as yet been any in-depth research into possible treatments, which generally remain experimental. This is true in ME in particular. Treatment usually involves counselling, coupled with measures that typically aim to boost the patient's overall performance level.

Complementary therapies

Nearly all complementary therapies promise to provide some relief for ME sufferers by directly tackling individual complaints, by detoxifying the body, or by taking a holistic treatment approach.

Treatment plan and limited trial

Before administering a complementary treatment, every therapist should propose a treatment plan (*see* page xxiii) that sets out a clear time frame and defines the goal that the treatment is designed to achieve. Treatment should then be tried for a limited term to test the patient's response.

Caution

Before any complementary treatment is attempted for chronic fatigue, the patient should be properly examined by a doctor to establish whether the condition has a possible physical or mental cause.

Complementary treatments for ME and chronic fatigue

Treatment	Rating	Point of delivery/risks
Acupressure This treatment (*see* page 769), otherwise known as pressure-point massage, is claimed to alleviate ME-related pain, ease tension, and improve general well-being. It is also used to impart vital energy (*see* Life force, page 928).	**May be of some use** as a short-term treatment attempt aimed at alleviating pain and relaxing the patient. Case reports claim efficacy; however, success is probably seen in only a proportion of patients (*see* Placebo, page xxi).	**Suitable for DIY** Qualified guidance is recommended. Practitioners should be properly qualified and should propose a treatment plan. **Risks:** Unlikely provided treatment is carried out competently.
Acupuncture Acupuncture in its various forms (*see* page 772) aims to encourage the flow of energy (*see* page 927) or to act directly to ease symptoms.	**May be of some use** as a short-term treatment attempt aimed at energizing the patient. Case reports and field studies claim efficacy; however, success is probably seen in only a proportion of patients (*see* Placebo, page xxi).	**Requires a qualified practitioner** Acupuncturists should be properly qualified and should propose a treatment plan. **Risks:** Probably rare provided treatment is carried out competently.
Anthroposophical medicine Art therapy and "biographical work" (*see* page 781) are said to motivate patients and encourage them to renew their interest in life.	**Of little use** Acceptable as a long-term treatment attempt when the patient accepts this form of treatment. Some studies claim efficacy; however, success is probably seen in only a small proportion of patients (*see* Placebo, page xxi).	**Requires a qualified practitioner** Practitioners should be properly qualified and should propose a treatment plan. **Risks:** Unlikely provided treatment is carried out competently.

Treatment	Rating	Point of delivery/risks
Aromatherapy Essential oils (*see* page 786), such as rosemary oil, are claimed to have an energizing effect. The essences may be taken orally, used externally as massage oils or bathing emulsions, or inhaled as vapors.	**Of little use** Acceptable as a short-term, supportive treatment attempt aimed at invigorating or relaxing the patient. Some case reports claim efficacy; however, success is probably seen in only a proportion of patients (*see* Placebo, page xxi).	**Suitable for DIY** Qualified guidance is recommended. The effects of individual essential oils differ widely. **Risks:** Allergies or intolerance are possible. Some oils are carcinogenic in test systems and possibly in humans.
Bioresonance therapy Bioresonance therapists use electrical devices in an attempt to discover the causes of illness and claim to be able to weaken or turn around pathogenic energies and disease related vibrations (*see* page 794).	**Of little use** Acceptable as a short-term treatment attempt for persistent or recurrent complaints when simpler, more established methods have been unsuccessful. Some case reports claim efficacy; however, success is probably seen, if at all, in only a small proportion of patients (*see* Placebo, page xxi).	**Requires a qualified practitioner** Practitioners should be properly qualified and should propose a treatment plan. No credence should be given to anyone promising immediate or total success. **Risks:** Fairly unlikely.
Cell therapy Injecting or ingesting products extracted from animal tissues or organs is said to have a rejuvenating effect and to enhance the healing of human tissues and organs (*see* page 796).	**Not advised** Based on present knowledge, there is little evidence of the efficacy and mode of action of these costly and relatively risky procedures.	**Risks:** Injecting foreign proteins into the body can provoke (possibly fatal) allergic reactions. Also, pathogens such as those that cause bovine spongiform encephalopathy (BSE) or other serious infections may be introduced.

Treatment	Rating	Point of delivery/risks
Electroacupuncture according to Voll By taking readings of the electrical conductivity of the skin (*see* page 802), therapists claim to be able to derive an insight into diseased areas of the body, pathogenic foci (*see* page 928), and stress factors (*see* Toxins, page 929). The factors that may be causing fatigue can then be addressed.	**Of little use** Acceptable as a short-term treatment attempt for persistent or recurrent complaints when simpler, more established methods have been unsuccessful. Some case reports claim efficacy; however, success is probably seen, if at all, in only a small proportion of patients (*see* Placebo, page xxi).	**Requires a qualified practitioner** Practitioners should be properly qualified and should propose a treatment plan. No credence should be given to anyone promising immediate or total success. **Risks:** A second opinion must always be obtained from a qualified physician before any attempt is made to "eliminate foci" (e.g. by surgery).
Electroneural therapy according to Croon According to the theory, readings taken at various reactive sites on the skin highlight diseased areas within the body. Based on these readings, electrostimulative therapy can then be used to address the factors that may be causing fatigue (*see* page 806).	**Of little use** Acceptable as a short-term treatment attempt for persistent or recurrent complaints when simpler, more established methods have been unsuccessful. Some case reports claim efficacy; however, success is probably seen, if at all, in only a small proportion of patients (*see* Placebo, page xxi).	**Requires a qualified practitioner** Practitioners should be properly qualified and should propose a treatment plan. No credence should be given to anyone promising immediate or total success. **Risks:** Proponents themselves warn that treatment should not be given in acute inflammatory conditions.
Eliminative methods, bloody Bloody cupping (*see* page 815) is said to alleviate pain and improve the body's own regulatory systems.	**Of little use** Acceptable as a short-term treatment attempt in chronic cases when more established, less invasive methods have been unsuccessful. Some case reports and field studies claim efficacy; however, success is probably seen in only a proportion of patients (*see* Placebo, page xxi).	**Requires a qualified practitioner** Practitioners should be properly qualified and should propose a treatment plan. **Risks:** Bloody cupping must not be practiced in persons with bleeding disorders.

Treatment	Rating	Point of delivery/risks
Eliminative methods, unbloody Unbloody cupping (*see* page 812) is claimed to improve the body's own regulatory systems and impart energy.	**May be of some use** as a short-term treatment attempt. Some case reports claim efficacy; however, success is probably seen in only a small proportion of patients (*see* Placebo, page xxi).	**Suitable for DIY** Unbloody cupping is best carried out under the guidance of a qualified practitioner. **Risks:** Unlikely provided treatment is carried out competently.
Flower remedies Flower remedies (*see* page 828) are said to restore emotional balance and assist the body's psychic ability to heal itself.	**Of little use** Acceptable as a short-term treatment attempt aimed at helping the patient come to terms with his/her condition. Some case reports claim efficacy; however, success is probably seen in only a proportion of patients (*see* Placebo, page xxi).	**Suitable for DIY** Qualified guidance is recommended. Practitioners should propose a treatment plan. **Risks:** Possible intolerance.
Homeopathy Highly diluted (potentized) solutions (*see* page 831) are believed to be able to encourage the body to regulate its disturbed vital energy. Organo- and functiotropic (*see* page 833) homeopathy is claimed to be effective for dealing with ME and chronic fatigue.	**May be of some use** as a short-term treatment attempt. Case reports and field studies claim efficacy; however, success is probably seen in only a proportion of patients (*see* Placebo, page xxi).	**Requires a qualified practitioner** Homeopaths should be properly qualified and should propose a treatment plan. Ready-formulated preparations are suitable for do-it-yourself. **Risks:** Possible intolerance.

Treatment	Rating	Point of delivery/risks
Manual therapies Chiropractors and osteopaths use a series of manipulations to realign allegedly displaced vertebrae and joints. This is said to release energy blockages (*see* page 927) and ease ME and chronic fatigue (*see* page 844).	**Of little use** Possibly acceptable in persistent cases as a short-term treatment attempt when less risky methods have been unsuccessful. Some case reports claim efficacy; however, success is probably seen, if at all, in only a small proportion of patients (*see* Placebo, page xxi).	**Requires a qualified practitioner** Practitioners should be properly qualified and should propose a treatment plan. **Risks:** Spinal manipulations can cause serious injury. Osteoporosis is one of several risk factors.
Massage Classical massage (*see* page 847) can invigorate the patient, as well as ease muscular and perhaps also emotional tension.	**Useful** as a short-term treatment attempt aimed at relaxing the patient and increasing general well-being. Case reports and field studies claim efficacy; however, success is probably seen in only a proportion of patients (*see* Placebo, page xxi).	**Suitable for DIY** Qualified guidance is recommended. Masseurs/masseuses should propose a treatment plan. **Risks:** Some people are sensitive to manual stimuli; others find it hard to tolerate close physical contact.
Nutritional therapies An organic diet (*see* page 4) provides the body with essential and secondary plant nutrients.	**Useful** as an individually directed general measure.	**Suitable for DIY** Qualified guidance is recommended though not essential. **Risks:** Avoid imbalanced or intolerable diets. They can cause deficiencies with serious consequences, particularly in children.

Treatment	Rating	Point of delivery/risks
Physical therapies Heat and cold treatments, various hydrotherapeutic techniques (*see* pages 871–8), and exercise therapy (*see* page 868) are said to relax and invigorate the system. Saunas (*see* page 876) are supposed to stimulate the circulation and improve the body's own regulatory systems.	**Useful** as a short-term treatment attempt aimed at invigorating the patient and giving a feeling of increased general well-being. Some case reports and field studies claim efficacy in the treatment of ME and chronic fatigue; however, success is probably seen in only a proportion of patients (*see* Placebo, page xxi). Saunas **may be of some use**; again, success is probably seen in only a proportion of patients.	**Suitable for DIY** An individual treatment program should be defined in association with the treating physician. **Risks:** Skin damage may be caused in persons with diminished temperature sensation when extreme temperatures are applied.
Reflex therapies Reflex zone massage (*see* page 883), reflexology (*see* page 883), and TENS (*see* page 886) are said to alleviate pain, relax, invigorate, and exercise a number of beneficial effects via reflex channels (*see* page 881).	**May be of some use** as a short-term treatment attempt for CFS-related muscular tension and pain. Some case reports and field studies claim efficacy; however, success is probably seen in only a proportion of patients (*see* Placebo, page xxi).	**Suitable for DIY** Qualified guidance is essential. Practitioners should be properly qualified and should propose a treatment plan. **Risks:** Some people are sensitive to manual stimuli; others find it hard to tolerate close physical contact.
Relaxation techniques Autogenic training (*see* page 888), muscle relaxation according to Jacobson (*see* page 893), and various biofeedback techniques (*see* page 891) are said to relieve muscle tension and inner unrest, and so might help the patient become more aware of his/her physical and emotional states.	**Useful** as a supportive treatment attempt aimed at relaxing the patient. Case reports claim efficacy; however, success is probably seen in only a proportion of patients (*see* Placebo, page xxi).	**Suitable for DIY** Once a sound understanding of the technique has been acquired from a trainer in group sessions or through individual tuition, patients can perform exercises themselves. Therapists should be properly qualified. **Risks:** Fairly unlikely.

Treatment	Rating	Point of delivery/risks
Vitamins and trace elements The painkilling properties of vitamin B6 are said to alleviate ME-related pain (*see* page 900). The antioxidative properties of beta-carotene, vitamins C and E, and selenium are thought to give a boost to the body's own defence against free radical formation and so modulate the immune system (*see* page 10).	**Useful** in vitamin deficiency. High doses of vitamins B, C, beta-carotene, and selenium **may be of some use** as a short-term treatment attempt. Recommended dosages vary widely but are probably set to rise. Field studies and initial controlled clinical studies ascribe a degree of success to high dosed vitamins in elderly patients.	**Suitable for DIY** Qualified guidance is recommended though not essential. **Risks:** Intolerance and overdosage are possible. Recent findings imply that beta-carotene might increase the risk of cancer. Vitamin B6 in high doses may cause serious side effects.

Herbal remedies for ME and chronic fatigue

Active ingredient/preparation	Rating
Ginseng, Asiatic (*Panax ginseng*)	Taken orally, Asiatic ginseng **may be of some use** as a treatment attempt in exhaustion, debility, and convalescence. In various tests it was seen to improve the ability of rodents to withstand stress, though the importance of these findings for humans is unclear. There is no effective difference between red and white ginseng. The red color of red ginseng comes from its being preserved with steam. **Daily dose:** Pour a cup or hot water over 1–2g root and infuse; equivalent to 25–30 mg ginsenosides or 200–400mg ginseng extract. **Duration of treatment:** Generally for a maximum of three weeks. Use ready-formulated preparations as instructed by the manufacturer/prescriber. **Risks:** Ginseng products should not be taken by persons with high blood pressure or arteriosclerosis (both common in the elderly), as they may increase blood pressure even further. High dosages may also lead to agitation and sleeplessness. Ginseng should be avoided by individuals who are highly energetic, nervous, manic, or schizophrenic, and it should not be taken with stimulants, including coffee and antipsychotic drugs.

Active ingredient/preparation	Rating

Ginseng, Siberian
(*Eleutherococcus senticosus*)

Taken orally, Siberian ginseng **may be of some use** as a treatment attempt in exhaustion, debility, and convalescence; also as an immune system stimulant.
Daily dose: As an infusion 0.6–3g dry root, generally for a maximum of three weeks. Use ready-formulated preparations as instructed by the manufacturer/prescriber.
Risks: Siberian ginseng may cause hypertension, headaches, and vertigo, possibly also vaginal bleeding and mastodynia through its estrogen-like action. Long-term use may result in loose morning stools, sleeplessness, depression, and menstrual disorders. Not to be taken by persons with high blood pressure. Not to be used for more than three weeks. Ginseng should be avoided by individuals who are highly energetic, nervous, manic, or schizophrenic, and it should not be taken with stimulants, including coffee and antipsychotic drugs.

Kola seeds
(*Cola nitida*)

Taken orally, kola seeds **may be of some use** as a treatment attempt for mental and physical exhaustion. Kola intensifies the effect of other central nervous stimulants, including caffeine.
Not advised in gastric ulcer.
Daily dose: 2–6g seeds, 0.25–0.75g extract, 2.5–8g fluid extract, 10–30g tincture, 60–180g kola wine. Use ready-formulated preparations as instructed by the manufacturer/prescriber.
Risks: Sleeplessness, hyperexcitability, nervous unrest, stomach problems.

Active ingredient/preparation	Rating
Lecithin in combination with vitamins	**Of little use**. Indiscriminate combination with vitamins is unnecessary; the lecithin dosage must be high for it to have any effect. Vitamin supplementation is only useful when there is a nutritional deficiency. **Dosage:** As instructed by the manufacturer/prescriber. **Risks:** Lecithin is not known to have any serious side effects.
Maté leaves (*Ilex paraguariensis*)	**Only suitable** as a central nervous stimulant (contains alkaloids, including caffeine). **Daily dose:** As an infusion 3g dried leaves. **Individual dose:** Pour a cup of boiling water over 1g of dried leaves and infuse. Use ready-formulated preparations as instructed by the manufacturer/prescriber. **Risks:** Nervousness, unrest. Do not take before retiring to bed. Maté tea should be used in moderation.
Pollen of various flowers	**May be of some use** for restoring vitality and appetite. **Dose:** As instructed by the manufacturer/prescriber. **Risks:** Pollen must not be taken by persons with pollen allergy, as it may cause intense allergic reactions (including asthma attacks).
Vitamin E in combination with herbal remedies	**Of little use**. Combination preparations of this type are chiefly advised for improving sexual performance, though there is little evidence that they have any effect. There is also little to corroborate claims that vitamin E can help with erection difficulties and ejaculation problems.

Neuropathy

Causes and symptoms

Neuropathy can have a variety of causes such as bacterial infection, alcoholism (*see* page 66), diabetes (*see* page 627), or contact with certain chemicals. Some drugs can also damage the nerves. Neuropathy may be caused, in addition, by liver or kidney disease, disturbed metabolism (*see* pages 627–41), or hormone imbalance.

Neuropathy is a general term denoting functional disturbances in the peripheral nervous system. In practice it means that the nerves no longer react as they should to stimuli. Initially, the patient feels "pins and needles" in the feet or legs, the soles of the feet become painful, the legs ache, and there are frequent cramps, especially at night. At a later stage the pain gives way to numbness, the patient can no longer feel heat and cold and, through lack of pain sensation, superficial injuries to the body go unnoticed. Even innocuous looking injuries may develop into raging sores that can destroy the soft tissues and even bone. The feet are at particular risk. If they turn black and become gangrenous, amputation is often the only way of stopping the whole body from being poisoned.

Sufferers must always have an understanding of the primary disease that is the cause of their neuropathy, and act appropriately. They should pay special attention to skin and foot care, and always choose properly fitting shoes.

Orthodox treatment

There is presently no cure for many types of nerve damage. Some clinics offer special advice on foot care.

Complementary therapies

Though not offering a cure, certain complementary therapies can offer pain relief and respite from certain symptoms.

Treatment plan and limited trial

Before administering a complementary treatment, every therapist should propose a treatment plan (*see* page xxiii) that sets out a clear time frame and defines the goal that the treatment is designed to achieve. Treatment should then be tried for a limited term to test the patient's response.

Caution

A proper medical diagnosis must be obtained before any complementary treatment is attempted for numbness or pain. Massage and needling techniques may simply exacerbate pain or endanger the limb.

Complementary treatments for neuropathy

Treatment	Rating	Point of delivery/risks
Acupressure This treatment (*see* page 769), otherwise known as pressure-point massage, is claimed to alleviate pain and ease tension when the appropriate points are stimulated.	**May be of some use** as a short-term treatment attempt aimed at alleviating pain and relaxing the patient. Case reports claim efficacy; however, success is probably seen in only a proportion of patients (*see* Placebo, page xxi).	**Suitable for DIY** Qualified guidance is recommended. **Risks:** Unlikely provided treatment is carried out competently. Acupressure should not be applied to areas in which the nerves have been damaged.
Acupuncture Acupuncture in its various forms (*see* page 772) aims to encourage the flow of energy (*see* page 927) or to act directly to alleviate pain. The acupuncture points chosen can vary from one practitioner to another.	**May be of some use** as a short-term treatment attempt aimed at alleviating pain. Some case reports claim efficacy; however, success is probably seen in only a proportion of patients (*see* Placebo, page xxi).	**Requires a qualified practitioner** Acupuncturists should be properly qualified and should propose a treatment plan. **Risks:** Probably rare provided treatment is carried out competently. Acupuncture should not be carried out on areas in which the nerves have been damaged.

Treatment	Rating	Point of delivery/risks
Aromatherapy Essential oils (*see* page 786) are used to soothe and relax, or to invigorate, thereby helping to relieve symptoms. The essences may be taken orally, used externally as massage oils or bathing emulsions, or inhaled as vapors.	**Of little use** Perhaps acceptable as a short-term, supportive treatment attempt aimed at soothing and relaxing the patient. Some case reports claim efficacy; however, success is probably seen in only a small proportion of patients (*see* Placebo, page xxi).	**Suitable for DIY** Qualified guidance is recommended. The effects of individual essential oils differ widely. **Risks:** Allergies or intolerance are possible. Some oils are carcinogenic in test systems and possibly in humans.
Bioresonance therapy Bioresonance therapists use electrical devices in an attempt to discover the causes of illness and claim to be able to weaken or turn around pathogenic energies and disease related vibrations (*see* page 794).	**Of little use** Acceptable as a short-term treatment attempt when simpler, more established methods have been unsuccessful. Some case reports claim efficacy; however, success is probably seen, if at all, in only a small proportion of patients (*see* Placebo, page xxi).	**Requires a qualified practitioner** Practitioners should be properly qualified and should propose a treatment plan. No credence should be given to anyone promising immediate or total success. **Risks:** Fairly unlikely.
Cell therapy Injecting or ingesting products extracted from the tissues of newborn animals or animal fetuses is said to have a rejuvenating and revitalizing effect and to enhance the healing of human tissues and organs (*see* page 796).	**Not advised** Based on present knowledge, there is inadequate evidence of the efficacy and mode of action of this costly and relatively risky procedure.	**Risks:** Injecting foreign proteins into the body can provoke (possibly fatal) allergic reactions. Also, pathogens such as those that cause bovine spongiform encephalopathy (BSE) or other serious infections may be introduced.

Treatment	Rating	Point of delivery/risks
Chelation therapy The chelating agent EDTA (*see* page 800) is able, it is claimed, to bind heavy metals and calcareous deposits in the bloodstream. These are subsequently eliminated from the body.	**Only useful** in heavy metal exposure and intoxication. Otherwise, this procedure is **not advised**.	**Requires a qualified practitioner** **Risks:** EDTA can, in extreme cases, cause cardiac arrhythmia, respiratory failure, cramps, and death.
Electroacupuncture according to Voll By taking readings of the electrical conductivity of the skin (*see* page 802), therapists claim to be able to derive an insight into diseased areas of the body, pathogenic foci (*see* page 928), and stress factors (*see* Toxins, page 929). The factors that may be causing neuropathy can then be addressed.	**Of little use** Possibly acceptable as a short-term, supportive treatment attempt when simpler, more established methods have been unsuccessful. Some case reports claim temporary efficacy; however, success is probably seen, if at all, in only a small proportion of patients (*see* Placebo, page xxi).	**Requires a qualified practitioner** Practitioners should be properly qualified and should propose a treatment plan. No credence should be given to anyone promising immediate or total success. **Risks:** A second opinion must always be obtained from a qualified physician before any attempt is made to "eliminate foci" (e.g. by surgery).
Electroneural therapy according to Croon According to the theory, readings taken at various reactive sites on the skin highlight diseased areas within the body. Based on these readings, electrostimulative therapy can then be used to address the factors that may be causing neuropathy (*see* page 806).	**Of little use** Possibly acceptable as a short-term, supportive treatment attempt when simpler, more established methods have been unsuccessful. Some case reports claim temporary efficacy; however, success is probably seen, if at all, in only a small proportion of patients (*see* Placebo, page xxi).	**Requires a qualified practitioner** Practitioners should be properly qualified and should propose a treatment plan. No credence should be given to anyone promising immediate or total success. **Risks:** Proponents themselves warn that treatment should not be given in acute inflammatory conditions.

Treatment	Rating	Point of delivery/risks
Eliminative methods, unbloody Unbloody cupping (*see* page 817) is supposed to improve the body's own regulatory systems, alleviate pain, and stimulate metabolism.	**Of little use** Acceptable as a short-term treatment attempt aimed at relieving pain. Some case reports claim efficacy; however, success is probably seen in only a small proportion of patients (*see* Placebo, page xxi).	**Suitable for DIY** Unbloody cupping is best carried out under the guidance of a qualified practitioner. **Risks:** Unlikely provided treatment is carried out competently.
Flower remedies Flower remedies (*see* page 828) are said to restore emotional balance and assist the body's psychic ability to heal itself.	**Of little use** Possibly acceptable as a short-term, supportive treatment attempt aimed at soothing and relaxing the patient. Some case reports claim efficacy; however, success is probably seen in only a small proportion of patients (*see* Placebo, page xxi).	**Suitable for DIY** Qualified guidance is recommended. **Risks:** Possible intolerance.
Homeopathy Highly diluted (potentized) solutions (*see* page 831) are believed to be able to encourage the body to regulate its disturbed vital energy. Organo- and functiotropic (*see* page 833) homeopathy is claimed to be effective for dealing symptomatically with neuropathy.	**Of little use** Possibly acceptable as a short-term, supportive treatment attempt aimed at addressing symptoms. Some case reports claim temporary success for homeopathic treatments; however, success is probably seen in only a proportion of patients (*see* Placebo, page xxi).	**Requires a qualified practitioner** Homeopaths should be properly qualified and should propose a treatment plan. Ready-formulated preparations are suitable for do-it-yourself. **Risks:** Possible intolerance.

Treatment	Rating	Point of delivery/risks
Hypnosis and self-hypnosis In the relaxed and generally altered state of awareness that is induced in hypnosis or self-hypnosis (*see* page 837), physical conditions can be addressed and pain relieved. Some professionally organized courses in self-hypnosis are now available. Hypnosis is often used in combination with other psycho- and behavioral therapies.	**Of little use** Possibly acceptable as a short-term, supportive treatment attempt aimed at relaxing the patient and helping him/her come to terms better with his/her condition. Some case reports claim efficacy; however, success is probably seen in only a proportion of patients (*see* Placebo, page xxi).	**Requires a qualified practitioner** Hypnotherapists should be properly qualified and should propose a treatment plan. **Risks:** Unlikely provided treatment is carried out competently.
Manual therapies Chiropractors and osteopaths use a series of manipulations to realign allegedly displaced vertebrae. This, it is believed, may ease pain and free blocked energy (*see* page 927); it can also allegedly remove the basis for other symptoms (*see* page 844).	**Of little use** Possibly acceptable as a short-term treatment attempt aimed at pain relief. Some case reports claim efficacy for this relatively risky procedure; however, success is probably seen, if at all, in only a small proportion of patients (*see* Placebo, page xxi).	**Requires a qualified practitioner** Practitioners should be properly qualified and should propose a treatment plan. **Risks:** Spinal manipulations can cause serious injury. Osteoporosis is one of several risk factors.
Massage Classical massage (*see* page 847) and lymphatic drainage (*see* page 850) can invigorate the patient, as well as ease muscular and perhaps also emotional tension.	**Of little use** Acceptable as a supportive treatment attempt aimed at relaxing the patient. Case reports claim efficacy; however, success is probably seen in only a proportion of patients (*see* Placebo, page xxi).	**Requires a qualified practitioner** Masseurs/masseuses should be properly qualified and should propose a treatment plan. **Risks:** Massaging areas affected by nerve damage may cause unpleasant sensations, or may actually exacerbate pain.

Treatment	Rating	Point of delivery/risks
Nutritional therapies An organic diet (*see* page 4) provides the body with essential and secondary plant nutrients (dietary fiber, antioxidants), which are believed to exercise a multitude of positive effects, such as boosting the immune system.	**Useful** as a basic measure in the treatment of alcohol-induced polyneuropathy. **May be of some use** as an individually directed supportive measure.	**Suitable for DIY** Qualified guidance is recommended though not essential. **Risks:** Avoid imbalanced or intolerable diets. They can cause deficiencies with serious consequences. Children are at particularly high risk.
Physical therapies Rising temperature partial immersion baths, full immersion baths with herbs added to the water, or exercising in warm water may provide relaxation, ease pain, and invigorate the patient (*see* pages 871–8).	**May be of some use** as a short-term treatment attempt aimed at pain relief. Some case reports claim efficacy; however, success is probably seen in only a proportion of patients (*see* Placebo, page xxi).	**Suitable for DIY** An individual treatment program should be defined in association with the treating physician. **Risks:** Skin damage may be caused to persons with diminished temperature sensation when extreme temperatures are applied. Treatment should not be carried out on areas affected by nerve damage.
Reflex therapies Reflexology (*see* page 883) and TENS (*see* page 886) are said to alleviate pain via reflex channels (*see* page 881)	**May be of some use** as a short-term treatment attempt aimed at reducing pain. Controlled clinical studies have shown TENS to offer a degree of efficacy in the relief of pain. Some case reports claim efficacy for the other procedures; however, success is probably seen in only a proportion of patients (*see* Placebo, page xxi).	**Requires a qualified practitioner** Practitioners should be properly qualified and should propose a treatment plan. **Risks:** Reflex therapies should not be carried out on areas affected by nerve damage.

Treatment	Rating	Point of delivery/risks
Relaxation techniques Autogenic training (*see* page 888), muscle relaxation according to Jacobson (*see* page 893), and various biofeedback techniques (*see* page 891) are said to relieve muscle tension and inner unrest, and might be instrumental in helping the patient come to terms better with his/her condition.	**May be of some use** as a supportive treatment attempt aimed at relaxing the patient and helping him/her come to terms better with his/her condition. Some case reports and field studies claim efficacy; however, success is probably seen in only a proportion of patients (*see* Placebo, page xxi).	**Suitable for DIY** Once a sound understanding of the technique has been acquired from a trainer in group sessions or through individual tuition, patients can perform exercises themselves. Therapists should be properly qualified. **Risks:** Fairly unlikely provided treatment is carried out competently.
Vitamins and trace elements Vitamin B6 is said to alleviate pain. The anti-oxidative properties of beta-carotene, vitamins C and E, and selenium are said to counter the formation of free radicals, to be instrumental in improving the body's own defence systems (*see* page 902), and to exercise a multitude of other beneficial effects (*see* page 900).	**Of little use** except in vitamin deficiency. No definitive recommendations can be given based on present knowledge.	**Suitable for DIY** Qualified guidance is recommended though not essential. **Risks:** Intolerance and overdosage are possible. Recent findings imply that beta-carotene might increase the risk of cancer. High doses of vitamin B6 can cause serious side effects.

Herbal remedies for neuropathy

There are no recommended herbal remedies for use in this indication.

Parkinson's disease

Causes and symptoms

Parkinson's disease is a condition involving the degeneration of brain nerve cells, leading to a deficit of dopamine, a nerve transmitter. The causes are varied and include genetic factors, inflammation, immune system disorders, and environmental influences. In most cases the precise cause is unknown. Parkinson's disease occurs mostly in persons aged over 60, and is more common in men than in women.

Symptoms similar to those in Parkinson's disease may be produced by certain types of poisoning (carbon monoxide intoxication, for instance) or brain tumor; they may also be drug-induced (e.g. by neuroleptin, which is used to treat schizophrenia).

A shortage of dopamine in the brain causes muscular rigidity, gradual loss of motor function, and tremors. Typical symptoms are: monotonous speech, a stooped posture, an uncontrolled gait, involuntary movements, and a tendency to fall over. Depression (*see* page 100) is a problem when sufferers start to find it increasingly difficult to deal with everyday situations and their mental state deteriorates. There is no effective cure for Parkinson's disease, though its symptoms can often be successfully controlled.

Orthodox treatment

Drug-based treatment normally concentrates on normalizing dopamine levels or countering the preponderance of acetylcholine, another nerve transmitter.

Counselling will play an important part in managing this disease, as will physio- and occupational therapy. These treatments can contribute significantly to helping sufferers cope with the rigors of everyday life.

Complementary therapies

Like orthodox treatments, complementary therapies will include various physical procedures. Complementary approaches frequently concentrate on alleviating symptoms. Some therapists believe Parkinson's disease to be triggered by exposure to toxins (*see* page 929) or by foci (*see* page 928); others see it as a constitutional problem (*see* Constitution, page 927) or as a manifestation of the patient's life force (*see* page 928) being out of balance.

Treatment plan and limited trial

Before administering a complementary treatment, every therapist should propose a treatment plan (*see* page xxiii) that sets out a clear time frame and defines the goal that the treatment is designed to achieve. Treatment should then be tried for a limited term to test the patient's response.

Cautions

Accurate diagnosis is essential and must involve orthodox neurological examination. Complementary treatments are no substitute for proper physio- or occupational therapy.

There is presently insufficient evidence to show whether, and to what extent, complementary treatments can replace state of the art drugs.

Complementary treatments for Parkinson's disease

Treatment	Rating	Point of delivery/risks
Acupressure This treatment (*see* page 769), otherwise known as pressure-point massage, is used to reduce symptoms such as nausea, excessive salivation, anxiety, or muscle pain. Acupressure is also used to impart vital energy (*see* Life force, page 928).	**Inappropriate** as a treatment for Parkinson's disease. **May be of some use** as a short-term, supportive attempt to treat concomitant conditions. Some case reports claim temporary efficacy; however, success is probably seen in only a small proportion of patients (*see* Placebo, page xxi).	**Suitable for DIY** Qualified guidance is recommended. **Risks:** Unlikely provided treatment is carried out competently.
Acupuncture Acupuncture in its various forms (*see* page 772) aims to encourage the flow of energy (*see* page 927) or to address tremors and the hardening of muscles directly.	**Inappropriate** as a treatment for Parkinson's disease. **May be of some use** as a short-term, supportive attempt to treat concomitant symptoms. Some case reports and field studies claim efficacy; however, success is probably seen in only a small proportion of patients (*see* Placebo, page xxi).	**Requires a qualified practitioner** Acupuncturists should be properly qualified and should propose a treatment plan. **Risks:** Probably rare provided treatment is carried out competently.
Anthroposophical medicine In the AM interpretation (*see* page 781) of degenerative diseases of the central nervous system, encroachment of the upper pole into the extremities is said to be normalized through curative eurhythmy, bathing, and potentized organ preparations.	**Inappropriate** as a treatment for Parkinson's disease. Acceptable as a supportive treatment attempt. Some studies claim efficacy; however, success is probably seen in only a proportion of patients (*see* Placebo, page xxi).	**Requires a qualified practitioner** Practitioners should be properly qualified and should propose a treatment plan. **Risks:** Allergies or intolerance are possible.

Treatment	Rating	Point of delivery/risks
Aromatherapy Essential oils (*see* page 786) are used to soothe and relax, or to invigorate. The essences may be taken orally, used externally as massage oils or bathing emulsions, or inhaled as vapors.	**Inappropriate** as a treatment for Parkinson's disease. **May be of some use** as a short-term, supportive treatment attempt aimed at soothing and relaxing. Some case reports claim slight and temporary efficacy; however, success is probably seen in only a small proportion of patients (*see* Placebo, page xxi).	**Suitable for DIY** Qualified guidance is recommended. The effects of individual essential oils differ widely. **Risks:** Allergies or intolerance are possible. Some oils are carcinogenic in test systems and possibly in humans.
Bioresonance therapy Bioresonance therapists use electrical devices in an attempt to discover the causes of illness and claim to be able to weaken or turn around pathogenic energies and disease related vibrations (*see* page 794).	**Inappropriate** as a treatment for Parkinson's disease. Possibly acceptable as a short-term, supportive attempt to treat concomitant conditions when more established methods have been unsuccessful. Some case reports claim efficacy; however, success is probably seen, if at all, in only a small proportion of patients (*see* Placebo, page xxi).	**Requires a qualified practitioner** Practitioners should be properly qualified and should propose a treatment plan. No credence should be given to anyone promising immediate or total success. **Risks:** Fairly unlikely.
Cell therapy Injecting or ingesting products extracted from the tissues of newborn animals or animal fetuses is said to have a rejuvenating and revitalizing effect and to enhance the healing of human tissues and organs (*see* page 796).	**Not advised** Based on present knowledge, there is inadequate evidence of the efficacy and mode of action of these costly and relatively risky procedures.	**Risks:** Injecting foreign proteins into the body can provoke (possibly fatal) allergic reactions. Also, pathogens such as those that cause bovine spongiform encephalopathy (BSE) or other serious infections may be introduced.

Treatment	Rating	Point of delivery/risks
Electroacupuncture according to Voll By taking readings of the electrical conductivity of the skin (*see* page 802), therapists claim to be able to derive an insight into diseased areas of the body, pathogenic foci (*see* page 928), and stress factors (*see* Toxins, page 929). The factors that may be causing Parkinson's disease can then be addressed.	**Inappropriate** as a treatment for Parkinson's disease. Possibly acceptable as a short-term, supportive treatment attempt aimed at improving general well-being when simpler, more established methods have been unsuccessful. Some case reports claim slight and temporary efficacy; however, success is probably seen, if at all, in only a small proportion of patients (*see* Placebo, page xxi).	**Requires a qualified practitioner** Practitioners should be properly qualified and should propose a treatment plan. No credence should be given to anyone promising immediate or total success. **Risks:** A second opinion must always be obtained from a qualified physician before any attempt is made to "eliminate foci" (e.g. by surgery).
Electroneural therapy according to Croon According to the theory, readings taken at various reactive sites on the skin highlight diseased areas within the body. Based on these readings, electrostimulative therapy can then be used to address the factors that may be causing Parkinson's disease (*see* page 806).	**Inappropriate** as a treatment for Parkinson's disease. Possibly acceptable as a short-term, supportive treatment attempt aimed at improving general well-being when simpler, more established methods have been unsuccessful. Some case reports claim slight and temporary efficacy; however, success is probably seen, if at all, in only a small proportion of patients (*see* Placebo, page xxi).	**Requires a qualified practitioner** Practitioners should be properly qualified and should propose a treatment plan. No credence should be given to anyone promising immediate or total success. **Risks:** Proponents themselves warn that treatment should not be given in acute inflammatory conditions.

Treatment	Rating	Point of delivery/risks
Flower remedies Flower remedies (*see* page 428) are said to restore emotional balance and assist the body's psychic ability to heal itself.	**Inappropriate** as a treatment for Parkinson's disease. **May be of some use** as a short-term, supportive treatment attempt aimed at soothing and relaxing. Some case reports claim slight and temporary efficacy; however, success is probably seen in only a small proportion of patients (*see* Placebo, page xxi).	**Suitable for DIY** Qualified guidance is recommended. Practitioners should propose a treatment plan. **Risks:** Possible intolerance.
Homeopathy Highly diluted (potentized) solutions (*see* page 831) are believed to encourage the body to regulate its disturbed vital energy. Organo- and functiotropic (*see* page 833) homeopathy is claimed to be effective for addressing the disease symptomatically.	**Inappropriate** as a treatment for Parkinson's disease. Possibly acceptable as a short-term, supportive treatment attempt aimed at the symptoms. Some case reports claim slight and temporary success for homeopathic treatments; however, success is probably seen in only a small proportion of patients (*see* Placebo, page xxi).	**Requires a qualified practitioner** Homeopaths should be properly qualified and should propose a treatment plan. Ready-formulated preparations are suitable for do-it-yourself. **Risks:** Possible intolerance.
Hypnosis and self-hypnosis In the relaxed and generally altered state of awareness that is induced in hypnosis or self-hypnosis (*see* page 837), physical conditions can be addressed. Hypnosis is often used in combination with other psycho- and behavioral therapies.	**Inappropriate** as a treatment for Parkinson's disease. Acceptable as a short-term, supportive treatment attempt aimed at relaxing the patient and helping him/her come to terms better with his/her disease. Some case reports claim efficacy; however, success is probably seen in only a proportion of patients treated (*see* Placebo, page xxi).	**Requires a qualified practitioner** Hypnotherapists should be properly qualified and should propose a treatment plan. **Risks:** Unlikely provided treatment is carried out competently.

Treatment	Rating	Point of delivery/risks
Massage Classical massage (*see* page 847) is said to invigorate the patient, as well as ease muscular and perhaps also emotional tension.	**Inappropriate** as a treatment for Parkinson's disease. **May be of some use** as a supportive measure aimed at relaxing the patient and improving general well-being. Some case reports claim efficacy; however, success is probably seen in only a proportion of patients (*see* Placebo, page xxi).	**Suitable for DIY** Qualified guidance is essential. Masseurs/masseuses should propose a treatment plan. **Risks:** Some people are sensitive to manual stimuli; others find it hard to tolerate close physical contact.
Nutritional therapies An organic diet (*see* page 4) provides the body with essential and secondary plant nutrients (dietary fiber, antioxidants), which are believed to exercise a multitude of positive effects.	**Inappropriate** as a treatment for Parkinson's disease. **Useful** as an individually directed supportive measure.	**Suitable for DIY** Qualified guidance is recommended though not essential. **Risks:** Avoid imbalanced or intolerable diets. They can cause deficiencies with serious consequences.
Physical therapies Warm baths, possibly with herbs added to the water, alternating washings, dry brushings, and exercise therapy (*see* pages 867–78) are said to induce relaxation, invigorate the patient, and improve various physical functions.	**Inappropriate** as a treatment for Parkinson's disease. **Useful** as an attempt to raise general well-being and improve various physical functions. Field studies ascribe a degree of efficacy to this treatment in some patients (*see* Placebo, page xxi).	**Suitable for DIY** Qualified guidance is recommended though not essential. **Risks:** Skin damage may be caused to persons with diminished temperature sensation when extreme temperatures are applied.

Treatment	Rating	Point of delivery/risks
Relaxation techniques Autogenic training (*see* page 888), muscle relaxation according to Jacobson (*see* page 893), and various biofeedback techniques (*see* page 891) are said to relieve muscle tension, anxiety, and inner unrest, and so might be instrumental in helping the patient come to terms better with his/her condition.	**Inappropriate** as a treatment for Parkinson's disease. **May be of some use** as a supportive treatment attempt aimed at relaxing the patient, relieving worries, and helping him/her come to terms better with his/her disease. Some case reports claim efficacy; however, success is probably seen in only a proportion of patients (*see* Placebo, page xxi).	**Suitable for DIY** Once a sound understanding of the technique has been acquired from a trainer in group sessions or through individual tuition, patients can perform exercises themselves. Therapists should be properly qualified. **Risks:** Fairly unlikely.
Vitamins and trace elements The anti-oxidative properties of vitamins C and E are thought to counter the formation of free radicals and boost the body's anti-oxidative defence systems, while also exercising a multitude of other beneficial effects (*see* page 900).	**Inappropriate** as a treatment for Parkinson's disease. **May be of some use** as a short-term supportive measure. Based on present knowledge, no definitive recommendations can be given.	**Suitable for DIY** Qualified guidance is recommended though not essential. **Risks:** Intolerance and overdosage are possible.

Herbal remedy for Parkinson's disease

Active ingredient/preparation	Rating
Deadly nightshade (*Atropa belladonna*)	Though formerly used for Parkinson's disease, deadly nightshade is **of little use** and should no longer be employed. **Caution:** This is a highly toxic remedy which, in the UK, can only be supplied by pharmacists and professional practitioners. It must never be used in pregnancy, prostatic disease, tachycardia, or glaucoma, nor in association with depressant drugs.

Psychotic disorders

Causes and symptoms

Psychotic disorders are characterized by the sufferer's inability to differentiate between his inner world and the "real world." Psychotic patients have delusions. Typical psychotic symptoms are: an inability to think rationally, to communicate effectively, to control impulses and obsessions, to behave "normally," to express one's feelings, or to maintain relationships with other people. For sufferers and their families the effect may be devastating.

There is a whole range of conditions, varying widely in severity, that qualify as being psychotic:

- Schizophrenic patients lose touch with reality—their sense of who they are and what is happening becomes distorted. Unrelated events may become illogically interlinked to form a new subjective reality. Sufferers may hallucinate: in other words, hear, see, and smell imaginary persons or objects.
- Manic depression is a condition in which the person experiences moods that alternate between highly euphoric and deeply depressive. During the manic phase sufferers may, for instance, have an exaggerated feeling of self-importance and, in this mood, may become provocative or go on spending sprees, may lose all sense of proportion and risk, and may become so driven on that they do not stop to contemplate their actions. During depression, however, they feel desperate, worthless, and guilty, possibly showing suicidal tendencies.

Orthodox treatment

Most psychotic disorders can be treated with antipsychotic drugs. Psychiatrists disagree, however, over the justification for resorting to drug therapy and over the doses that should be given and for how long. Antipsychotic drugs often cause side effects such as drowsiness, apathy, dry mouth, muscular rigidity, tremor, dyskinesia, and impairment of mental function.

Complementary therapies

Various complementary treatments are believed to cure, alleviate, or prevent psychotic behavior. These are chiefly used against mild forms of psychosis. No complementary treatment has ever been researched to the standards required by modern mainstream medicine. Most procedures would appear to be incapable of addressing psychotic illness in any meaningful way. There are certain complementary practitioners who believe psychotic behavior to be produced, *inter alia*, by food intolerance, food additives, environmental pollutants, allergies, or sensitivity to a variety of chemicals. To date there have been no controlled studies into these environment implicating theories.

Treatment plan and limited trial

Before administering a complementary treatment, every therapist should propose a treatment plan (*see* page xxiii) that sets out a clear time frame and defines the goal that the treatment is designed to achieve. Treatment should then be tried for a limited term to test the patient's response.

Cautions

Psychotic disorders must be properly diagnosed and evaluated by a qualified doctor to enable possible causes such as a brain tumor and inflammation, metabolic disease (*see* pages 627–41), and poisoning to be detected and appropriately treated. Certain complementary treatments, especially those involving electrical stimulation, vibration, or needling, may be perceived by some sufferers as a threat to their person and so induce or exacerbate paranoia.

Complementary treatments for psychotic disorders

Treatment	Rating	Point of delivery/risks
Acupuncture Acupuncture in its various forms (*see* page 772) is used in mild to moderate psychotic disorders to ease symptoms such as delusions and hallucinations; also, to alleviate adverse side effects of neuroleptic agents, such as tremors, restlessness, and muscular rigidity (*see* page 157).	**Inappropriate** as a treatment for psychotic disorders. **May be of some use** as a short-term attempt to treat symptoms. Some field studies claim efficacy in the reduction of adverse side effects of neuroleptic drugs; however, success is probably seen in only a proportion of patients (*see* Placebo, page xxi).	**Requires a qualified practitioner** Acupuncturists should be properly qualified and should propose a treatment plan. **Risks:** Probably rare provided treatment is carried out competently and the patient does not perceive it as menacing.
Anthroposophical medicine AM (*see* page 781) interprets psychotic disorders as an expression of impaired cardiac, hepatic, renal, or pulmonary function. Once the cause has been found, the organ in question is treated with various drugs specific to AM.	**Inappropriate** as a treatment for psychotic disorders. **May be of some use** as a short-term, supportive treatment attempt for chronic conditions when the patient accepts this form of treatment. Case reports claim efficacy; however, success is probably seen in only a proportion of patients (*see* Placebo, page xxi).	**Requires a qualified practitioner** Practitioners should be properly qualified and should propose a treatment plan. No credence should be given to anyone promising immediate or total success. **Risks:** Allergies or intolerance are possible.

Treatment	Rating	Point of delivery/risks
Aromatherapy Essential oils (*see* page 786) are used to soothe and relax, or to invigorate, thereby helping ease psychotic symptoms. The essences may be taken orally, used externally as massage oils or bathing emulsions, or inhaled as vapors.	**Inappropriate** as a treatment for psychotic disorders. **May be of some use** as a short-term, supportive treatment attempt aimed at soothing and relaxing. Some case reports claim efficacy; however, success is probably seen in only a proportion of patients (*see* Placebo, page xxi).	**Suitable for DIY** Qualified guidance is recommended. The effects of individual essential oils differ widely. **Risks:** Allergies or intolerance are possible. Some oils are carcinogenic in test systems and possibly in humans. Certain aromas may be perceived as menacing or may actually exacerbate symptoms.
Bioresonance therapy Bioresonance therapists use electrical devices in an attempt to discover the causes of illness and claim to be able to weaken or turn around pathogenic energies and disease related vibrations (*see* page 794).	**Inappropriate** as a treatment for psychotic disorders. Possibly acceptable as a short-term, supportive treatment attempt when simpler, more established methods have been unsuccessful. Some case reports claim efficacy; however, success is probably seen, if at all, in only a small proportion of patients (*see* Placebo, page xxi).	**Requires a qualified practitioner** Practitioners should be properly qualified and should propose a treatment plan. **Risks:** Fairly unlikely provided that the patient does not perceive the treatment as menacing; otherwise treatment may trigger or reinforce delusions.
Cell therapy Products extracted from the tissues of newborn animals or animal fetuses are said to have a rejuvenating and revitalizing effect and to enhance the healing of human tissues and organs (*see* page 796).	**Not advised** Based on present knowledge, there is a lack of convincing evidence of the efficacy and mode of action of this costly and relatively risky procedure.	**Risks:** Injecting foreign proteins into the body can provoke (possibly fatal) allergic reactions. Also, pathogens such as those that cause bovine spongiform encephalopathy (BSE) or other serious infections may be introduced.

Treatment	Rating	Point of delivery/risks
Electroacupuncture according to Voll By taking readings of the electrical conductivity of the skin (*see* page 902), therapists claim to be able to derive an insight into diseased areas of the body, pathogenic foci (*see* page 928), and stress factors (*see* Toxins, page 929). Subsequently, factors causing psychosis can be addressed, and treatment attempted with homeopathic remedies and eliminative procedures (*see* below).	**Inappropriate** as a treatment for psychotic disorders. **Of little use** based on present knowledge. Possibly acceptable as a short-term, supportive treatment attempt when simpler, more established methods have been unsuccessful. Some case reports claim efficacy; however, success is probably seen, if at all, in only a small proportion of patients (*see* Placebo, page xxi).	**Requires a qualified practitioner** Practitioners should be properly qualified and should propose a treatment plan. No credence should be given to anyone promising immediate or total success. **Risks:** A second opinion must always be obtained from a qualified physician before any attempt is made to "eliminate foci" (e.g. by surgery). Recommendation of this form of treatment may feed some patients' delusions of being poisoned and intensify their self-aggression. Also, the equipment used may trigger or reinforce delusions.
Eliminative methods, bloody Bloody cupping (*see* page 815) is said to improve the body's own regulatory systems and ease symptoms.	**Not advised** There is no evidence for the efficacy and mode of action of this invasive and sometimes risky procedure.	**Risks:** Bloody cupping may lead to infection or scarring. Furthermore, it should not be practiced on patients with bleeding disorders.
Eliminative methods, unbloody Mild emetics, sweating (*see* page 877), colonic irrigation (*see* page 819), or unbloody cupping (*see* page 817) are said to improve the body's own regulatory systems and ease symptoms.	**Inappropriate** as a treatment for psychotic disorders. Possibly acceptable as a short-term, supportive treatment attempt. Some case reports claim efficacy; however, success is probably seen in only a small proportion of patients (*see* Placebo, page xxi).	**Suitable for DIY** Unbloody cupping should be carried out by friends or relatives of the patient, preferably under the guidance of a qualified practitioner. **Risks:** Unlikely provided treatment is carried out competently and the patient does not perceive it as menacing.

Treatment	Rating	Point of delivery/risks
Flower remedies Flower remedies (*see* page 828) are said to restore emotional balance and assist the body's psychic ability to heal itself.	**Inappropriate** as a treatment for psychotic disorders. **May be of some use** as a short-term, supportive treatment attempt aimed at soothing and relaxing the patient. Some case reports claim efficacy; however, success is probably seen in only a small proportion of patients (*see* Placebo, page xxi).	**Suitable for DIY** Qualified guidance is recommended. Practitioners should propose a treatment plan. **Risks:** Possible intolerance.
Homeopathy Highly diluted (potentized) solutions (*see* page 831) are believed to be able to redress vital energy imbalances. Organo- and functiotropic (*see* page 833) homeopathy is claimed to be effective for dealing with psychotic symptoms. Recently, there has been a tendency for homeopathic approaches to be applied against alleged untoward side effects of some neuroleptic drugs (*see* page 157).	**Inappropriate** as a treatment for psychotic disorders. **May be of some use** as a short-term, supportive treatment attempt; also for reducing side effects of neuroleptic drugs. Some case reports claim success for homeopathic treatments; however, success is probably seen in only a proportion of patients (*see* Placebo, page xxi).	**Requires a qualified practitioner** Homeopaths should be properly qualified and should propose a treatment plan. Ready-formulated preparations are suitable for do-it-yourself. **Risks:** Possible intolerance.
Massage Classical massage (*see* page 847) is said to invigorate the patient, as well as ease muscular and perhaps also emotional tension.	**Inappropriate** as a treatment for psychotic disorders. **May be of some use** as a supportive measure aimed at relaxing the patient and improving general well-being. Some case reports claim efficacy; however, success is probably seen in only a proportion of patients (*see* Placebo, page xxi).	**Suitable for DIY** Qualified guidance is essential. Masseurs/masseuses should propose a treatment plan. **Risks:** Some patients perceive massage as menacing.

Treatment	Rating	Point of delivery/risks
Nutritional therapies An organic diet (*see* page 4) provides the body with essential and secondary plant nutrients (dietary fiber, antioxidants). In psychotic patients this type of diet may also allay any delusions that their food is poisoned. Orthomolecular medicine and clinical oncology see psychoses as being associated with food intolerance.	**Inappropriate** as a treatment for psychotic disorders. **Useful** as an individually directed general measure. Owing to the relative lack of information, it is not possible at present to give a definitive judgment of the recommendations put forward by orthomolecular medicine and clinical oncology. Some case reports claim efficacy for these methods in the treatment of psychotic disorders; however, success is probably seen in only a proportion of patients (*see* Placebo, page xxi).	**Suitable for DIY** Qualified guidance is recommended though not essential. Possible food intolerance can be discovered through elimination and rotation diets. These time-consuming and costly nutritional therapies must be medically supervised. **Risks:** Avoid imbalanced or intolerable diets. They can cause deficiencies with serious consequences, particularly in children.
Physical therapies Heat and cold treatments, bathing, and exercise therapy (*see* pages 867–78) are said to relax and invigorate.	**Inappropriate** as a treatment for psychotic disorders. **May be of some use** as a short-term, supportive treatment attempt aimed at relaxing the patient and improving general well-being. Case reports claim efficacy; however, success is probably seen in only a proportion of patients (*see* Placebo, page xxi).	**Suitable for DIY** Qualified guidance is recommended though not essential. A treatment plan should be defined in collaboration with the treating physician. **Risks:** Patients may perceive these treatments as menacing.

Treatment	*Rating*	*Point of delivery/risks*
Reflex therapies Reflex zone massage (*see* page 883) and reflexology (*see* page 883) are said to act via reflex channels (*see* page 881) to ease the pain, muscle tensions, and tremors sometimes associated with the use of neuroleptic drugs (*see* page 157).	**Inappropriate** as a treatment for psychotic disorders. **May be of some use** as a short-term, supportive treatment attempt for pain or muscle tension. Case reports claim efficacy; however, success is probably seen in only a proportion of patients (*see* Placebo, page xxi).	**Requires a qualified practitioner** Practitioners should be properly qualified and should propose a treatment plan. **Risks:** Patients may perceive these treatments as menacing.
Relaxation techniques Autogenic training (*see* page 888), muscle relaxation according to Jacobson (*see* page 893), and various biofeedback techniques (*see* page 891) are said to relieve muscle tension and inner unrest, and might be instrumental in helping patients become more aware of their mental and emotional states.	**Inappropriate** as a treatment for psychotic disorders. **May be of some use** as a supportive treatment attempt aimed at relaxing the patient and making him/her more aware of his/her physical and emotional states. Some case reports and field studies claim efficacy; however, success is probably seen in only a small proportion of patients (*see* Placebo, page xxi).	**Suitable for DIY** Once a sound understanding of the technique has been acquired from a trainer in group sessions or through individual tuition, patients can perform exercises themselves. Therapists should be properly qualified. **Risks:** Fairly unlikely provided treatment is carried out competently.
TENS The use of low frequency electrical currents (*see* page 886) on the surface of the skin is said to counter the adverse side effects of neuroleptic drugs (e.g. tremors) (*see* page 157).	**Inappropriate** as a treatment for psychotic disorders. **May be of some use** as a short-term treatment attempt for tremors or the involuntary movement of muscles, such as occur as a side effect of neuroleptic drugs. Field studies and initial controlled clinical studies ascribe a degree of efficacy to this treatment.	**Requires a qualified practitioner** Practitioners should be properly qualified and should propose a treatment plan. **Risks:** Patients may perceive TENS as menacing.

Treatment	Rating	Point of delivery/risks
Vitamins and trace elements In the treatment of psychotic disorders, orthomolecular medicine makes use primarily of vitamins C, B6 and E, as well as folic acid and trace elements such as manganese and zinc. Dosages are generally defined individually (*see* page 900).	**Inappropriate** as a treatment for psychotic disorders. **May be of some use** as a short-term, supportive treatment attempt. Owing to the relative lack of information, it is not possible at present to give a definitive judgment of the recommendations put forward by orthomolecular medicine and clinical oncology. Some case reports claim efficacy for these methods in the treatment of psychotic disorders; however, success is probably seen in only a small proportion of patients (*see* Placebo, page xxi).	**Requires a qualified practitioner** Treating psychiatrists should have a knowledge of the principles of orthomolecular medicine and should propose a treatment plan. **Risks:** Intolerance and overdosage are possible. Long-term treatment with manganese may cause severe intoxication, e.g. of the central nervous system. Vitamin B6 in high doses can have serious side effects.

Herbal remedies for psychotic disorders

Active ingredient/preparation	Rating
Kava root (*Piper methysticum*)	Taken orally, kava root **may be of some use** as a treatment attempt for slight to moderate forms of nervous anxiety, tension, and restlessness accompanying some psychotic disorders. **Daily dose:** 1.5–2g root. **Individual dose:** infuse 0.5g root with 1 cup of boiling water. **Risks:** Not to be taken during pregnancy or lactation. Not to be taken in depression. The action of kava may be potentiated when it is taken with alcohol, barbiturates, or psychotropic drugs. Not to be taken for longer than three months except on a doctor's advice. Even in recommended dosages, kava affects vision and the ability to drive and operate machinery. Prolonged use may result in yellowing of the skin, allergic skin reactions, difficulty in focusing the eyes, and pupil dilation. Use of kava root extracts is not advised in children under 12 years.
St. John's wort (*Hypericum perforatum*)	**Of little use**. Taken orally, St. John's wort is possibly acceptable as a potential treatment for moderate anxiety associated with some psychotic disorders. **Daily dose:** 2–4g dried herb. **Individual dose:** Infuse 1–2g of dried herb with 1 cup of hot water. **Risks:** Photosensitization (persons with a light complexion should avoid bright sunlight after taking St. John's wort, or they may suffer allergic skin irritation).

Muscle, bones and joints

Back pain

Causes and symptoms

Nine people out of ten experience back pain at least once in their lives. Half of the people applying for early retirement quote back problems as the reason. Approximately every second orthopedic consultation and every fourth visit to a doctor can be attributed to a back problem in one form or another. The financial cost runs into the millions. Back pain can originate through any number of causes, including severe organ dysfunction. It also often has an emotional or psychological component. Sitting for long periods and lifting or carrying heavy objects are other possible causes.

Poor posture can lead to increased wearing of the spine, causing lumbago and sciatica. Damaged, displaced, or prolapsed discs can press on the spinal nerves, ligaments, and blood vessels and lead to referred pain in other regions of the body, causing headaches, pain in the lower arm or leg, disturbed vision, hearing and balance, and the classic signs of paralysis. A damaged disc can nowadays be successfully treated with drugs, or by surgical intervention or physiotherapy.

Having strong back and stomach muscles does provide the spine with greater support. Mattresses should give enough so that they adapt to your spine, and not vice versa. Have a good look at your workplace and, if you think there is a problem, ask for a full ergonomic assessment.

Some health centers now offer "back schools" that teach people how to strengthen their muscles and take better care of their backs.

Orthodox treatment

Increasingly, mainstream doctors are working in unison with certain complementary practitioners, notably osteopaths and chiropractors. Painkillers, though addressing the symptoms in the short term, may, if used to excess, cause a possible organic disease to be missed during diagnosis. Muscle-relaxing tranquilizers are sometimes prescribed in addition to painkillers. Owing to the risk of habituation, these should only be used briefly to deal with persistent symptoms.

In cases where previous treatments have been unsuccessful or the problem is recurrent, a disc that has slipped and is causing partial paralysis by pressing on a spinal nerve will often be surgically removed. Nowadays, laser treatment to evaporate the damaged disc is becoming more commonplace and is replacing the traditional scalpel. Pain sometimes returns, however, despite surgery.

If back pain is thought to be of psychological or emotional origin, counselling or behavioral therapy may be used as a prophylactic measure, and relaxation exercises may also be beneficial.

Complementary therapies

Complementary therapies aim to stop back pain from occurring in the first place but, once it has, to deal with the pain either directly or by improving relaxation.

Treatment plan and limited trial

Before administering a complementary treatment, every therapist should propose a treatment plan (*see* page xxiii) that sets out a clear time frame and defines the goal that the treatment is designed to achieve. Treatment should then be tried for a limited term to test the patient's response.

Cautions

Before any attempt is made to treat recurrent or persistent back pain by a complementary procedure, the patient must be examined by a qualified doctor to exclude a possible physical cause such as a diseased internal organ.

Most complementary treatments are more appropriate in a supportive role than as the sole treatment.

Complementary treatments for back pain

Treatment	Rating	Point of delivery/risks
Acupressure This treatment (*see* page 769), otherwise known as pressure-point massage, is claimed to reduce pain and ease tension. The pressure points chosen can vary from one practitioner to another.	**Useful** as a short-term treatment attempt aimed at reducing pain. Case reports claim efficacy; however, success is probably seen in only a proportion of patients (*see* Placebo, page xxi).	**Suitable for DIY** Qualified guidance is essential. **Risks:** Significant risks are unlikely provided treatment is carried out competently.
Acupuncture Acupuncture in its various forms (*see* page 772) aims to encourage the flow of energy (*see* page 927) or to act directly to reduce pain and ease tension.	**Useful** as a short-term treatment attempt aimed at reducing pain. Controlled clinical studies, case reports, and field studies ascribe a certain efficacy to this treatment in some patients.	**Requires a qualified practitioner** Acupuncturists should be properly qualified and should propose a treatment plan. **Risks:** Probably rare provided treatment is carried out competently.

Treatment	Rating	Point of delivery/risks
Anthroposophical medicine Physicians who practice AM (*see* page 781) inject organ extracts or bamboo preparations depending on the nature of the symptoms, or carry out rhythmic massage, curative eurhythmy, or special exercises.	Curative eurhythmy is **useful** as a preventive measure. The various "compositions" are acceptable as a short-term, supportive treatment attempt. Some studies claim efficacy; however, success is probably seen in only a proportion of patients (*see* Placebo, page xxi).	**Requires a qualified practitioner** Practitioners should be properly qualified and should propose a treatment plan. **Risks:** Allergies and intolerance are possible.
Aromatherapy Essential oils (*see* page 786) are used to soothe and relax, thereby alleviating pain. The essences may be taken orally, used externally as massage oils or bathing emulsions, or inhaled as vapors.	**Of little use** Acceptable as a short-term treatment attempt aimed at invigorating and relaxing the patient. Some case reports claim efficacy; however, success is probably seen in only a proportion of patients (*see* Placebo, page xxi).	**Suitable for DIY** Qualified guidance is recommended. The effects of individual essential oils differ widely. **Risks:** Allergies or intolerance are possible. Some oils are carcinogenic in test systems and possibly in humans.
Bioresonance therapy Bioresonance therapists use electrical devices in an attempt to discover the causes of illness and claim to be able to regulate pathogenic energies and disease related vibrations (*see* page 794).	**Of little use** Possibly acceptable as a short-term treatment attempt aimed at relieving chronic pain when simpler, more established methods have been unsuccessful. Some case reports claim efficacy; however, success is probably seen, if at all, in only a small proportion of patients (*see* Placebo, page xxi).	**Requires a qualified practitioner** Practitioners should be properly qualified and should propose a treatment plan. No credence should be given to anyone promising immediate or total success. **Risks:** Fairly unlikely.

Treatment	Rating	Point of delivery/risks

Cell therapy
Injecting or ingesting products extracted from animal tissues or organs is said to have an immune system modulating effect (*see* page 10) and to enhance the healing of human tissues and organs (*see* page 796).

Not advised
The administration of organ extracts is, at most, acceptable as a limited treatment attempt for chronic or recurrent pain when less risky, better established methods have been unsuccessful. Field studies claim efficacy; however, success is probably seen in only a proportion of patients (*see* Placebo, page xxi). Fresh cell therapy is **not advised**.

Requires a qualified practitioner
Practitioners should be properly qualified and should propose a treatment plan. No credence should be given to anyone promising immediate or total success.
Risks: Injecting foreign proteins into the body can provoke (possibly fatal) allergic reactions. Also, pathogens such as those that cause bovine spongiform encephalopathy (BSE) or other serious infections may be introduced.

Electroacupuncture according to Voll
By taking readings of the electrical conductivity of the skin (*see* page 802), therapists claim to be able to derive an insight into diseased areas of the body, pathogenic foci (*see* page 928), and stress factors (*see* Toxins, page 929). The supposed causes of back pain can then be addressed.

Of little use
Possibly acceptable as a short-term, supportive treatment attempt aimed at relief of chronic pain when simpler, more established methods have been unsuccessful. Some case reports claim efficacy; however, success is probably seen, if at all, in only a small proportion of patients (*see* Placebo, page xxi).

Requires a qualified practitioner
Practitioners should be properly qualified and should propose a treatment plan. No credence should be given to anyone promising immediate or total success.
Risks: A second opinion must always be obtained from a qualified physician before any attempt is made to "eliminate foci"(e.g. by surgery).

Treatment	Rating	Point of delivery/risks
Electroneural therapy according to Croon According to the theory, readings taken at various reactive sites on the skin highlight diseased areas within the body. Based on these readings, electrostimulative therapy can then be used to address the supposed causes of back pain (*see* page 806).	**Of little use** Possibly acceptable as a short-term, supportive treatment attempt at addressing chronic and persistent pain when simpler, more established methods have been unsuccessful. Some case reports and field studies claim efficacy; however, success is probably seen, if at all, in only a small proportion of patients (*see* Placebo, page xxi).	**Requires a qualified practitioner** Practitioners should be properly qualified and should propose a treatment plan. No credence should be given to anyone promising immediate or total success. **Risks:** Proponents themselves warn that treatment should not be given in acute inflammatory conditions.
Eliminative methods, bloody Bloody cupping (*see* page 815) is said to reduce pain in the skeletomuscular system and to ease other symptoms too.	**Of little use** Possibly acceptable as a short-term, supportive treatment attempt aimed at easing chronic pain when less invasive, more established methods have been unsuccessful. Some case reports claim efficacy; however, success is probably seen in only a small proportion of patients (*see* Placebo, page xxi).	**Requires a qualified practitioner** Practitioners should be properly qualified and should propose a treatment plan. No credence should be given to anyone promising immediate or total success. **Risks:** Bloody cupping can cause infection and scarring. Furthermore, it should not be carried out in persons with bleeding disorders.
Eliminative methods, unbloody Unbloody cupping (*see* page 817) is said to ease pain in the skeletomuscular system and to ease other symptoms too.	**May be of some use** as a short-term, supportive treatment attempt aimed at relief of pain. Some case reports claim efficacy; however, success is probably seen in only a proportion of patients (*see* Placebo, page xxi).	**Suitable for DIY** Unbloody cupping is best carried out under the guidance of a qualified practitioner. **Risks:** Unlikely provided treatment is carried out competently.

Treatment	Rating	Point of delivery/risks
Enzyme therapy The enzymes used reportedly dispell and destroy "immune complexes" that course in the blood and are responsible, for instance, for sustaining inflammatory processes (*see* page 824) such as those that occur in arthrosis and soft tissue rheumatism (*see* page 174).	**Of little use** Some case reports claim efficacy for this little researched and relatively costly treatment; however, success is probably seen in only a small proportion of patients (*see* Placebo, page xxi).	**Requires a qualified practitioner** Practitioners should propose a treatment plan. Non-prescription formulations are suitable for do-it-yourself. **Risks:** Allergies or intolerance are possible.
Flower remedies Flower remedies (*see* page 828) are said to restore emotional balance and to assist the body's psychic ability to heal itself.	**Of little use** Acceptable as a short-term, supportive treatment attempt aimed at soothing and relaxing. Some case reports claim efficacy; however, success is probably seen in only a small proportion of patients (*see* Placebo, page xxi).	**Suitable for DIY** Qualified guidance is recommended. Practitioners should propose a treatment plan. **Risks:** Possible intolerance.
Homeopathy Highly diluted (potentized) solutions (*see* page 831) are believed to be able to redress vital energy imbalances. Organo- and functiotropic (*see* page 833) homeopathy is claimed to be effective for dealing with pain in the skeletomuscular system.	**Of little use** Possibly acceptable as a short-term, supportive treatment attempt aimed at dealing with chronic symptoms. Initial (controversial) controlled studies and various field studies claim success for homeopathic treatments; however, success is probably seen in only a proportion of patients (*see* Placebo, page xxi).	**Requires a qualified practitioner** Homeopaths should be properly qualified and should propose a treatment plan. Ready-formulated preparations are suitable for do-it-yourself. **Risks:** Allergies and intolerance are possible.

Treatment	Rating	Point of delivery/risks
Hypnosis and self-hypnosis In the relaxed and generally altered state of awareness that is induced in hypnosis or self-hypnosis (*see* page 837), physical conditions can be addressed and pain relieved. Hypnosis is sometimes used in combination with other psycho- and behavioral therapies to encourage behavioral changes.	**May be of some use** as a short-term, supportive treatment attempt aimed at relieving persistent symptoms. Some case reports and field studies claim efficacy; however, success is probably seen in only a proportion of patients treated (*see* Placebo, page xxi).	**Requires a qualified practitioner** Hypnotherapists should be properly qualified and should propose a treatment plan. No credence should be given to anyone promising immediate or total success. **Risks:** Unlikely provided treatment is carried out competently.
Magnetic field therapy The use of magnetic field generators, magnetic strips, bracelets, and other objects (*see* page 841) allegedly encourages cell metabolism and so relieves pain.	**Inappropriate** Based on present knowledge, there is inadequate evidence of the efficacy and mode of action of magnetic field therapy in the treatment of back pain.	Operation of magnetic field equipment **requires a qualified practitioner**. **Risks:** Magnetic field equipment can cause implanted cardiac pacemakers to malfunction.
Manual therapies Chiropractors and osteopaths use a series of manipulations to realign allegedly displaced vertebrae and joints which, it is believed, are responsible for a number of diseases and complaints (*see* page 844).	**Useful** as a short-term treatment attempt for addressing acute low back pain. Initial controlled clinical studies and case reports have shown that some patients with acute or chronic back pain may find at least partial relief from pain (*see* Placebo, page xxi).	**Requires a qualified practitioner** Practitioners should be properly qualified and should propose a treatment plan. **Risks:** Spinal manipulations can cause serious injury. Osteoporosis is one of several risk factors.

Treatment	Rating	Point of delivery/risks
Massage Classical massage (*see* page 847) can ease muscular and emotional tension; some techniques aim to induce counterirritation to obscure pain at least temporarily. Ice massage is said to ease the pain of a slipped disc.	**Useful** as a supportive treatment attempt aimed at providing relief from pain and improving general well-being. Case reports claim efficacy in the treatment of acute and chronic back pain; however, success is probably seen in only a proportion of patients (*see* Placebo, page xxi).	**Requires a qualified practitioner** or a sufficiently adept partner. Masseurs/masseuses should be properly qualified and should propose a treatment plan. **Risks:** Some people are sensitive to cold or manual stimuli; others find it hard to tolerate close physical contact.
Nutritional therapies An organic diet (*see* page 4) provides the body with essential and secondary plant nutrients that are believed to exercise a multitude of positive effects.	**May be of some use** as an individually directed general measure for dealing with recurrent and persistent problems, e.g. obesity.	**Suitable for DIY** Qualified guidance is recommended though not essential. **Risks:** Avoid imbalanced or intolerable diets. They can cause deficiencies with serious consequences. Children are at particular risk.
Physical therapies Hot packs and various forms of hydrotherapy (*see* page 871) are said to alleviate pain. Some forms of exercise therapy (*see* page 868) will improve posture. Warm packs (*see* page 878) are said to ease the pain of a slipped disc.	**Useful** as a treatment attempt and/or as a standard physical therapy. The effects of the various treatments can differ widely from one person to another. Case studies, case reports, and field studies claim efficacy; however, success is probably seen in only a proportion of patients (*see* Placebo, page xxi).	**Suitable for DIY** Qualified guidance is essential. Practitioners should be properly qualified and should propose a treatment plan. **Risks:** Skin damage may be caused to persons with diminished temperature sensation when extreme temperatures are applied.

Treatment	Rating	Point of delivery/risks
Probiotics The introduction of certain bacteria into the gut is claimed to bring the intestinal flora back into balance and to have a beneficial effect on other parts of the immune system (*see* page 878).	**Of little use** Possibly acceptable as a short-term treatment attempt for dealing with inflammation when more established methods have been unsuccessful. Some case reports claim efficacy; however, success is probably seen in only a proportion of patients (*see* Placebo, page xxi).	**Requires a qualified practitioner** Practitioners should be properly qualified and should propose a treatment plan. Non-prescription formulations are suitable for do-it-yourself. **Risks:** Fairly unlikely provided treatment is carried out competently.
Reflex therapies Reflex zone massage (*see* page 883), reflexology (*see* page 883), and TENS (*see* page 886) are said to act via so-called reflex channels (*see* page 881) to ease pain and relax the patient.	**Useful** as a short-term attempt to ease pain. Controlled clinical studies and numerous field studies ascribe a certain efficacy to these treatments in some patients (*see* Placebo, page xxi).	**Suitable for DIY** Qualified guidance is essential. **Risks:** Some people are sensitive to electrical or manual stimuli; others find it hard to tolerate close physical contact or rubber electrodes.
Relaxation techniques Autogenic training (*see* page 888), muscle relaxation according to Jacobson (*see* page 893), and various biofeedback techniques (*see* page 891) are said to relieve muscle tension and inner unrest, and might be instrumental in bringing relief from pain in the skeletomuscular system.	**Useful** as a short-term, supportive treatment attempt aimed at relaxing the patient. Clinical and field studies claim efficacy for these procedures in addressing pain in the skeletomuscular system; however, success is probably seen in only a proportion of patients (*see* Placebo, page xxi).	**Suitable for DIY** Once a sound understanding of the technique has been acquired from a trainer, patients can perform exercises themselves. Therapists should be properly qualified. **Risks:** Fairly unlikely.
Vitamins and trace elements The painkilling properties of vitamin B6 or (in the case of rheumatic pain) of vitamin E are thought to contribute to pain relief (*see* page 900).	**Of little use** There is no evidence of an unequivocal painkilling action. No definitive recommendations can be made based on present knowledge.	**Suitable for DIY** Qualified guidance is recommended though not essential. **Risks:** Intolerance and overdosage are possible. Vitamin B6 in high doses can have serious side effects.

Herbal remedies for back pain

Active ingredient/preparation	Rating
Cajeput oil (*Melaleuca leucadendron*)	Used externally, cajeput oil **may be of some use** as a treatment attempt for back problems and pain. It contains the rubefacient and skin-warming ingredient cineol. **Dosage:** Use externally as a 5 percent alcoholic solution. **Risks:** Be careful not to get the oil into the eyes, as it will cause them to sting painfully. Do not apply to the face and nostrils of infants. Not to be used in sensitive persons. Inhalation may lead to inflammation of the respiratory system. Extensive external use may lead to kidney problems and disorders of the central nervous system. Cajeput oil can irritate the mucous membranes and cause skin allergies.
Camphor (*Cinnamomum camphora*)	Camphor is **only useful** as a treatment attempt for back problems and pain (used locally in an alcoholic solution). It produces a cooling effect and stimulates blood flow. **Dosage:** To apply, spread on the palm of the hand and massage in. Use ready-formulated preparations as instructed by the manufacturer/prescriber. **Risks:** Camphor can cause contact eczema. Do not use on damaged skin. Do not apply to the nose or face of infants and young children (at risk of collapse).
Devil's claw (*Harpagophytum procumbens*)	Devil's claw **may be of some use** as a treatment attempt for degenerative diseases of the joints and muscular apparatus. It also has a slight painkilling effect. **Daily dose:** As an infusion, 4.5g of rhizome. **Individual dose:** Pour a cup of boiling water over 1.5g of dried rhizome, allow it to stand for eight hours, then heat again before drinking. **Risks:** Not to be used by persons with a gastric or duodenal ulcer; persons with gallstones should ask their doctor first. Not to be used during pregnancy on account of its presumed abortifacient and labor-inducing properties.

Active ingredient/preparation	Rating

Eucalyptus oil
(*Eucalyptus globulus*)

Only useful as an external treatment attempt for back problems and pain. Eucalyptus oil is a rubefacient which stimulates blood flow.
Dosage: To apply, rub in externally, 5–20 percent in oily formulations, 5–10 percent in alcoholic formulations. Use ready-formulated preparations as instructed by the manufacturer/prescriber.
Risks: Eucalyptus oil can cause skin allergies. Do not apply to the face and nose of infants and young children. Not to be used on sensitive persons. Inhalation may lead to inflammation of the respiratory system. Extensive external use may lead to kidney problems and disorders of the central nervous system.

Hayseeds
(*Graminis flos*)

Only useful as an attempted local heat treatment for back problems and pain. Hayseeds have a rubefacient effect and stimulate blood flow.
Dosage: Apply once or twice daily as a compress, 108 °F, leaving it in place for 40–50 minutes.
Risks: Do not use in acute episodes of rheumatic disease.

Horseradish root
(*Armoracia rusticana*)

Horseradish is **only useful** as an attempted external treatment for back problems and pain. It contains mustard oil.
Daily dose: 10g fresh root or preparations thereof with 2 percent mustard oil. To prepare, press fresh roots.
Risks: Horseradish may cause severe allergic reactions. Taken orally, it also tends to depress the function of the thyroid, so it should not be used when thyroid levels are low.

Active ingredient/preparation	*Rating*
Mistletoe (*Viscum album*)	**May be of some use** when attempted as an adjunct to other treatments for conditions affecting the joints, e.g. degenerative arthropathy. **Risks:** Shivering attacks, raised temperature (a slight rise is desirable for interferon induction), headaches, angina pectoris, circulatory disorders, allergic reactions. Do not use in protein allergy, chronic infection, or acute, highly febrile, inflammatory disease. **Caution:** The berries must not be used.
Mustard seeds for compresses (*Sinapis alba*)	**Only useful** as a treatment attempt for back problems and pain (in the form of warm compresses), problems with the locomotor system, chronic degenerative arthropathy (in the form of poultices), and rheumatism of the soft tissues. Acts as a skin and circulatory stimulant. **Dosage:** 4 dessertspoons of powdered mustard seeds as a watery paste (poultice). **Risks:** Protracted use at the same site may damage the nerves and skin. For external use only. Not to be used in children under six years or in persons with kidney disease (mustard oils are absorbed through the skin).
Paprika-containing poultices or ointments (*Capsicum frutescens*)	**Only useful** as a treatment attempt for back problems when used externally near the spine (in adults and children). Has a stimulating and warming effect on the skin. **Dosage:** As instructed by the manufacturer/prescriber. **Risks:** Mucosal irritation and hypersensitive reactions are possible. Not to be used on damaged skin or if the person suffers allergic reactions. Not to be used for longer than two days. Wait 14 days before using again. Sensitive nerves may be damaged if plasters are used at the same site for protracted periods.

Active ingredient/preparation	Rating
Pine needle oil (*Pinus pinaster*)	Rubbed in externally, pine needle oil is **useful** as a treatment attempt for back problems and pain. **Dosage:** Best used externally in a 10–50 percent concentration in liquid and semi-liquid formulations. Use ready-formulated preparations as instructed by the manufacturer/prescriber. **Risks:** Be careful not to get the oil into the eyes, as it will cause them to sting painfully. Do not apply to the face and nostrils of infants. Not to be used on sensitive persons. Inhalation may lead to inflammation of the respiratory system. Extensive external use may lead to kidney problems and disorders of the central nervous system. Pine needle oil can cause skin allergies.
Rosemary leaves and oil (*Rosmarinus officinalis*)	**Only useful** (rosemary oil) as an external treatment attempt for back problems and pain. Acts as a skin and circulatory stimulant. **Dosage:** For external use, apply a 10 percent oily preparation or, in a bathtub, use 2.0ml oil or 2oz rosemary leaves. Use ready-formulated preparations as instructed by the manufacturer/prescriber. **Risks:** Rosemary oil may provoke allergic skin reactions.

Gout

Causes and symptoms

Gout is a condition caused by a high level of uric acid in the blood or by the body's inefficiency in processing and removing uric acid. It occurs when crystals of uric acid are deposited in the lining of the joints, causing swelling, redness, and severe pain. Gout usually starts with just individual joints affected (the big toe, for instance), but can go on to affect other joints, such as the knuckles, knees, and elbows. The disease may become chronic unless suitable medication is given (e.g. allopurinol) to reduce the level of uric acid in the blood.

Orthodox treatment

Gout is mostly treated with drugs. Normally, an anti-inflammatory agent (a so-called non-steroidal antirheumatic) is prescribed for the acute phase, followed by a drug to reduce the level of uric acid in the blood and so prevent the buildup of crystallized uric acid.

Complementary therapies

Whether complementary treatments can address the causes of gout is debatable. However, certain remedies may be useful in alleviating symptoms. Colchicine, an alkaloid obtained from the meadow saffron, *Colchicum autumnale*, is used as a suppressant for gout in complementary as well as in mainstream medicine.

Treatment plan and limited trial

Before administering a complementary treatment, every therapist should propose a treatment plan (*see* page xxiii) that sets out a clear time frame and defines the goal that the treatment is designed to achieve. Treatment should then be tried for a limited term to test the patient's response.

Caution

Anyone seeking a complementary therapy as the sole treatment for the acute phase of gout must appreciate that pain relief will not be as effective and the pain may last longer than with an orthodox treatment.

Complementary treatments for gout

Treatment	Rating	Point of delivery/risks
Acupressure This treatment (*see* page 769), otherwise known as pressure-point massage, is used to reduce pain and ease tension. The pressure points chosen can vary from one practitioner to another.	**May be of some use** as a short-term treatment attempt aimed at reducing pain. Some case reports claim efficacy; however, success is probably seen in only a small proportion of patients (*see* Placebo, page xxi).	**Suitable for DIY** Qualified guidance is recommended. **Risks:** Unlikely provided treatment is carried out competently.
Acupuncture Acupuncture in its various forms (*see* page 772) aims to encourage the flow of energy (*see* page 927) or to act directly to ease pain and reduce inflammation.	**May be of some use** as a short-term, supportive treatment attempt aimed at alleviating pain. Some case reports claim efficacy; however, success is probably seen in only a proportion of patients (*see* Placebo, page xxi).	**Requires a qualified practitioner** Acupuncturists should be properly qualified and should propose a treatment plan. **Risks:** Probably rare provided treatment is carried out competently.
Anthroposophical medicine In AM (*see* page 781), gout is treated with a "constitutional therapy" that is supposed to support metabolism and encourage elimination.	**Of little use** Acceptable as a short-term, supportive treatment attempt for chronic symptoms. Case studies claim efficacy; however, success is probably seen in only a proportion of patients (*see* Placebo, page xxi).	**Requires a qualified practitioner** Practitioners should be properly qualified and should propose a treatment plan. **Risks:** Allergies or intolerance are possible.

Treatment	Rating	Point of delivery/risks

Aromatherapy
Essential oils (*see* page 786) are used to soothe and relax, or to invigorate, thereby improving general well-being. The essences may be taken orally, used externally as massage oils or bathing emulsions, or inhaled as vapors.

Of little use
Acceptable as a short-term, supportive treatment attempt aimed at soothing and relaxing. Some case reports claim efficacy; however, success is probably seen in only a proportion of patients (*see* Placebo, page xxi).

Suitable for DIY
Qualified guidance is recommended. The effects of individual essential oils differ widely.
Risks: Allergies or intolerance are possible. Some oils are carcinogenic in test systems and possibly in humans.

Bioresonance therapy
Bioresonance therapists use electrical devices in an attempt to discover the causes of illness and claim to be able to weaken or turn around pathogenic energies and disease related vibrations (*see* page 794).

Of little use
Possibly acceptable as a short-term, supportive treatment attempt for chronic and persistent complaints when simpler, more established methods have been unsuccessful. Some case reports claim efficacy; however, success is probably seen, if at all, in only a small proportion of patients (*see* Placebo, page xxi).

Requires a qualified practitioner
Practitioners should be properly qualified and should propose a treatment plan. No credence should be given to anyone promising immediate or total success.
Risks: Fairly unlikely.

Cell therapy
Injecting or ingesting products extracted from the tissues of newborn animals or animal fetuses is said to have a rejuvenating and revitalizing effect and to enhance the healing of human tissues and organs (*see* page 796).

Not advised
The efficacy and mode of action of these costly and relatively risky procedures remain unproven.

Risks: Injecting foreign proteins into the body can provoke (possibly fatal) allergic reactions. Also, pathogens such as those that cause bovine spongiform encephalopathy (BSE) or other serious infections may be introduced.

Treatment	*Rating*	*Point of delivery/risks*
Electroneural therapy according to Croon According to the theory, readings taken at various reactive sites on the skin highlight diseased areas within the body. Based on these readings, electrostimulative treatment can be carried out to ease gout (*see* page 806).	**Of little use** Possibly acceptable as a short-term, supportive treatment attempt at addressing chronic and persistent complaints when simpler, more established methods have been unsuccessful. Some case reports claim efficacy; however, success is probably seen, if at all, in only a small proportion of patients (*see* Placebo, page xxi).	**Requires a qualified practitioner** Practitioners should be properly qualified and should propose a treatment plan. No credence should be given to anyone promising immediate or total success. **Risks:** Proponents themselves warn that treatment should not be given in acute inflammatory conditions.
Eliminative methods, bloody Gout is occasionally treated with leeches (*see* page 822), bloodletting (*see* page 810), or bloody cupping (*see* page 815). These treatments are generally for improving the patient's outlook rather than addressing pain directly.	**Of little use** Possibly acceptable as a short-term, supportive treatment attempt for persistent symptoms when less invasive, more established methods have been unsuccessful. Some case reports claim efficacy; however, success is probably seen in only a proportion of patients (*see* Placebo, page xxi).	**Requires a qualified practitioner** Practitioners should be properly qualified and should propose a treatment plan. No credence should be given to anyone promising immediate or total success. **Risks:** Bloody cupping can cause infection and scarring. Furthermore, it should not be carried out in persons with bleeding disorders.
Eliminative methods, unbloody Gout is sometimes treated with sweating (*see* page 877) or colonic irrigation (*see* page 819) to improve the body's own regulatory systems, or by unbloody cupping (*see* page 817) to ease pain and improve the body's own regulatory systems.	**Of little use** Acceptable as a short-term, supportive treatment attempt. Some case reports claim efficacy; however, success is probably seen in only a proportion of patients (*see* Placebo, page xxi).	**Suitable for DIY** Unbloody cupping is best carried out under the guidance of a qualified practitioner. **Risks:** Unlikely provided treatment is carried out competently.

Treatment	Rating	Point of delivery/risks
Enzyme therapy The enzymes used reportedly dispel and destroy "immune complexes" that course in the blood and are responsible, for instance, for sustaining inflammatory processes such as those in arthrosis or soft-tissue rheumatism (*see* page 824).	**Of little use** Some case reports claim efficacy for this little researched therapy; however, success is probably seen in only a small proportion of patients (*see* Placebo, page xxi).	**Requires a qualified practitioner** Practitioners should propose a treatment plan. Non-prescription formulations are suitable for do-it-yourself. **Risks:** Allergies or intolerance are possible.
Flower remedies Flower remedies (*see* page 828) are said to restore emotional balance and assist the body's psychic ability to heal itself.	**Of little use** Acceptable as a short-term, supportive treatment attempt aimed at soothing and relaxing. Some case reports claim efficacy; however, success is probably seen in only a small proportion of patients (*see* Placebo, page xxi).	**Suitable for DIY** Qualified guidance is recommended. Practitioners should propose a treatment plan. **Risks:** Possible intolerance.
Homeopathy Highly diluted (potentized) solutions (*see* page 831) are believed to be able to redress vital energy imbalances. Organo- and functiotropic (*see* page 833) homeopathy is claimed to be effective in the treatment of gout.	**Of little use** Possibly acceptable as a short-term, supportive treatment attempt for chronic gout. Some case reports claim success for homeopathic treatments; however, success is probably seen in only a small proportion of patients (*see* Placebo, page xxi).	**Requires a qualified practitioner** Homeopaths should be properly qualified and should propose a treatment plan. Ready-formulated preparations are suitable for do-it-yourself. **Risks:** Allergies and intolerance are possible.

Treatment	Rating	Point of delivery/risks
Massage Classical massage (*see* page 847) can invigorate the patient and ease muscular and emotional tension.	**May be of some use** as a supportive measure aimed at easing pain and improving general well-being. Case reports claim efficacy; however, success is probably seen in only a proportion of patients (*see* Placebo, page xxi).	**Requires a qualified practitioner** Masseurs/masseuses should be properly qualified and should propose a treatment plan. **Risks:** Some people are sensitive to manual stimuli; others find it hard to tolerate close physical contact.
Nutritional therapies An organic diet (*see* page 4) provides the body with essential and secondary plant nutrients that are believed to exercise a multitude of positive effects and to be capable, *inter alia*, of strengthening the immune system.	**Useful** as an individually directed supportive measure. Avoiding certain foods may assist in preventing relapses.	**Suitable for DIY** Qualified guidance is recommended though not essential. **Risks:** Avoid imbalanced or intolerable diets. They can cause deficiencies with serious consequences. Children are at particular risk.
Physical therapies Cold treatments (*see* pages 871–8) for acute gout and various therapeutic techniques and Kneipp treatments (*see* page 871) for chronic gout are said to ease pain and encourage the metabolism. Saunas are sometimes used to improve the body's own regulatory systems.	**Useful** as a short-term treatment attempt aimed at alleviating pain. Case reports and field studies claim efficacy; however, success is probably seen in only a proportion of patients (*see* Placebo, page xxi). Saunas are **of little use**, but are acceptable as a short-term supportive treatment attempt.	**Suitable for DIY** Qualified guidance is recommended. Practitioners should be properly qualified and should propose a treatment plan. **Risks:** Skin damage may be caused to persons with diminished temperature sensation when extreme temperatures are applied.

Treatment	Rating	Point of delivery/risks
Reflex therapies Reflexology (*see* page 883) and TENS (*see* page 886) are thought to be good for easing pain and inflammation and relaxing the patient.	**May be of some use** as a short-term treatment attempt aimed at alleviating pain. Some case reports claim efficacy; however, success is probably seen in only a proportion of patients (*see* Placebo, page xxi).	**Suitable for DIY** Qualified guidance is essential. Practitioners should propose a treatment plan. **Risks:** Some people are sensitive to electrical or manual stimuli and rubber electrodes; others find it hard to tolerate close physical contact.

Herbal remedies for gout

There are no recommended herbal remedies for use in this indication.

Muscle soreness

Causes and symptoms

Muscle soreness is usually the painful result of unaccustomed muscular activity. The precise mechanism is not fully understood but may be due to minor muscular tears or the buildup of lactic acid in the muscle tissue. In severe cases the sufferer may barely be able to move.

The condition improves spontaneously after a day or two.

Orthodox treatment

Various physical treatments are recommended to alleviate the pain: for example, a warm bath or contrast baths followed by limbering-up exercises. A painkiller (*see* page 24) may be prescribed if pain is intense.

Complementary therapies

Several complementary treatments for aching muscles are claimed to work, including ones that act directly on the site of the pain and others that provide pain relief through potentiated or non-potentiated drugs.

Caution

Muscle soreness improves spontaneously. There is not usually any need for ambitious complementary treatments.

Complementary treatments for muscle soreness

Treatment	Rating	Point of delivery/risks
Acupuncture Acupuncture in its various forms (*see* page 772) is used to ease severe muscle pain. The acupuncture points chosen can vary from one practitioner to another.	**Of little use** Some case reports claim efficacy for this relatively involved procedure; however, success is probably seen in only a proportion of patients (*see* Placebo, page xxi).	**Requires a qualified practitioner** Practitioners should be properly qualified and should propose a treatment plan. **Risks:** Probably rare provided treatment is carried out competently.
Flower remedies Bach Rescue Remedy (*see* page 829) is reported to ease muscle pain.	**Of little use** Acceptable as a treatment attempt aimed at relaxing the patient. Some case reports claim efficacy; however, success is probably seen in only a proportion of patients (*see* Placebo, page xxi).	**Suitable for DIY** Qualified guidance is recommended. **Risks:** Possible intolerance.

Treatment	Rating	Point of delivery/risks
Homeopathy The highly diluted (potentized) solutions (see page 831) that are used in organo- and functiotropic (*see* page 833) homeopathy are claimed to ease muscle pain.	**Of little use** Acceptable as a treatment attempt. The majority of controlled trials refutes the notion that homeopathy is helpful. Success is probably seen in only a small proportion of patients (*see* Placebo, page xxi).	**Suitable for DIY** **Risks:** Allergies and intolerance are possible.
Massage Local massage (*see* page 847) is claimed to improve the circulation and ease muscle pain.	**May be of some use** as a treatment attempt. Case reports and field studies claim efficacy; however, success is probably seen in only a proportion of patients (*see* Placebo, page xxi).	**Suitable for DIY** Qualified guidance is recommended. **Risks:** Unlikely provided treatment is carried out competently.
Physical therapies Heat treatments (*see* pages 871–8), hot baths and showers, loosening-up or stretching exercises, especially when muscle soreness first appears, are claimed to prevent and ease pain.	**Useful** as a treatment attempt. Some case reports and field studies claim efficacy; however, success is probably seen in only a proportion of patients (*see* Placebo, page xxi).	**Suitable for DIY** **Risks:** Skin damage may be caused to persons with diminished temperature sensation when extreme temperatures are applied.
Reflex therapies Various techniques such as reflex zone massage (*see* page 883) and TENS (*see* page 886) are claimed to act via reflex channels (*see* page 881) to ease pain and tense muscles.	**May be of some use** as a treatment attempt. Some case reports claim efficacy; however, success is probably seen in only a proportion of patients (*see* Placebo, page xxi).	**Suitable for DIY** **Risks:** Fairly unlikely provided treatment is carried out competently. Some people are sensitive to electrodes.

Treatment	Rating	Point of delivery/risks
Vitamins and trace elements Vitamin and electrolyte cocktails are claimed to ease muscle pain (*see* page 900).	**Of little use** Based on present knowledge, no definitive recommendations can be given. Case reports claim efficacy; however, success is probably seen in only a proportion of patients (*see* Placebo, page xxi).	**Suitable for DIY** Qualified guidance is recommended though not essential. **Risks:** Intolerance and overdosage are possible. Vitamin B6 in high doses can cause serious side effects. Recent findings imply that beta-carotene and vitamin A might increase the risk of cancer.

Herbal remedies for muscle soreness

Active ingredient/preparation	Rating
Cajeput oil (*Melaleuca leucadendron*)	Used externally, cajeput oil **may be of some use** as a treatment attempt for muscular aches and pains. It contains the rubefacient and skin-warming ingredient cineol. **Dosage:** Use externally as a 5 percent alcoholic solution. **Risks:** Be careful not to get the oil into the eyes, as it will cause them to sting painfully. Do not apply to the face and nostrils of infants. Not to be used on sensitive persons. Inhalation may lead to inflammation of the respiratory system. Extensive external use may lead to kidney problems and disorders of the central nervous system. Cajeput oil can irritate the mucous membranes and cause skin allergies.

Active ingredient/preparation	*Rating*
Camphor (*Cinnamomum camphora*)	Camphor is **only useful** as an external treatment attempt for muscular pain. It has a painkilling and locally anesthetizing effect on the skin. **Dosage:** To apply, rub in externally. Use ready-formulated preparations as instructed by the manufacturer/prescriber. **Risks:** Camphor can cause contact eczema. Do not use on damaged skin. Do not apply to the nose and face of young children as it may cause collapse.
Carmelite water (spirit of melissa) (*Spiritus melissae*)	**May be of some use** when used as an external treatment attempt for muscular aches and pains. **Risks:** Used externally, spirit of melissa is not known to have any serious side effects.
Devil's claw (*Harpagophytum procumbens*)	Devil's claw **may be of some use** as a treatment attempt for degenerative diseases of the joints and muscular apparatus. It also has a slight painkilling effect. **Daily dose:** As an infusion, 4.5g of rhizome. **Individual dose:** pour a cup of boiling water over 1.5g of dried rhizome, allow it to stand for eight hours, then heat again before drinking. Use ready-formulated preparations as instructed by the manufacturer/prescriber. **Risks:** Not to be used by persons with a gastric or duodenal ulcer; persons with gall stones should ask their doctor first. Not to be used during pregnancy on account of its presumed abortifacient and labor-inducing properties.

Active ingredient/preparation	Rating

Eucalyptus oil
(*Eucalyptus globulus*)

Only useful as an external treatment attempt for muscular aches and pains. Eucalyptus oil is a local skin stimulant.
Dosage: To apply, rub in externally, 5–20 percent in oily formulations, 5–10 percent in alcoholic formulations. Use ready-formulated preparations as instructed by the manufacturer/prescriber.
Risks: Eucalyptus oil can cause skin allergies. Do not apply to the face and nose of infants and young children. Not to be used on sensitive persons. Inhalation may lead to inflammation of the respiratory system. Extensive external use may lead to kidney problems and disorders of the central nervous system.

Fir needle oil
(*Abies sibirica*)

Fir needle oil is **only useful** as an external treatment attempt for muscular aches and pains. It produces a warm sensation on the skin and stimulates blood flow.
Dosage: To apply, rub in externally in a 10–50 percent concentration. Use ready-formulated preparations as instructed by the manufacturer/prescriber.
Risks: Be careful not to get the oil into the eyes, as it will cause them to sting painfully. This oil may irritate the mucous membranes if incorrectly used; because of this irritant effect, it must not be used by persons with asthma or whooping cough.

Hayseeds
(*Graminis flos*)

Only useful as an attempted local heat treatment for muscular aches and pains. Hayseeds have a rubefacient effect and stimulate blood flow.
Dosage: Apply once or twice daily as a compress, 108 °F, leaving it in place for 40–50 minutes.
Risks: Do not use in acute episodes of rheumatic disease.

Active ingredient/preparation	*Rating*
Horseradish root (*Armoracia rusticana*)	Horseradish is **only useful** as an external treatment attempt for muscular aches and pains. It contains mustard oil. **Daily dose:** 10g fresh root or preparations thereof with 2 percent mustard oil. **Risks:** Horseradish may cause allergic skin reactions. Taken orally, it also tends to depress the function of the thyroid, so it should not be used when thyroid levels are low.
Mustard seeds for compresses (*Sinapis alba*)	**Only useful** as an external treatment attempt for pain in the joints and muscular apparatus (in the form of poultices). Acts as a skin and circulatory stimulant. **Dosage:** 4 dessertspoons of powdered mustard seeds as a watery paste (poultice). **Risks:** Protracted use at the same site may damage the nerves and skin. For external use only. Not to be used on children under six years or on persons with kidney disease (mustard oils are absorbed through the skin).
Paprika-containing poultices or ointments (*Capsicum frutescens*)	**Only useful** as an external treatment attempt for painful joints and muscular aches and pains, e.g. in shoulder–arm syndrome, for use near the spine (in adults and children of school age). Apply to the painful area. Has a stimulating and warming effect on the skin. **Dosage:** As instructed by the manufacturer/prescriber. **Risks:** Mucosal irritation and hypersensitive reactions are possible. Not to be used on damaged skin or if the person suffers allergic reactions. Not to be used for longer than two days. Wait 14 days before using it again. Sensitive nerves may be damaged if plasters are used on the same site for protracted periods.

Active ingredient/preparation	*Rating*
Pine needle oil (*Pinus pinaster*)	Pine needle oil is **only useful** as a treatment attempt for muscular aches and pains. It has a warming effect and stimulates blood flow. **Dosage:** To apply, massage in a 10–50 percent concentration. Use ready-formulated preparations as instructed by the manufacturer/prescriber. **Risks:** Be careful not to get the oil into the eyes, as it will cause them to sting painfully. Do not apply to the face and nostrils of infants. Not to be used on sensitive persons. Inhalation may lead to inflammation of the respiratory system. Extensive external use may lead to kidney problems and disorders of the central nervous system. Pine needle oil can cause skin allergies.
Rosemary leaves and oil (*Rosmarinus officinalis*)	**Only useful** (rosemary oil) as an external treatment attempt for muscular aches and pains. Stimulates the skin and promotes blood flow. **Dosage:** Apply a 10 percent oily preparation externally or, in a bathtub, use 2.0ml oil or 2oz rosemary leaves. Use ready-formulated preparations as instructed by the manufacturer/prescriber. **Risks:** Rosemary oil may provoke allergic skin reactions.
Willow bark (*Salix fragilis*)	Taken orally, willow bark **may be of some use** as a treatment attempt for muscular pain. Willow bark is a febrifuge, analgesic and anti-inflammatory agent. **Individual dose:** 2.0g willow bark contains about 20mg total salicin. Use ready-formulated preparations as instructed by the manufacturer/prescriber. **Daily dose:** 60–120mg total salicin. **Risks:** Skin allergies, asthmatic symptoms (bronchospasm), and gastrointestinal complaints may occur in persons sensitive to aspirin or other salicylates.

Osteoporosis (brittle bone disease)

Causes and symptoms

Osteoporosis (brittle bones) is a condition that occurs when bone density is reduced owing to loss of calcium and other minerals. Rarefication of bone tissue is confirmed when two bone density measurements taken on the same bone three months apart using the same measuring equipment show a difference of more than 3.5 percent.

Osteoporosis progresses swiftly; even when still in their sixties, sufferers may present with pain and restricted movement. The bones become porous and brittle and are unable to regenerate themselves. The condition is more common in women than in men. The onset is gradual and symptom-free. Severe back pain may be the first sign of a weakened spine, when the vertebrae collapse through softening of the bone, culminating in curvature of the spine (dowager's hump).

Several factors contribute to the disease, including diet. A calcium-rich diet that includes plenty of dairy products encourages the growth of strong bones. Another factor is exercise (or rather lack of it). People with a healthy diet who take lots of exercise in the fresh air have a lower risk of developing osteoporosis.

Orthodox treatment

Dietary supplements of calcium, magnesium, and vitamin D are useful in warding off and treating the disease. Regular exercise is suggested as a preventive measure. If there is a strong family history of osteoporosis, or the patient's childhood diet was deficient in calcium and other minerals, or if bone density measurements suggest that bone demineralization has already occurred, then treatment with a calcium-retaining hormone will usually be advised.

Complementary therapies

Certain complementary treatments (such as reflexology) focus on pain relief. Complementary therapists sometimes regard osteoporosis as being caused by toxins (*see* page 929), foci (*see* page 928), or a poor energy balance (*see* page 927), and aim to restore a normal body situation.

Treatment plan and limited trial

Before administering a complementary treatment, every therapist should propose a treatment plan (*see* page xxiii) that sets out a clear time frame and defines the goal that the treatment is designed to achieve. Treatment should then be tried for a limited term to test the patient's response.

Cautions

There is no evidence that any complementary procedure is an appropriate substitute for modern mainstream diagnosis and therapy. Complementary treatments have at most a supportive function: for example, as a means of providing pain relief.

Complementary treatments for osteoporosis

Treatment	Rating	Point of delivery/risks
Acupressure This treatment (*see* page 769), otherwise known as pressure-point massage, is used to ease pain and alleviate tension. The pressure points chosen may differ from one practitioner to another.	**Inappropriate** as the sole treatment for advanced osteoporosis. **May be of some use** as a short-term, supportive treatment attempt aimed at alleviating pain. Case reports and field studies claim efficacy; however, success is probably seen in only a small proportion of patients (*see* Placebo, page xxi).	**Requires a qualified practitioner** Therapists should be properly qualified and should propose a treatment plan. **Risks:** Unlikely provided treatment is carried out competently.

Treatment	Rating	Point of delivery/risks
Acupuncture Acupuncture in its various forms (*see* page 772) is used to ease painful bones and relieve tension. The acupuncture points chosen can vary from one practitioner to another.	**Inappropriate** as the sole treatment for advanced osteoporosis. **May be of some use** as a short-term, supportive treatment attempt aimed at alleviating pain. Case reports and field studies claim efficacy; however, success is probably seen in only a proportion of patients (*see* Placebo, page xxi).	**Requires a qualified practitioner** Acupuncturists should be properly qualified and should propose a treatment plan. **Risks:** Probably rare provided treatment is carried out competently.
Aromatherapy Essential oils (*see* page 786) are used to soothe and relax, or to invigorate, so contributing to an improvement in general well-being. The essences may be taken orally, used externally as massage oils or bathing emulsions, or inhaled as vapors.	**Inappropriate** as the sole treatment for advanced osteoporosis. **May be of some use** as a short-term, supportive treatment attempt when the patient perceives the treatment as being soothing and relaxing.	**Suitable for DIY** Qualified guidance is recommended. The effects of individual essential oils differ widely. Therapists should propose a treatment plan. **Risks:** Allergies or intolerance are possible. Some oils are carcinogenic in test systems and possibly in humans.
Bioresonance therapy Bioresonance therapists use electrical devices in an attempt to discover the causes of illness and claim to be able to weaken or turn around pathogenic energies and disease related vibrations (*see* page 794).	**Of little use** Possibly acceptable as a short-term, supportive treatment attempt when simpler, more established methods have been unsuccessful. Some case reports claim efficacy; however, success is probably seen, if at all, in only a small proportion of patients (*see* Placebo, page xxi).	**Requires a qualified practitioner** Practitioners should be properly qualified and should propose a treatment plan. No credence should be given to anyone promising immediate or total success. **Risks:** Fairly unlikely.

Treatment	Rating	Point of delivery/risks
Cell therapy Injecting or ingesting products extracted from the tissues of newborn animals or animal fetuses is said to have a rejuvenating and revitalizing effect and to enhance the healing of human tissues and organs (*see* page 796).	**Not advised** Based on present knowledge, there is inadequate evidence of the efficacy and mode of action of these costly and relatively risky procedures.	**Risks:** Injecting foreign proteins into the body can provoke (possibly fatal) allergic reactions. Also, pathogens such as those that cause bovine spongiform encephalopathy (BSE) or other serious infections may be introduced.
Electroacupuncture according to Voll By taking readings of the electrical conductivity of the skin (*see* page 802), therapists claim to be able to derive an insight into diseased areas of the body, pathogenic foci (*see* page 928), and stress factors (*see* Toxins, page 929). The factors supposedly responsible for osteoporosis can then be addressed.	**Of little use** Possibly acceptable as a short-term, supportive treatment attempt when simpler, more established methods have been unsuccessful. Some case reports claim efficacy; however, success is probably seen, if at all, in only a small proportion of patients (*see* Placebo, page xxi).	**Requires a qualified practitioner** Practitioners should be properly qualified and should propose a treatment plan. No credence should be given to anyone promising immediate or total success. **Risks:** A second opinion must always be obtained from a qualified physician before any attempt is made to "eliminate foci" (e.g. by surgery).
Electroneural therapy according to Croon According to the theory, readings taken at various reactive sites on the skin highlight diseased areas within the body. Based on these readings, targeted electrostimulative measures can be undertaken to address the factors underlying osteoporosis (*see* page 806).	**Of little use** Possibly acceptable as a short-term treatment attempt for severe anxiety and unrest when simpler, more established methods have been unsuccessful. Some case reports claim efficacy; however, success is probably seen, if at all, in only a small proportion of patients (*see* Placebo, page xxi).	**Requires a qualified practitioner** Practitioners should be properly qualified and should propose a treatment plan. No credence should be given to anyone promising immediate or total success. **Risks:** Proponents themselves warn that treatment should not be given in acute inflammatory conditions.

Treatment	Rating	Point of delivery/risks
Eliminative methods, unbloody Unbloody cupping (*see* page 817) is claimed to ease pain in patients with osteoporosis, improve the body's own regulatory systems, and influence the metabolic processes.	**Inappropriate** as the sole treatment for advanced osteoporosis. **Of little use** as a short-term, supportive treatment attempt aimed at alleviating pain. Case reports claim efficacy; however, success is probably seen in only a proportion of patients (*see* Placebo, page xxi).	**Suitable for DIY** Qualified guidance is recommended. **Risks:** Unlikely provided treatment is carried out competently.
Flower remedies Flower remedies (*see* page 828) are said to restore emotional balance and assist the body's psychic ability to heal itself.	**Inappropriate** as the sole treatment for advanced osteoporosis. **May be of some use** as a short-term, supportive treatment attempt aimed at soothing and relaxing the patient. Case reports claim efficacy; however, success is probably seen in only a proportion of patients (*see* Placebo, page xxi).	**Suitable for DIY** Qualified guidance is recommended. Practitioners should propose a treatment plan. **Risks:** Possible intolerance.
Homeopathy Highly diluted (potentized) solutions (*see* page 831) are believed to be able to redress vital energy imbalances. Organo- and functiotropic (*see* page 833) homeopathy is claimed to be effective for dealing with the symptoms of osteoporosis.	**Inappropriate** as the sole treatment for advanced osteoporosis. **May be of some use** as a short-term, supportive treatment attempt. Case reports claim success for homeopathic treatments; however, success is probably seen in only a proportion of patients (*see* Placebo, page xxi).	**Requires a qualified practitioner** Homeopaths should be properly qualified and should propose a treatment plan. Ready-formulated preparations are suitable for do-it-yourself. **Risks:** Allergies and intolerance are possible.

Treatment	Rating	Point of delivery/risks
Magnetic field therapy The use of magnetic field generators, magnetic strips, bracelets, and other objects (*see* page 841) allegedly encourages cell metabolism.	**Of little use** Based on present knowledge, there is inadequate evidence of the efficacy and mode of action of magnetic field therapy in osteoporosis.	Operation of magnetic field equipment **requires a qualified practitioner**. **Risks:** Magnetic field equipment can cause implanted cardiac pacemakers to malfunction.
Manual therapies Chiropractors and osteopaths use a series of manipulations to realign allegedly displaced vertebrae in an attempt to ease pain (*see* page 844).	**Inappropriate** for the treatment of advanced osteoporosis on account of the high risk of injury and complications.	**Risks:** Osteoporosis increases the risk of injury through manual therapies.
Massage Classical massage (*see* page 847) is said to invigorate the patient and to ease muscular and emotional tension.	**Inappropriate** as the sole treatment for advanced osteoporosis. **Useful** as a short-term, supportive treatment attempt aimed at relaxing the patient and improving general well-being.	**Requires a qualified practitioner** Masseurs/masseuses should be properly qualified and should propose a treatment plan. **Risks:** Only light massage should be applied to areas affected by osteoporosis.
Nutritional therapies An organic diet (*see* page 4) provides the body with essential and secondary nutrients. An adequate supply of vitamin D, fluoride, calcium, and magnesium should be guaranteed; intake of phosphates should be reduced.	**Inappropriate** as the sole treatment for advanced osteoporosis. **Useful** as a preventive and supportive measure. Controlled clinical studies ascribe a degree of efficacy to nutritional therapies in the prevention and treatment of osteoporosis.	**Suitable for DIY** Qualified guidance is recommended though not essential. Sugar, alcohol, and nicotine should be avoided. **Risks:** Avoid imbalanced or intolerable diets. They can cause deficiencies with serious consequences. Children are particularly at risk.

Treatment	Rating	Point of delivery/risks
Physical therapies Exercise therapy (*see* page 868) and regular bone strengthening exercises are claimed to be effective in the prevention of osteoporosis and in slowing down or reversing the condition. Bathing, wraps, and heat treatments (*see* pages 871–8) are claimed to alleviate pain and improve the circulation.	**Useful** as a treatment attempt. Regular exercise and bone strengthening measures may prevent or slow down progression of the disease. Controlled trials and field studies ascribe a certain efficacy to this procedure. Bathing, wraps, and heat treatments may be beneficial when used supportively.	**Suitable for DIY** An individual plan of treatment should be defined in association with the treating physician. **Risks:** Exercise programs must be individually tailored so as not to put excessive demands on the patient or put him/her at risk of injury.
Reflex therapies Reflex zone massage (*see* page 883), reflexology (*see* page 883), and TENS (*see* page 886) are claimed to act via reflex channels (*see* page 881) to alleviate pain.	**Inappropriate** as the sole treatment for advanced osteoporosis. **May be of some use** as a short-term, supportive treatment attempt aimed at alleviating pain. Case reports claim efficacy; however, success is probably seen in only a proportion of patients (*see* Placebo, page xxi).	**Suitable for DIY** Qualified guidance is essential. **Risks:** Some people are sensitive to electrical stimuli and rubber electrodes; others find it hard to tolerate manual stimulation or close physical contact. Only light massage should be applied to regions affected by osteoporosis.
Relaxation techniques Autogenic training (*see* page 888), muscle relaxation according to Jacobson (*see* page 893), and various biofeedback techniques (*see* page 891) are said to relieve muscle tension and inner unrest, and thus may be instrumental in helping the patient become more aware of his/her physical and emotional states.	**Inappropriate** as the sole treatment for advanced osteoporosis. **May be of some use** as a short-term, supportive treatment attempt aimed at alleviating pain and improving general well-being. Case reports claim efficacy; however, success is probably seen in only a proportion of patients (*see* Placebo, page xxi).	**Suitable for DIY** Once a sound understanding of the technique has been acquired from a trainer, patients can perform exercises themselves. Therapists should be properly qualified. **Risks:** Fairly unlikely.

Treatment	Rating	Point of delivery/risks

Vitamins and trace elements
(*see* Nutritional therapies, page 200)

Herbal remedies for osteoporosis

Active ingredient/preparation	Rating
Black cohosh (*Cimicifuga racemosa*)	**Of little use** as a hormone-free alternative to estrogen replacement therapy. Black cohosh has estrogenic effects. **Dosage:** As instructed by the manufacturer/prescriber. **Risks:** Black cohosh may increase menstrual blood loss as well as cause intermediate or perpetual bleeding. Not to be used by persons with tumors (e.g. many forms of breast cancer) described as estrogen-binding. Black cohosh is potentially dangerous in high doses. It must not be used during pregnancy.
Willow bark (*Salix fragilis*)	**May be of some use** as a treatment attempt for osteoporosis when the aim is to alleviate pain. **Individual dose:** 2.0g willow bark contains about 20mg total salicin. Use ready-formulated preparations as instructed by the manufacturer/prescriber. **Daily dose:** 60–120mg total salicin. **Risks:** Skin allergies, asthmatic symptoms (bronchospasm), and gastrointestinal complaints may occur in persons sensitive to aspirin and other salicylates.

Rheumatism

Causes and symptoms

"Rheumatism" denotes any of a variety of disorders affecting the joints and/or connective tissue structures. The two most common rheumatic disorders are osteoarthritis and rheumatoid arthritis, though other inflammatory or degenerative diseases also fall under the general umbrella: rheumatic fever, chronic arthritis, muscular rheumatism, and arthrosis. Typical rheumatic symptoms are joint pain, stiffness, and swelling. In osteoarthritis (basically the result of "wear and tear"), the spinal and other weight-bearing joints are often affected. Rheumatoid arthritis is a systemic inflammatory disease that can affect not only the joints but other structures too. The causation of rheumatoid arthritis is not fully understood. Sufferers should consult their doctor, who will propose a treatment designed to alleviate pain and stop the disease from progressing.

Joining a support group may be beneficial.

Orthodox treatment

The treatments that doctors usually suggest for rheumatic disorders include some of the procedures used in complementary medicine, notably physical treatments such as physiotherapy, hydrotherapy, etc.

Patients who do not respond to simple painkillers may be given non-steroidal antirheumatics. As these preparations differ widely in effect from one patient to another, there may be a need to try out several before a suitable one is found. As many as four in ten patients receiving non-steroidal anti-inflammatories complain of side effects and, in some cases, of permanent damage. Side effects include stomach and bowel problems (perforated ulcer in extreme cases), kidney damage (occasionally renal failure), skin disorders, and liver damage. Cortisone is often prescribed and, in severe rheumatoid arthritis, gold injections or methotrexate may be appropriate. Doctors disagree, however, about the point at which this type of treatment becomes appropriate. Surgery to remove the synovial membrane is now an option, as is replacement hip and knee surgery.

Complementary therapies

Complementary therapies concentrate on the relief of pain, either directly or through relaxation and stress reduction. Some therapists also claim to be able to treat the cause of the problem, e.g. with diets.

Treatment plan and limited trial

Before administering a complementary treatment, every therapist should propose a treatment plan (*see* page xxiii) that sets out a clear time frame and defines the goal that the treatment is designed to achieve. Treatment should then be tried for a limited term to test the patient's response.

Cautions

Before any treatment is attempted for persistent or recurrent pain, a doctor must be consulted for a thorough medical examination. Most nonorthodox procedures are more appropriately used in a supportive role than as the sole treatment. None can cure rheumatism.

Complementary treatments for rheumatism

Treatment	Rating	Point of delivery/risks
Acupressure This treatment (*see* page 769), otherwise known as pressure-point massage, is claimed to ease tension and alleviate pain. The pressure points chosen may differ from one practitioner to another.	**Of little use** as the sole treatment for advanced rheumatism. **May be of some use** as a short-term treatment attempt aimed at easing pain. Case reports and field studies claim efficacy; however, success is probably seen in only a proportion of patients (*see* Placebo, page xxi).	**Suitable for DIY** Qualified guidance is essential. Therapists should propose a treatment plan. **Risks:** Unlikely provided treatment is carried out competently.
Acupuncture Acupuncture in its various forms (*see* page 772) aims to encourage the flow of energy (*see* page 927) or to act directly to ease rheumatic pain and tension. The acupuncture points chosen can vary from one practitioner to another.	**Inappropriate** as the sole treatment for advanced rheumatism. **May be of some use** as a short-term treatment attempt aimed at alleviating pain. Controlled clinical studies and case reports ascribe a degree of efficacy to this treatment; however, success is probably seen in only a proportion of patients (*see* Placebo, page xxi).	**Requires a qualified practitioner** Acupuncturists should be properly qualified and should propose a treatment plan. **Risks:** Probably rare provided treatment is carried out competently.

Treatment	Rating	Point of delivery/risks
Anthroposophical medicine Substances deposited as a result of hardening tendencies in the nerve–sense system are said to be removed through the use of specific preparations, rhythmic massage, hydrotherapy, ointments, or embrocations (*see* page 781).	**Inappropriate** as the sole treatment for advanced rheumatism. **May be of some use** as a short-term treatment attempt. Case reports claim efficacy; however, success is probably seen in only a proportion of patients (*see* Placebo, page xxi).	**Requires a qualified practitioner** Practitioners should be properly qualified and should propose a treatment plan. Ointments and embrocations are suitable for DIY. **Risks:** Allergies and intolerance are possible.
Aromatherapy Essential oils (*see* page 786) are used to soothe and relax, thereby helping to ease rheumatic pain. The essences may be taken orally, used externally as massage oils or bathing emulsions, or inhaled as vapors.	**Inappropriate** as the sole treatment for advanced rheumatism. **May be of some use** as a short-term, supportive treatment attempt aimed at soothing and relaxing. Some case reports claim efficacy; however, success is probably seen in only a small proportion of patients (*see* Placebo, page xxi).	**Suitable for DIY** Qualified guidance is recommended. Therapists should propose a treatment plan. The effects of individual essential oils differ widely. No credence should be given to anyone promising immediate or total success. **Risks:** Allergies or intolerance are possible. Some oils are carcinogenic in test systems and possibly in humans.
Bioresonance therapy Bioresonance therapists use electrical devices in an attempt to discover the causes of illness and claim to be able to weaken or turn around pathogenic energies and disease related vibrations (*see* page 794).	**Inappropriate** as the sole treatment for advanced rheumatism. Possibly acceptable as a short-term treatment attempt for persistent or recurrent symptoms when simpler, more established methods have been unsuccessful. Some case reports claim efficacy; however, success is probably seen, if at all, in only a small proportion of patients (*see* Placebo, page xxi).	**Requires a qualified practitioner** Practitioners should be properly qualified and should propose a treatment plan. No credence should be given to anyone promising immediate or total success. **Risks:** Fairly unlikely.

Treatment	Rating	Point of delivery/risks
Cell therapy Injecting or ingesting products extracted from animal tissues or organs is said to have an immune system modulating effect (*see* page 10) and to enhance the healing of human tissues and organs (*see* page 796). Products extracted from cartilage or joint structures are sometimes administered as a treatment for rheumatism.	**Inappropriate** as the sole treatment for advanced rheumatism. Fresh cell therapy is **not advised**. Organ extracts are acceptable at most as a short-term treatment attempt for persistent or recurrent symptoms when less risky, more established treatments have been unsuccessful. Some reports and studies ascribe a degree of efficacy to this procedure in the relief of pain and the reversal of inflammation; however, success is probably seen in only a proportion of patients (*see* Placebo page xxi). Initial field studies and small-scale controlled clinical studies suggest that most thymus preparations have a degree of efficacy in rheumatoid arthritis.	Administration of organ extracts **requires a qualified practitioner**. Practitioners should be properly qualified and should propose a treatment plan. **Risks:** Injecting foreign proteins into the body can provoke (possibly fatal) allergic reactions. Also, pathogens such as those that cause bovine spongiform encephalopathy (BSE) or other serious infections may be introduced.
Electroacupuncture according to Voll By taking readings of the electrical conductivity of the skin (*see* page 802), therapists claim to be able to derive an insight into diseased areas of the body, pathogenic foci (*see* page 928), and stress factors (*see* Toxins, page 929). The supposed causes of rheumatism can then be addressed.	**Inappropriate** as the sole treatment for advanced rheumatism. Possibly acceptable as a short-term, supportive treatment attempt for persistent or recurrent symptoms when simpler, more established methods have been unsuccessful. Some case reports claim efficacy; however, success is probably seen, if at all, in only a small proportion of patients (*see* Placebo, page xxi).	**Requires a qualified practitioner** Practitioners should be properly qualified and should propose a treatment plan. No credence should be given to anyone promising immediate or total success. **Risks:** A second opinion must always be obtained from a qualified physician before any attempt is made to "eliminate foci" (e.g. by surgery).

Treatment	Rating	Point of delivery/risks
Electroneural therapy according to Croon According to the theory, readings taken at various reactive sites on the skin highlight diseased areas within the body. Based on these readings, targeted electrostimulative measures can be undertaken to eliminate rheumatic pain (*see* page 806).	**Inappropriate** as the sole treatment for advanced rheumatism. Possibly acceptable as a short-term, supportive treatment attempt for persistent or recurrent symptoms when simpler, more established methods have been unsuccessful. Some case reports claim efficacy; however, success is probably seen, if at all, in only a small proportion of patients (*see* Placebo, page xxi).	**Requires a qualified practitioner** Practitioners should be properly qualified and should propose a treatment plan. No credence should be given to anyone promising immediate or total success. **Risks:** Proponents themselves warn that treatment should not be given in acute inflammatory conditions.
Eliminative methods, bloody Bloody cupping (*see* page 815) is said to improve the body's own regulatory systems and ease symptoms in patients with rheumatic pain.	**Inappropriate** as the sole treatment for advanced rheumatism. Possibly acceptable as a short-term, supportive treatment attempt when more established, less invasive methods have been unsuccessful. Some case reports and field studies claim efficacy; however, success is probably seen in only a small proportion of patients (*see* Placebo, page xxi).	**Requires a qualified practitioner** Practitioners should be properly qualified and should propose a treatment plan. No credence should be given to anyone promising immediate or total success. **Risks:** Bloody cupping can cause infection and scarring. Furthermore, it should not be carried out in persons with bleeding disorders.
Eliminative methods, unbloody Enemas (*see* page 819) and unbloody cupping (*see* page 817) are supposed to improve the body's own regulatory systems and ease symptoms in persons with rheumatic pain.	**Inappropriate** as the sole treatment for advanced rheumatism. **May be of some use** as a short-term, supportive treatment attempt aimed at alleviating pain. Case reports and field studies claim efficacy; however, success is probably seen in only a proportion of patients (*see* Placebo, page xxi).	**Suitable for DIY** Qualified guidance is recommended. **Risks:** Unlikely provided treatment is carried out competently.

Treatment	Rating	Point of delivery/risks
Enzyme therapy The enzymes used are said to dispel and destroy "immune complexes" (*see* page 824) that course in the blood and that are responsible, for instance, for sustaining inflammatory processes (as in arthrosis and soft-tissue rheumatism).	**May be of some use** as a short-term treatment attempt. Some case reports claim efficacy for this little researched therapy; however, success is probably seen in only a small proportion of patients (*see* Placebo, page xxi).	**Requires a qualified practitioner** Practitioners should propose a treatment plan. Non-prescription preparations are suitable for do-it-yourself. **Risks:** Allergies or intolerance are possible.
Flower remedies Flower remedies (*see* page 828) are said to restore emotional balance and assist the body's psychic ability to heal itself.	**Inappropriate** as the sole treatment for advanced rheumatism. **May be of some use** as a short-term, supportive treatment attempt aimed at soothing and relaxing. Some case reports claim efficacy; however, success is probably seen in only a small proportion of patients (*see* Placebo, page xxi).	**Suitable for DIY** Qualified guidance is recommended. Practitioners should propose a treatment plan. **Risks:** Possible intolerance.
Homeopathy Highly diluted (potentized) solutions (*see* page 831) are believed to be able to redress vital energy imbalances. Organo- and functiotropic (*see* page 833) homeopathy is claimed to be effective for dealing with rheumatic pain.	**Inappropriate** as the sole treatment for advanced rheumatism. **May be of some use** as a short-term, supportive treatment attempt. Some studies and numerous case reports claim efficacy for homeopathic treatments; however, success is probably seen in only a proportion of patients (*see* Placebo, page xxi).	**Requires a qualified practitioner** Homeopaths should be properly qualified and should propose a treatment plan. Ready-formulated preparations are suitable for do-it-yourself. **Risks:** Allergies and intolerance are possible.

Treatment	Rating	Point of delivery/risks
Hypnosis and self-hypnosis In the relaxed and generally altered state of awareness that is induced in hypnosis or self-hypnosis (*see* page 837), physical conditions can be addressed and pain alleviated.	**Inappropriate** as the sole treatment for advanced rheumatism. **May be of some use** as a short-term, supportive treatment. Some case reports claim efficacy; however, success is probably seen in only a proportion of patients treated (*see* Placebo, page xxi).	**Requires a qualified practitioner** Hypnotherapists should be properly qualified and should propose a treatment plan. **Risks:** Unlikely provided treatment is carried out competently.
Magnetic field therapy The use of magnetic field generators, magnetic strips, bracelets, and other objects (*see* page 841) allegedly encourages cell metabolism and so relieves pain.	**Of little use** Based on present knowledge, there is inadequate evidence of the efficacy and mode of action of magnetic field therapy on rheumatism.	Operation of magnetic field equipment **requires a qualified practitioner**. **Risks:** Magnetic field equipment can cause implanted cardiac pacemakers to malfunction.
Manual therapies Chiropractors and osteopaths use a series of manipulations to realign allegedly displaced vertebrae which, it is believed, are responsible for a number of pathological conditions (*see* page 844).	**Inappropriate** as the sole treatment for advanced rheumatism. **May be of some use** as a short-term treatment attempt aimed at alleviating pain. Case reports and initial controlled clinical studies suggest that some patients with acute or chronic pain may enjoy temporary alleviation of symptoms.	**Requires a qualified practitioner** Practitioners should be properly qualified and should propose a treatment plan. **Risks:** Spinal manipulations can cause serious injury. Osteoporosis is one of several risk factors. These procedures should not be used in massively affected areas, e.g. when parts of the spinal column have become inflamed.

Treatment	Rating	Point of delivery/risks
Massage Classical massage (*see* page 847) can ease muscular and perhaps also emotional tension. Certain techniques can be used to induce counterirritation to obscure existing pain, if only temporarily. Ice massage (*see* page 878) is claimed to ease pain and provide relaxation, as well as exercising a number of other beneficial effects.	**Inappropriate** as the sole treatment for advanced rheumatism. **Useful** as a supportive treatment attempt aimed at rehabilitation and improving general well-being. The easing of acute and chronic pain described in case reports and field studies is probably seen in only a proportion of patients (*see* Placebo, page xxi).	**Requires a qualified practitioner** or a sufficiently adept partner. Masseurs/masseuses should be properly qualified and should propose a treatment plan. **Risks:** Some people are sensitive to manual stimuli; others find it hard to tolerate close physical contact.
Nutritional therapies Organic and vegetarian diets (*see* pages 2–4), through their high content of dietary fiber, vitamins, and secondary plant constituents, exercise a multitude of positive effects within the body. Curative fasting is claimed to help reduce swelling, stiffness, and pain.	**Inappropriate** as the sole treatment for advanced rheumatism. Organic or vegetarian diets are **useful** as an individually directed supportive measure. Field studies report that fasting and curative fasting have a beneficial effect in reducing swelling of the joints, stiffness, and pain, e.g. as in rheumatoid arthritis.	**Suitable for DIY** Qualified guidance is recommended though not essential. Curative fasts must be medically supervised. **Risks:** Avoid imbalanced or intolerable diets. They can cause deficiencies with serious consequences. Children are particularly at risk. Intense fasting may cause the body to lose fluids and electrolytes.
Physical therapies Certain forms of hydrotherapy (*see* page 871) and physical exercise (*see* page 868) are claimed to ease symptoms and maintain physical functions in patients with rheumatism.	**Inappropriate** as the sole treatment for advanced rheumatism. **Useful** as a supportive treatment attempt. Controlled clinical studies suggest that sulphur or mud baths may have a painkilling action. Case reports and field studies suggest that physiotherapy can alleviate pain in most patients.	**Suitable for DIY** Qualified guidance is essential. Practitioners should be properly qualified and should propose a treatment plan. **Risks:** Skin damage may be caused to persons with diminished temperature sensation when extreme temperatures are applied.

Treatment	Rating	Point of delivery/risks
Probiotics The introduction of certain bacteria into the gut is claimed to bring the intestinal flora back into balance and to have a beneficial effect on other parts of the immune system, e.g. those associated with the synovial membrane (*see* page 878).	**Inappropriate** as the sole treatment for advanced rheumatism. **Of little use** Possibly acceptable as a short-term treatment attempt for persistent and recurrent symptoms when more established methods have been unsuccessful. Some case reports claim efficacy; however, success is probably seen in only a proportion of patients (*see* Placebo, page xxi).	**Requires a qualified practitioner** Practitioners should be properly qualified and should propose a treatment plan. Non-prescription formulations are suitable for do-it-yourself. **Risks:** Fairly unlikely provided treatment is carried out competently.
Reflex therapies Reflex zone massage (*see* page 883), reflexology (*see* page 883), and TENS (*see* page 886) are claimed to act via reflex channels (*see* page 881) to ease pain and provide relaxation, as well as exercise a number of other beneficial effects.	**Inappropriate** as the sole treatment for advanced rheumatism. **Useful** as a short-term, supportive treatment attempt aimed at alleviating pain. Case reports and field studies claim efficacy; however, success is probably seen in only a proportion of patients (*see* Placebo, page xxi). When compared, the various techniques appear to be equally effective, though the benefits they provide vary greatly from person to person.	**Suitable for DIY** Qualified guidance is essential. Therapists should be properly qualified and should propose a treatment plan. **Risks:** Some people are sensitive to electrical stimuli and rubber electrodes; others find it hard to tolerate manual stimulation or close physical contact.

Treatment	Rating	Point of delivery/risks
Relaxation techniques Autogenic training (*see* page 888), muscle relaxation according to Jacobson (*see* page 893), and various biofeedback techniques (*see* page 891) are said to relieve muscle tension and inner unrest, and might be instrumental in reducing pain.	**Inappropriate** as the sole treatment for advanced rheumatism. **May be of some use** as a supportive treatment attempt aimed at relaxing the patient and reducing the intake of painkillers. Some studies report a reduction in the amount of painkillers needed. Case reports claim efficacy in the easing of pain; however, success is probably seen in only a proportion of patients (*see* Placebo, page xxi).	**Suitable for DIY** Once a sound understanding of the technique has been acquired from a trainer, patients can perform exercises themselves. Therapists should be properly qualified. **Risks:** Fairly unlikely.
Vitamins and trace elements The painkilling properties of vitamin B6 are thought to contribute to pain relief. The antioxidative properties of beta-carotene, vitamins C and E, and selenium are, it is supposed, instrumental in boosting the body's defences and suppressing inflammation (*see* page 900).	**Inappropriate** as the sole treatment for advanced rheumatism. **May be of some use** as a treatment attempt when a patient receiving treatment for pain cannot tolerate the full dose of painkillers needed. Field studies ascribe a degree of efficacy to vitamin B6 in the treatment of pain, especially in combination with antirheumatic drugs. In some patients it is suggested that vitamin B6 on its own can alleviate pain. Evidence that vitamin E and selenium might have antirheumatic properties is contradictory.	**Suitable for DIY** Medical supervision is recommended, though not essential. **Risks:** Intolerance and overdosage are possible. Vitamin B6 in high doses can cause serious side effects. Recent findings imply that beta-carotene might increase the risk of cancer.

Herbal remedies for rheumatism

Active ingredient/preparation	Rating
Cajeput oil (*Melaleuca leucadendron*)	Used externally, cajeput oil **may be of some use** as a treatment attempt for rheumatic pain. It contains the rubefacient and skin-warming ingredient cineol. **Dosage:** Use externally as a 5 percent alcoholic solution. To apply, massage a few drops into the painful area several times daily. **Risks:** Be careful not to get the oil into the eyes, as it will cause them to sting painfully. Do not apply to the face and nostrils of infants. Not to be used on sensitive persons. Inhalation may lead to inflammation of the respiratory system. Extensive external use may lead to kidney problems and disorders of the central nervous system. Cajeput oil can irritate the mucous membranes and cause skin allergies.
Camphor (*Cinnamomum camphora*)	Camphor is **only useful** as an external treatment attempt for muscular rheumatism. It has a painkilling effect and anesthetizes the skin. **Dosage:** To apply, rub in externally. Use ready-formulated preparations as instructed by the manufacturer/prescriber. **Risks:** Camphor can cause contact eczema. Do not use on damaged skin. Do not apply to the nose and face of infants and young children.

Active ingredient/preparation	Rating
Eucalyptus oil (*Eucalyptus globulus*)	**Only useful** as an external treatment attempt for rheumatic pain and problems of the musculature. Eucalyptus oil stimulates blood flow. **Dosage:** Externally, 5–20 percent in oily formulations, 5–10 percent in alcoholic formulations. To apply, massage a few drops into the painful area several times daily. Use ready-formulated preparations as instructed by the manufacturer/prescriber. **Risks:** Eucalyptus oil can cause skin allergies. Do not apply to the face and nose of infants and young children. Not to be used on sensitive persons. Inhalation may lead to inflammation of the respiratory system. Extensive external use may lead to kidney problems and disorders of the central nervous system.
Hayseeds (*Graminis flos*)	**Only useful** as an attempted local heat treatment for rheumatic pain. Hayseeds have a rubefacient effect and stimulate blood flow. **Not advised** in acute episodes of rheumatic disease. **Dosage:** Apply once or twice daily as a compress, 108 °F, leaving it in place for 40–50 minutes. **Risks:** Do not use in acute episodes of rheumatic disease.
Mustard seeds for compresses (*Sinapis alba*)	**Only useful** as an external treatment attempt for chronic degenerative joint disease and rheumatism of the soft tissues. Acts as a skin and circulatory stimulant. **Dosage:** Prepare 4 dessertspoons of powdered mustard seeds as a watery paste (poultice). **Risks:** Protracted use at the same site may damage the nerves and skin. For external use only. Not to be used on children under six years or on persons with kidney disease (mustard oils are absorbed through the skin).

Active ingredient/preparation	*Rating*

Peppermint oil
(*Mentha piperita*)

Only useful as an external treatment attempt for rheumatic pain or problems with the musculature.
Dosage: To apply, massage a few drops into the part that is hurting. Use ready-formulated preparations as instructed by the manufacturer/prescriber.
Risks: Be careful not to get the oil into the eyes, as it will cause them to sting painfully. Peppermint oil can cause allergic reactions. Do not apply to the nose and face of infants and young children.

Pine needle oil
(*Pinus pinaster*)

Pine needle oil is **only useful** as an external treatment attempt for rheumatic pain in the muscles and joints.
Dosage: Best used externally in a 10–50 percent concentration in liquid and semi-liquid formulations. To apply, massage a few drops into the painful area several times daily. Use ready-formulated preparations as instructed by the manufacturer/prescriber.
Risks: Be careful not to get the oil into the eyes, as it will cause them to sting painfully. Do not apply to the face and nostrils of infants. Not to be used on sensitive persons. Inhalation may lead to inflammation of the respiratory system. Extensive external use may lead to kidney problems and disorders of the central nervous system. Pine needle oil can cause skin allergies.

Rosemary leaves and oil
(*Rosmarinus officinalis*)

Only useful (rosemary oil) as an external treatment attempt for joint problems and rheumatism. Acts as a skin and circulatory stimulant.
Dosage: For external use, apply a 10 percent oily preparation or, in a bathtub, use 2.0ml oil or 2oz rosemary leaves. Use ready-formulated preparations as instructed by the manufacturer/prescriber.
Risks: Rosemary oil may provoke allergic skin reactions.

Active ingredient/preparation	Rating
Turpentine oil (*Terebinthina laricina*)	**Only useful** as an external treatment attempt for rheumatism and neuralgia. Turpentine oil has a warming effect and stimulates blood flow through the skin. **Dosage:** In liquid and semi-solid formulations 10–20 percent (e.g. mixed with isopropyl alcohol). **Risks:** Be careful not to get the oil into the eyes, as it will cause them to sting painfully. Oil should be used fresh. Do not apply to the face and nostrils of infants. Hypersensitivity and allergies are possible; inhalation may cause acute inflammation of the respiratory tract.
Willow bark (*Salix fragilis*)	Willow bark, taken orally, **may be of some use** as a treatment attempt for rheumatic pain. **Individual dose:** 2.0g willow bark contains about 20mg total salicin. Use ready-formulated preparations as instructed by the manufacturer/prescriber. **Daily dose:** 60–120mg total salicin. **Risks:** Skin allergies, asthmatic symptoms (bronchospasm), and gastrointestinal complaints may occur in persons sensitive to aspirin and other salicylates.

Sprains and strains

Causes and symptoms

Sprains and strains most commonly result from sporting activities and, in the elderly, from falls. In addition to the above mentioned causes, muscle strain can also be the result of a dull blow and is often accompanied by painful swelling and bruising.

A sprain is a joint injury in which the supporting ligaments become overstretched or even rupture. Ligamental sprains vary in severity from being just moderately painful to involving complete failure of the joint.

Orthodox treatment

Doctors will generally prescribe anti-inflammatory ointments and various forms of physical treatment, including ice packs.

Following a sprain the affected limb should immediately be rested, and then immobilized through a pressure or support bandage, through splinting, or by setting in plaster. Ruptured flexor or extensor tendons will generally require surgery. Following a suitable period of immobilization, the doctor may suggest underwater exercises and/or medical gymnastics to bring the joint back up to strength.

Complementary therapies

Most complementary procedures focus on pain relief. Local use of essential oils and various physical therapies are reportedly effective in reducing pain, as are reflexology and acupuncture. Properly designed exercises can also speed recovery.

Treatment plan and limited trial

Before administering a complementary treatment, every therapist should propose a treatment plan (*see* page xxiii) that sets out a clear time frame and defines the goal that the treatment is designed to achieve. Treatment should then be tried for a limited term to test the patient's response.

Cautions

Always consult an orthodox doctor if the pain persists for more than just a few days. Complementary medicine can offer nothing as effective as modern surgical methods for treating torn ligaments.

Complementary treatments for sprains and strains

Treatment	Rating	Point of delivery/risks
Acupressure This treatment (*see* page 769), otherwise known as pressure-point massage, is used to alleviate pain and ease tension. The acupressure points chosen can vary from one practitioner to another.	**May be of some use** as a treatment attempt. Case reports and field studies claim efficacy; however, success is probably seen in only a proportion of patients (*see* Placebo, page xxi).	**Suitable for DIY** Qualified guidance is recommended. Therapists should be properly qualified. **Risks:** Unlikely provided treatment is carried out competently.
Acupuncture Acupuncture in its various forms (*see* page 772) aims to alleviate pain and ease tension. The acupuncture points chosen can vary from one practitioner to another.	**May be of some use** as a treatment attempt. Case reports and field studies claim efficacy; however, success is probably seen in only a proportion of patients (*see* Placebo, page xxi).	**Requires a qualified practitioner** Practitioners should be properly qualified and should propose a treatment plan. **Risks:** Probably rare provided treatment is carried out competently.
Anthroposophical medicine AM (*see* page 781) uses poultices and ointments with arnica or comfrey to ease symptoms and reduce swelling.	**May be of some use** as a treatment attempt. Case reports claim efficacy; however, success is probably seen in only a proportion of patients (*see* Placebo, page xxi).	**Suitable for DIY** **Risks:** Unlikely provided treatment is carried out competently.
Enzyme therapy Enzymes (*see* page 824) can be swallowed or applied externally. They are reported to ease pain and speed up the healing process.	**May be of some use** as a short-term treatment attempt. Some case reports claim efficacy for this little researched therapy; however, success is probably seen in only a proportion of patients (*see* Placebo, page xxi).	**Requires a qualified practitioner** Practitioners should propose a treatment plan. Non-prescription preparations are suitable for do-it-yourself. **Risks:** Allergies or intolerance are possible.

Treatment	Rating	Point of delivery/risks
Flower remedies Bach Rescue Remedy (*see* page 829) is claimed to reduce pain.	**Of little use** Acceptable as a short-term treatment attempt. Some case reports claim efficacy; however, success is probably seen in only a small proportion of patients (*see* Placebo, page xxi).	**Suitable for DIY** **Risks:** Possible intolerance.
Homeopathy The highly diluted (potentized) solutions (*see* page 831) of organo- and functiotropic (*see* page 833) homeopathy are claimed to alleviate pain, speed up healing, and improve the circulation.	**Of little use** Acceptable as a supportive treatment attempt for persistent or recurrent symptoms. Some case reports claim efficacy; however, success is probably seen, if at all, in only a small proportion of patients (*see* Placebo, page xxi).	**Suitable for DIY** **Risks:** Allergies and intolerance are possible.
Massage Lymphatic drainage (*see* page 850) is claimed to clear fluids from the affected area and speed up healing.	**May be of some use** as a treatment attempt aimed at alleviating pain. Case reports and field studies claim efficacy; however, success is probably seen in only a proportion of patients (*see* Placebo, page xxi).	**Requires a qualified practitioner** Masseurs/masseuses should be properly qualified and should propose a treatment plan. **Risks:** Some people are sensitive to manual stimuli; others find it hard to tolerate close physical contact.

Treatment	Rating	Point of delivery/risks
Physical therapies In the early stages, ice and cold treatments (*see* pages 871–8) can, it is claimed, prevent swelling and inflammation and ease pain. In later stages, cold moisture treatments or heat treatments are said to alleviate pain and cause swellings to subside.	**May be of some use** as a treatment attempt. Case reports and field studies claim efficacy; however, success is probably seen in only a proportion of patients (*see* Placebo, page xxi).	**Suitable for DIY** Qualified guidance is recommended. **Risks:** Skin damage may be caused to persons with diminished temperature sensation when extreme temperatures are applied.
Reflex therapies Reflex zone massage (*see* page 883) and TENS (*see* page 886) are claimed to act via reflex channels (*see* page 881) to ease muscle tension and alleviate pain.	**May be of some use** as a treatment attempt aimed at alleviating pain. Case reports and field studies claim efficacy; however, success is probably seen in only a proportion of patients (*see* Placebo, page xxi).	**Suitable for DIY** Qualified guidance is recommended. **Risks:** Some people are sensitive to electrical stimuli and rubber electrodes; others find it hard to tolerate manual stimulation or close physical contact.

Herbal remedies for sprains and strains

Active ingredient/preparation	Rating
Arnica flowers (*Arnica montana*)	**Only useful** as a treatment attempt for rheumatic joint and muscular pain (external use only). Has a painkilling and decongestant effect. **Dosage:** For externally applied infusions: 2g flower heads to 4fl oz hot water; for compresses: use tincture and dilute three- to tenfold; ointments should contain 20–25 percent tincture or a maximum of 15 percent oil. To apply, massage a few drops into the area causing pain several times daily. Use ready-formulated preparations as instructed by the manufacturer/prescriber. **Risks:** Do not use internally. Do not use on broken skin. Arnica can damage skin and cause blistering.

Active ingredient/preparation	Rating

Comfrey herb, leaves, and root
(*Symphytum officinale*)

Only useful as an external treatment attempt for sprains, strains, and bruising. Comfrey is an anti-inflammatory.
Dosage: Ointments must not contain more than 10–20 percent dried root and leaves. Use ready-formulated preparations as instructed by the manufacturer/prescriber.
Risks: Use on intact skin only; ask your doctor about its use during pregnancy. Do not use for longer than four to six weeks per year. Comfrey must not be used internally, as it contains hepatotoxic and possibly carcinogenic pyrrolizidine alkaloids. These are also absorbed when ointment is applied extensively to the skin.

Horse chestnut
(*Aesculus hippocastanum*)

Used externally, horse chestnut **may be of some use** as a treatment attempt for soft-tissue swellings and swollen ankles.
Dosage: As instructed by the manufacturer/prescriber.
Risks: Horse chestnut may cause gastric irritation, nausea, and itchiness. Be sure to persist with other medically prescribed measures, such as pressure dressings, support hosiery, and bathing with cold water.

Pineapple enzyme
(Bromelain from *Ananas comosus*)

May be of some use as a treatment attempt for swelling following surgery and accidental injury, particularly to the nose and sinuses.
Not advised in hypersensitive persons.
Daily dose: Use ready-formulated preparations as instructed by the manufacturer/prescriber. Use for 8–20 days, or for longer where justifiable.
Risks: Bromelain may cause gastric problems, diarrhea, and allergic reactions.

Shepherd's myrtle root
(*Ruscus aculeatus*)

Used externally, shepherd's myrtle **may be of some use** as a treatment attempt for swellings.
Dosage: As instructed by the manufacturer/prescriber.
Risks: Allergic irritation is possible.

Active ingredient/preparation	Rating
Sweet clover (*Melilotus officinalis*)	**Only useful** as an external treatment attempt for sprains, strains, and superficial bruising (in the form of compresses with a sweet clover infusion). **Dosage:** 5g to 1 pint of lukewarm water for compresses several times daily. Use ready-formulated preparations as instructed by the manufacturer/prescriber. **Risks:** Sweet clover can cause skin irritation, as well as headaches if applied extensively.

Tendons and ligaments

Causes and symptoms

Tendons are cords of fibrous tissue that connect muscles to the bones and joints and are generally surrounded by a sheath. Synovial bursae are interposed between surfaces to ensure the smooth working of tendons, muscles, and skin tissue. Ligaments, on the other hand, are rigid structures that hold the joint in place. Though tendons and ligaments are fairly resilient, they have little elastic "give." Overstretching may lead to rupturing (*see* Sprains and Strains, page 216) or tearing. Excessive or repetitive use of these connective structures can lead to tenosynovitis and bursitis (a characteristic feature of repetitive strain injury), though bursitis may also be of bacterial origin. The conditions outlined here can be extremely painful.

Orthodox treatment

Doctors usually suggest painkillers and antirheumatic ointments, as well as certain physical treatments such as ice packs. Cortisone may also be given when tenosynovitis and bursitis have failed to respond to other treatments.

Sprains and tenosynovitis should be treated by resting the affected limb and immobilizing it with a pressure or support bandage, through splinting, or by setting it in plaster. Ruptured flexor or extensor tendons will generally require surgery. Following a suitable period of immobilization the doctor may suggest underwater exercises and/or medical gymnastics to bring the joint back up to strength.

Complementary therapies

Most complementary procedures that are used for damaged tendons and ligaments focus on pain relief. Essential oils used locally and various physical therapies are reportedly effective in reducing pain, as are reflexology and acupuncture. Properly designed exercises can also speed recovery once the underlying disorder has been successfully treated.

Treatment plan and limited trial

Before administering a complementary treatment, every therapist should propose a treatment plan (*see* page xxiii) that sets out a clear time frame and defines the goal that the treatment is designed to achieve. Treatment should then be tried for a limited term to test the patient's response.

Cautions

Complementary medicine can offer nothing as effective as modern surgical methods for treating torn ligaments. Tenosynovitis can also be the first sign of chronic arthritis. Always consult an orthodox doctor if pain persists for more than just a few days.

Complementary treatments for problems with tendons and ligaments

Treatment	Rating	Point of delivery/risks
Acupressure This treatment (*see* page 769), otherwise known as pressure-point massage, is claimed to alleviate pain, ease tension, and improve general well-being.	**May be of some use** as a short-term treatment attempt aimed at easing pain. Case reports claim efficacy; however, success is probably seen in only a proportion of patients (*see* Placebo, page xxi).	**Suitable for DIY** Qualified guidance is recommended. Therapists should be properly qualified. **Risks:** Unlikely provided treatment is carried out competently.
Acupuncture Acupuncture in its various forms (*see* page 772) aims to alleviate pain and reduce inflammation. The acupuncture points chosen can vary from one practitioner to another.	**May be of some use** as a short-term treatment attempt for pain and inflammation. Various studies and reports ascribe a degree of efficacy to this procedure in some patients (*see* Placebo, page xxi).	**Requires a qualified practitioner** Practitioners should be properly qualified and should propose a treatment plan. **Risks:** Probably rare provided treatment is carried out competently.
Cell therapy Injecting or ingesting products extracted from the tissues of newborn animals or animal fetuses is said to have a rejuvenating and revitalizing effect and to enhance the healing of human tissues and organs (*see* page 796).	**Not advised** Based on present knowledge, there is inadequate evidence of the efficacy and mode of action of these costly and relatively risky procedures.	**Risks:** Injecting foreign proteins into the body can provoke (possibly fatal) allergic reactions. Also, pathogens such as those that cause bovine spongiform encephalopathy (BSE) or other serious infections may be introduced.

Treatment	Rating	Point of delivery/risks
Eliminative methods, unbloody Unbloody cupping (*see* page 817) and cantharide poultices (*see* page 812) are often used for pain relief in persons with damaged tendons and ligaments.	Unbloody cupping **may be of some use** as a short-term treatment attempt aimed at relieving pain. Cantharide poultices, on the other hand, are **of little use**, except in the small number of persistent cases in which more established, less invasive methods have been unsuccessful. Some case reports claim efficacy; however, success is probably seen in only a proportion of patients (*see* Placebo, page xxi).	**Suitable for DIY** Unbloody cupping is best carried out under the guidance of a qualified practitioner. Treatment with cantharide poultices requires a qualified practitioner. **Risks:** Cantharide poultices can cause second-degree burns.
Enzyme therapy Enzymes that are swallowed or applied locally as ointments are said to lessen pain and swelling and accelerate healing (*see* page 824).	**May be of some use** as a short-term treatment attempt. Some case reports claim efficacy for this little researched therapy; however, success is probably seen in only a small proportion of patients (*see* Placebo, page xxi).	**Requires a qualified practitioner** Practitioners should propose a treatment plan. Non-prescription preparations are suitable for do-it-yourself. **Risks:** Allergies or intolerance are possible.

Treatment	*Rating*	*Point of delivery/risks*
Homeopathy The highly diluted (potentized) solutions (*see* page 831) of organo- and functiotropic (*see* page 833) homeopathy are claimed to be effective for easing pain and inflammation and speeding up recovery.	**Of little use** Acceptable as a short-term, supportive treatment attempt for chronic complaints. Case reports claim success for homeopathic treatments; however, success is probably seen in only a proportion of patients (*see* Placebo, page xxi).	**Suitable for DIY** Qualified guidance is recommended. Homeopaths should be properly qualified and should propose a treatment plan. No credence should be given to anyone promising immediate or total success. **Risks:** Allergies and intolerance are possible.
Manual therapies Chiropractors and osteopaths use a series of manipulations to realign allegedly displaced vertebrae to ease pain (*see* page 844).	**May be of some use** as a short-term treatment attempt for persistent pain when less risky, more established methods have been unsuccessful. Case reports and field studies claim efficacy; however, success is probably seen, if at all, in only a proportion of patients (*see* Placebo, page xxi).	**Requires a qualified practitioner** Practitioners should be properly qualified and should propose a treatment plan. **Risks:** Spinal manipulations can cause serious injury. Osteoporosis is one of several risk factors.
Massage Local massage (see page 847) is claimed to ease muscular tension and alleviate pain.	**May be of some use** as a short-term, supportive treatment attempt aimed at relaxing the patient and easing pain. Case reports and field studies claim efficacy; however, success is probably seen in only a proportion of patients (*see* Placebo, page xxi).	**Requires a qualified practitioner** Masseurs/masseuses should be properly qualified and should propose a treatment plan. **Risks:** Some people are sensitive to manual stimuli; others find it hard to tolerate close physical contact.

Treatment	Rating	Point of delivery/risks
Physical therapies In the acute stage, cold treatments such as compresses and packs (*see* page 878) and ice treatments are said to alleviate pain and reduce oedema. In chronic conditions, warm packs or wraps (*see* pages 877–8) are claimed to relax hardened muscles and reduce pain.	**Useful** as a short-term treatment attempt aimed at alleviating pain and relaxing the patient. Case reports and field studies claim efficacy; however, success is probably seen in only a proportion of patients (*see* Placebo, page xxi).	**Suitable for DIY** Qualified guidance is recommended. Practitioners should be properly qualified and should propose a treatment plan. **Risks:** Skin damage may be caused to persons with diminished temperature sensation when extreme temperatures are applied.
Reflex therapies Reflex zone massage (*see* page 883) and TENS (*see* page 886) are claimed to act via reflex channels (*see* page 881) to ease pain and relieve muscular tension.	**Useful** as a short-term treatment attempt aimed at alleviating pain. Case reports and field studies claim efficacy; however, success is probably seen in only a proportion of patients (*see* Placebo, page xxi).	**Suitable for DIY** Qualified guidance is essential. **Risks:** Unlikely provided treatment is carried out competently.

Herbal remedies for problems with tendons and ligaments

Active ingredient/preparation	Rating
Camphor (*Cinnamomum camphora*)	Camphor is **only useful** in an alcoholic solution as an external treatment attempt for damaged tendons and ligaments. It has a cooling effect and stimulates blood flow through the skin. **Dosage:** To apply, rub in externally. Use ready-formulated preparations as instructed by the manufacturer/prescriber. **Risks:** Camphor can cause contact eczema. Do not use on damaged skin. Do not apply to the nose and face of infants and young children (at risk of collapse).

Active ingredient/preparation	Rating
Menthol	Menthol is **only useful** as an external treatment attempt for diseased muscles, tendons, and ligaments. It has a cooling effect. **Dosage:** To apply, massage in as a 0.5–1 percent alcoholic solution. **Risks:** Menthol can cause contact eczema. Do not use on damaged skin. Do not apply to the nose and face of infants and young children.
Mint oil (essential oil of *Mentha arvensis*)	Mint oil is **useful** as an external treatment attempt for diseased tendons and ligaments. It has a cooling effect. **Dosage:** Apply externally as a 5–10 percent concentration in the case of oily preparations, and also in the case of aqueous–alcoholic formulations. Use ready-formulated preparations as instructed by the manufacturer/prescriber. **Risks:** Be careful not to get the oil into the eyes, as it will cause them to sting painfully. Do not apply to the face and nostrils of infants. This oil may irritate the mucous membranes if incorrectly used and can cause skin allergies.
Peppermint oil (*Mentha piperita*)	**Only useful** as an external treatment attempt for rheumatic pain or problems with the musculature. To apply, massage into the painful area. **Dosage:** As instructed by the manufacturer/prescriber. **Risks:** Be careful not to get the oil into the eyes, as it will cause them to sting painfully. Peppermint oil can cause allergic reactions. Do not apply to the nose and face of infants and young children.

Respiratory ailments

Asthma

Causes and symptoms

Bronchial asthma is a disease of the respiratory system in which the bronchial mucosa become extremely sensitive. A key causative role is played by inflammatory, immunological, toxicological, infectious, and psychosocial factors. An asthma attack may be triggered off by infection of the airways, by irritants such as pollen, animal fur or house dust, or by physical exercise.

Asththma is characterized by breathlessness and wheezing, with exhaling being particularly difficult. Asthma, at least in its early stages, does not permanently affect the lungs although, with time, it may become chronic and cause secondary lung problems.

Orthodox treatment

General preventive measures are usually applied in association with orthodox medications for acute or long-term treatment. Medications will include anti-allergics and anti-inflammatories, beta-sympathomimetics and sometimes corticosteriods in inhalers. Modern orthodox drugs enable even potentially life-threatening situations to be mastered.

Complementary therapies

No complementary approach is suitable as the sole treatment in severe, acute asthma attacks. The role of complementary therapies is thus to be seen as supportive. Whether and to what extent complementary therapies are useful for prevention or long-term treatment is still unclear.

Treatment plan and limited trial

Before administering a complementary treatment, every therapist should propose a treatment plan (see page xxiii) that sets out a clear time frame and defines the goal that the treatment is designed to achieve. Treatment should then be tried for a limited term to test the patient's response.

Cautions

All asthma sufferers receiving complementary treatment should be kept under medical review. For example, the efficacy of (or resistance to) prescribed medications should be closely monitored and a careful watch kept for any inflammatory symptoms. In acute asthma attacks, complementary procedures are no substitute for the effective methods of modern mainstream medicine.

Complementary treatments for asthma

Treatment	Rating	Point of delivery/risks
Acupressure This treatment (*see* page 769), otherwise known as pressure-point massage, is claimed to soothe the patient during asthma attacks and reduce the resistance to respiration. Acupressure is also used for its restorative action.	**Inappropriate** as the sole treatment for acute asthma attacks. Acceptable as a short-term treatment attempt. Various case reports and field studies claim efficacy; however, success is probably seen in only a small proportion of patients (*see* Placebo, page xxi).	**Suitable for DIY** Qualified guidance is recommended. Therapists should be properly qualified. **Risks:** Unlikely provided treatment is carried out competently.
Acupuncture Acupuncture in its various forms (*see* page 772) aims to encourage the flow of energy (*see* page 727) or to act directly to ease asthma attacks and reduce the intake of medication. The acupuncture points chosen can vary from one practitioner to another.	**Inappropriate** as the sole treatment for acute asthma attacks. **May be of some use** as a short-term, supportive treatment attempt for prevention, for easing symptoms and inflammatory reactions, and for improving general well-being. Controlled clinical studies, case reports, and field studies ascribe a degree of efficacy to this procedure as asthma prophylaxis in some patients (*see* Placebo, page xxi).	**Requires a qualified practitioner** Practitioners should be properly qualified and should propose a treatment plan. **Risks:** Probably rare provided treatment is carried out competently.

Treatment	Rating	Point of delivery/risks
Anthroposophical medicine Depending on the presumed cause of asthma, anthroposophical medicine (*see* page 781) offers various compositions and psychotherapeutic approaches.	**May be of some use** as a longer-term preventive measure. Some case reports claim efficacy; however, success is probably seen in only a proportion of patients (*see* Placebo, page xxi).	**Requires a qualified practitioner** Practitioners should be properly qualified and should propose a treatment plan. **Risks:** Allergies and intolerance are possible.
Aromatherapy Essential oils (*see* page 786) are used to soothe and relax, or to invigorate the patient, and so possibly alleviate symptoms. The essences may be taken orally, used externally as massage oils or bathing emulsions, or inhaled as vapors.	**Inappropriate** as the sole treatment for acute asthma attacks. Acceptable as a short-term, supportive treatment attempt aimed at soothing and relaxing the patient. Some case reports claim efficacy; however, success is probably seen in only a small proportion of patients (*see* Placebo, page xxi).	**Suitable for DIY** Qualified guidance is recommended. The effects of individual essential oils differ widely. **Risks:** Allergies or intolerance are possible. Some oils are carcinogenic in test systems and possibly in humans.
Bioresonance therapy Bioresonance therapists use electrical devices in an attempt to discover the causes of illness and claim to be able to weaken or turn around pathogenic energies and disease related vibrations (*see* page 794).	**Of little use** Possibly acceptable as a short-term, supportive treatment attempt when simpler, more established methods have been unsuccessful. Despite the relative popularity of this procedure in the treatment of asthma, the efficacy described in case reports (and nowhere else) is probably seen, if at all, in only a small proportion of patients (*see* Placebo, page xxi).	**Requires a qualified practitioner** Practitioners should be properly qualified and should propose a treatment plan. No credence should be given to anyone promising immediate or total success. **Risks:** Fairly unlikely.

Treatment	Rating	Point of delivery/risks
Cell therapy Injecting or ingesting products extracted from the tissues of newborn animals or animal fetuses is said to have a rejuvenating and revitalizing effect and to enhance the healing of human tissues and organs (*see* page 796).	**Not advised** Based on present knowledge, there is inadequate evidence of the efficacy and mode of action of these costly and relatively risky procedures.	**Risks:** Injecting foreign proteins into the body can provoke (possibly fatal) allergic reactions. Also, pathogens such as those that cause bovine spongiform encephalopathy (BSE) or other serious infections may be introduced.
Electroacupuncture according to Voll By taking readings of the electrical conductivity of the skin (*see* page 802), therapists claim to be able to derive an insight into diseased areas of the body, pathogenic foci (*see* page 928), and stress factors (*see* Toxins, page 929). The supposed causes of asthma can then be addressed.	**Of little use** Possibly acceptable as a short-term, supportive treatment attempt when simpler, more established methods have been unsuccessful. Some case reports claim efficacy; however, success is probably seen, if at all, in only a small proportion of patients (*see* Placebo, page xxi).	**Requires a qualified practitioner** Practitioners should be properly qualified and should propose a treatment plan. No credence should be given to anyone promising immediate or total success. **Risks:** A second opinion must always be obtained from a qualified physician before any attempt is made to "eliminate foci" (e.g. by surgery).
Electroneural therapy according to Croon According to the theory, readings taken at various reactive sites on the skin highlight diseased areas within the body. Based on these readings, targeted electrostimulative measures can be undertaken to address the presumed causes of asthma (*see* page 806).	**Of little use** Possibly acceptable as a short-term, supportive treatment attempt when simpler, more established methods have been unsuccessful. Some case reports claim efficacy; however, success is probably seen, if at all, in only a small proportion of patients (*see* Placebo, page xxi).	**Requires a qualified practitioner** Practitioners should be properly qualified and should propose a treatment plan. No credence should be given to anyone promising immediate or total success. **Risks:** Proponents themselves warn that treatment should not be given in acute inflammatory conditions.

Treatment	Rating	Point of delivery/risks
Eliminative methods, bloody Bloody cupping (*see* page 815) is said to energize the patient and improve the body's own regulatory systems (*see* page 927).	**Not advised** The efficacy of this relatively invasive procedure is lacking.	**Risks:** Bloody cupping can cause infection and scarring. Furthermore, it should not be carried out in persons with bleeding disorders.
Eliminative methods, unbloody Unbloody cupping (*see* page 817) is supposed to alleviate soreness, improve the body's own regulatory systems, and energize (*see* page 927) the patient.	**Inappropriate** as the sole treatment for acute asthma attacks. **May be of some use** as a short-term, supportive treatment attempt. Some case reports claim efficacy; however, success is probably seen in only a small proportion of patients (*see* Placebo, page xxi).	**Suitable for DIY** Unbloody cupping is best carried out under the guidance of a qualified practitioner. **Risks:** Unlikely provided treatment is carried out competently.
Flower remedies Some flower therapists see asthma as an expression of emotional disharmony. Flower remedies (*see* page 828) are said to restore emotional balance and assist the body's psychic ability to heal itself.	**Inappropriate** as the sole treatment for acute asthma attacks. **May be of some use** as a short-term, supportive treatment attempt aimed at soothing and relaxing the patient. Some case reports claim efficacy; however, success is probably seen in only a small proportion of patients (*see* Placebo, page xxi).	**Suitable for DIY** Qualified guidance is recommended. Practitioners should propose a treatment plan. **Risks:** Possible intolerance.

Treatment	Rating	Point of delivery/risks
Homeopathy Highly diluted (potentized) solutions (*see* page 831) are believed able to redress vital energy imbalances. Organo- and functiotropic (*see* page 833) homeopathy is claimed to be effective for a symptomatic treatment of asthma.	**Inappropriate** as the sole treatment for acute asthma attacks. **May be of some use** as a short-term, supportive treatment attempt. Some case reports and minor studies claim efficacy for homeopathic treatments; however, success is probably seen in only a proportion of patients (*see* Placebo, page xxi).	**Requires a qualified practitioner** Homeopaths should be properly qualified and should propose a treatment plan. Ready-formulated preparations are suitable for do-it-yourself. **Risks:** Allergies and intolerance are possible.
Hypnosis and self-hypnosis In the relaxed and generally altered state of awareness that is induced in hypnosis or self-hypnosis (*see* page 837), physical conditions can be addressed and pain alleviated. Some professionally organized courses in self-hypnosis are now available. Hypnosis is often used in combination with other psycho- and behavioral therapies to help patients come to terms with their condition.	**Inappropriate** as the sole treatment for acute asthma attacks. **May be of some use** as a short-term, supportive treatment attempt aimed at relaxing the patient and helping him/her come to terms better with his/her condition. Some case reports and field studies claim efficacy; however, success is probably seen in only a proportion of patients (*see* Placebo, page xxi).	**Requires a qualified practitioner** Hypnotherapists should be properly qualified and should propose a treatment plan. No credence should be given to anyone promising immediate or total success. **Risks:** Unlikely provided treatment is carried out competently.

Treatment	Rating	Point of delivery/risks
Manual therapies Chiropractors and osteopaths use a series of manipulations to realign allegedly displaced vertebrae. This is said to reduce pain, release energy blockages (*see* page 927), and improve the mechanics of respiration (*see* page 844).	**Inappropriate** as the sole treatment for acute asthma attacks. Possibly acceptable as a short-term treatment attempt when less risky, more established methods have been unsuccessful. Some case reports claim efficacy for this potentially risky procedure; however, success is probably seen, if at all, in only a small proportion of patients (*see* Placebo, page xxi).	**Requires a qualified practitioner** Practitioners should be properly qualified and should propose a treatment plan. **Risks:** Spinal manipulations can cause serious injury. Osteoporosis is one of several risk factors.
Massage Classical massage (*see* page 847) and lymphatic drainage (*see* page 850), are said to have an invigorating effect and to ease muscular and emotional tension.	**Inappropriate** as the sole treatment for acute asthma attacks. **Useful** as a short-term, supportive treatment attempt aimed at relaxing the patient and improving his/her general well-being. Some case reports claim efficacy; however, success is probably seen in only a proportion of patients (*see* Placebo, page xxi).	**Requires a qualified practitioner** Masseurs/masseuses should be properly qualified and should propose a treatment plan. **Risks:** Some people are sensitive to manual stimuli; others find it hard to tolerate close physical contact.
Nutritional therapies An organic diet (*see* page 4) provides the body with essential and secondary nutrients that are believed to exercise a multitude of positive effects and to be capable, *inter alia*, of boosting the immune system.	**Useful** as an individually directed supportive measure. Elimination and rotation diets may be of some assistance in identifying the cause of chronic food allergy induced asthma.	**Suitable for DIY** Qualified guidance is recommended. See your doctor before starting an elimination or rotation diet. **Risks:** Avoid imbalanced or intolerable diets. They can cause deficiencies with serious consequences. Children are particularly at risk.

Treatment	Rating	Point of delivery/risks
Physical therapies Chest wraps (*see* page 877), semi-immersion baths with or without herbal additives, ascending temperature arm baths, hot compresses on the chest and back, cold and heat treatments (*see* pages 871–8) and breathing exercises are said to reduce the frequency of asthma attacks and also alleviate symptoms.	**Inappropriate** as the sole treatment for acute asthma attacks. **Useful** as a supportive measure aimed at reducing symptoms and improving the patient's quality of life. Case reports and field studies claim efficacy; however, success is probably seen in only a proportion of patients (*see* Placebo, page xxi).	**Suitable for DIY** Qualified guidance is recommended though not essential. **Risks:** Skin damage (scalding, frostbite) may be caused to persons with diminished temperature sensation when extreme temperatures are applied.
Probiotics The introduction of certain bacteria into the gut is claimed to bring the intestinal flora back into balance and to have a beneficial effect on the immune system (*see* page 878).	**Of little use** Possibly acceptable as a short-term, supportive treatment attempt when more established methods have been unsuccessful. Case reports claim efficacy; however, success is probably seen in only a proportion of patients (*see* Placebo, page xxi).	**Requires a qualified practitioner** Practitioners should be properly qualified and should propose a treatment plan. Non-prescription formulations are suitable for do-it-yourself. **Risks:** Fairly unlikely provided treatment is carried out competently.
Reflex therapies Reflex zone massage (*see* page 883), reflexology (*see* page 883), and TENS (*see* page 886) are claimed to act via reflex channels (*see* page 881) to relax the patient and alleviate other symptoms.	**Inappropriate** as the sole treatment for acute asthma attacks. Acceptable as a short-term, supportive treatment attempt aimed at alleviating symptoms. Some case reports claim efficacy; however, success is probably seen in only a proportion of patients (*see* Placebo, page xxi).	**Suitable for DIY** Qualified guidance is essential. **Risks:** Some people are sensitive to cold, electrical stimuli, and rubber electrodes; others find it hard to tolerate manual stimulation, close physical contact, or the pressure applied during massage.

Treatment	Rating	Point of delivery/risks
Relaxation techniques Autogenic training (*see* page 888), muscle relaxation according to Jacobson (*see* page 893), and various biofeedback techniques (*see* page 891) are said to relieve muscle tension, anxiety, and inner unrest, and might be instrumental in preventing asthma attacks.	**Inappropriate** as the sole treatment for acute asthma attacks. Acceptable as a supportive treatment attempt aimed at relaxing the patient, reducing anxiety, and preventing asthma attacks. Case reports claim efficacy; however, success is probably seen in only a proportion of patients (*see* Placebo, page xxi).	**Suitable for DIY** Once a sound understanding of the technique has been acquired from a trainer in groups or through individual tuition, patients can perform exercises themselves. Therapists should be properly qualified. **Risks:** Fairly unlikely.
Vitamins and trace elements The antioxidative properties of beta-carotene, vitamins C and E, and selenium are, it is supposed, instrumental in countering the formation of free radicals and boosting the body's anti-oxidative defence systems, exercising a multitude of beneficial effects (*see* page 900).	**Inappropriate** as the sole treatment for acute asthma attacks. It is not possible to make any definitive statements with respect to efficacy in the long term.	**Suitable for DIY** Medical supervision is recommended though not essential. **Risks:** Intolerance and overdosage are possible. Recent reports imply that beta-carotene might increase the risk of cancer.

Herbal remedies for asthma

Active ingredient/preparation	Rating
Remedies containing **Ephedra** (*Ephedra sinica*)	Taken orally, remedies containing ephedra **may be of some use** as a treatment attempt alongside other measures. Ephedra can play a supportive role, for instance, in asthma-like bronchitis, emphysema, and whooping cough. **Dosage:** Use as instructed by the manufacturer/prescriber. **Risks:** Ephedra preparations can cause sleeplessness and tachycardia. They may also interact with commonly used hypotensive drugs. In the UK, ephedra is controlled under the Medicines Act 1968.

Colds

Causes and symptoms

The common cold is an acute viral infection of the upper respiratory tract that is characterized by increased temperature, a runny nose, hoarseness, a sore throat, watery eyes, a cough, and sometimes a mild fever. Sufferers may also complain of a headache as well as general muscular aches and pains. The name "cold" probably arose through the popular belief that it was caused by inclement wintry weather, and is thus a misnomer.

Orthodox treatment

The usual suggested remedies for colds are medicines and various forms of physical treatment, such as "sweating it out," vapor inhalations, etc. Suitable painkillers and nasal decongestants are also sometimes used. Antibiotic treatment is generally inappropriate, as antibiotics are ineffective for viral infections.

Complementary therapies

Complementary therapists make wide use of physical therapies and herbal remedies. In recurrent infection they may also seek to stimulate the immune system. Various forms of reflexology and similar practices are applied to provide relief from pain and other symptoms. Inhalations may alleviate symptoms, as they ease congestion and make breathing easier. Teas and infusions not containing an essential oil are generally not as effective when inhaled.

Treatment plan and limited trial

Before administering a complementary treatment, every therapist should propose a treatment plan (*see* page xxiii) that sets out a clear time frame and defines the goal that the treatment is designed to achieve. Treatment should then be tried for a limited term to test the patient's response.

Caution

Chronic hoarseness may also be caused by a serious disorder such as a malignant tumor. If hoarseness persists, you must see your doctor.

Complementary treatments for colds

Treatment	Rating	Point of delivery/risks
Acupressure This treatment (*see* page 769), otherwise known as pressure-point massage, is claimed to reduce nausea and local symptoms such as headaches when the appropriate pressure points are stimulated. The pressure points chosen may differ from one practitioner to another.	**May be of some use** as a short-term treatment attempt for symptoms such as headaches. Case reports and field studies claim efficacy; however, success is probably seen in only a proportion of patients (*see* Placebo, page xxi).	**Suitable for DIY** Qualified guidance is recommended. Therapists should be properly qualified. **Risks:** Unlikely provided treatment is carried out competently.

Treatment	Rating	Point of delivery/risks

Acupuncture
Acupuncture in its various forms (*see* page 272) aims to encourage the flow of energy (*see* page 927) or to bring direct relief of symptoms. The acupuncture points chosen can vary from one practitioner to another.

May be of some use as a treatment attempt in the initial stages of the common cold, aimed at easing symptoms. Case reports claim efficacy; however, success is probably seen in only a proportion of patients (*see* Placebo, page xxi).

Requires a qualified practitioner
Practitioners should be properly qualified and should propose a treatment plan.
Risks: Probably rare provided treatment is carried out competently.

Anthroposophical medicine
Inflamed tissues, it is claimed, respond to foot baths, compresses around the lower legs, or sweating from the extremities. AM also uses specially tailored drugs (*see* pages 781–6).

May be of some use as a short-term treatment attempt. Some studies claim efficacy; however, success is probably seen in only a small proportion of patients (*see* Placebo, page xxi).

Requires a qualified practitioner
Practitioners should be properly qualified and should propose a treatment plan.
Risks: Allergies and intolerance are possible.

Aromatherapy
Essential oils (*see* page 786) are used to soothe and relax, or to invigorate, thereby helping to ease symptoms. The essences may be taken orally, used externally as massage oils or bathing emulsions, or inhaled as vapors.

Of little use
Acceptable as a short-term, supportive treatment attempt aimed as soothing and relaxing. Some case reports claim efficacy; however, success is probably seen in only a proportion of patients (*see* Placebo, page xxi).

Suitable for DIY
Qualified guidance is recommended. The effects of individual essential oils differ widely.
Risks: Allergies or intolerance are possible. Some oils are carcinogenic in test systems and possibly in humans.

Treatment	Rating	Point of delivery/risks
Bioresonance therapy Bioresonance therapists use electrical devices in an attempt to discover the causes of illness and claim to be able to weaken or turn around pathogenic energies and disease related vibrations (*see* page 794).	**Of little use** Possibly acceptable as a short-term, supportive treatment attempt for frequent colds when simpler, more established methods have been unsuccessful. Some case reports claim efficacy; however, success is probably seen, if at all, in only a small proportion of patients (*see* Placebo, page xxi).	**Requires a qualified practitioner** Practitioners should be properly qualified and should propose a treatment plan. No credence should be given to anyone promising immediate or total success. **Risks:** Fairly unlikely.
Cell therapy Injecting or ingesting products extracted from the tissues of newborn animals or animal fetuses is said to have a rejuvenating and revitalizing effect and to enhance the healing of human tissues and organs (*see* page 796).	**Not advised** Based on present knowledge, there is inadequate evidence of the efficacy and mode of action of these costly and relatively risky procedures.	**Risks:** Injecting foreign proteins into the body can provoke (possibly fatal) allergic reactions. Also, pathogens such as those that cause bovine spongiform encephalopathy (BSE) or other serious infections may be introduced.
Electroacupuncture according to Voll By taking readings of the electrical conductivity of the skin (*see* page 802), therapists claim to be able to derive an insight into diseased areas of the body, pathogenic foci (*see* page 928), and stress factors (*see* Toxins, page 929). The supposed causative factors can then be addressed.	**Of little use** Possibly acceptable as a short-term, supportive treatment attempt for frequent colds when simpler, more established methods have been unsuccessful. Some case reports claim efficacy; however, success is probably seen, if at all, in only a small proportion of patients (*see* Placebo, page xxi).	**Requires a qualified practitioner** Practitioners should be properly qualified and should propose a treatment plan. No credence should be given to anyone promising immediate or total success. **Risks:** A second opinion must always be obtained from a qualified physician before any attempt is made to "eliminate foci" (e.g. by surgery).

Treatment	Rating	Point of delivery/risks
Electroneural therapy according to Croon According to the theory, readings taken at various reactive sites on the skin highlight diseased areas within the body. Based on these readings, targeted electrostimulative measures can be undertaken to address the causative factors (*see* page 806).	**Of little use** Possibly acceptable as a short-term, supportive treatment attempt for frequent colds when simpler, more established methods have been unsuccessful. Some case reports claim efficacy; however, success is probably seen, if at all, in only a small proportion of patients (*see* Placebo, page xxi).	**Requires a qualified practitioner** Practitioners should be properly qualified and should propose a treatment plan. No credence should be given to anyone promising immediate or total success. **Risks:** Proponents themselves warn that treatment should not be given in acute inflammatory conditions.
Eliminative methods, bloody Bloody cupping (*see* page 815) is said to improve mental outlook and modulate the immune system (*see* page 10).	**Not advised** There is no conclusive evidence of the efficacy and mode of action of bloody eliminative methods.	**Risks:** Bloody cupping can cause infection and scarring. Furthermore, it should not be carried out in persons with bleeding disorders.
Eliminative methods, unbloody Sweating, colonic irrigation (*see* page 819), and unbloody cupping (*see* page 817) are said to improve mental outlook, ease symptoms, and detoxify the body.	Cupping and enemas **may be of some use** as a treatment attempt. Some case reports claim efficacy; however, success is probably seen in only a proportion of patients (*see* Placebo, page xxi).	**Suitable for DIY** Unbloody cupping and enemas are best administered under the guidance of a qualified practitioner. **Risks:** Frequent enemas may cause the body to absorb too much fluid. If not applied competently, enemas can damage the colonic mucosa.

Treatment	Rating	Point of delivery/risks
Enzyme therapy The enzymes used are said to dispel and destroy "immune complexes" (*see* page 824) that course in the blood and that are responsible, for instance, for sustaining inflammatory processes. Enzyme preparations are also claimed to kill bacteria and viruses.	**Of little use** Case reports claim efficacy for this little researched therapy; however, success is probably seen in only a proportion of patients (*see* Placebo, page xxi).	**Requires a qualified practitioner** Practitioners should propose a treatment plan. Non-prescription preparations are suitable for do-it-yourself. **Risks:** Allergies or intolerance are possible.
Flower remedies Flower remedies (*see* page 828) are said to restore emotional balance and assist the body's psychic ability to heal itself. Bach Rescue Remedy is recommended for severe symptoms.	**Of little use** Acceptable as a short-term, supportive treatment attempt aimed at soothing and relaxing. Some case reports claim efficacy; however, success is probably seen in only a proportion of patients (*see* Placebo, page xxi).	**Suitable for DIY** Qualified guidance is recommended. Practitioners should propose a treatment plan. **Risks:** Possible intolerance.
Homeopathy Highly diluted (potentized) solutions (*see* page 831) are believed to be able to redress vital energy imbalances. Organo- and functiotropic (*see* page 833) homeopathy is claimed to be effective for dealing directly with the common cold.	**Of little use** Acceptable as a short-term treatment attempt. Some case reports claim efficacy; however, success is probably seen in only a proportion of patients (*see* Placebo, page xxi).	**Requires a qualified practitioner** Homeopaths should be properly qualified and should propose a treatment plan. Ready-formulated preparations are suitable for do-it-yourself. **Risks:** Allergies and intolerance are possible.

Treatment	Rating	Point of delivery/risks
Hypnosis and self-hypnosis In the relaxed and generally altered state of awareness that is induced in hypnosis or self-hypnosis (*see* page 837), physical and mental conditions can be addressed. The relaxation and emotional balance thus achieved is claimed to have a certain preventive effect.	**Of little use** Possibly acceptable as a relaxing and preventive measure in persons suffering from frequent or persistent colds. Case reports claim efficacy; however, success is probably seen in only a small proportion of patients (*see* Placebo, page xxi).	**Requires a qualified practitioner** Hypnotherapists should be properly qualified and should propose a treatment plan. **Risks:** Unlikely provided treatment is carried out competently.
Manual therapies Chiropractors and osteopaths use a series of manipulations to realign allegedly displaced vertebrae which, it is believed, might be associated with high susceptibility to infection. Treatment is also said to reduce pain, release energy blockages (*see* page 927), and address factors that may be at the root of the common cold (*see* page 844).	**Of little use** Some case reports claim efficacy; however, success is probably seen, if at all, in only a small proportion of patients (*see* Placebo, page xxi).	**Requires a qualified practitioner** Practitioners should be properly qualified and should propose a treatment plan. No credence should be given to anyone promising immediate or total success. **Risks:** Manipulation of the cervical vertebrae can cause serious injury. Osteoporosis is one of several risk factors.

Treatment	Rating	Point of delivery/risks
Massage Classical massage (*see* page 847) can invigorate the patient, as well as ease muscular and perhaps also emotional tension. Lymphatic drainage (*see* page 850) is claimed to boost the body's defences.	**Of little use** Acceptable as a treatment attempt aimed at soothing and relaxing the patient. Whether lymphatic drainage does boost the body's defences is unclear. Case reports claim efficacy; however, success is probably seen in only a proportion of patients (*see* Placebo, page xxi).	**Suitable for DIY** Qualified guidance is essential. Masseurs/masseuses should be properly qualified. Lymphatic drainage requires a qualified practitioner. **Risks:** Some people are sensitive to manual stimuli; others find it hard to tolerate close physical contact.
Nutritional therapies An organic diet (*see* page 4) provides the body with essential and secondary plant nutrients that are believed to exercise a multitude of positive effects and to be capable, *inter alia*, of strengthening the immune system.	**Useful** as an individually directed supportive measure. There are suggestions that an organic diet can reduce the frequency and severity of colds.	**Suitable for DIY** Qualified guidance is recommended though not essential. **Risks:** Avoid imbalanced or intolerable diets. They can cause deficiencies with serious consequences. Children are particularly at risk.

Treatment	Rating	Point of delivery/risks
Physical therapies Steam inhalation, sweating, and local wraps (*see* pages 871–8) are claimed to alleviate symptoms and shorten the course of the common cold. Cold chest or torso wraps several times daily can be used to bring down high temperatures. If there is no fever, ascending temperature arm and foot baths, partial immersion baths with chest wraps, or packs may be beneficial.	**Useful** as an individually directed treatment attempt and as a preventive measure. Studies have shown vapor inhalation to achieve a degree of efficacy. Field studies also ascribe a degree of efficacy to the other procedures in some patients (*see* Placebo, page xxi). Regular saunas are **useful** as a preventive measure. Studies indicate that they have an undisputed beneficial effect. Once cold symptoms have developed, sweating is useful as an attempted treatment. Case reports claim efficacy; however, success is probably seen in only a proportion of patients (*see* Placebo, page xxi).	**Suitable for DIY** Qualified guidance is recommended though not essential. Therapists should be properly qualified. **Risks:** Persons running a temperature should not take a sauna. Skin damage may be caused in persons with diminished temperature sensation when extreme temperatures are applied.
Probiotics The introduction of certain bacteria into the gut is claimed to bring the intestinal flora back into balance and to have a beneficial effect on the immune system (*see* page 878).	Preparations that act specifically on the respiratory system **may be of some use**. Other preparations are possibly acceptable as a preventive measure in patients suffering from frequent or persistent colds. Case reports claim efficacy; however, success is probably seen in only a proportion of patients (*see* Placebo, page xxi).	**Requires a qualified practitioner** Practitioners should be properly qualified and should propose a treatment plan. Non-prescription formulations are suitable for do-it-yourself. **Risks:** Fairly unlikely provided treatment is carried out competently.

Treatment	*Rating*	*Point of delivery/risks*
Reflex therapies Heat treatments, reflex zone massage (*see* page 883), reflexology (*see* page 883), and TENS (*see* page 886) are claimed to act via reflex channels (*see* page 881) to ease pain, relax the patient, and exert a number of other beneficial effects.	**Of little use** Acceptable as a short-term treatment attempt aimed at alleviating pain. Field studies claim efficacy; however, success is probably seen in only a proportion of patients (*see* Placebo, page xxi). When compared, the various techniques appear to be equally effective, though the benefits they provide vary greatly from one person to another.	**Suitable for DIY** Qualified guidance is essential. Therapists should be properly qualified and should propose a treatment plan. **Risks:** Some people are sensitive to cold, electrical stimuli, and rubber electrodes; others find it hard to tolerate manual stimulation or close physical contact.
Relaxation techniques Autogenic training (*see* page 888), muscle relaxation according to Jacobson (*see* page 893), and various biofeedback techniques (*see* page 891) are said to relieve muscle tension and inner unrest, and might be instrumental in easing symptoms of the common cold.	**May be of some use** as a prevention against frequent colds and as a supportive treatment attempt. Case reports claim efficacy; however, success is probably seen in only a proportion of patients (*see* Placebo, page xxi).	**Suitable for DIY** Once a sound understanding of the technique has been acquired from a trainer in groups or through individual tuition, patients can perform exercises themselves. Therapists should be properly qualified. **Risks:** Fairly unlikely.
Vitamins and trace elements The antioxidative properties of beta-carotene, vitamins C and E, and selenium are, it is supposed, instrumental in countering the formation of free radicals and in boosting the body's antioxidative defence systems (*see* page 900).	**May be of some use** as a preventive measure. No definitive recommendations can be made based on present knowledge. The efficacy ascribed to these vitamins is probably seen in only a proportion of patients (*see* Placebo, page xxi).	**Suitable for DIY** Medical supervision is recommended though not essential. **Risks:** Intolerance and overdosage are possible. Recent reports imply that beta-carotene might increase the risk of cancer.

Herbal remedies for bronchitis

Active ingredient/preparation	Rating
Ivy leaves (*Hedera helix*)	Taken orally, ivy leaves **may be of some use** as a treatment attempt for chronic inflammation of the bronchial system. Antispasmodic and expectorant action. **Daily dose:** 0.3g herb. **Individual dose:** Pour 1 cup of hot water over 0.1–0.2g of the herb and infuse. Use ready-formulated preparations as instructed by the manufacturer/prescriber. **Risks:** Consult your doctor so as not to miss out on more appropriate treatments. There are no reports of serious side effects.
Thyme, common (*Thymus vulgaris*)	Common thyme taken orally **may be of some use** as a treatment for symptoms of bronchitis, whooping cough, and catarrh of the upper airways. It eases the expulsion of phlegm. **Daily dose:** 1–2g herb. **Individual dose:** Pour 1 cup of hot water over 1–2g of the herb and infuse. Use ready-formulated preparations as instructed by the manufacturer/prescriber. **Risks:** Common thyme can cause reversible gastrointestinal irritation.
Thyme, wild (*Thymus serpyllum*)	**May be of some use** for treating symptoms of bronchitis, whooping cough, and catarrh of the upper airways. Its action is antitussive. **Daily dose:** 1–2g herb. **Individual dose:** Pour 1 cup of hot water over 2g of the herb and infuse. For chest poultices use a 5 percent solution. **Risks:** Wild thyme can cause reversible gastrointestinal irritation.

Active ingredient/preparation	Rating
Turpentine oil (purified essential oil from *Pinus pinaster* or *Pinus australis*)	**Only useful** as an external treatment attempt for chronic bronchial infection producing copious amounts of phlegm. For use as an inhalation or embrocation. **Dosage:** In liquid and semi-solid formulations use in a 10–50 percent concentration. **Risks:** Turpentine oil must not be used by hypersensitive persons. Not to be inhaled in acute inflammation of the respiratory system. Extensive external use at high dosages can produce kidney and nerve damage. Do not apply to the nose and face of infants and young children.

Herbal remedies for coughs

Active ingredient/preparation	Rating
Coltsfoot flowers, aerial parts, and roots (*Tussilago farfara*)	**Not advised.** Coltsfoot flowers, aerial parts, and roots are given a negative assessment because there is no adequate proof of efficacy. **Risks:** Coltsfoot contains hepatotoxic and potentially carcinogenic substances (pyrrolizidine alkaloids).
Coltsfoot leaves (*Tussilago farfara*)	**Of little use.** Taken orally, coltsfoot may be acceptable as a treatment attempt for acute respiratory catarrh with coughing. **Daily dose:** 4.5–6g herb. **Individual dose:** Pour 1 cup of hot water over 2g of the dried leaves and infuse. Use ready-formulated preparations as instructed by the manufacturer/prescriber. **Risks:** Pyrrolizidine alkaloids contained in coltsfoot leaves are hepatotoxic and potentially carcinogenic. Do not use coltsfoot for more than four to six weeks per year.

Active ingredient/preparation	Rating
Cowslip root (*Primula veris*)	Taken orally, cowslip **may be of some use** as a treatment attempt for respiratory catarrh. Has a mucolytic and expectorant action. **Daily dose:** 0.5–1.5g herb. **Individual dose:** To prepare a decoction, bring 0.3g of the root to a boil with 1 cup of water. Use ready-formulated preparations as instructed by the manufacturer/prescriber. **Risks:** Cowslip may cause reversible gastrointestinal problems, and allergic reactions in sensitive individuals.
Ephedra root and aerial parts (*Ephedra sinica*)	**Useful** for treating conditions attended by slight bronchial spasm in adults and children of school age. **Dosage:** Use ready-formulated preparations as instructed by the manufacturer/prescriber. **Risks:** Sleeplessness, nausea, vomiting, difficulty in passing water, cardiac arrhythmia, and dependence at high dosages. Ephedra root and aerial parts contain ephedrine (in the UK ephedra is controlled under the Medicines Act 1968). Not to be taken by persons with high blood pressure, anxiety and restlessness, cataracts, circulatory problems, enlargement of the prostate with formation of residual urine in the bladder, adrenomedullary tumors, or an overactive thyroid.
Grindelia (*Grindelia robusta*)	**May be of some use** as a relaxing expectorant for respiratory catarrh. **Daily dose:** 4–6g herb. **Individual dose:** Pour 1 cup of hot water over 2g of the dried herb and infuse. Use ready-formulated preparations as instructed by the manufacturer/prescriber. **Risks:** May irritate the lining of the stomach. Large doses of grindelia may irritate the kidneys.

Active ingredient/preparation	Rating
Iceland moss (*Cetraria islandica*)	Taken orally, Iceland moss **may be of some use** as a treatment attempt for an irritable dry cough. Has a soothing and mildly antibacterial action. **Daily dose:** 4–6g herb. **Individual dose:** Pour 1 cup of hot water over 2g of shredded moss and infuse. Use ready-formulated preparations as instructed by the manufacturer/prescriber. **Risks:** Iceland moss is not known to have any serious side effects.
Ivy leaves (*Hedera helix*)	Taken orally, ivy leaves **may be of some use** as a treatment attempt for respiratory catarrh and for symptomatic treatment of chronic bronchial inflammation. **Daily dose:** 0.3g herb. **Individual dose:** Pour 1 cup of hot water over 0.2–0.3g of the herb and infuse. Use ready-formulated preparations as instructed by the manufacturer/prescriber. **Risks:** There are no reports of serious side effects. Many cough syrups contain sorbitol as a sweetener, which has a slight laxative effect.
Limeflowers (*Tilia cordata*)	Taken orally, limeflowers **may be of some use** as a treatment attempt for the common cold. Has a mucolytic action. **Daily dose:** 2–4g herb. **Individual dose:** Pour 1 cup of hot water over 1–2g of dried flowers and infuse. Use ready-formulated preparations as instructed by the manufacturer/prescriber. **Risks:** Limeflowers are not known to have any serious side effects.

Active ingredient/preparation	Rating

Licorice root (*Glycyrrhiza glabra* and other species)

May be of some use as a treatment attempt for upper respiratory catarrh. Has an expectorant and mucolytic action.
Daily dose: 5–15g root. **Individual dose:** As a decoction, 2–3g (½ teaspoon) of root to 1 cup of boiling water. Use ready-formulated preparations as instructed by the manufacturer/prescriber.
Risks: Prolonged use and high dosages may lead to edema, potassium deficiency, and high blood pressure. These effects can be amplified by simultaneous administration of diuretics. Not to be taken during pregnancy or by persons with liver disease, hypertension, or potassium deficiency. Do not take for longer than four to six weeks without consulting a doctor. Caution: Licorice increases sensitivity to digitalis.

Mallow leaves and flowers (*Malva sylvestris* and *neglecta*)

May be of some use for an irritable dry cough. Has a soothing effect.
Daily dose: 5g herb (leaves and flowers).
Individual dose: Pour 1 cup of hot water over 1–2g of the dried herb and infuse.
Risks: Mallow is not known to have any serious side effects.

Marsh mallow root and leaves (*Althaea officinalis*)

Taken orally, marsh mallow **may be of some use** as a treatment attempt for a dry cough. Has a soothing action.
Daily dose: 5g dried leaf or 6g dried root.
Individual dose: 1 cup of cold water to a dessertspoon of dried leaf or root. Allow it to stand for one to two hours, then heat and drink. Use ready-formulated preparations as instructed by the manufacturer/prescriber.
Risks: Marsh mallow may slow down the absorption and action of other drugs taken simultaneously.

Active ingredient/preparation	*Rating*

Mullein
(*Verbascum densiflorum*)

May be of some use as a treatment attempt for catarrh of the airways attended by coughing. Has a soothing action.
Daily dose: 3–4g herb.
Individual dose: Pour 1 cup of hot water over 1g of the herb and infuse.
Risks: Mullein is not known to have any serious side effects.

Ribwort
(*Plantago lanceolata*)

Taken orally, ribwort **may be of some use** as a treatment attempt for upper respiratory catarrh (attended by coughing).
It has a soothing expectorant action as well as being mildly antibacterial and astringent.
Daily dose: 3–6g herb. **Individual dose:** Pour 1 cup of hot water over 2–3g of the dried herb and infuse. Use ready-formulated preparations as instructed by the manufacturer/prescriber.
Risks: Ribwort is not known to have any serious side effects.

Snake root
(*Polygala senega*)

Taken orally, snake root **may be of some use** as an expectorant for upper respiratory catarrh.
Daily dose: 1.5–3g herb.
Individual dose: To prepare a decoction, pour 1 cup of hot water over 0.5–1g of the dried root. Use ready-formulated preparations as instructed by the manufacturer/prescriber.
Risks: Snake root taken for too long may cause gastrointestinal irritation.

Soapbark
(*Quillaja saponaria*)

Taken orally, soapbark **may be of some use** as an expectorant (irritation of the gastric mucosa stimulates production of mucus).
Daily dose: 1.5g bark. **Individual dose:** As a decoction, 0.5g bark to 1 cup of hot water.
Risks: Soapbark may cause unpleasant gastric irritation.

Active ingredient/preparation	Rating

Soapwort root
(*Saponaria officinalis*)

Taken orally, soapwort **may be of some use** as an expectorant for respiratory catarrh. **Daily dose:** 1.5g herb. **Individual dose:** Bring 0.5g of the root to a boil with water and simmer.
Risks: Soapwort may occasionally cause gastric irritation. Avoid high dosages: cytotoxic risk.

Sundew
(*Drosera rotundifolia*)

Taken orally, sundew **may be of some use** as a treatment attempt for a dry and paroxysmal cough. Has an antispasmodic and demulcent action.
Daily dose: 3g herb. **Individual dose:** Pour 1 cup of hot water over 1g of the dried herb and infuse. Use ready-formulated preparations as instructed by the manufacturer/prescriber.
Risks: Sundew is not known to have any serious side effects.

Thyme, common
(*Thymus vulgaris*)

May be of some use as a treatment attempt for symptoms of bronchitis, whooping-cough, and catarrh of the upper airways. Has an expectorant action.
Daily dose: 1–2g herb. **Individual dose:** Pour 1 cup of hot water over 1–2g of the dried herb and infuse. Use ready-formulated preparations as instructed by the manufacturer/prescriber.
Risks: Common thyme can cause reversible gastrointestinal irritation.

Vervain
(*Verbena officinalis*)

Of little use for coughs. Adequate proof of efficacy is lacking. It may have an expectorant action on upper respiratory catarrh.
Daily dose: 4.5–6g dried herb. **Individual dose:** Pour 1 cup of hot water over 1.5g of the dried herb and infuse.
Risks: Vervain is not known to have any serious side effects.

Herbal remedies for sniffles and sneezes

Active ingredient/preparation	Rating
Elderflowers (*Sambucus nigra*)	**Only useful** as a diaphoretic in the feverish patient. Also promotes bronchial secretion. **Daily dose:** 6–12g herb. Pour 1 pint of boiling water over 5 heaped teaspoons of dried or fresh blossoms, infuse for 10 minutes, then add the juice of half a lemon and 2 teaspoons of honey. This should be drunk hot. **Individual dose:** 3g. Use ready-formulated preparations as instructed by the manufacturer/prescriber. **Risks:** Elderflowers are not known to have any serious side effects.
Eucalyptus leaves (*Eucalyptus globulus*)	**May be of some use** as a treatment attempt for symptoms of the common cold. The action and side effects are the same as for eucalyptus oil (*see* below). **Daily dose:** 4–6g herb. **Individual dose:** Pour 1 cup of hot water over 2g of leaves and infuse. Use ready-formulated preparations as instructed by the manufacturer/prescriber. As eucalyptus leaves infused in hot water release only a small amount of their volatile oil, inhalation with an isolated oil or tincture is to be preferred. **Risks:** Nausea, vomiting, and diarrhea are possible, but reversible.

Active ingredient/preparation	Rating

Eucalyptus oil
(*Eucalyptus globulus*)

Only useful as a treatment attempt for colds when inhaled or rubbed into the chest. It is a mucolytic, mild antispasmodic, and local circulatory stimulant.
Daily dose: Used internally, 0.05–0.2ml oil; externally, 5–20 percent in oily preparations, 5–10 percent in alcoholic formulations. To prepare an inhalation, place 1 dessertspoon of the dried herb, 1 teaspoon of cream or balsam, or 15 drops of volatile oil in a bowl of hot water, cover the head and bowl with a towel, and inhale the vapors alternately through the mouth and nose. Use ready-formulated preparations as instructed by the manufacturer/prescriber.
Risks: Nausea, vomiting, diarrhea, and allergic skin reactions are possible. Not to be used internally by persons with gastritis, enteritis, gall bladder disease, or severe liver disease. Do not apply to the nose and face of infants and young children. Undiluted eucalyptus oil is toxic and should not be taken internally unless suitably diluted.

German camomile
(*Chamomilla recutita*)

Only useful as a supportive treatment attempt for bacterial inflammation of the oral cavity, gums, and lungs; also as an inhalation.
Daily dose: 10–12g herb. **Individual dose:** Pour 1 cup of hot water over 3g of dried leaves and infuse. Use ready-formulated preparations as instructed by the manufacturer/prescriber.
Risks: German camomile may provoke powerful allergic reactions.

Active ingredient/preparation	Rating
Herbal remedies in combination with chemical ingredients	**Of little use**. Pure herbal or pure chemical remedies should be used in preference, as the nasal mucosa may be damaged by long-term use of combination preparations containing chemical ingredients. Combination preparations with ephedrine, xylometazoline, or oxymetazoline are **not advised**.
Hibiscus flowers (*Hibiscus sabdarifla*)	**Of little use** as a remedy for respiratory catarrh; proof of efficacy is lacking. Not suitable as a vitamin C reserve. **Daily dose:** 4–6g herb. **Individual dose:** 1–2g of dried flowers to 1 cup of hot water. **Risks:** Hibiscus is not known to have any serious side effects.
Limeflowers (*Tilia cordata*)	**Only useful** as a supportive treatment attempt for symptoms of the common cold in the feverish patient. **Daily dose:** 2–4g herb. **Individual dose:** Pour 1 cup of hot water over 1–2g of flowers and infuse. Use ready-formulated preparations as instructed by the manufacturer/prescriber. **Risks:** Limeflowers are not known to have any serious side effects.
Meadowsweet flowers and leaves (*Filipendula ulmaria*)	**Only useful** as a supportive treatment attempt for the common cold. **Daily dose:** 2.5–3.5g meadowsweet flowers or 4–5g leaves. **Individual dose:** Pour 1 cup of hot water over 1g of flowers or leaves and infuse. Use ready-formulated preparations as instructed by the manufacturer/prescriber. **Risks:** Meadowsweet should not be taken by aspirin-sensitive persons.

Active ingredient/preparation	Rating

Mint oil
(*Mentha arvensis* var.
piperascens)

Only useful as a treatment attempt for the common cold in the form of an inhalation.
Daily dose: 3–4 drops as an inhalation twice or three times a day. Use ready-formulated preparations as instructed by the manufacturer/prescriber.
Risks: Gastric problems are possible. Not to be used in inflammation or occlusion of the gall bladder or serious liver disease. If you have gall stones or gravel, ask your GP before using mint oil. Do not apply to the nose and face of infants and young children.

Peppermint oil
(*Mentha piperita*)

Only useful as a treatment attempt in the form of an inhalation or as an externally applied remedy for upper respiratory catarrh.
Daily dose: 3–4 drops as an inhalation twice or three times a day. Use ready-formulated preparations as instructed by the manufacturer/prescriber.
Risks: Allergic skin reactions are possible. Do not apply to the nose and face of infants and young children.

Rose hips
(*Rosae pseudofructus*)

Of little use for the common cold; the vitamin C content decreases rapidly during storage.
Daily dose: 8–10g hips. **Individual dose:** For a decoction, 2g of rose hips to 1 cup of hot water.
Risks: Rose hips are not known to have any serious side effects.

Herbal remedies used supportively in colds

Active ingredient/preparation	Rating
Elderflowers (*Sambucus nigra*)	**Only useful** as a diaphoretic in the feverish patient. Also promotes bronchial secretion. **Daily dose:** 10–15g herb. Pour 1 pint of boiling water over 5 heaped teaspoons of dried or fresh blossoms, infuse for 10 minutes, then add the juice of half a lemon and 2 teaspoons of honey. This should be drunk hot. **Individual dose:** 3g. Use ready-formulated preparations as instructed by the manufacturer/prescriber. **Risks:** Elderflowers are not known to have any serious side effects.
Limeflowers (*Tilia cordata*)	**Only useful** as a supportive treatment attempt for symptoms of the common cold in the feverish patient who needs to "sweat it out." **Daily dose:** 2–4g herb. **Individual dose:** Pour 1 cup of hot water over 1–2g of flowers and infuse. Use ready-formulated preparations as instructed by the manufacturer/prescriber. **Risks:** Limeflowers are not known to have any serious side effects.
Meadowsweet (*Filipendula ulmaria*)	**Only useful** as a supportive treatment attempt for the common cold. **Daily dose:** 2.5–3.5g meadowsweet flowers or 4–5g leaves. **Individual dose:** Pour 1 cup of hot water over 1g of flowers or leaves and infuse for 20 minutes. Use ready-formulated preparations as instructed by the manufacturer/prescriber. **Risks:** Meadowsweet should not be taken by aspirin-sensitive persons.

Active ingredient/preparation	Rating
Willow bark (*Salix fragilis*)	**May be of some use** as a treatment attempt for cold symptoms, aching limbs, and headaches in the feverish patient. Willow bark is a febrifuge, analgesic, and anti-inflammatory agent. **Daily dose:** 6–12g bark. **Individual dose:** For a decoction, 1 cup of hot water to 2g of bark. Use ready-formulated preparations as instructed by the manufacturer/prescriber. **Risks:** Skin allergies, asthmatic symptoms (bronchospasm), and gastrointestinal problems are possible. Precautions associated with salicylate are also applicable to willow.

Hoarseness and laryngitis

Causes and symptoms

Laryngitis is acute inflammation of the voicebox (larynx), usually caused by a viral infection but due in some cases to bacterial inflammation. In addition, hoarseness can be brought on by airborne pollutants, cigarette smoke, chemicals that irritate the mucosa, or overuse of the voice through loud singing or shouting.

Orthodox treatment

Treatment mostly involves various forms of therapy including inhalations and fomentations. Suitable painkillers and nasal decongestants are also sometimes used. Antibiotic treatment is only appropriate when the condition is caused by bacterial infection.

Complementary therapies

Non-orthodox therapists make wide use of physical therapies and herbal remedies. In recurrent infection they may also seek to stimulate the immune system. Various forms of reflexology and similar practices are applied to provide relief from pain and other symptoms. Inhalations will possibly alleviate symptoms.

Treatment plan and limited trial

Before administering a complementary treatment, every therapist should propose a treatment plan (*see* page xxiii) that sets out a clear time frame and defines the goal that the treatment is designed to achieve. Treatment should then be tried for a limited term to test the patient's response.

Caution

Chronic hoarseness may also be caused by a serious disorder such as a malignant tumor. If hoarseness persists, you must see your doctor.

Complementary treatments for hoarseness and laryngitis

Treatment	Rating	Point of delivery/risks
Acupuncture Acupuncture in its various forms (*see* page 772) aims to encourage the flow of energy (*see* page 927) or to relieve symptoms directly. The acupuncture points chosen can vary from one practitioner to another.	**Of little use** Possibly acceptable as a short-term treatment attempt for frequent or recurrent hoarseness. Case reports claim efficacy; however, success is probably seen in only a proportion of patients (*see* Placebo, page xxi).	**Requires a qualified practitioner** Practitioners should be properly qualified and should propose a treatment plan. **Risks:** Probably rare provided treatment is carried out competently.
Anthroposophical medicine Inflammation is treated with foot baths, compresses around the lower legs, or sweating from the extremities. AM also uses specially tailored drugs (*see* page 781).	**May be of some use** as a short-term treatment attempt. Some studies claim efficacy; however, success is probably seen in only a proportion of patients (*see* Placebo, page xxi).	**Requires a qualified practitioner** Practitioners should be properly qualified and should propose a treatment plan. **Risks:** Allergies and intolerance are possible.

Treatment	Rating	Point of delivery/risks
Aromatherapy Essential oils (*see* page 786) are used to soothe and relax, or to invigorate the patient, thereby helping to ease symptoms. The essences may be taken orally, used externally as massage oils or bathing emulsions, or inhaled as vapors.	**Of little use** Acceptable as a short-term, supportive treatment attempt aimed as soothing and relaxing the patient. Some case reports claim efficacy; however, success is probably seen in only a proportion of patients (*see* Placebo, page xxi).	**Suitable for DIY** Qualified guidance is recommended. The effects of individual essential oils differ widely. **Risks:** Allergies or intolerance are possible. Some oils are carcinogenic in test systems and possibly in humans.
Bioresonance therapy Bioresonance therapists use electrical devices in an attempt to discover the causes of illness and claim to be able to weaken or turn around pathogenic energies and disease related vibrations (*see* page 794).	**Of little use** Possibly acceptable as a short-term, supportive treatment attempt for recurrent or persistent hoarseness when simpler, more established methods have been unsuccessful. Some case reports claim efficacy; however, success is probably seen, if at all, in only a small proportion of patients (*see* Placebo, page xxi).	**Requires a qualified practitioner** Practitioners should be properly qualified and should propose a treatment plan. No credence should be given to anyone promising immediate or total success. **Risks:** Fairly unlikely.
Electroneural therapy according to Croon According to the theory, readings taken at various reactive sites on the skin highlight diseased areas within the body. Based on these readings, targeted electrostimulative measures can be undertaken to address the causes of hoarseness (*see* page 806).	**Of little use** Possibly acceptable as a short-term treatment attempt for recurrent or persistent hoarseness when simpler, more established methods have been unsuccessful. Some case reports claim efficacy; however, success is probably seen, if at all, in only a small proportion of patients (*see* Placebo, page xxi).	**Requires a qualified practitioner** Practitioners should be properly qualified and should propose a treatment plan. No credence should be given to anyone promising immediate or total success. **Risks:** Proponents themselves warn that treatment should not be given in acute inflammatory conditions.

Treatment	Rating	Point of delivery/risks
Flower remedies Flower remedies (*see* page 828) are said to restore emotional balance and assist the body's psychic ability to heal itself. Bach Rescue Remedy is recommended for severe symptoms.	**Of little use** Acceptable as a short-term, supportive treatment attempt aimed at soothing and relaxing the patient. Case reports claim efficacy; however, success is probably seen in only a proportion of patients (*see* Placebo, page xxi).	**Suitable for DIY** Qualified guidance is recommended. Practitioners should propose a treatment plan. **Risks:** Possible intolerance.
Homeopathy Highly diluted (potentized) solutions (*see* page 831) are believed to be able to redress vital energy imbalances. Organo- and functiotropic (*see* page 833) homeopathy is claimed to be effective for dealing directly with hoarseness.	**May be of some use** as a short-term treatment attempt for recurrent hoarseness. Some case reports claim efficacy for homeopathic treatments; however, success is probably seen in only a proportion of patients (*see* Placebo, page xxi).	**Requires a qualified practitioner** Homeopaths should be properly qualified and should propose a treatment plan. Ready-formulated preparations are suitable for do-it-yourself. **Risks:** Allergies and intolerance are possible.
Hypnosis and self-hypnosis In the relaxed and generally altered state of awareness that is induced in hypnosis or self-hypnosis (*see* page 837), physical and mental conditions can be addressed. The relaxation and emotional balance thus achieved is claimed to be instrumental in alleviating psychosomatically induced hoarseness.	**Of little use** Possibly acceptable as a short-term treatment attempt for recurrent and persistent hoarseness when simpler, more established methods have been unsuccessful. Some case reports claim efficacy; however, success is probably seen in only a proportion of patients treated (*see* Placebo, page xxi).	**Requires a qualified practitioner** Hypnotherapists should be properly qualified and should propose a treatment plan. No credence should be given to anyone promising immediate or total success. **Risks:** Unlikely provided treatment is carried out competently.

Treatment	Rating	Point of delivery/risks
Manual therapies Chiropractors and osteopaths use a series of manipulations to realign allegedly displaced vertebrae which, it is believed, might be responsible for hoarseness. This is said to release energy blockages (*see* page 927) and address factors that may be at the root of hoarseness (*see* page 844).	**Of little use** Possibly acceptable as a short-term treatment attempt for chronic and persistent hoarseness when less risky, more established methods have been unsuccessful. Some case reports claim efficacy for this potentially risky procedure; however, success is probably seen, if at all, in only a small proportion of patients (*see* Placebo, page xxi).	**Requires a qualified practitioner** Practitioners should be properly qualified and should propose a treatment plan. **Risks:** Manipulation of the cervical vertebrae can cause serious injury. Osteoporosis is one of several risk factors.
Physical therapies Gargling with teas (e.g. sage, camomile), ascending temperature arm baths, chest and neck wraps, alternating temperature washes, ascending and alternating temperature foot baths, arm and knee douches, and saunas (*see* pages 871–8) are claimed to tone up the system and alleviate hoarseness.	**Useful** as an individually tailored treatment attempt. Case reports and field studies claim efficacy; however, success is probably seen in only a proportion of patients (*see* Placebo, page xxi).	**Suitable for DIY** Qualified guidance is recommended though not essential. Therapists should be properly qualified. **Risks:** Skin damage may be caused to persons with diminished temperature sensation when extreme temperatures are applied.
Reflex therapies Reflex zone massage (*see* page 883), reflexology (*see* page 883), and TENS (*see* page 886) are claimed act via so-called reflex channels (*see* page 881) to relax the patient and provide a multitude of other benefits.	**Of little use** Possibly acceptable as a short-term treatment attempt for recurrent or persistent hoarseness when more established methods have been unsuccessful. Some case reports claim efficacy; however, success is probably seen in only a proportion of patients (*see* Placebo, page xxi).	**Suitable for DIY** Qualified guidance is essential. Therapists should be properly qualified and should propose a treatment plan. **Risks:** Some people are sensitive to electrical stimuli and rubber electrodes; others find it hard to tolerate manual stimulation or close physical contact.

Treatment	Rating	Point of delivery/risks
Relaxation techniques Autogenic training (*see* page 888), muscle relaxation according to Jacobson (*see* page 893), and various biofeedback techniques (*see* page 891) are said to relieve muscle tension and inner unrest, and might be instrumental in alleviating psychosomatically induced hoarseness.	**May be of some use** as a preventive measure and as a supportive treatment attempt. Some case reports claim efficacy; however, success is probably seen in only a proportion of patients (*see* Placebo, page xxi).	**Suitable for DIY** Once a sound understanding of the technique has been acquired from a trainer in groups or through individual tuition, patients can perform exercises themselves. Therapists should propose a treatment plan. **Risks:** Fairly unlikely.

Herbal remedies for hoarseness and laryngitis

Active ingredient/preparation	Rating
Coltsfoot leaves (*Tussilago farfara*)	**Of little use** as a locally administered treatment attempt for hoarseness (as a gargle) and acute mouth and throat infections (as a mouthwash). Do not swallow. **Individual dose:** Take 0.6–2g of the dried herb by decoction three times daily. **Risks:** Pyrrolizidine alkaloids contained in coltsfoot leaves are hepatotoxic and potentially carcinogenic. Do not use for longer than four to six weeks per year.
Rhatany root (*Krameria triandra*)	**Only useful** as a gargle for local treatment of mild inflammatory infections of the mouth and throat. Has an astringent action. **Daily dose:** 1–2g root to 1 cup of warm water or 5–10 drops of tincture to a glass of water for gargling; gargle or rinse two or three times daily. **Risks:** Rhatany root may cause allergic mucosal reactions. Do not use for longer than two weeks except on a doctor's advice.

Active ingredient/preparation	Rating

Sage leaves
(*Salvia officinalis*)

Only useful as a gargle for inflammation of the mouth and throat or as an infusion. Has an astringent and antibacterial action, as well as supposedly inhibiting viral growth. **Individual dose:** 1–1.5g leaves to 5fl oz water. **Daily dose:** 4–6g herb or 2.7–7.5g tincture diluted in water.
Risks: Alcoholic extracts of the herb may lead to cramps if used for long periods of time. Caution: Use sage remedies carefully and avoid altogether during pregnancy. Avoid overdosage (more than 15g per dose); sage leaves contain small quantities of thujone, which is toxic.

Tormentil root
(*Potentilla erecta*)

Only useful as a mouthwash and gargle for oral and pharyngeal affections and hoarseness. Has an astringent action.
Daily dose: 4–6g herb. **Individual dose:** As a decoction for gargling, 1–2g of rhizome to 1 cup of hot water. Use ready-formulated preparations as instructed by the manufacturer/prescriber.
Risks: Tormentil may cause reversible gastric problems.

Mouth ulcers

Causes and symptoms

Mouth ulcers are tiny sores that appear on the tongue, the inside of the cheeks, and gums, and are usually associated with viral, bacterial, or fungal infection, stress, mechanical problems of dentition, antibiotics, chemotherapy, radiation therapy, alcohol, poisoning, nicotine, or vitamin deficiency. Occasionally mouth ulcers are the result of diabetes, cancer, leukemia, rheumatic disease, or diseases of the liver or gut. They are often a sign that the person is run down. The sores can be extremely painful and may, on occasion, make eating difficult.

Mouth ulcers may lead to a number of problems ranging from loss of appetite (*see* page 583) and halitosis to cancerous growths (*see* Cancer, page 701). Always consult a doctor or dentist if mouth ulcers fail to heal or become a recurrent problem.

Orthodox treatment

Where there is an underlying disease, this will be addressed. Treatment also concentrates on alleviating acute symptoms, for which a number of approaches are adopted: analgesic and disinfecting mouthwashes, various locally applied medications, and vitamin supplements. Prophylactic measures to discourage superinfection (with fungi, for instance) are sometimes undertaken. Doctors will generally encourage smokers to cut down.

Counselling or behavioral therapy is sometimes recommended when mouth ulcers are persistent.

Complementary therapies

Some complementary procedures focus on pain relief or address a presumed immune deficiency. Others aim to promote relaxation and to eliminate stress and emotional conflicts as a precipitating factor.

Certain therapies interpret mouth ulcers as being caused by environmental pollutants or disease-causing foci (*see* page 928), as a constitutional problem (*see* Constitution, page 927) or as a life force imbalance (*see* Life force, page 929).

Treatment plan and limited trial

Before administering a complementary treatment, every therapist should propose a treatment plan (*see* page xxiii) that sets out a clear time frame and defines the goal that the treatment is designed to achieve. Treatment should then be tried for a limited term to test the patient's response.

Caution

Before receiving a complementary treatment for chronic mouth ulcers, see a doctor to rule out a possible serious disease as the root cause.

Complementary treatments for mouth ulcers

Treatment	Rating	Point of delivery/risks
Acupuncture Acupuncture in its various forms (*see* page 772) aims to encourage the flow of energy (*see* page 927) or to act directly to prevent mouth ulcers and relieve symptoms.	**May be of some use** as a short-term treatment attempt aimed at alleviating pain. Case reports and field studies claim efficacy; however, success is probably seen in only a proportion of patients (*see* Placebo, page xxi).	**Requires a qualified practitioner** Practitioners should be properly qualified and should propose a treatment plan. **Risks:** Probably rare provided treatment is carried out competently.
Aromatherapy Essential oils (*see* page 786) are used to soothe and relax, or to invigorate, so assisting in the relief of symptoms. The essences may be taken orally, used externally as massage oils or bathing emulsions, or inhaled as vapors.	**Of little use** Acceptable as a short-term, supportive treatment attempt aimed at soothing and relaxing the patient. Some case reports claim efficacy for this procedure in the treatment of inflammation of the oral cavity; however, success is probably seen in only a small proportion of patients (*see* Placebo, page xxi).	**Suitable for DIY** Qualified guidance is recommended. The effects of individual essential oils differ widely. **Risks:** Allergies or intolerance are possible. Some oils are carcinogenic in test systems and possibly in humans.
Bioresonance therapy Bioresonance therapists use electrical devices in an attempt to discover the causes of illness and claim to be able to weaken or turn around pathogenic energies and disease related vibrations (*see* page 794).	**Of little use** Possibly acceptable as a short-term treatment attempt for chronic, recurrent, and persistent inflammation and when simpler, more established methods have been unsuccessful. Some case reports claim efficacy; however, success is probably seen, if at all, in only a small proportion of patients (*see* Placebo, page xxi).	**Requires a qualified practitioner** Practitioners should be properly qualified and should propose a treatment plan. No credence should be given to anyone promising immediate or total success. **Risks:** Fairly unlikely.

Treatment	Rating	Point of delivery/risks
Cell therapy Injecting or ingesting products extracted from the tissues of newborn animals or animal fetuses is said to have a rejuvenating and revitalizing effect and to enhance the healing of human tissues and organs (*see* page 796).	**Not advised** Based on present knowledge, there is inadequate evidence of the efficacy and mode of action of these costly and relatively risky procedures.	**Risks:** Injecting foreign proteins into the body can provoke (possibly fatal) allergic reactions. Also, pathogens such as those that cause bovine spongiform encephalopathy (BSE) or other serious infections may be introduced.
Electroacupuncture according to Voll By taking readings of the electrical conductivity of the skin (*see* page 802), therapists claim to be able to derive an insight into diseased areas of the body, pathogenic foci (*see* page 928), and stress factors (*see* Toxins, page 929). The supposed causes of inflammation can then be addressed.	**Of little use** Possibly acceptable as a short-term, supportive treatment attempt for chronic, recurrent, and persistent inflammation and when simpler, more established methods have been unsuccessful. Some case reports claim efficacy; however, success is probably seen, if at all, in only a small proportion of patients (*see* Placebo, page xxi).	**Requires a qualified practitioner** Practitioners should be properly qualified and should propose a treatment plan. No credence should be given to anyone promising immediate or total success. **Risks:** A second opinion must always be obtained from a qualified physician before any attempt is made to "eliminate foci" (e.g. by surgery).
Electroneural therapy according to Croon According to the theory, readings taken at various reactive sites on the skin highlight diseased areas within the body. Based on these readings, targeted electrostimulative measures can be undertaken to address the causes of inflammation (*see* page 806).	**Of little use** Possibly acceptable as a short-term, supportive treatment attempt when simpler, more established methods have been unsuccessful. Some case reports claim efficacy; however, success is probably seen, if at all, in only a small proportion of patients (*see* Placebo, page xxi).	**Requires a qualified practitioner** Practitioners should be properly qualified and should propose a treatment plan. No credence should be given to anyone promising immediate or total success. **Risks:** Proponents themselves warn that treatment should not be given in acute inflammatory conditions.

Treatment	Rating	Point of delivery/risks
Enzyme therapy The enzymes used are said to dispel and destroy "immune complexes" (*see* page 824) that course in the blood and that are responsible, for instance, for sustaining inflammatory processes.	**Of little use** Some case reports claim efficacy for this little researched therapy; however, success is probably seen in only a small proportion of patients (*see* Placebo, page xxi).	**Requires a qualified practitioner** Practitioners should propose a treatment plan. Non-prescription preparations are suitable for do-it-yourself. **Risks:** Allergies or intolerance are possible.
Flower remedies Flower remedies (*see* page 828) are said to restore emotional balance and assist the body's psychic ability to heal itself.	**Of little use** Acceptable as a short-term treatment attempt aimed at soothing and relaxing. Some case reports claim efficacy for this procedure in the treatment of inflammation of the oral cavity; however, success is probably seen in only a small proportion of patients (*see* Placebo, page xxi).	**Suitable for DIY** Qualified guidance is recommended. Practitioners should propose a treatment plan. **Risks:** Possible intolerance.
Homeopathy Highly diluted (potentized) solutions (*see* page 831) are believed to be able to redress vital energy imbalances. Organo- and functiotropic (*see* page 833) homeopathy is claimed to be effective for dealing with mouth ulcers.	**Of little use** Possibly acceptable as a short-term, supportive treatment attempt. Some case reports claim success for homeopathic treatments; however, success is probably seen in only a proportion of patients (*see* Placebo, page xxi).	**Requires a qualified practitioner** Homeopaths should be properly qualified and should propose a treatment plan. Ready-formulated preparations are suitable for do-it-yourself. **Risks:** Allergies and intolerance are possible.

Treatment	Rating	Point of delivery/risks
Manual therapies Chiropractors and osteopaths use a series of manipulations to realign allegedly displaced vertebrae. This, it is believed, stops dysfunctions, releases energy blockages (*see* page 927), and eliminates factors presumed to be instrumental in the causation of mouth ulcers (*see* page 841).	**Of little use** Possibly acceptable as a short-term treatment attempt for chronic complaints when less risky, more established methods have been unsuccessful. Some case reports claim efficacy for this potentially risky procedure; however, success is probably seen, if at all, in only a small proportion of patients (*see* Placebo, page xxi).	**Requires a qualified practitioner** Practitioners should be properly qualified and should propose a treatment plan. **Risks:** Spinal manipulations can cause serious injury. Osteoporosis is one of several risk factors.
Nutritional therapies An organic diet (*see* page 4) provides the body with essential and secondary plant nutrients that are believed to exercise a multitude of positive effects and to be capable, *inter alia*, of boosting the immune system (*see* page 10).	**Useful** as an individually directed supportive measure. Elimination and rotation diets may be of some assistance in identifying the cause of food allergy induced ulcers.	**Suitable for DIY** Qualified guidance is recommended. See your doctor before starting an elimination or rotation diet. **Risks:** Avoid imbalanced or intolerable diets. They can cause deficiencies with serious consequences. Children are particularly at risk.
Physical therapies Neck wraps, tongue brushing, cold face douches, gargles, mouth rinses, and inhalations with herbal additives are said to inhibit inflammation and ease symptoms (*see* page 867).	**Useful** as a short-term treatment attempt. Some case reports and field studies claim efficacy; however, success is probably seen in only a proportion of patients (*see* Placebo, page xxi).	**Suitable for DIY** Qualified guidance is recommended though not essential. **Risks:** Skin damage may be caused to persons with diminished temperature sensation when extreme temperatures are applied.

Treatment	Rating	Point of delivery/risks
Probiotics The introduction of certain bacteria into the gut is claimed to bring the intestinal flora back into balance and to have a beneficial effect on the immune system (*see* page 878).	**Of little use** Possibly acceptable as a short-term treatment attempt aimed at persistent complaints when more established methods have been unsuccessful. Some case reports claim efficacy; however, success is probably seen in only a small proportion of patients (*see* Placebo, page xxi).	**Requires a qualified practitioner** Practitioners should be properly qualified and should propose a treatment plan. Non-prescription formulations are suitable for do-it-yourself. **Risks:** Fairly unlikely provided treatment is carried out competently.
Relaxation techniques Autogenic training (*see* page 888), muscle relaxation according to Jacobson (*see* page 893), and various biofeedback techniques (*see* page 891) are said to relieve muscle tension and inner unrest, and might be instrumental in helping the patient become more aware of his/her physical and emotional states.	**May be of some use** as a treatment attempt for persistent symptoms. Some case reports claim efficacy for this procedure in the treatment of inflammation of the oral cavity; however, success is probably seen in only a small proportion of patients (*see* Placebo, page xxi).	**Suitable for DIY** Once a sound understanding of the technique has been acquired from a trainer in groups or through individual tuition, patients can perform exercises themselves. Therapists should propose a treatment plan. **Risks:** Fairly unlikely.
TENS The use of low frequency electrical currents on the surface of the skin is said to act through so-called reflex channels (*see* page 886) to ease the soreness of mouth inflammation and ulcers.	**May be of some use** as a short-term treatment attempt aimed at alleviating pain. Case reports and field studies claim efficacy; however, success is probably seen in only a proportion of patients (*see* Placebo, page xxi).	**Requires a qualified practitioner** Practitioners should be properly qualified and should propose a treatment plan. **Risks:** Some people react sensitively to electrical stimuli or rubber electrodes.

Treatment	Rating	Point of delivery/risks
Vitamins and trace elements The antioxidative properties of beta-carotene, vitamins C and E, and selenium are, it is supposed, instrumental in countering the formation of free radicals and boosting the body's defences (*see* page 900).	**May be of some use** as a short-term treatment attempt. Case reports and field studies claim efficacy; however, success is probably seen in only a proportion of patients (*see* Placebo, page xxi).	**Suitable for DIY** Medical supervision is recommended though not essential. **Risks:** Intolerance and overdosage are possible. Recent findings imply that beta-carotene might increase the risk of cancer.

Herbal remedies for mouth ulcers

Active ingredient/preparation	Rating
Tincture of camomile in combination with other herbal or chemical ingredients	**Of little use**. Pure camomile extract is sufficient on its own. **Dosage:** Use ready-formulated preparations as instructed by the manufacturer/ prescriber. **Risks:** Allergic skin reactions are possible.
Coltsfoot leaves (*Tussilago farfara*)	**Of little use** as a locally administered treatment attempt for hoarseness (as a gargle) and acute mild inflammation of the mouth and throat (as a mouthwash). **Daily dose:** 4.5–6g herb. **Individual dose:** Pour 1 cup of hot water over 1.5g of dried leaves, infuse, and use as a mouthwash or gargle. **Risks:** Pyrrolizidine alkaloids contained in coltsfoot leaves are hepatotoxic and potentially carcinogenic. Do not use for longer than four to six weeks per year. Do not swallow.

Active ingredient/preparation	*Rating*

Marsh mallow leaves and root
(*Althaea officinalis*)

Only useful as a gargle for treating oral and pharyngeal irritation. Has a soothing effect.
Daily dose: 5g leaves or 6g root. **Individual dose:** For use as a gargle, 2g to 1 cup of water (prepare cold, wait one to two hours, then use).
Risks: Marsh mallow may slow down the absorption and action of other drugs taken simultaneously.

Mint oil
(*Mentha arvensis* var. *piperascens*)

Only useful as a mouthwash for treating inflammation of the mouth and throat. Mint oil is a mild antibacterial agent.
Dosage: Use ready-formulated preparations as instructed by the manufacturer/prescriber; otherwise dissolve a few drops in warm water and rinse.
Risks: Gastric problems are possible. May also irritate the skin, in particular the mucosa. If you have gallstones or gravel, ask your doctor before using mint oil. Not to be used by persons with gall bladder occlusion, cholecystitis, or severe liver disease. Do not apply to the nose and face of infants and young children.

Myrrh
(*Commiphora molmol*)

Only useful as a locally administered treatment for slight inflammation of the mouth and throat. Has an astringent action.
Dosage: Apply diluted two to three times a day or, as a mouthwash or gargle, use 5–10 drops in 150ml of water.
Risks: Myrrh can cause skin irritation.

Rhatany root
(*Krameria triandra*)

Only useful for the treatment of mild inflammation of the mouth and throat. Has an astringent action.
Daily dose: 3g root. **Individual dose:** As a decoction for gargling or rinsing, 1g root to 1 cup of hot water, or 5–10 drops of tincture to a glass of water for gargling; gargle or rinse two to three times daily. Use ready-formulated preparations as instructed by the manufacturer/prescriber.
Risks: Rhatany root may cause allergic mucosal reactions. Do not use for longer than two weeks except on a doctor's advice.

Active ingredient/preparation	*Rating*
Ribwort (*Plantago lanceolata*)	**Only useful** as a gargle for local treatment of inflammation of the mouth and throat. Ribwort is an astringent. **Daily dose:** 3–6g herb. **Individual dose:** as an infusion for gargling, 2g of dried herb to 1 cup of hot water. **Risks:** Ribwort is not known to have any serious side effects.
Sage leaves (*Salvia officinalis*)	**Only useful** as a mouthwash for inflammation of the mouth and throat or as an infusion. Has an astringent and antibacterial action, as well as supposedly inhibiting viral growth. **Daily dose:** 4–6g herb. **Individual dose:** 1–1.5g leaves to 1 cup of warm water. Use ready-formulated preparations as instructed by the manufacturer/prescriber. **Risks:** Alcoholic extracts of the herb may lead to cramps if used for long periods of time. Caution: Use sage remedies carefully and avoid altogether in pregnancy. Avoid overdosage (more than 15g per dose); sage leaves contain small quantities of thujone, which is toxic.
Preparations containing Sage oil together with various other herbal ingredients	**Of little use.** Such preparations often contain more than ten ingredients, the need for which is questionable. **Dosage:** Use ready-formulated preparations as instructed by the manufacturer/ prescriber. **Risks:** The pure oil and alcoholic extracts of the herb may lead to cramps if used for long periods of time. Caution: Use these remedies carefully and avoid altogether during pregnancy. Avoid overdosage.
Tormentil root (*Potentilla erecta*)	**Only useful** for local treatment of inflammation of the mouth and throat. Has an astringent action. **Daily dose:** 4–6g herb. **Individual dose:** as a decoction for gargling, 2g of herb to 1 cup of hot water; or 10–20 drops of tincture three to four times daily. **Risks:** Tormentil may cause gastric problems.

Active ingredient/preparation	Rating
White dead nettle flowers (*Lamium album*)	**Only useful** for local treatment of inflammation of the mouth and throat. **Daily dose:** 3g herb. **Individual dose:** As a gargle or mouthwash, 1g dried flowering tops to 1 cup of hot water. **Risks:** White dead nettle is not known to have any serious side effects.
Witch hazel leaves (*Hamamelis virginiana*)	**Only useful** as a mouth and throat rinse. It is an astringent, mild anti-inflammatory agent, and anti-hemorrhagic. **Daily dose:** 0.1–1g dried leaves. **Individual dose:** Pour 1 cup of hot water over 0.5g of leaves and infuse. **Risks:** Witch hazel is not known to have any serious side effects.

Pneumonia

Causes and symptoms

Pneumonia is inflammation of one or both lungs through bacterial, viral, or fungal infection, through a foreign body, or through exposure to a chemical irritant. If the immune system is suppressed for any reason (e.g. in AIDS), the person's chances of contracting pneumonia increase.

Symptoms vary widely depending on the causative agent and frequently include high temperature, shivering attacks, malaise, headache, and general aches and pains. Typically, sufferers will have a painful dry cough producing phlegm that is sometimes specked with blood.

Where pneumonia is due to bacterial infection (the most frequent scenario), an otherwise healthy patient will generally recover within two to three weeks after a course of antibiotics, and suffer no complications.

Orthodox treatment

Bacterial pneumonia is generally treated with antibiotics. With other pneumonias the doctor aims to treat the underlying cause—for example, with anti-fungal or anti-viral drugs.

Complementary therapies

An attempt is sometimes made to strengthen the immune system. Various forms of reflexology and similar techniques are used to alleviate pain and other symptoms.

Treatment plan and limited trial

Before administering a complementary treatment, every therapist should propose a treatment plan (see page xxiii) that sets out a clear time frame and defines the goal that the treatment is designed to achieve. Treatment should then be tried for a limited term to test the patient's response.

Caution

In pneumonia caused by bacteria, no complementary medical procedure can adequately replace state of the art antibiotics.

Complementary treatments for pneumonia

Treatment	Rating	Point of delivery/risks
Acupressure This treatment (*see* page 769), otherwise known as pressure-point massage, is used in pneumonia to ease pain, facilitate breathing, and improve general well-being.	**Inappropriate** as the sole treatment for pneumonia. **May be of some use** as a short-term treatment attempt aimed at easing pain and facilitating breathing. Some case reports claim efficacy; however, success is probably seen in only a small proportion of patients (*see* Placebo, page xxi).	**Suitable for DIY** Qualified guidance is recommended. Therapists should be properly qualified. **Risks:** Unlikely provided treatment is carried out competently.

Treatment	Rating	Point of delivery/risks
Acupuncture Acupuncture in its various forms (*see* page 772) aims to act directly to ease pain and other symptoms and to facilitate breathing. The acupuncture points chosen can vary from one practitioner to another.	**Inappropriate** as the sole treatment for pneumonia. **May be of some use** as a short-term, supportive treatment attempt aimed at easing pain and other symptoms, and facilitating breathing. Case reports claim efficacy; however, success is probably seen in only a proportion of patients (*see* Placebo, page xxi).	**Requires a qualified practitioner** Practitioners should be properly qualified and should propose a treatment plan. **Risks:** Probably rare provided treatment is carried out competently.
Anthroposophical medicine Inflammation, it is claimed, can be eliminated through the extremities by means of foot baths, compresses around the lower legs, or sweating (*see* page 781). In addition, AM uses specially tailored remedies, including potentized "Pneumodoron."	**Inappropriate** as the sole treatment for pneumonia. **May be of some use** as a supportive treatment attempt for bacterial pneumonia or as a treatment attempt for viral pneumonia. Case reports claim efficacy; however, success is probably seen in only a proportion of patients (*see* Placebo, page xxi).	**Requires a qualified practitioner** Practitioners should be properly qualified and should propose a treatment plan. **Risks:** Allergies and intolerance are possible.
Aromatherapy Essential oils (*see* page 786) are reported to exercise an invigorating or relaxing effect on patients. The essences may be taken orally, used externally as massage oils or bathing emulsions, or inhaled as vapors.	**Inappropriate** as the sole treatment for pneumonia. **May be of some use** as a short-term, supportive treatment attempt aimed at soothing and relaxing the patient and improving his/her general well-being. Case reports claim efficacy; however, success is probably seen in only a proportion of patients (*see* Placebo, page xxi).	**Suitable for DIY** Qualified guidance is recommended. The effects of individual essential oils differ widely. **Risks:** Allergies or intolerance are possible. Some oils are carcinogenic in test systems and possibly in humans.

Treatment	Rating	Point of delivery/risks
Bioresonance therapy Bioresonance therapists use electrical devices in an attempt to discover the causes of illness and claim to be able to weaken or turn around pathogenic energies and disease related vibrations (*see* page 794).	**Inappropriate** as the sole treatment for pneumonia. Possibly acceptable as a short-term, supportive treatment attempt for individual persistent symptoms when simpler, more established methods have been unsuccessful. Some case reports claim efficacy; however, success is probably seen, if at all, in only a small proportion of patients (*see* Placebo, page xxi).	**Requires a qualified practitioner** Practitioners should be properly qualified and should propose a treatment plan. No credence should be given to anyone promising immediate or total success. **Risks:** Fairly unlikely.
Cell therapy Injecting or ingesting products extracted from animal tissues or organs is said to have an immune system modulating effect and to enhance the healing of human tissues and organs (*see* page 796).	**Inappropriate** as the sole treatment for pneumonia. **Not advised**. Case reports claim efficacy (e.g. for thymus therapy in the alleviation of symptoms); however, success is probably seen in only a proportion of patients (*see* Placebo, page xxi). Fresh cell therapy is **not advised**.	**Requires a qualified practitioner** Practitioners should be properly qualified and should propose a treatment plan. No credence should be given to anyone promising immediate or total success. **Risks:** Injecting foreign proteins into the body can provoke (possibly fatal) allergic reactions. Also, pathogens such as those that cause bovine spongiform encephalopathy (BSE) or other serious infections may be introduced.

Treatment	Rating	Point of delivery/risks
Electroacupuncture according to Voll By taking readings of the electrical conductivity of the skin (*see* page 802), therapists claim to be able to derive an insight into diseased areas of the body, pathogenic foci (*see* page 928), and stress factors (*see* Toxins, page 929). The causative factors at the root of pneumonia can then be addressed.	**Inappropriate** as the sole treatment for pneumonia. Possibly acceptable as a short-term, supportive treatment attempt for individual persistent symptoms when simpler, more established methods have been unsuccessful. Some case reports claim efficacy; however, success is probably seen, if at all, in only a small proportion of patients (*see* Placebo, page xxi).	**Requires a qualified practitioner** Practitioners should be properly qualified and should propose a treatment plan. No credence should be given to anyone promising immediate or total success. **Risks:** A second opinion must always be obtained from a qualified physician before any attempt is made to "eliminate foci" (e.g. by surgery).
Electroneural therapy according to Croon According to the theory, readings taken at various reactive sites on the skin highlight diseased areas within the body. Based on these readings, targeted electrostimulative measures can be undertaken to address the factors presumed to be conducive to pneumonia (*see* page 806).	**Inappropriate** as the sole treatment for pneumonia. Possibly acceptable as a short-term, supportive treatment attempt for individual persistent symptoms when simpler, more established methods have been unsuccessful. Some case reports claim efficacy; however, success is probably seen, if at all, in only a small proportion of patients (*see* Placebo, page xxi).	**Requires a qualified practitioner** Practitioners should be properly qualified and should propose a treatment plan. No credence should be given to anyone promising immediate or total success. **Risks:** Proponents themselves warn that treatment should not be given in acute inflammatory conditions.

Treatment	Rating	Point of delivery/risks
Eliminative methods, bloody Bloody cupping (*see* page 815) is sometimes used in pneumonia. This treatment is said to improve the body's own regulatory systems and energize the patient and, as a reflex therapy (*see* page 881), to alleviate pain.	**Inappropriate** as the sole treatment for pneumonia. Possibly acceptable as a short-term, supportive treatment attempt for pain when more established, less invasive methods have been unsuccessful. Some case reports and field studies claim efficacy; however, success is probably seen in only a proportion of patients (*see* Placebo, page xxi).	**Requires a qualified practitioner** Practitioners should be properly qualified and should propose a treatment plan. No credence should be given to anyone promising immediate or total success. **Risks:** Bloody cupping can cause infection and scarring. Furthermore, it should not be carried out in persons with bleeding disorders.
Eliminative methods, unbloody Unbloody cupping (*see* page 817) is supposed to improve the body's own regulatory systems and energize the patient and, as a reflex therapy, to alleviate pain.	**Inappropriate** as the sole treatment for pneumonia. **May be of some use** as a short-term, supportive treatment attempt aimed at alleviating pain. Some case reports claim efficacy; however, success is probably seen in only a proportion of patients (*see* Placebo, page xxi).	**Suitable for DIY** Unbloody cupping is best carried out under the guidance of a qualified practitioner. **Risks:** Unlikely provided treatment is carried out competently.
Enzyme therapy Enzymes extracted from plant and animal tissues are claimed to have an anti-inflammatory and immune system modulating action (*see* page 824).	**Inappropriate** as the sole treatment for pneumonia. Some case reports claim efficacy for this treatment, which is aimed at improving general well-being; however, success is probably seen in only a small proportion of patients (*see* Placebo, page xxi).	**Requires a qualified practitioner** Practitioners should propose a treatment plan. Non-prescription preparations are suitable for do-it-yourself. **Risks:** Allergies or intolerance are possible.

Treatment	Rating	Point of delivery/risks
Flower remedies Flower remedies (*see* page 828) are said to restore emotional balance and assist the body's psychic ability to heal itself.	**Inappropriate** as the sole treatment for pneumonia. **May be of some use** as a short-term, supportive treatment attempt aimed at soothing and relaxing. Some case reports claim efficacy; however, success is probably seen in only a proportion of patients (*see* Placebo, page xxi).	**Suitable for DIY** Qualified guidance is recommended. Practitioners should propose a treatment plan. **Risks:** Possible intolerance.
Homeopathy Highly diluted (potentized) solutions (*see* page 831) are believed to be able to redress vital energy imbalances. Organo- and functiotropic (*see* page 833) homeopathy is claimed to be effective for dealing directly with symptoms.	**Inappropriate** as the sole treatment for pneumonia. **May be of some use** as a short-term, supportive treatment attempt. Some case reports claim efficacy for homeopathic treatments; however, success is probably seen in only a small proportion of patients (*see* Placebo, page xxi).	**Requires a qualified practitioner** Homeopaths should be properly qualified and should propose a treatment plan. Ready-formulated preparations are suitable for do-it-yourself. **Risks:** Allergies and intolerance are possible.
Manual therapies Chiropractors and osteopaths use a series of manipulations to realign allegedly displaced vertebrae, as well as the head joints and jaw (*see* page 844). This is said to reduce pain. Sometimes these procedures are used holistically (*see* page 928) to free energy blockages (*see* page 927).	**Inappropriate** as the sole treatment for pneumonia. Possibly acceptable as a short-term, supportive treatment attempt aimed at alleviating persistent pain when less risky, more established methods have been unsuccessful. Some case reports claim efficacy for these potentially risky procedures; however, success is probably seen, if at all, in only a small proportion of patients (*see* Placebo, page xxi).	**Requires a qualified practitioner** Practitioners should be properly qualified and should propose a treatment plan. **Risks:** Spinal manipulations and manipulations to the head and neck can cause serious injury. Osteoporosis is one of several risk factors.

Treatment	Rating	Point of delivery/risks
Massage Classical massage (*see* page 817) and lymphatic drainage (*see* page 850) can, it is claimed, invigorate the patient and ease muscular and perhaps also emotional tension, as well as alleviate pain and help with the ejection of mucus.	**Inappropriate** as the sole treatment for pneumonia. **May be of some use** as a short-term, supportive treatment attempt aimed at relaxing the patient and easing discomfort. Some case reports claim efficacy in the treatment of muscle pain; however, success is probably seen in only a proportion of patients (*see* Placebo, page xxi).	**Requires a qualified practitioner** Masseurs/masseuses should be properly qualified. **Risks:** Some people are sensitive to manual stimuli; others find it hard to tolerate close physical contact.
Nutritional therapies An organic diet (*see* page 4) provides the body with essential and secondary plant nutrients that are believed to exercise a multitude of positive effects.	**Inappropriate** as the sole treatment for pneumonia. **Useful** as an individually directed supportive measure provided that the diet is tolerated.	**Suitable for DIY** Qualified guidance is recommended though not essential. Fresh fruit or fruit juice may be beneficial in patients lacking appetite. **Risks:** Avoid imbalanced or intolerable diets. They can cause deficiencies with serious consequences. Children are particularly at risk.
Physical therapies Warm wraps (*see* page 877), e.g. with mustard powder, are said to ease pain, reduce fever, loosen secretions, and facilitate the ejection of mucus.	**Inappropriate** as the sole treatment for pneumonia. **Useful** as a short-term treatment attempt. Case reports and field studies claim efficacy; however, success is probably seen in only a proportion of patients (*see* Placebo, page xxi).	**Suitable for DIY** Qualified guidance is recommended though not essential. **Risks:** Unlikely provided treatment is carried out competently.

Treatment	Rating	Point of delivery/risks
Probiotics The introduction of certain bacteria into the gut is claimed to bring the intestinal flora back into balance and to have a beneficial effect on the immune system (*see* page 878).	**Inappropriate** as the sole treatment for pneumonia. Possibly acceptable as a supportive treatment attempt aimed at persistent symptoms. Some case reports claim efficacy; however, success is probably seen in only a proportion of patients (*see* Placebo, page xxi).	**Requires a qualified practitioner** Practitioners should be properly qualified. Non-prescription formulations are suitable for do-it-yourself. **Risks:** Fairly unlikely provided treatment is carried out competently.
Reflex therapies Heat treatments, reflex zone massage (*see* page 883), reflexology (*see* page 883), and TENS (*see* page 886) are claimed to act via reflex channels (*see* page 881) to relax the patient, ease pain, and facilitate the ejection of mucus.	**Inappropriate** as the sole treatment for pneumonia. **Useful** as a short-term, supportive treatment attempt aimed at alleviating pain, providing relaxation, or facilitating the expulsion of mucus. Case reports and field studies claim efficacy; however, success is probably seen in only a proportion of patients (*see* Placebo, page xxi).	**Suitable for DIY** Qualified guidance is essential. Practitioners should be properly qualified and should propose a treatment plan. **Risks:** Some people are sensitive to electrical stimuli and rubber electrodes; others find it hard to tolerate manual stimulation or close physical contact.
Relaxation techniques Autogenic training (*see* page 888), muscle relaxation according to Jacobson (*see* page 893), and various biofeedback techniques (*see* page 891) are said to relieve muscle tension and inner unrest, and might be instrumental in alleviating pain.	**Inappropriate** as the sole treatment for pneumonia. **Useful** as a short-term, supportive treatment attempt aimed at relaxing the patient and easing pain. Case reports claim efficacy; however, success is probably seen in only a proportion of patients (*see* Placebo, page xxi).	**Suitable for DIY** Once a sound understanding of the technique has been acquired from a trainer, patients can perform exercises themselves. Therapists should propose a treatment plan. **Risks:** Fairly unlikely.

Treatment	Rating	Point of delivery/risks
Vitamins and trace elements The painkilling properties of vitamin B6 are thought to contribute to pain relief. The antioxidative properties of beta-carotene and vitamins C and E are, it is supposed, instrumental in countering free radical formation and in boosting the body's antioxidative defences (*see* page 900).	**Inappropriate** as the sole treatment for pneumonia. **Useful** in vitamin deficiency. High doses of vitamins (vitamins B6, C, E, beta-carotene) may be of some use as a preventive measure. No definitive recommendations can be made based on present knowledge. Field studies ascribe a degree of success to vitamin B6 in the treatment of pain.	**Suitable for DIY** Medical supervision is recommended though not essential. Recommended dosages vary widely but are probably set to rise. **Risks:** Intolerance and overdosage are possible. Vitamin B6 in high doses can cause serious side effects. Recent findings imply that beta-carotene might increase the risk of cancer.

Herbal remedies for pneumonia

Self-treatment is not a viable option in pneumonia. There are no suitable herbal remedies available for this indication. The use of antibiotics is generally required. Whenever pneumonia is suspected, see your doctor.

Sinusitis

Causes and symptoms

Sinusitis manifests itself as a powerful pressure headache in the cheekbones, over the eyes, or over the forehead. It is particularly intense on stooping or after standing up. The chief causes of sinusitis are bacterial or viral infection and an allergic response. The risk of sinusitis occurring is raised when nasal polyps are present or when the tiny tubes that connect the various bony cavities become blocked as a result of a displaced nasal septum.

Orthodox treatment

Acute bacterial infections will normally respond to antibiotics. Antihistamine preparations can be used in sinusitis if an allergy is believed to be the root cause. Nasal decongestants or a salt solution may be useful in freeing up, or keeping open, the tubes between the nose and sinuses. Surgery might be an option to remove polyps or deal with a displaced septum.

Complementary therapies

Depending on individual philosophies, various complementary practitioners see sinusitis as being caused by foci (*see* page 928) or as a manifestation of toxins (*see* page 929), of a weakened immune system, or of an imbalanced vital force, and offer corresponding treatments. The proponents of reflexology (*see* page 883) and similar techniques claim to be able to alleviate pain and other symptoms.

Treatment plan and limited trial

Before administering a complementary treatment, every therapist should propose a treatment plan (*see* page xxiii) that sets out a clear time frame and defines the goal that the treatment is designed to achieve. Treatment should then be tried for a limited term to test the patient's response.

Complementary treatments for sinusitis

Treatment	Rating	Point of delivery/risks
Acupressure This treatment (*see* page 769), otherwise known as pressure-point massage, is claimed to alleviate symptoms and improve general well-being when the appropriate pressure points are stimulated.	**Of little use** Acceptable as a short-term, supportive treatment attempt aimed at alleviating symptoms. Some case reports and field studies claim efficacy; however, success is probably seen in only a proportion of patients (*see* Placebo, page xxi).	**Suitable for DIY** Qualified guidance is recommended. Therapists should be properly qualified. **Risks:** Unlikely provided treatment is carried out competently.
Acupuncture Acupuncture in its various forms (*see* page 772) aims to encourage the flow of energy (*see* page 927) or to act directly to alleviate pain and facilitate the drainage of secretions. The acupuncture points chosen can vary from one practitioner to another.	**May be of some use** as a short-term treatment attempt aimed at alleviating pain and facilitating the drainage of secretions. Case reports and field studies claim efficacy; however, success is probably seen in only a proportion of patients (*see* Placebo, page xxi).	**Requires a qualified practitioner** Acupuncturists should be properly qualified and should propose a treatment plan. **Risks:** Probably rare provided treatment is carried out competently.
Anthroposophical medicine Inflammation, it is claimed, can be eliminated through the extremities by means of foot baths, compresses around the lower legs, or sweating (*see* page 781). In addition, AM uses a number of specially tailored remedies.	**May be of some use** as a short-term treatment attempt. Some case reports claim efficacy; however, success is probably seen in only a proportion of patients (*see* Placebo, page xxi).	**Requires a qualified practitioner** Practitioners should be properly qualified and should propose a treatment plan. **Risks:** Allergies and intolerance are possible.

Treatment	*Rating*	*Point of delivery/risks*
Aromatherapy Essential oils (*see* page 786) are used to soothe and relax, or to invigorate the patient, exercising a beneficial effect on the mucosa and facilitating breathing. The essences may be taken orally, used externally as massage oils or bathing emulsions, or inhaled as vapors.	**Of little use** Acceptable as a short-term, supportive treatment attempt aimed at facilitating breathing, as well as soothing and relaxing the patient. Some case reports claim efficacy; however, success is probably seen in only a proportion of patients (*see* Placebo, page xxi).	**Suitable for DIY** Qualified guidance is recommended. The effects of individual essential oils differ widely. **Risks:** Allergies or intolerance are possible. Some oils are carcinogenic in test systems and possibly in humans.
Bioresonance therapy Bioresonance therapists use electrical devices in an attempt to discover the causes of illness and claim to be able to weaken or turn around pathogenic energies and disease related vibrations (*see* page 794).	**Of little use** Possibly acceptable as a short-term, supportive treatment attempt for recurrent symptoms when simpler, more established methods have been unsuccessful. Some case reports claim efficacy; however, success is probably seen, if at all, in only a small proportion of patients (*see* Placebo, page xxi).	**Requires a qualified practitioner** Practitioners should be properly qualified and should propose a treatment plan. No credence should be given to anyone promising immediate or total success. **Risks:** Fairly unlikely.
Cell therapy Injecting or ingesting products extracted from the tissues of newborn animals or animal fetuses is said to have a rejuvenating and revitalizing effect and to enhance the healing of human tissues and organs (*see* page 796).	**Not advised** Based on present knowledge, there is inadequate evidence of the efficacy and mode of action of these costly and relatively risky procedures.	**Risks:** Injecting foreign proteins into the body can provoke (possibly fatal) allergic reactions. Also, pathogens such as those that cause bovine spongiform encephalopathy (BSE) or other serious infections may be introduced.

Treatment	Rating	Point of delivery/risks
Electroacupuncture according to Voll By taking readings of the electrical conductivity of the skin (*see* page 802), therapists claim to be able to derive an insight into diseased areas of the body, pathogenic foci (*see* page 928), and stress factors (*see* Toxins, page 929). The factors that are presumed to be at the root of sinusitis can then be addressed.	**Of little use** Possibly acceptable as a short-term, supportive treatment attempt for recurrent symptoms when simpler, more established methods have been unsuccessful. Some case reports claim efficacy; however, success is probably seen, if at all, in only a small proportion of patients (*see* Placebo, page xxi).	**Requires a qualified practitioner** Practitioners should be properly qualified and should propose a treatment plan. No credence should be given to anyone promising immediate or total success. **Risks:** A second opinion must always be obtained from a qualified physician before any attempt is made to "eliminate foci" (e.g. by surgery).
Electroneural therapy according to Croon According to the theory, readings taken at various reactive sites on the skin highlight diseased areas within the body. Based on these readings, targeted electrostimulative measures can be undertaken to address factors presumed to be at the root of sinusitis (*see* page 806).	**Of little use** Possibly acceptable as a short-term, supportive treatment attempt for persistent sinusitis when simpler, more established methods have been unsuccessful. Some case reports claim efficacy; however, success is probably seen, if at all, in only a small proportion of patients (*see* Placebo, page xxi).	**Requires a qualified practitioner** Practitioners should be properly qualified and should propose a treatment plan. No credence should be given to anyone promising immediate or total success. **Risks:** Proponents themselves warn that treatment should not be given in acute inflammatory conditions.
Eliminative methods, bloody Bloody cupping (*see* page 815) is said to alleviate symptoms and improve the body's own regulatory systems.	**Not advised** There is little evidence of the efficacy of this relatively invasive procedure.	**Risks:** Bloody cupping can cause infection and scarring. Furthermore, it should not be carried out in persons with bleeding disorders.

Treatment	Rating	Point of delivery/risks
Eliminative methods, unbloody Unbloody cupping (*see* page 817) is said to ease the pain of sinusitis and improve the body's own regulatory systems.	**Of little use** Acceptable as a short-term, supportive treatment attempt for recurrent sinusitis. Some case reports claim efficacy; however, success is probably seen in only a proportion of patients (*see* Placebo, page xxi).	**Suitable for DIY** Unbloody cupping is best carried out under the guidance of a qualified practitioner. **Risks:** Unlikely provided treatment is carried out competently.
Enzyme therapy The enzymes used are said to dispel and destroy "immune complexes" (*see* page 824) that course in the blood and that are responsible, for instance, for sustaining inflammatory processes.	**Of little use** Some case reports claim efficacy for this little researched therapy; however, success is probably seen in only a small proportion of patients (*see* Placebo, page xxi).	**Requires a qualified practitioner** Practitioners should propose a treatment plan. Non-prescription preparations are suitable for do-it-yourself. **Risks:** Allergies or intolerance are possible.
Flower remedies Flower remedies (*see* page 828) are said to restore emotional balance and assist the body's psychic ability to heal itself.	**May be of some use** as a short-term, supportive treatment attempt aimed at soothing and relaxing. Some case reports claim efficacy; however, success is probably seen in only a proportion of patients (*see* Placebo, page xxi).	**Suitable for DIY** Qualified guidance is recommended. Practitioners should propose a treatment plan. **Risks:** Possible intolerance.

Treatment	Rating	Point of delivery/risks
Homeopathy Highly diluted (potentized) solutions (*see* page 831) are believed to be able to redress vital energy imbalances and strengthen the body's defences. Organo- and functiotropic (*see* page 833) homeopathy is claimed to be effective for dealing with sinusitis.	**May be of some use** as a short-term treatment attempt for chronic sinusitis. Some case reports, field studies, and other studies ascribe a degree of efficacy to this procedure in some patients (*see* Placebo, page xxi).	**Requires a qualified practitioner** Homeopaths should be properly qualified and should propose a treatment plan. Ready-formulated preparations are suitable for do-it-yourself. **Risks:** Allergies and intolerance are possible.
Manual therapies Chiropractors and osteopaths use a series of manipulations to re-align allegedly displaced vertebrae. This is said to reduce pain, release energy blockages (*see* page 927), and speed up healing (*see* page 844).	**Of little use** Possibly acceptable as a short-term treatment attempt in persistent cases when less risky, more established methods have been unsuccessful. Some case reports claim efficacy for this potentially risky procedure; however, success is probably seen, if at all, in only a small proportion of patients (*see* Placebo, page xxi).	**Requires a qualified practitioner** Practitioners should be properly qualified and should propose a treatment plan. **Risks:** Manipulation of the head and cervical vertebrae can cause serious injury. Osteoporosis is one of several risk factors.
Nutritional therapies An organic diet (*see* page 4) provides the body with essential and secondary plant nutrients that are believed to exercise a multitude of positive effects and to be capable, *inter alia*, of boosting the immune system (*see* page 10).	**May be of some use** as an individually directed supportive measure for the treatment of persistent symptoms. Elimination and rotation diets may be of some assistance in identifying the cause of food allergy induced sinusitis.	**Suitable for DIY** Qualified guidance is recommended though not essential. See your doctor before starting an elimination or rotation diet. **Risks:** Avoid imbalanced or intolerable diets. They can cause deficiencies with serious consequences. Children are particularly at risk.

Treatment	Rating	Point of delivery/risks
Physical therapies Ascending temperature arm and foot baths, chest wraps, gargling with sage tea, cold face douches (*see* pages 871–8) following chamomile vapor inhalation, and moist warm compresses with healing earth applied to the sinuses and neck are said to improve the circulation and the function of the mucous membranes.	**Useful** as a short-term treatment attempt for acute and chronic sinusitis. Some case reports claim efficacy; however, success is probably seen in only a proportion of patients (*see* Placebo, page xxi).	**Suitable for DIY** Qualified guidance is recommended though not essential. **Risks:** Skin damage may be caused to persons with diminished temperature sensation when extreme temperatures are applied.
Probiotics The introduction of certain bacteria into the gut is claimed to bring the intestinal flora back into balance and to have a beneficial effect on the immune system (*see* page 878).	**Of little use** Acceptable as a short-term, supportive treatment attempt in chronic or persistent cases when more established methods have been unsuccessful. Case reports claim efficacy; however, success is probably seen in only a proportion of patients (*see* Placebo, page xxi).	**Requires a qualified practitioner** Practitioners should be properly qualified and should propose a treatment plan. Non-prescription formulations are suitable for do-it-yourself. **Risks:** Fairly unlikely provided treatment is carried out competently.
Reflex therapies Reflex zone massage (*see* page 883), nose massage, reflexology (*see* page 883), heat and cold treatments, and TENS (*see* page 886) are claimed to act via reflex channels (*see* page 881) to ease pain and other symptoms.	**May be of some use** as a short-term treatment attempt aimed at alleviating symptoms. Some case reports claim efficacy; however, success is probably seen in only a proportion of patients (*see* Placebo, page xxi).	**Suitable for DIY** Qualified guidance is essential. **Risks:** Some people are sensitive to electrical stimuli and rubber electrodes; others find it hard to tolerate manual stimulation or close physical contact.

Treatment	Rating	Point of delivery/risks
Relaxation techniques Autogenic training (*see* page 888), muscle relaxation according to Jacobson (*see* page 893), and various biofeedback techniques (*see* page 891) are said to relieve muscle tension and inner unrest, and might be instrumental in helping the patient become more aware of his/her physical and emotional states.	**Of little use** Acceptable as a short-term treatment attempt for persistent sinusitis, for soothing and relaxing, and for helping the patient to become more aware of his/her physical and emotional states. Case reports claim efficacy; however, success is probably seen in only a proportion of patients (*see* Placebo, page xxi).	**Suitable for DIY** Once a sound understanding of the technique has been acquired from a trainer in groups or through individual tuition, patients can perform exercises themselves. Therapists should propose a treatment plan. **Risks:** Fairly unlikely.
Vitamins and trace elements The antioxidative properties of beta-carotene, vitamins C and E, and selenium are, it is supposed, instrumental in countering the formation of free radicals and in boosting the body's defence systems (*see* page 900).	**Of little use** Evidence of efficacy is lacking. Based on present knowledge, no definitive recommendations can be made.	**Suitable for DIY** Qualified guidance is recommended though not essential. **Risks:** Intolerance and overdosage are possible. Recent findings imply that beta-carotene might increase the risk of cancer.

Herbal remedies for sinusitis

Active ingredient/preparation	Rating
Cineol (1,8-cineol from essential oil of myrtle)	Used internally, cineol **may be of some use** as a treatment attempt. **Dosage:** Use ready-formulated preparations as instructed by the manufacturer/prescriber. **Risks:** Cineol can cause transient gastrointestinal problems.
Eucalyptus leaves (*Eucalyptus globulus*)	**May be of some use** as a treatment attempt for sinusitis. The action and side effects are the same as for eucalyptus oil. **Daily dose:** 4–6g herb. **Individual dose:** Pour 1 cup of hot water over 2g of leaves and infuse. Use ready-formulated preparations as instructed by the manufacturer/prescriber. As eucalyptus leaves infused with hot water release only a small amount of their volatile oil, inhalation with the isolated oil or a tincture is to be preferred. **Risks:** Nausea, vomiting, and diarrhea are possible.
Eucalyptus oil (*Eucalyptus globulus*)	**Only useful** as a treatment attempt for sinusitis when inhaled or rubbed into the chest. It is a mucolytic, mild antispasmodic, and local circulatory stimulant. **Daily dose:** Used internally, 0.05–0.2ml oil; externally, 5–20 percent in oily preparations, 5–10 percent in alcoholic formulations. To prepare an inhalation, place 1 dessertspoon of the dried herb, 1 teaspoon of cream or balsam, or 15 drops of volatile oil in a bowl of hot water, cover the head and bowl with a towel, and inhale the vapors alternately through the mouth and nose. Use ready-formulated preparations as instructed by the manufacturer/prescriber. **Risks:** Nausea, vomiting, diarrhea, and allergic skin reactions are possible. Not to be used internally by persons with gastritis, enteritis, gall bladder disease, or severe liver disease. Do not apply to the nose and face of infants and young children. Undiluted oil is toxic and should not be taken internally unless suitably diluted.

Active ingredient/preparation	Rating
Peppermint oil (*Mentha piperita*)	**Only useful** as a treatment attempt in the form of an inhalation or as an externally applied remedy for upper respiratory catarrh. **Daily dose:** 3–4 drops as an inhalation twice or three times a day. Use ready-formulated preparations as instructed by the manufacturer/prescriber. **Risks:** Allergic skin reactions are possible. Do not apply to the nose and face of infants and young children.
Pineapple enzyme (bromelain from *Ananas comosus*)	**May be of some use** as a treatment attempt for acute swelling of the nose and sinuses. **Dosage:** Use ready-formulated preparations as instructed by the manufacturer/prescriber. Do not use for longer than 8–20 days unless there is good reason. **Risks:** Pineapple enzyme can cause transient gastric problems, diarrhea, and allergic reactions. Not to be used in hypersensitive persons.

Sore throat

Causes and symptoms

A sore throat may be a condition *per se* or the result of another condition such as flu. A sore throat can have a number of causes, including viral or bacterial infection and immune deficiency. Symptoms associated with a sore throat are: difficulty in swallowing, pain radiating from the back of the nose and mouth, swelling of the cervical lymph nodes, inflamed and swollen tonsils, a temperature, and general malaise.

Orthodox treatment

Mainstream doctors directly address the causes of a sore throat, for example by prescribing antibiotics—often without due reason (antibiotics should only be prescribed for a bacterial sore throat). Often the treatment is only palliative.

Complementary therapies

Complementary practitioners aim to alleviate the symptoms and/or help the body to help itself. There is no evidence that such treatments are effective in preventing the "knock-on" effects of certain throat infections which, following a streptococcal infection, may include rheumatic fever or nephritis.

Treatment plan and limited trial

Before administering a complementary treatment, every therapist should propose a treatment plan (*see* page xxiii) that sets out a clear time frame and defines the goal that the treatment is designed to achieve. Treatment should then be tried for a limited term to test the patient's response.

Cautions

In the case of bacterial throat infection the procedures suggested by non-orthodox practitioners are no substitute for a properly prescribed course of antibiotics.

Complementary treatments for sore throat

Treatment	Rating	Point of delivery/risks
Acupressure This treatment (*see* page 769), otherwise known as pressure-point massage, is claimed to ease a sore throat. The pressure points chosen may differ from one practitioner to another.	**Of little use** Acceptable as a short-term treatment attempt for acute and chronic pain and inflammation. Case reports claim efficacy; however, success is probably seen in only a proportion of patients (*see* Placebo, page xxi).	**Suitable for DIY** Qualified guidance is recommended. Therapists should be properly qualified. **Risks:** Unlikely provided treatment is carried out competently.
Acupuncture Acupuncture in its various forms (*see* page 772) aims to encourage the flow of energy (*see* page 927) and boost the immune system, or to act directly to ease a sore throat. The acupuncture points chosen can vary from one practitioner to another.	**Of little use** Acceptable as a short-term treatment attempt for acute or chronic pain and inflammation. Case reports and field studies claim efficacy; however, success is probably seen in only a proportion of patients (*see* Placebo, page xxi).	**Requires a qualified practitioner** Practitioners should be properly qualified and should propose a treatment plan. **Risks:** Probably rare provided treatment is carried out competently.
Anthroposophical medicine Inflammation can, it is believed, be reversed through the use of foot baths, wet compresses around the lower legs, or by sweating from the extremities (*see* page 781). Also, AM uses specially tailored drugs and the basic remedy, Erysidoron 1 and 2.	**May be of some use** as a short-term treatment attempt. Some studies claim efficacy; however, success is probably seen in only a proportion of patients (*see* Placebo, page xxi).	**Requires a qualified practitioner** Practitioners should be properly qualified and should propose a treatment plan. **Risks:** Allergies and intolerance are possible.

Treatment	Rating	Point of delivery/risks
Aromatherapy Essential oils (*see* page 786) are used to soothe and relax, or to invigorate. The essences may be taken orally, used externally as massage oils or bathing emulsions, or inhaled as vapors.	**Of little use** Acceptable as a short-term treatment attempt aimed at soothing and relaxing. Some case reports claim efficacy; however, success is probably seen in only a small proportion of patients (*see* Placebo, page xxi).	**Suitable for DIY** Qualified guidance is recommended. The effects of individual essential oils differ widely. **Risks:** Allergies or intolerance are possible. Some oils are carcinogenic in test systems and possibly in humans.
Bioresonance therapy Bioresonance therapists use electrical devices in an attempt to discover the causes of a chronic sore throat and claim to be able to weaken or turn around pathogenic energies and disease related vibrations (*see* page 794).	**Of little use** Possibly acceptable as a short-term, supportive treatment attempt for a persistent or recurrent sore throat when simpler, more established methods have been unsuccessful. Some case reports claim efficacy; however, success is probably seen, if at all, in only a small proportion of patients (*see* Placebo, page xxi).	**Requires a qualified practitioner** Practitioners should be properly qualified and should propose a treatment plan. No credence should be given to anyone promising immediate or total success. **Risks:** Fairly unlikely.
Electroacupuncture according to Voll By taking readings of the electrical conductivity of the skin (*see* page 802), therapists claim to be able to derive an insight into diseased areas of the body, pathogenic foci (*see* page 928), and stress factors (*see* Toxins, page 929). The supposed causes of the sore throat can then be addressed.	**Of little use** Possibly acceptable as a short-term, supportive treatment attempt for a recurrent or persistent sore throat when simpler, more established methods have been unsuccessful. Some case reports claim efficacy; however, success is probably seen, if at all, in only a small proportion of patients (*see* Placebo, page xxi).	**Requires a qualified practitioner** Practitioners should be properly qualified and should propose a treatment plan. No credence should be given to anyone promising immediate or total success. **Risks:** A second opinion must always be obtained from a qualified physician before any attempt is made to "eliminate foci" (e.g. by surgery).

Treatment	Rating	Point of delivery/risks
Electroneural therapy according to Croon According to the theory, readings taken at various reactive sites on the skin highlight diseased areas within the body. Based on these readings, targeted electrostimulative measures can be undertaken to address the causes of the sore throat (*see* page 806).	**Of little use** Possibly acceptable as a short-term, supportive treatment attempt for a persistent or recurrent sore throat when simpler, more established methods have been unsuccessful. Some case reports claim efficacy; however, success is probably seen, if at all, in only a small proportion of patients (*see* Placebo, page xxi).	**Requires a qualified practitioner** Practitioners should be properly qualified and should propose a treatment plan. No credence should be given to anyone promising immediate or total success. **Risks:** Proponents themselves warn that treatment should not be given in acute inflammatory conditions.
Eliminative methods, bloody Bloody cupping (*see* page 815) is sometimes used to alleviate pain and improve the body's own regulatory systems in patients with chronic sore throats.	**Not advised** The efficacy and mode of action of this relatively invasive procedure are unproven.	**Risks:** Bloody cupping can cause infection and scarring. Furthermore, it should not be carried out in persons with bleeding disorders.
Eliminative methods, unbloody Cantharide poultices (*see* page 812) are occasionally used to ease a sore throat.	**Of little use** The efficacy and mode of action of this relatively risky procedure are unproven.	**Requires a qualified practitioner** **Risks:** Cantharide poultices can cause second-degree burns. Sensitivity and irritation of the kidneys and efferent urinary tract are possible.

Treatment	*Rating*	*Point of delivery/risks*
Flower remedies Flower remedies (*see* page 828) are said to restore emotional balance and assist the body's psychic ability to heal itself.	**Of little use** Acceptable as a short-term, supportive treatment attempt aimed at soothing and improving general well-being. Some case reports claim efficacy; however, success is probably seen in only a proportion of patients (*see* Placebo, page xxi).	**Suitable for DIY** Qualified guidance is recommended. Practitioners should propose a treatment plan. **Risks:** Possible intolerance.
Homeopathy Highly diluted (potentized) solutions (*see* page 831) are believed to be able to redress vital energy imbalances and strengthen the body's defences. Organo- and functiotropic (*see* page 833) homeopathy is claimed to be effective for dealing symptomatically with a sore throat.	**May be of some use** as a short-term, supportive treatment attempt for a recurrent or persistent sore throat. Case reports and field studies claim efficacy; however, success is probably seen in only a proportion of patients (*see* Placebo, page xxi).	**Requires a qualified practitioner** Homeopaths should be properly qualified and should propose a treatment plan. Ready-formulated preparations are suitable for do-it-yourself. **Risks:** Allergies and intolerance are possible.
Manual therapies Chiropractors and osteopaths use a series of manipulations to realign allegedly displaced cervical vertebrae. This is said to have a beneficial effect in patients with a chronic sore throat (*see* page 844).	**Of little use** Possibly acceptable as a short-term treatment attempt for a persistent or recurrent sore throat when more established, less risky procedures have been unsuccessful. Some case reports claim efficacy for this potentially risky procedure; however, success is probably seen, if at all, in only a small proportion of patients (*see* Placebo, page xxi).	**Requires a qualified practitioner** Practitioners should be properly qualified and should propose a treatment plan. **Risks:** Manipulation of the cervical vertebrae can cause serious injury. Osteoporosis is one of several risk factors.

Treatment	Rating	Point of delivery/risks
Physical therapies Neck wraps (*see* page 877), foot baths (*see* pages 873–4), ice collars (in particularly acute cases), and inhalations are said to ease pain, inhibit inflammation, and lower fever.	**Useful** as a treatment attempt. Case reports and field studies claim efficacy; however, success is probably seen in only a proportion of patients (*see* Placebo, page xxi).	**Suitable for DIY** Qualified guidance is recommended though not essential. **Risks:** Skin damage may be caused to persons with diminished temperature sensation when extreme temperatures are applied.
Probiotics The introduction of certain bacteria into the gut is claimed to bring the intestinal flora back into balance and to have a beneficial effect on the immune system (*see* page 878).	**Of little use** Possibly acceptable as a short-term treatment attempt for a persistent sore throat when more established methods have been unsuccessful. Case reports claim efficacy; however, success is probably seen in only a proportion of patients (*see* Placebo, page xxi).	**Requires a qualified practitioner** Practitioners should be properly qualified and should propose a treatment plan. Non-prescription formulations are suitable for do-it-yourself. **Risks:** Fairly unlikely provided treatment is carried out competently.
Reflex therapies Reflex zone massage (*see* page 883), reflexology (*see* page 883), heat and cold treatments, and TENS (*see* page 886) are claimed to act via reflex channels (*see* page 881) to ease pain, soreness, and other symptoms.	**May be of some use** as a treatment attempt Case reports and field studies claim efficacy; however, success is probably seen in only a proportion of patients (*see* Placebo, page xxi).	**Suitable for DIY** Qualified guidance is essential. **Risks:** Some people are sensitive to electrical stimuli and rubber electrodes; others find it hard to tolerate manual stimulation or close physical contact.

Treatment	Rating	Point of delivery/risks
Vitamins and trace elements The antioxidative properties of beta-carotene, vitamins C and E, and selenium are, it is supposed, instrumental in countering the formation of free radicals and boosting the body's antioxidative defence systems (*see* page 900).	**May be of some use** as a general treatment attempt. No definitive recommendations can be made based on present knowledge.	**Suitable for DIY** Qualified supervision is recommended though not essential. **Risks:** Intolerance and overdosage are possible. Recent findings imply that beta-carotene might increase the risk of cancer.

Herbal remedies for a sore throat

Active ingredient/preparation	Rating
For a sore throat not associated with furring of the tonsils, high temperature, and lassitude, the herbal remedies suggested for hoarseness (*see* page 266) and mouth ulcers (*see* page 274) can be used.	**Of little use** when there are signs of furring of the tonsils and lassitude. In this case, treatment with penicillin will be required to prevent complications such as rheumatic disease and endocarditis.

Allergies

Causes and symptoms

"Allergy" is a term for any of a number of conditions that can arise in any part of the body when the immune system over-reacts, or becomes hypersensitive to certain stimuli. Psychological and emotional factors may also be contributing factors. Hypersensitivity varies in degree from mild hayfever on the one hand to severe life-threatening anaphylactic shock on the other, with the middle ground being occupied by numerous food allergies and forms of asthma (*see* page 229).

Modern medicine places allergies into four main categories and the approach taken in treating them will differ widely according to the reaction mechanism involved. An allergologist will be able to assign a particular allergy to one of these four types.

Orthodox treatment

Orthodox treatment will start with an exact medical diagnosis. By identifying the agent that is causing the allergy, a doctor can help the sufferer steer clear of that particular allergen in future. Various types of medication (mostly antihistamines) are used to suppress allergic reactions, to reverse swelling, and to alleviate and prevent symptoms. Desensitizing treatments are sometimes useful, although they should only be given by a medically qualified allergologist, owing to the severe shock reactions (requiring emergency medical attention) that might be induced.

Complementary therapies

Complementary approaches are partly based on the orthodox view of allergy. However, there are therapists who confuse allergy with intolerance and offer their own diagnostic procedures.

Claims by some practitioners that they have developed effective new techniques for identifying and treating allergies have not been corroborated by clinical studies. Many practitioners also claim to be able to control the body's allergic response (*see* Constitution, page 927) and thereby counteract, or even prevent, allergic reactions.

Treatment plan and limited trial

Before administering a complementary treatment, every therapist should propose a treatment plan (*see* page xxiii) that sets out a clear time frame and defines the goal that the treatment is designed to achieve. Treatment should then be tried for a limited term to test the patient's response.

Cautions

Anyone receiving treatment for an allergy from a complementary practitioner should be kept under medical review by a physician.

Anaphylactic shock is life threatening and requires prompt and effective countermeasures. No complementary technique can provide the speed of action required.

Complementary treatments for allergies

Treatment	Rating	Point of delivery/risks
Acupressure This treatment (*see* page 769), otherwise known as pressure-point massage, is claimed to boost the immune system and alleviate symptoms when pressure is applied to the appropriate points.	**Of little use** Acceptable as a short-term, supportive treatment attempt aimed at alleviating symptoms. Some case reports claim efficacy; however, success is probably seen in only a minority of patients (*see* Placebo, page xxi).	**Suitable for DIY** Qualified guidance is recommended. Therapists should be properly qualified. **Risks:** Unlikely provided treatment is carried out competently.
Acupuncture Acupuncture in its various forms (*see* page 772) aims to encourage the flow of energy (*see* page 927) or to act directly against allergies. The acupuncture points chosen can vary from one practitioner to another.	**May be of some use** as a short-term treatment attempt for hayfever and as a means of reducing the intake of drugs. Controlled clinical studies, case reports, and field studies ascribe a degree of efficacy to this treatment in some patients (*see* Placebo, page xxi).	**Requires a qualified practitioner** Practitioners should be properly qualified and should propose a treatment plan. **Risks:** Probably rare provided treatment is carried out competently.
Anthroposophical medicine To the anthroposophical physician (*see* page 781), allergies are the result of a poorly organized ego, which manifests itself in the skin and mucosal region.	**May be of some use** as a short-term treatment. Some studies claim efficacy; however, success is probably seen in only a proportion of patients (*see* Placebo, page xxi).	**Requires a qualified practitioner** Practitioners should be properly qualified and should propose a treatment plan. **Risks:** Allergies and intolerance are possible.

Treatment	Rating	Point of delivery/risks
Aromatherapy Essential oils (*see* page 786) are used to soothe and relax, or to invigorate, thereby contributing to the relief of discomfort. The essences may be taken orally, used externally as massage oils or bathing emulsions, or inhaled as vapors.	**Of little use** Acceptable as a short-term, supportive treatment attempt aimed at soothing and relaxing. Some case reports claim efficacy; however, success is probably seen in only a proportion of patients (*see* Placebo, page xxi).	**Suitable for DIY** Qualified guidance is recommended. The effects of individual essential oils differ widely. **Risks:** Allergies or intolerance are possible. Some oils are carcinogenic in test systems and possibly in humans.
Bioresonance therapy Bioresonance therapists use electrical devices in an attempt to discover the causes of illness and claim to be able to weaken or turn around pathogenic energies and disease related vibrations (*see* page 794).	**Of little use** Possibly acceptable as a short-term, supportive treatment attempt. The efficacy of this widely used procedure is unproven. Some case reports claim efficacy; however, success is probably seen in only a proportion of patients (*see* Placebo, page xxi).	**Requires a qualified practitioner** Practitioners should be properly qualified and should propose a treatment plan. No credence should be given to anyone promising immediate or total success. **Risks:** Fairly unlikely.
Cell therapy Injecting or ingesting products extracted from the tissues of newborn animals or animal fetuses is said to have a rejuvenating and revitalizing effect and to enhance the healing of human tissues and organs (*see* page 796).	**Not advised** Based on present knowledge, there is inadequate evidence of the efficacy and mode of action of these costly and relatively risky procedures.	**Risks:** Injecting foreign proteins into the body can provoke (possibly fatal) allergic reactions. Also, pathogens such as those that cause bovine spongiform encephalopathy (BSE) or other serious infections may be introduced.

Treatment	Rating	Point of delivery/risks
Electroacupuncture according to Voll By taking readings of the electrical conductivity of the skin (*see* page 862), therapists claim to be able to derive an insight into diseased areas of the body, pathogenic foci (*see* page 928), and stress factors (*see* Toxins, page 929). The supposed causes of allergies can then be addressed.	**Of little use** Possibly acceptable as a short-term, supportive treatment attempt when simpler, more established methods have been unsuccessful. Some case reports claim efficacy; however, success is probably seen, if at all, in only a small proportion of patients (*see* Placebo, page xxi).	**Requires a qualified practitioner** Practitioners should be properly qualified and should propose a treatment plan. No credence should be given to anyone promising immediate or total success. **Risks:** A second opinion must always be obtained from a qualified physician before any attempt is made to "eliminate foci" (e.g. by surgery).
Electroneural therapy according to Croon According to the theory, readings taken at various reactive sites on the skin highlight diseased areas within the body. Based on these readings, targeted electrostimulative measures can be undertaken to address the presumed causes of allergies (*see* page 806).	**Of little use** Possibly acceptable as a short-term, supportive treatment attempt when simpler, more established methods have been unsuccessful. Some case reports claim efficacy; however, success is probably seen, if at all, in only a small proportion of patients (*see* Placebo, page xxi).	**Requires a qualified practitioner** Practitioners should be properly qualified and should propose a treatment plan. No credence should be given to anyone promising immediate or total success. **Risks:** Proponents themselves warn that treatment should not be given in acute inflammatory conditions.
Eliminative methods, bloody Bloody cupping (*see* page 815) is said to encourage the immune system and alleviate symptoms.	**Not advised** The efficacy and mode of action of this relatively invasive procedure are unproven.	**Risks:** Bloody cupping can cause infection and scarring. Furthermore, it should not be carried out in persons with bleeding disorders.

Treatment	Rating	Point of delivery/risks
Eliminative methods, unbloody Unbloody cupping (*see* page 817) is supposed to improve the body's own regulatory systems and to energize (*see* page 927) the patient, stimulate the immune system, and alleviate symptoms.	**Of little use** Possibly acceptable as an additional preventive measure against hayfever and asthma. Some case reports claim efficacy; however, success is probably seen in only a small proportion of patients (*see* Placebo, page xxi).	**Suitable for DIY** Qualified guidance is recommended. **Risks:** Unlikely provided treatment is carried out competently.
Flower remedies Flower remedies (*see* page 828) are said to restore emotional balance in persons with allergies and to assist the body's psychic ability to heal itself.	**Of little use** Acceptable as a short-term, supportive treatment attempt aimed at soothing and relaxing. Some case reports claim efficacy; however, success is probably seen in only a small proportion of patients (*see* Placebo, page xxi).	**Suitable for DIY** Qualified guidance is recommended. Practitioners should propose a treatment plan. **Risks:** Possible intolerance.
Homeopathy Highly diluted (potentized) solutions (*see* page 831) are believed to be able to redress vital energy imbalances. Organo- and functiotropic (*see* page 833) homeopathy is claimed to be effective for dealing with allergies.	**May be of some use** as a short-term treatment attempt. The majority of controlled clinical studies ascribe a degree of efficacy to homeopathy in persons with allergic asthma and hayfever.	**Requires a qualified practitioner** Homeopaths should be properly qualified and should propose a treatment plan. Ready-formulated preparations are suitable for do-it-yourself. **Risks:** Allergies and intolerance are possible.

Treatment	Rating	Point of delivery/risks
Hypnosis and self-hypnosis In the relaxed and generally altered state of awareness that is induced in hypnosis or self-hypnosis (*see* page 837), physical and emotional conditions can be addressed. Some professionally organized courses in self-hypnosis are now available. Hypnosis is often used in combination with other psycho- and behavioral therapies.	**Of little use** Acceptable as a short-term treatment attempt for chronic allergies when simpler, more established methods have been unsuccessful. Some case reports claim efficacy; however, success is probably seen in only a proportion of patients treated (*see* Placebo, page xxi).	**Requires a qualified practitioner** Hypnotherapists should be properly qualified and should propose a treatment plan. No credence should be given to anyone promising immediate or total success. **Risks:** Unlikely provided treatment is carried out competently.
Manual therapies Chiropractors and osteopaths use a series of manipulations to realign allegedly displaced vertebrae. This is said to release energy blockages (*see* page 927) and to eliminate the basis on which allergies are presumed to exist (*see* page 844).	**May be of some use** as a short-term, supportive treatment attempt in chronic cases when less risky methods have been unsuccessful. Some case reports claim efficacy for this potentially risky procedure; however, success is probably seen, if at all, in only a small proportion of patients (*see* Placebo, page xxi).	**Requires a qualified practitioner** Practitioners should be properly qualified and should propose a treatment plan. **Risks:** Manipulation of the head and cervical vertebrae can cause serious injury. Osteoporosis is one of several risk factors.

Treatment	Rating	Point of delivery/risks
Nutritional therapies An organic diet (*see* page 4) provides the body with essential and secondary plant nutrients that are believed to exercise a multitude of positive effects and to be capable, *inter alia*, of boosting the immune system.	**May be of some use** as an individually directed supportive measure. Elimination and rotation diets may be of some assistance in identifying food allergies.	**Suitable for DIY** Qualified guidance is recommended though not essential. See your doctor before starting an elimination or rotation diet. **Risks:** Avoid imbalanced or intolerable diets. They can cause deficiencies with serious consequences. Children are particularly at risk.
Physical therapies Kneipp treatments (*see* page 871) are said to improve the body's own regulatory systems, modulate the immune system (*see* page 10), and alleviate allergies.	**Of little use** Acceptable as a short-term treatment attempt. Some case reports claim efficacy; however, success is probably seen in only a small proportion of patients (*see* Placebo, page xxi).	**Suitable for DIY** Qualified guidance is recommended though not essential. **Risks:** Unlikely provided treatment is carried out competently.
Probiotics The introduction of certain bacteria into the gut is claimed to bring the intestinal flora back into balance and to have a beneficial effect on the immune system (*see* page 878).	**Of little use** Possibly acceptable as a short-term treatment attempt and prophylaxis in people with food intolerance. Some case reports claim efficacy; however, success is probably seen in only a proportion of patients (*see* Placebo, page xxi).	**Requires a qualified practitioner** Practitioners should be properly qualified and should propose a treatment plan. Non-prescription formulations are suitable for do-it-yourself. **Risks:** Fairly unlikely provided treatment is carried out competently.

Treatment	Rating	Point of delivery/risks
Reflex therapies Reflex zone massage (*see* page 883) and reflexology (*see* page 883) are claimed to act via reflex channels (*see* page 881) to boost the immune system and alleviate symptoms.	**Of little use** Acceptable as a short-term, supportive treatment attempt aimed at alleviating symptoms. Some case reports claim efficacy; however, success is probably seen in only a small proportion of patients (*see* Placebo, page xxi).	**Suitable for DIY** Qualified guidance is essential. **Risks:** Some people are sensitive to pressure; others find it hard to tolerate manual stimulation or close physical contact.
Relaxation techniques Autogenic training (*see* page 888), muscle relaxation according to Jacobson (*see* page 893), and various biofeedback techniques (*see* page 891) are said to relieve muscle tension and inner unrest, and might be effective in helping patients to become better aware of their physical and emotional states.	**Useful** as a short-term treatment attempt aimed at soothing and relaxing. Some case reports claim efficacy; however, success is probably seen in only a small proportion of patients (*see* Placebo, page xxi).	**Suitable for DIY** Once a sound understanding of the technique has been acquired from a trainer in groups or through individual tuition, patients can perform exercises themselves. Therapists should be properly qualified. **Risks:** Fairly unlikely.
Vitamins and trace elements The antioxidative properties of beta-carotene, vitamins C and E, and selenium are, it is supposed, instrumental in countering the formation of free radicals and in boosting the body's antioxidative defence systems (*see* page 900).	**Of little use** Some case reports claim efficacy; however, success is probably seen in only a proportion of patients (*see* Placebo, page xxi).	**Suitable for DIY** Medical supervision is recommended though not essential. **Risks:** Intolerance and overdosage are possible. Recent findings imply that beta-carotene might increase the risk of cancer.

Herbal remedies for allergies

Active ingredient/preparation	Rating
Cardiospermum ointment	**May be of some use** as a potentized treatment for itchy eczema and skin allergies. **Dosage** and application as instructed by the manufacturer/prescriber.
Echinacin ointment (from *Echinacea purpurea*)	**May be of some use** as a treatment attempt for slow to heal surface wounds, possibly also as a treatment attempt for skin allergies. Echinacin ointment is an immune stimulant and vulnerary. **Dosage:** As instructed by the manufacturer/prescriber. **Risks:** In isolated cases the ointment may exacerbate existing skin allergies.
Marigold ointment (*Calendula officinalis*)	**May be of some use** as a treatment attempt for skin allergies, slow to heal superficial wounds and suppurating sores. Marigold is a vulnerary and anti-inflammatory. **Dosage:** As instructed by the manufacturer/prescriber. **Risks:** Skin irritation may occur.

Herbal remedies for hayfever

Active ingredient/preparation	Rating
Echinacea with or without added calcium	**Of little use**. The benefit of adding calcium is in doubt; there is no proof that this type of preparation is effective for hayfever or other allergic conditions or symptoms. **Dosage:** As instructed by the manufacturer/prescriber. **Risks:** In isolated cases existing skin allergies may be exacerbated.

Skin

Acne

Causes and symptoms

Acne (*Acne vulgaris*) is a chronic, mainly adolescent affliction, though it may continue into middle age. It affects the skin in areas of the body where large amounts of sebum (the oily secretion of the sebaceous glands) are produced. Over-production of sebum causes the sebaceous ducts to become blocked, forming a comedo or blackhead, which may become inflamed. Inflammation varies in intensity and, in extreme cases, may produce pustules that burst and cause scarring.

Acne has numerous causes. As well as a possible hereditary component, the main factors are over-production of sebum (seborrhea), disturbed hornification, immunological processes, changing hormone levels, certain bacteria, stress, anxiety, and nutritional factors.

Orthodox treatment

As well as suggesting the use of one of the many available skin cleansing preparations, orthodox doctors may prescribe a medication to remove the horny layer, disinfect the skin, inhibit bacterial growth, and ease inflammation.

Complementary therapies

Some practitioners use treatments that are very similar in nature to those of orthodox medicine. Some take a more constitutional approach (*see* Constitution, page 927), while others aim to remove foci (*see* page 928) or toxins (*see* page 929), or aim to redress an energy imbalance (*see* page 927) or change the diet.

Clinical studies are beginning to confirm that some herbal preparations are possibly efficacious to a degree.

Treatment plan and limited trial

Before administering a complementary treatment, every therapist should propose a treatment plan (*see* page xxiii) that sets out a clear time frame and defines the goal that the treatment is designed to achieve. Treatment should then be tried for a limited term to test the patient's response.

Caution

Promises of quick cures often seen in the media are clearly unrealistic.

Complementary treatments for acne

Treatment	Rating	Point of delivery/risks
Acupuncture Acupuncture in its various forms (*see* page 772) aims to encourage the flow of energy (*see* page 927) and to encourage metabolic processes, or to act directly to alleviate symptoms and speed up healing.	**Of little use** Acceptable as a short-term treatment attempt. Case reports and field studies claim efficacy; however, success is probably seen in only a proportion of patients (*see* Placebo, page xxi).	**Requires a qualified practitioner** Acupuncturists should be properly qualified and should propose a treatment plan. **Risks:** Probably rare provided treatment is carried out competently.
Anthroposophical medicine For proponents of AM (*see* page 781), acne is a sign that metabolic processes in the upper pole have overshot the mark. Therefore, elimination via the liver and kidneys must be encouraged. Medications used include potentized drugs and the remedy Dermatodoron.	**May be of some use** as a short-term treatment attempt. Some studies claim efficacy; however, success is probably seen in only a proportion of patients (*see* Placebo, page xxi).	**Requires a qualified practitioner** Practitioners should be properly qualified and should propose a treatment plan. **Risks:** Allergies and intolerance are possible.
Bioresonance therapy Bioresonance therapists use electrical devices in an attempt to discover the causes of illness and claim to be able to weaken or turn around pathogenic energies and disease related vibrations (*see* page 794).	**Of little use** Possibly acceptable as a short-term, supportive treatment attempt when simpler, more established methods have been unsuccessful. Some case reports claim efficacy; however, success is probably seen in only a small proportion of patients (*see* Placebo, page xxi).	**Requires a qualified practitioner** Practitioners should be properly qualified and should propose a treatment plan. No credence should be given to anyone promising immediate or total success. **Risks:** Fairly unlikely.

Treatment	*Rating*	*Point of delivery/risks*
Cell therapy Injecting or ingesting products extracted from the tissues of newborn animals or animal fetuses is said to have a rejuvenating and revitalizing effect and to enhance the healing of human tissues and organs (*see* page 796).	**Not advised** Based on present knowledge, there is inadequate evidence of the efficacy and mode of action of these costly and relatively risky procedures.	**Risks:** Injecting foreign proteins into the body can provoke (possibly fatal) allergic reactions. Also, pathogens such as those that cause bovine spongiform encephalopathy (BSE) or other serious infections may be introduced.
Electroacupuncture according to Voll By taking readings of the electrical conductivity of the skin (*see* page 802), therapists claim to be able to derive an insight into diseased areas of the body, pathogenic foci (*see* page 928), and stress factors (*see* Toxins, page 929). The factors supposedly instrumental in the causation of acne can then be addressed.	**Of little use** Possibly acceptable as a short-term, supportive treatment attempt when simpler, more established methods have been unsuccessful. Some case reports claim efficacy; however, success is probably seen, if at all, in only a small proportion of patients (*see* Placebo, page xxi).	**Requires a qualified practitioner** Practitioners should be properly qualified and should propose a treatment plan. No credence should be given to anyone promising immediate or total success. **Risks:** A second opinion must always be obtained from a qualified physician before any attempt is made to "eliminate foci" (e.g. by surgery).

Treatment	Rating	Point of delivery/risks
Electroneural therapy according to Croon According to the theory, readings taken at various reactive sites on the skin highlight diseased areas within the body. Based on these readings, targeted electrostimulative measures can be undertaken to address the factors that are supposedly instrumental in the causation of acne (*see* page 806).	**Of little use** Possibly acceptable as a short-term, supportive treatment attempt when simpler, more established methods have been unsuccessful. Some case reports claim efficacy; however, success is probably seen, if at all, in only a small proportion of patients (*see* Placebo, page xxi).	**Requires a qualified practitioner** Practitioners should be properly qualified and should propose a treatment plan. No credence should be given to anyone promising immediate or total success. **Risks:** Proponents themselves warn that treatment should not be given in acute inflammatory conditions.
Eliminative methods, bloody Bloody cupping (*see* page 815) is said to improve the body's own regulatory systems and detoxify the body.	**Not advised** The mode of action and efficacy of this invasive procedure are unproven.	**Risks:** Bloody cupping can cause infection and scarring. Furthermore, it should not be carried out in persons with bleeding disorders.
Eliminative methods, unbloody Unbloody cupping (*see* page 817) is supposed to improve the body's own regulatory systems, modulate the immune system (*see* page 10), and ease symptoms.	**Of little use** Possibly acceptable as a short-term treatment attempt when more established methods have been unsuccessful. Some case reports claim efficacy; however, success is probably seen in only a small proportion of patients (*see* Placebo, page xxi).	**Suitable for DIY** Qualified guidance is recommended. **Risks:** Unlikely provided treatment is carried out competently.

Treatment	Rating	Point of delivery/risks
Enzyme therapy The enzymes used are said to dispel and destroy "immune complexes" (*see* page 824) that course in the blood and that are responsible, for instance, for sustaining inflammatory processes.	**Of little use** Some case reports claim efficacy for this little researched therapy; however, success is probably seen in only a small proportion of patients (*see* Placebo, page xxi).	**Requires a qualified practitioner** Practitioners should propose a treatment plan. Non-prescription preparations are suitable for do-it-yourself. **Risks:** Allergies or intolerance are possible.
Flower remedies Flower remedies (*see* page 828) are said to restore emotional balance and assist the body's psychic ability to heal itself.	**Of little use** Acceptable as a short-term treatment attempt aimed at soothing and relaxing. Some case reports claim efficacy; however, success is probably seen in only a proportion of patients (*see* Placebo, page xxi).	**Suitable for DIY** Qualified guidance is recommended. Practitioners should propose a treatment plan. **Risks:** Possible intolerance.
Homeopathy Highly diluted (potentized) solutions (*see* page 831) are believed to be able to redress vital energy imbalances. Organo- and functiotropic (*see* page 833) homeopathy is claimed to be effective for dealing symptomatically with acne.	**May be of some use** as a short-term treatment attempt. Initial clinical studies, field studies, and case reports ascribe a degree of efficacy to this treatment in some patients (*see* Placebo, page xxi).	**Requires a qualified practitioner** Homeopaths should be properly qualified and should propose a treatment plan. Ready-formulated preparations are suitable for do-it-yourself. **Risks:** Allergies and intolerance are possible.

Treatment	Rating	Point of delivery/risks
Manual therapies Chiropractors and osteopaths use a series of manipulations to realign allegedly displaced vertebrae. This is said to rectify dysfunctions, release energy blockages (*see* page 927), and remove the presumed basis on which acne can exist (*see* page 844).	**Of little use** Possibly acceptable in chronic cases as a short-term, supportive treatment attempt when less risky, more established methods have been unsuccessful. Some case reports claim efficacy for this potentially risky procedure; however, success is probably seen, if at all, in only a small proportion of patients (*see* Placebo, page xxi).	**Requires a qualified practitioner** Practitioners should be properly qualified and should propose a treatment plan. **Risks:** Manipulation of the head and cervical vertebrae can cause serious injury. Osteoporosis is one of several risk factors.
Nutritional therapies An organic diet (*see* page 4) provides the body with essential and secondary plant nutrients that are believed to be capable, *inter alia*, of boosting the immune system. Patients are sometimes advised to cut down on fats, sugar, alcohol, and hot, spicy foods.	**Useful** as an individually directed supportive measure. Case reports claim efficacy; however, success is probably seen in only a proportion of patients (*see* Placebo, page xxi).	**Suitable for DIY** Qualified guidance is recommended though not essential. **Risks:** Avoid imbalanced or intolerable diets. They can cause deficiencies with serious consequences. Children are particularly at risk.
Physical therapies Various physical therapies including vapor inhalation, steam douches, packs (*see* page 878) with bran or horsetail, dry brushing, and sunlight are claimed to alleviate symptoms and speed up the healing process.	**Useful** as a short-term treatment attempt. Case reports and field studies claim efficacy; however, success is probably seen in only a proportion of patients (*see* Placebo, page xxi).	**Suitable for DIY** Qualified guidance is recommended though not essential. **Risks:** Skin damage may be caused to persons with diminished temperature sensation when extreme temperatures are applied.

Treatment	Rating	Point of delivery/risks
Probiotics The introduction of certain bacteria into the gut is claimed to bring the intestinal flora back into balance and to have a beneficial effect on the immune system (*see* page 878).	**Of little use** Possibly acceptable as a short-term, supportive treatment attempt for chronic acne when more established methods have been unsuccessful. Some case reports claim efficacy; however, success is probably seen in only a small proportion of patients (*see* Placebo, page xxiii).	**Requires a qualified practitioner** Practitioners should be properly qualified and should propose a treatment plan. Non-prescription formulations are suitable for do-it-yourself. **Risks:** Fairly unlikely provided treatment is carried out competently.
Vitamins and trace elements Vitamin E, derivatives of vitamin A (retinoids), and zinc are claimed to alleviate symptoms and speed up the healing process (*see* page 900).	**Of little use** Based on present knowledge, it is not possible to make any definitive recommendations. Use of vitamin A derivatives, vitamin D, and zinc is a conventional treatment for certain skin conditions.	**Suitable for DIY** Qualified guidance is recommended. Any proposed treatments with retinoids should be discussed with your doctor or dermatologist. **Risks:** Intolerance and overdosage are possible.

Herbal remedies for acne

Active ingredient/preparation	Rating
Agnus castus fruits (*Vitex agnus-castus*)	**May be of some use** to girls and women suffering from acne. Agnus castus has estrogenic activity. The substance is slow to act and must be taken over a period of weeks (up to six months). **Daily dose:** 1–1.5oz dried fruits, 1 tablet/capsule or 40 drops of tincture once a day. **Risks:** Agnus castus may occasionally cause skin itchiness. It must not be taken by women who are pregnant or breastfeeding.

Active ingredient/preparation	Rating
Brewer's yeast (*Saccharomyces cerevisiae*)	Taken orally, brewer's yeast **may be of some use** as a treatment attempt for chronic acne. However, its use may actually exacerbate the condition. **Daily dose:** 750mg. **Individual dose:** Take 250mg with water. Use ready-formulated preparations as instructed by the manufacturer/prescriber. **Risks:** Has a hypertensive action when taken with MAO inhibitors (a type of antidepressant drug). May cause flatulence and, rarely, hypersensitivity with itching or even Quincke's edema.
Tea tree oil (*Melaleuca alternifolia*)	**May be of some use** as an alternative to exfoliating agents such as benzoyl peroxide, and for skin care for acne. **Dosage:** As instructed by the manufacturer/prescriber. **Risks:** Tea tree oil can cause allergic skin reactions.

Herpes

Causes and symptoms

Herpes is a viral infection that presents as small, painful blisters on the skin. There are several strains of the virus, the most common being *Herpes zoster* (the chicken pox and shingles virus) and *Herpes simplex* (responsible also for genital herpes).

Herpes simplex is mostly caught in early childhood, though it remains dormant and symptomless until being activated when the immune system is at a low ebb. The first signs are localized itchiness, followed by the formation of small blisters or sores, which are usually grouped around the mouth and nose; occasionally also around the genitalia or cornea of the eye. Lack of prompt treatment if the condition affects the meninges (lining of the brain) or the brain itself can be severely damaging or even fatal. Genital herpes can be caught by sexual contact. Herpes infections may also be secondary to other forms of skin disease, such as neurodermatitis (*see* page 341).

Orthodox treatment

Conventional doctors aim to ease irritation and, through suitable anti-viral medications, to shorten the duration of the disease and stop the symptoms from spreading to other parts of the body. Some doctors see immunomodulation (*see* page 10) as a way of controlling the disease.

Complementary therapies

Some complementary practitioners seek to ease symptoms by acting directly through energy links (*see* page 928). Some see herpes as being caused by a weak immune system, by environmental pollutants or foci (*see* page 928), or as the result of an energy imbalance (*see* page 929). Treatment is offered accordingly.

Treatment plan and limited trial

Before administering a complementary treatment, every therapist should propose a treatment plan (*see* page xxiii) that sets out a clear time frame and defines the goal that the treatment is designed to achieve. Treatment should then be tried for a limited term to test the patient's response.

Cautions

If meningitis or encephalitis is suspected, the patient must be immediately admitted to a hospital. An eye specialist must be seen immediately if the cornea is affected.

Complementary treatments for herpes

Treatment	Rating	Point of delivery/risks
Acupressure This treatment (*see* page 769), otherwise known as pressure-point massage, is claimed to alleviate soreness associated with herpes.	**May be of some use** as a short-term treatment attempt aimed at alleviating soreness. Some case reports claim efficacy; however, success is probably seen in only a proportion of patients (*see* Placebo, page xxi).	**Suitable for DIY** Qualified guidance is recommended. Therapists should be properly qualified. **Risks:** Unlikely provided treatment is carried out competently.
Acupuncture Acupuncture in its various forms (*see* page 772) aims to encourage the flow of energy (*see* page 927) or to act directly to alleviate symptoms and prevent herpes.	**May be of some use** as a short-term treatment attempt aimed at alleviating soreness. Some case reports and field studies claim efficacy; however, success is probably seen in only a proportion of patients (*see* Placebo, page xxi).	**Requires a qualified practitioner** Acupuncturists should be properly qualified and should propose a treatment plan. **Risks:** Probably rare provided treatment is carried out competently.
Anthroposophical medicine AM (*see* page 781) sees herpes as a condition in which the body responds locally to various stress factors. In persons with a weakened immune system, a general constitutional therapy will be provided.	**May be of some use** as a short-term treatment attempt. Case reports claim efficacy; however, success is probably seen in only a proportion of patients (*see* Placebo, page xxi).	**Requires a qualified practitioner** Practitioners should be properly qualified and should propose a treatment plan. **Risks:** Allergies and intolerance are possible.

Treatment	Rating	Point of delivery/risks
Aromatherapy Essential oils (*see* page 786) are used to soothe and relax the patient. The essences may be taken orally, used externally as massage oils or bathing emulsions, or inhaled as vapors.	**Of little use** Acceptable as a short-term, supportive measure aimed at soothing and relaxing, or invigorating. Some case reports claim efficacy; however, success is probably seen in only a small proportion of patients (*see* Placebo, page xxi).	**Suitable for DIY** Qualified guidance is recommended. The effects of individual essential oils differ widely. **Risks:** Allergies or intolerance are possible. Some oils are carcinogenic in test systems and possibly in humans.
Bioresonance therapy Bioresonance therapists use electrical devices in an attempt to discover the causes of illness and claim to be able to weaken or turn around pathogenic energies and disease related vibrations (*see* page 794).	**Of little use** Possibly acceptable as a short-term treatment attempt in persistent cases when simpler, more established methods have been unsuccessful. Some case reports claim efficacy; however, success is probably seen, if at all, in only a small proportion of patients (*see* Placebo, page xxi).	**Requires a qualified practitioner** Practitioners should be properly qualified and should propose a treatment plan. No credence should be given to anyone promising immediate or total success. **Risks:** Fairly unlikely.
Cell therapy Injecting or ingesting products extracted from the tissues of newborn animals or animal fetuses is said to have a rejuvenating and revitalizing effect and to enhance the healing of human tissues and organs (*see* page 796).	**Not advised** Based on present knowledge, there is inadequate evidence of the efficacy and mode of action of these costly and relatively risky procedures. Study findings for the immune system modulating action of thymus therapy (*see* page 798) are contradictory.	**Risks:** Injecting foreign proteins into the body can provoke (possibly fatal) allergic reactions. Also, pathogens such as those that cause bovine spongiform encephalopathy (BSE) or other serious infections may be introduced.

Treatment	*Rating*	*Point of delivery/risks*
Electroacupuncture according to Voll By taking readings of the electrical conductivity of the skin (*see* page 802), therapists claim to be able to derive an insight into diseased areas of the body, pathogenic foci (*see* page 928), and stress factors (*see* Toxins, page 929). The factors presumed to be instrumental in the causation of herpes can then be addressed.	**Of little use** Possibly acceptable as a short-term, supportive treatment attempt in persistent cases when simpler, more established methods have been unsuccessful. Some case reports claim efficacy; however, success is probably seen, if at all, in only a small proportion of patients (*see* Placebo, page xxi).	**Requires a qualified practitioner** Practitioners should be properly qualified and should propose a treatment plan. **Risks:** A second opinion must always be obtained from a qualified physician before any attempt is made to "eliminate foci" (e.g. by surgery).
Electroneural therapy according to Croon According to the theory, readings taken at various reactive sites on the skin highlight diseased areas within the body. Based on these readings, targeted electrostimulative measures can be undertaken to address the factors presumed to be instrumental in the causation of herpes (*see* page 806).	**Of little use** Possibly acceptable as a short-term treatment attempt in persistent cases when simpler, more established methods have been unsuccessful. Some case reports claim efficacy; however, success is probably seen, if at all, in only a small proportion of patients (*see* Placebo, page xxi).	**Requires a qualified practitioner** Practitioners should be properly qualified and should propose a treatment plan. **Risks:** Proponents themselves warn that treatment should not be given in acute inflammatory conditions.
Eliminative methods, unbloody Unbloody cupping (*see* page 817) is supposed to improve the body's own regulatory systems, ease pain, and energize the patient (*see* page 927). Cantharide poultices (*see* page 812) are said to detoxify the body.	**May be of some use** as a short-term treatment attempt for chronic pain. Some case reports claim efficacy; however, success is probably seen in only a small proportion of patients (*see* Placebo, page xxi).	**Suitable for DIY** Unbloody cupping is best carried out under the guidance of a qualified practitioner. Treatment with cantharide poultices requires a qualified practitioner. **Risks:** Cantharide poultices can cause second-degree burns.

Treatment	Rating	Point of delivery/risks
Enzyme therapy The enzymes used are said to dispel and destroy "immune complexes" (*see* page 824) that course in the blood and that are responsible, for instance, for causing autoimmune disorders and for sustaining inflammatory processes.	**Of little use** Possibly acceptable as a short-term treatment attempt. Some case reports claim efficacy for this little researched therapy; however, success is probably seen in only a small proportion of patients (*see* Placebo, page xxi).	**Requires a qualified practitioner** Practitioners should propose a treatment plan. Non-prescription preparations are suitable for do-it-yourself. **Risks:** Allergies or intolerance are possible.
Flower remedies Flower remedies (*see* page 828) are said to restore emotional balance and assist the body's psychic ability to heal itself.	**Of little use** Acceptable as a short-term treatment attempt aimed at soothing and relaxing. Some case reports claim efficacy; however, success is probably seen in only a proportion of patients (*see* Placebo, page xxi).	**Suitable for DIY** Qualified guidance is recommended. Practitioners should propose a treatment plan. **Risks:** Possible intolerance.
Homeopathy Highly diluted (potentized) solutions (*see* page 831) are believed to be able to redress vital energy imbalances and strengthen the body's defences. Organo- and functiotropic (*see* page 833) homeopathy is claimed to be effective for dealing with symptoms.	**May be of some use** as a short-term treatment attempt. Some case reports and field studies claim efficacy; however, success is probably seen in only a small proportion of patients (*see* Placebo, page xxi).	**Requires a qualified practitioner** Homeopaths should be properly qualified and should propose a treatment plan. Ready-formulated preparations are suitable for do-it-yourself. **Risks:** Allergies and intolerance are possible.

Treatment	Rating	Point of delivery/risks
Hypnosis and self-hypnosis In the relaxed and generally altered state of awareness that is induced in hypnosis or self-hypnosis (*see* page 837), physical conditions can be influenced and pain alleviated.	**Of little use** Acceptable as an additional treatment attempt in persistent cases. Case reports suggest that some patients experience an easing of symptoms (*see* Placebo, page xxi).	**Requires a qualified practitioner** Hypnotherapists should be properly qualified and should propose a treatment plan. **Risks:** Unlikely provided treatment is carried out competently.
Manual therapies Chiropractors and osteopaths use a series of manipulations to realign allegedly displaced vertebrae. This is said to release energy blockages (*see* page 927) and remove factors that are presumed to be instrumental in the causation of herpes (*see* page 844).	**Of little use** Possibly acceptable as a short-term treatment attempt in persistent cases. Some case reports claim efficacy for this relatively risky, little researched procedure; however, success is probably seen, if at all, in only a small proportion of patients (*see* Placebo, page xxi).	**Requires a qualified practitioner** Practitioners should be properly qualified and should propose a treatment plan. **Risks:** Manipulation of the head and cervical vertebrae can cause serious injury. Osteoporosis is one of several risk factors.
Nutritional therapies An organic diet (*see* page 4) provides the body with essential and secondary plant nutrients that are believed to exercise a multitude of positive effects and to be capable, *inter alia*, of boosting the immune system.	**Useful** as an individually directed supportive measure. Some case reports claim efficacy for this treatment in the prevention and treatment of herpes; however, success is probably seen in only a proportion of patients (*see* Placebo, page xxi).	**Suitable for DIY** Qualified guidance is recommended though not essential. **Risks:** Avoid imbalanced or intolerable diets. They can cause deficiencies with serious consequences. Children are particularly at risk.

Treatment	Rating	Point of delivery/risks
Physical therapies Cold stimuli are said to tone up the body, improve the body's own regulatory systems, and modulate the immune system (*see* page 10). Ice massage is also used to alleviate the pain of shingles. Electrotherapies are claimed to kill viruses (*see* pages 867–78).	**May be of some use** as a supportive treatment attempt aimed at toning up the body. Some case reports claim efficacy; however, success is probably seen in only a proportion of patients (*see* Placebo, page xxi).	**Suitable for DIY** Qualified guidance is recommended though not essential. **Risks:** Skin damage may be caused to persons with diminished temperature sensation when extreme temperatures are applied.
Probiotics The introduction of certain bacteria into the gut is claimed to bring the intestinal flora back into balance and to have a beneficial effect on other parts of the immune system (*see* page 878).	**Of little use** Possibly acceptable as a preventive measure and as a short-term treatment attempt when more established methods have been unsuccessful. Some case reports claim efficacy; however, success is probably seen in only a small proportion of patients (*see* Placebo, page xxi).	**Requires a qualified practitioner** Practitioners should be properly qualified and should propose a treatment plan. Non-prescription formulations are suitable for do-it-yourself. **Risks:** Fairly unlikely provided treatment is carried out competently.
Reflex therapies Reflex zone massage (*see* page 883), reflexology (*see* page 883), and TENS (*see* page 886) are claimed to act via reflex channels (*see* page 881) to release energy blockages (*see* page 927) and ease pain.	**May be of some use** as a short-term treatment attempt aimed at alleviating pain. Case reports claim efficacy; however, success is probably seen in only a proportion of patients (*see* Placebo, page xxi).	**Suitable for DIY** Qualified guidance is essential. **Risks:** Some people are sensitive to electrical stimuli and rubber electrodes; others find it hard to tolerate manual stimulation or close physical contact.

Treatment	Rating	Point of delivery/risks
Relaxation techniques Autogenic training (*see* page 888), muscle relaxation according to Jacobson (*see* page 893), and various biofeedback techniques (*see* page 891) are said to relieve muscle tension and inner unrest, alleviate pain, and help the patient to become more aware of his/her physical and emotional states.	**May be of some use** as a supportive treatment attempt aimed at soothing and relaxing. Some case reports claim efficacy; however, success is probably seen in only a proportion of patients (*see* Placebo, page xxi).	**Suitable for DIY** Once a sound understanding of the technique has been acquired from a trainer, patients can perform exercises themselves. Therapists should propose a treatment plan. **Risks:** Fairly unlikely.
Vitamins and trace elements The antioxidative properties of beta-carotene and vitamins C and E are, it is supposed, instrumental in boosting the body's antioxidative defence systems and modulating the immune system (*see* page 10). High doses of vitamin B12 are claimed to help ease herpes (*see* page 900).	**Of little use** Some case reports claim efficacy for this poorly documented treatment; however, success is probably seen in only a small proportion of patients (*see* Placebo, page xxi).	**Suitable for DIY** Qualified guidance is recommended though not essential. **Risks:** Intolerance and overdosage are possible. Recent findings imply that beta-carotene might increase the risk of cancer.

Herbal remedy for herpes

Active ingredient/preparation	Rating
Lemon balm leaves (*Melissa officinalis*)	In formulations for external use, lemon balm **may be of some use** as a treatment attempt for herpes. Early use is important. Symptomatic treatment is usually ineffective once sores have formed. **Daily dose:** 8–10g dried leaves or as instructed by the manufacturer/prescriber. **Risks:** Lemon balm is not known to have any serious side effects.

Itching

Causes and symptoms

Itching is a condition that can involve the autonomic nervous system, the peripheral blood circulation, the internal organs, and psychological factors. Chronic itching can have many causes: it may be a symptom of skin disease, an expression of emotional problems or stress, or (especially in the elderly) a result of having dry skin. It may also be caused, however, by serious internal disease, including various forms of cancer. Compulsive scratching in response to itchiness can damage the skin and produce scarring.

Orthodox treatment

Conventional doctors aim first to identify the cause of itching and then to eliminate it. If itching is drug-induced, the preparation that precipitates the symptoms should be discontinued and replaced with a chemically unrelated drug substance.

Complementary therapies

Depending on their particular standpoint, complementary practitioners believe chronic itching to be caused by constitutional factors (*see* Constitution, page 927), foci (*see* page 928), toxins (*see* page 929), or energy imbalances (*see* 927), and attempt to treat it accordingly. Certain practitioners claim to act directly on the symptoms by exploiting energy links (*see* page 928).

Treatment plan and limited trial

Before administering a complementary treatment, every therapist should propose a treatment plan (*see* page xxiii) that sets out a clear time frame and defines the goal that the treatment is designed to achieve. Treatment should then be tried for a limited term to test the patient's response.

Caution

Before any attempt is made to treat recurrent or chronic itching by nonorthodox means, the patient must be examined by a qualified doctor to exclude a serious physical disease as the possible cause.

Complementary treatments for itching

Treatment	Rating	Point of delivery/risks
Acupressure This treatment (*see* page 769), otherwise known as pressure-point massage, is claimed to improve the circulation and ease itching.	**May be of some use** as a short-term treatment attempt. Case reports and field studies claim efficacy; however, success is probably seen in only a proportion of patients (*see* Placebo, page xxi).	**Suitable for DIY** Qualified guidance is recommended. Therapists should be properly qualified. **Risks:** Unlikely provided treatment is carried out competently.
Acupuncture Acupuncture in its various forms (*see* page 772) aims to encourage the flow of energy (*see* page 927) or to ease itching directly (symptomatically). The acupuncture points chosen can vary from one practitioner to another.	**May be of some use** as a short-term treatment attempt aimed at easing itchiness. Case reports and field studies claim efficacy; however, success is probably seen in only a proportion of patients (*see* Placebo, page xxi).	**Requires a qualified practitioner** Practitioners should be properly qualified and should propose a treatment plan. **Risks:** Probably rare provided treatment is carried out competently.

Treatment	Rating	Point of delivery/risks
Aromatherapy Essential oils (*see* page 786) are used to soothe and relax, or to invigorate, thereby helping to ease itchiness. The essences may be taken orally, used externally as massage oils or bathing emulsions, or inhaled as vapors.	**Of little use** Acceptable as a short-term treatment attempt aimed at soothing and relaxing. Some case reports claim efficacy in alleviating itchiness; however, success is probably seen in only a proportion of patients (*see* Placebo, page xxi).	**Suitable for DIY** Qualified guidance is recommended. The effects of individual essential oils differ widely. **Risks:** Allergies or intolerance are possible. Some oils are carcinogenic in test systems and possibly in humans.
Bioresonance therapy Bioresonance therapists use electrical devices in an attempt to discover the causes of illness and claim to be able to weaken or turn around pathogenic energies and disease related vibrations, and so remove the causes of itchiness (*see* page 794).	**Of little use** Possibly acceptable as a short-term treatment attempt for persistent itchiness when simpler, more established methods have been unsuccessful. Some case reports claim efficacy; however, success is probably seen, if at all, in only a small proportion of patients (*see* Placebo, page xxi).	**Requires a qualified practitioner** Practitioners should be properly qualified and should propose a treatment plan. No credence should be given to anyone promising immediate or total success. **Risks:** Fairly unlikely.

Treatment	Rating	Point of delivery/risks
Electroacupuncture according to Voll By taking readings of the electrical conductivity of the skin (*see* page 802), therapists claim to be able to derive an insight into diseased areas of the body, pathogenic foci (*see* page 928), and stress factors (*see* Toxins, page 929). The factors presumed to be instrumental in the causation of itchiness can then be eliminated.	**Of little use** Possibly acceptable as a short-term treatment attempt when simpler, more established methods have been unsuccessful. Some case reports claim efficacy; however, success is probably seen, if at all, in only a small proportion of patients (*see* Placebo, page xxi).	**Requires a qualified practitioner** Practitioners should be properly qualified and should propose a treatment plan. No credence should be given to anyone promising immediate or total success. **Risks:** A second opinion must always be obtained from a qualified physician before any attempt is made to "eliminate foci" (e.g. by surgery).
Eliminative methods, bloody Bloody cupping (*see* page 815) is said to improve the body's own regulatory systems and so ease itchiness.	**Not advised** The efficacy of this relatively invasive and sometimes risky procedure is unproven.	**Risks:** Bloody cupping can cause infection and scarring. Furthermore, it should not be carried out on persons with bleeding disorders.
Eliminative methods, unbloody Unbloody cupping (*see* page 817) is supposed to improve the body's own regulatory systems and so ease itchiness.	**Of little use** Possibly acceptable as a short-term treatment attempt when simpler, more established methods have been unsuccessful. Some case reports claim efficacy; however, success is probably seen in only a small proportion of patients (*see* Placebo, page xxi).	**Suitable for DIY** Qualified guidance is recommended. **Risks:** Unlikely provided treatment is carried out competently.

Treatment	Rating	Point of delivery/risks
Flower remedies Flower remedies (*see* page 828) are said to restore emotional balance and assist the body's psychic ability to heal itself.	**Of little use** Acceptable as a short-term, supportive treatment attempt aimed at soothing and relaxing. Some case reports claim efficacy in easing itchiness; however, success is probably seen in only a small proportion of patients (*see* Placebo, page xxi).	**Suitable for DIY** Qualified guidance is recommended. Practitioners should propose a treatment plan. **Risks:** Possible intolerance.
Homeopathy Highly diluted (potentized) solutions (*see* page 831) are believed to be able to redress vital energy imbalances and strengthen the body's defences. Organo- and functiotropic (*see* page 833) homeopathy is claimed to be effective for treating itchiness.	**Of little use** Acceptable as a short-term treatment attempt when more established methods have been unsuccessful. Some case reports and field studies claim efficacy for organotropic preparations; however, success is probably seen in only a proportion of patients (*see* Placebo, page xxi).	**Requires a qualified practitioner** Homeopaths should be properly qualified and should propose a treatment plan. Ready-formulated preparations are suitable for do-it-yourself. **Risks:** Allergies and intolerance are possible.
Hypnosis and self-hypnosis In the relaxed and generally altered state of awareness that is induced in hypnosis or self-hypnosis (*see* page 837), physical conditions can be influenced and itchiness eased. Hypnosis is often used in combination with other psycho- and behavioral therapies.	**Of little use** Acceptable as a short-term treatment attempt in persistent cases when simpler, more established methods have been unsuccessful. Case reports claim efficacy; however, success is probably seen in only a proportion of patients treated (*see* Placebo, page xxi).	**Requires a qualified practitioner** Hypnotherapists should be properly qualified and should propose a treatment plan. **Risks:** Unlikely provided treatment is carried out competently.

Treatment	Rating	Point of delivery/risks
Nutritional therapies An organic diet (*see* page 4) provides the body with essential and secondary plant nutrients that are believed to exercise a multitude of positive effects.	**Useful** as an individually directed supportive measure.	**Suitable for DIY** Qualified guidance is recommended though not essential. **Risks:** Avoid imbalanced or intolerable diets. They can cause deficiencies with serious consequences. Children are particularly at risk.
Physical therapies Dry brushing is said to improve the circulation and ease itchiness (*see* pages 867–78).	**May be of some use** as a treatment attempt. Case reports claim efficacy; however, success is probably seen in only a proportion of patients (*see* Placebo, page xxi).	**Suitable for DIY** **Risks:** Unlikely provided treatment is carried out competently.
Probiotics The introduction of certain bacteria into the gut is claimed to bring the intestinal flora back into balance, to have a beneficial effect on various physical reactions, and so to ease itching (*see* page 878).	**Of little use** Possibly acceptable as a short-term treatment attempt for persistent itchiness when more established methods have been unsuccessful. Some case reports claim efficacy; however, success is probably seen in only a proportion of patients (*see* Placebo, page xxi).	**Requires a qualified practitioner** Practitioners should be properly qualified and should propose a treatment plan. Non-prescription formulations are suitable for do-it-yourself. **Risks:** Fairly unlikely provided treatment is carried out competently.

Treatment	Rating	Point of delivery/risks
Relaxation techniques Autogenic training (*see* page 888), muscle relaxation according to Jacobson (*see* page 893), and various biofeedback techniques (*see* page 891) are said to relieve muscle tension and inner unrest, and might be instrumental in helping the patient to become more aware of his/her physical and emotional states.	**May be of some use** as a treatment attempt in persistent cases. Some case reports ascribe a degree of efficacy to this treatment; however, success is probably seen in only a proportion of patients (*see* Placebo, page xxi).	**Suitable for DIY** Once a sound understanding of the technique has been acquired from a trainer in groups or through individual tuition, patients can perform exercises themselves. **Risks:** Fairly unlikely.

Herbal remedies for itching

Active ingredient/preparation	Rating
Menthol (constituent of the volatile oil from peppermint)	**May be of some use** as a treatment attempt for itchiness. Has a cooling, soothing action. **Dosage:** Apply several drops to a hand and rub into the skin. **Risks:** Allergic reactions are possible. Gastrointestinal problems may occur when high doses are absorbed through the skin. Do not apply to the nose and face of infants and young children.
Oat straw (*Avena sativa*)	**Only useful** as a supportive treatment attempt for inflammatory and scaly skin conditions, especially when there is itchiness. **Dosage:** 100g herb to a full immersion bath. **Risks:** Allergic skin reactions are possible.
Shepherd's myrtle root (*Ruscus aculeatus*)	**May be of some use** as a supportive external treatment attempt for chronic circulatory problems involving painful, heavy legs and itchiness, and for itchy hemorrhoids. **Dosage:** As instructed by the manufacturer/prescriber. **Risks:** Occasional skin intolerance, which quickly subsides once the remedy has been discontinued.

Active ingredient/preparation	Rating
Sweet clover (*Melilotus officinalis*)	**May be of some use** as a treatment attempt for itchiness caused by chronic circulatory disorders. **Dosage:** As instructed by the manufacturer/prescriber. **Risks:** Extensive use of ointments, creams, liniments, etc., can cause headaches.

Lice and mites

Causes and symptoms

Head, body, and crab lice are caught by direct physical contact as well as from infested clothing, bedding, communally used towels, and stuffed animals. They cause symptoms which include itchiness (*see* Itching, page 331) and skin irritation. Violent scratching can cause skin lesions. Lice and their eggs (nits) need to be physically removed, as they do not usually disappear of their own accord.

Mites are minute parasitic arachnids, mostly with an oval body form. Itch mites can be transferred by close personal contact. Female itch mites gouge out $^3/_8$-inch long cuniculi or burrows in the stratum corneum, the outermost layer of the epidermis, causing scabies, a disease that is attended with intense itching (*see* page 331).

Orthodox treatment

Orthodox treatment with anti-louse and anti-mite shampoos is very effective, especially when used in conjunction with a steel comb to remove the nits. All bedclothes, towels, undergarments, and (where possible) outer garments should be hot washed. If this is not possible, lice can also be killed by placing infested articles in a plastic bag for a day at a temperature above 95°F/35°C. Combs and hairbrushes should be discarded.

Complementary therapies

Some complementary practitioners claim to offer effective treatment against lice and mites. Such claims cannot be corroborated, however. Complementary procedures are, as a whole, inferior to the modern anti-louse, anti-mite, and anti-nit shampoos.

Attempted treatment

If an attempt at removing lice or mites by alternative means has not succeeded within a day or so, a modern anti-louse, anti-mite, and anti-nit shampoo should be used instead.

Caution

If you are not sure how to deal with lice or mites or have not already been given instructions (for example, by a school nurse) on how to tackle an infestation, seek a doctor's advice. Effective treatment will be required to stop the infestation spreading and lice from becoming established in hair, clothes, combs, bedding, stuffed animals and furnishings, from where they are extremely difficult to remove.

Complementary treatments for lice and mites

Treatment	Rating	Point of delivery/risks
Aromatherapy (*see* page 786) and **herbal remedies** Used locally, essential oils, e.g. of garlic, lavender, or rosemary, are said to dispel lice and mites.	**Of little use** Possibly acceptable as a short-term treatment attempt. Case reports claim efficacy; however, success is probably seen in only a proportion of patients (*see* Placebo, page xxi).	**Suitable for DIY** The essences should be massaged in and rinsed out after 15–20 minutes. The hair should then be combed with a nit comb. **Risks:** Allergies or intolerance are possible.
Homeopathy Some homeopaths report that highly diluted (potentized) solutions (*see* page 831) are capable of ridding the hair of lice and mites.	**Of little use** There is no evidence that this treatment works. Case reports claim efficacy; however, success is probably seen in only a small proportion of patients (*see* Placebo, page xxi).	**Requires a qualified practitioner** Homeopaths should be properly qualified and should propose a treatment plan. Ready-formulated preparations are suitable for do-it-yourself. **Risks:** Allergies and intolerance are possible.
Washing with vinegar Washing the scalp with dilute vinegar is said to make it easier to comb out live lice and nits.	**May be of some use** as a short-term treatment attempt. Some case reports claim efficacy; however, success is probably seen in only a small proportion of patients (*see* Placebo, page xxi).	**Suitable for DIY** A dilute water/vinegar mixture should be massaged into the scalp. After a few minutes the lice and nits should be combed out with a fine-toothed nit comb. **Risks:** Fairly unlikely.

Herbal remedy for lice and mites

Active ingredient/preparation	Rating
Pyrethrins from *Chrysanthemum cineraria*	**May be of some use** as a treatment attempt. **Dosage and use:** As instructed by the manufacturer/prescriber. **Risks:** The pyrethrins contained in this flower may cause irritation and reddening of the scalp. Keep well away from the eyes and mucous membranes. Do not use during breastfeeding or in the first three months of pregnancy. Do not use on infants and young children.

Neurodermatitis

Causes and symptoms

Neurodermatitis is chronic, itchy irritation of the epidermis. It varies in severity and may present in a number of ways. Neurodermatitis often begins in early childhood. Symptoms include itchiness, redness, dry scaliness, blistering, and encrustation. Possible complications include bacterial and viral inflammation.

Neurodermatitis has a wide range of causes: intolerance of certain substances, temperature changes, and genetic, emotional, and social factors. The effect of food allergens as a trigger is probably overestimated.

Orthodox treatment

Thorough skin care will be the mainstay of treatment. Drugs will also be used—some in the form of locally applied preparations, including corticosteroid ointments, and some as tablets (anti-inflammatory and anti-pruritic preparations). Various types of physical therapy (climatic therapy and hydrotherapy) may also be used to alleviate the symptoms. Persistent cases may respond well to a change in diet or to counselling and stress management.

Complementary therapies

Practitioners of complementary therapies often suggest that neurodermatitis is a constitutional problem (*see* Constitution, page 927), or the result of a weakened immune system, an expression of disturbed life force (*see* page 928), or a consequence of airborne pollutants, food allergens, or toxic damage. Some treatments directly address the symptoms.

Treatment plan and limited trial

Before administering a complementary treatment, every therapist should propose a treatment plan (*see* page xxiii) that sets out a clear time frame and defines the goal that the treatment is designed to achieve. Treatment should then be tried for a limited term to test the patient's response.

Note

Orthodox and complementary therapies can be suitably combined in an overall program of treatment specially tailored to the individual's needs.

Complementary treatments for neurodermatitis

Treatment	Rating	Point of delivery/risks
Acupressure This treatment (*see* page 769), otherwise known as pressure-point massage, is claimed to alleviate pain, ease itching, and improve general well-being when pressure is applied to the appropriate points. It is also used as a means of imparting vital energy to the body (*see* Life force, page 928).	**Of little use** Acceptable as a short-term treatment attempt in persistent cases. Some case reports claim efficacy; however, success is probably seen in only a small proportion of patients (*see* Placebo, page xxi).	**Suitable for DIY** Qualified guidance is essential. **Risks:** Unlikely provided treatment is carried out competently.

Treatment	*Rating*	*Point of delivery/risks*
Acupuncture Acupuncture in its various forms (*see* page 772) aims to encourage the flow of energy (*see* page 927), to alleviate symptoms directly, or to prolong the intervals between acute phases.	**Of little use** Acceptable as a short-term treatment attempt and as a measure for alleviating symptoms and preventing the condition from worsening. Case reports claim efficacy; however, success is probably seen in only a proportion of patients (*see* Placebo, page xxi).	**Requires a qualified practitioner** Acupuncturists should be properly qualified and should propose a treatment plan. **Risks:** Probably rare provided treatment is carried out competently.
Anthroposophical medicine Once it has been established whether the symptoms are of an allergic, psychosomatic, or genetic nature, AM practitioners carry out individual "constitutional therapies" (*see* page 781).	**May be of some use** as a short-term treatment attempt when other treatments have been unsuccessful. Case reports claim efficacy; however, success is probably seen in only a proportion of patients (*see* Placebo, page xxi).	**Requires a qualified practitioner** Practitioners should be properly qualified and should propose a treatment plan. **Risks:** Allergies and intolerance are possible.
Aromatherapy Essential oils (*see* page 786) are used to soothe and relax, or to invigorate, thereby helping to ease symptoms. The essences may be taken orally, used externally as massage oils or bathing emulsions, or inhaled as vapors.	**Of little use** Acceptable as a short-term, supportive treatment attempt aimed at soothing and relaxing. Some case reports claim efficacy; however, success is probably seen in only a proportion of patients (*see* Placebo, page xxi).	**Suitable for DIY** Qualified guidance is recommended. The effects of individual essential oils differ widely. **Risks:** Allergies or intolerance are possible. Some oils are carcinogenic in test systems and possibly in humans.

Treatment	Rating	Point of delivery/risks
Bioresonance therapy Bioresonance therapists use electrical devices in an attempt to discover the causes of illness and claim to be able to weaken or turn around pathogenic energies and disease related vibrations (*see* page 794).	**Of little use** Possibly acceptable as a short-term, supportive treatment attempt when simpler, more established methods have been unsuccessful. Despite the fairly widespread use of this treatment for neurodermatitis, there are hardly any recorded data. Some case reports claim efficacy; however, success is probably seen, if at all, in only a small proportion of patients (*see* Placebo, page xxi).	**Requires a qualified practitioner** Practitioners should be properly qualified and should propose a treatment plan. No credence should be given to anyone promising immediate or total success. **Risks:** Fairly unlikely.
Cell therapy Injecting or ingesting products extracted from the tissues of newborn animals or animal fetuses is said to have a rejuvenating and revitalizing effect and to enhance the healing of human tissues and organs (*see* page 796).	**Not advised** Based on present knowledge, there is inadequate evidence of the efficacy and mode of action of these costly and relatively risky procedures.	**Risks:** Injecting foreign proteins into the body can provoke (possibly fatal) allergic reactions. Also, pathogens such as those that cause bovine spongiform encephalopathy (BSE) or other serious infections may be introduced.
Electroacupuncture according to Voll By taking readings of the electrical conductivity of the skin (*see* page 802), therapists claim to be able to derive an insight into diseased areas of the body, pathogenic foci (*see* page 928), and stress factors (*see* Toxins, page 929). The factors presumed to be instrumental in the causation of neurodermatitis can then be addressed.	**Of little use** Possibly acceptable as a short-term, supportive treatment attempt when simpler, more established methods have been unsuccessful. Some case reports claim efficacy; however, success is probably seen, if at all, in only a small proportion of patients (*see* Placebo, page xxi).	**Requires a qualified practitioner** Practitioners should be properly qualified and should propose a treatment plan. No credence should be given to anyone promising immediate or total success. **Risks:** A second opinion must always be obtained from a qualified physician before any attempt is made to "eliminate foci" (e.g. by surgery).

Treatment	Rating	Point of delivery/risks
Electroneural therapy according to Croon According to the theory, readings taken at various reactive sites on the skin highlight diseased areas within the body. Based on these readings, targeted electrostimulative measures can be undertaken to address the presumed causative factors (*see* page 806).	**Of little use** Possibly acceptable as a short-term, supportive treatment attempt when simpler, more established methods have been unsuccessful. Some case reports claim efficacy; however, success is probably seen, if at all, in only a small proportion of patients (*see* Placebo, page xxi).	**Requires a qualified practitioner** Practitioners should be properly qualified and should propose a treatment plan. No credence should be given to anyone promising immediate or total success. **Risks:** Proponents themselves warn that treatment should not be given in acute inflammatory conditions.
Eliminative methods, unbloody Unbloody cupping (*see* page 815) is supposed to ease symptoms and improve the body's own regulatory systems. Cantharide poultices (*see* page 812) are claimed to detoxify the body.	**Of little use** Unbloody cupping is possibly acceptable as a short-term treatment attempt when more established methods have been unsuccessful. Case reports claim efficacy; however, success is probably seen in only a small proportion of patients (*see* Placebo, page xxi).	**Suitable for DIY** Unbloody cupping is best carried out under the guidance of a qualified practitioner. Treatment with cantharide poultices requires a qualified practitioner. **Risks:** Cantharide poultices can cause second-degree burns.
Enzyme therapy The enzymes used are said to dispel and destroy "immune complexes" (*see* page 824) that course in the blood and that are responsible, for instance, for sustaining inflammatory processes.	**Of little use** Some case reports claim efficacy for this little researched therapy; however, success is probably seen, if at all, in only a small proportion of patients (*see* Placebo, page xxi).	**Requires a qualified practitioner** Practitioners should propose a treatment plan. Non-prescription preparations are suitable for do-it-yourself. **Risks:** Allergies or intolerance are possible.

Treatment	Rating	Point of delivery/risks
Flower remedies Flower remedies (*see* page 828) are said to restore emotional balance and assist the body's psychic ability to heal itself.	**Of little use** Acceptable as a short-term, supportive treatment attempt aimed at soothing and relaxing. Some case reports claim efficacy; however, success is probably seen in only a small proportion of patients (*see* Placebo, page xxi).	**Suitable for DIY** Qualified guidance is recommended. Practitioners should propose a treatment plan. **Risks:** Possible intolerance.
Homeopathy Highly diluted (potentized) solutions (*see* page 831) are believed to be able to redress vital energy imbalances and strengthen the body's defences. Organo- and functiotropic (*see* page 833) homeopathy is claimed to be effective for dealing with symptoms.	**May be of some use** as a treatment attempt. Controlled clinical studies, field studies, and case reports ascribe a degree of efficacy to homeopathy in some patients (*see* Placebo, page xxi).	**Requires a qualified practitioner** Homeopaths should be properly qualified and should propose a treatment plan. Ready-formulated preparations are suitable for do-it-yourself. **Risks:** Allergies and intolerance are possible.
Hypnosis and self-hypnosis In the relaxed and generally altered state of awareness that is induced in hypnosis or self-hypnosis (*see* page 837), physical conditions can be addressed and pain alleviated. Hypnosis is often used in combination with other psycho- and behavioral therapies.	**May be of some use** as a short-term, supportive treatment attempt aimed at relaxing the patient and helping him/her come to terms better with his/her condition. Some case reports claim efficacy; however, success is probably seen in only a proportion of patients treated (*see* Placebo, page xxi).	**Requires a qualified practitioner** Hypnotherapists should be properly qualified and should propose a treatment plan. **Risks:** Unlikely provided treatment is carried out competently.

Treatment	Rating	Point of delivery/risks
Nutritional therapies An organic diet (*see* page 4) provides the body with essential and secondary plant nutrients that are believed to exercise a multitude of positive effects and to be capable, *inter alia*, of boosting the immune system (*see* page 10).	**Useful** as an individually directed supportive measure. Elimination and rotation diets may be of some assistance in identifying the cause of chronic food allergy induced neurodermatitis.	**Suitable for DIY** Qualified guidance is recommended though not essential. See your doctor before starting an elimination or rotation diet. **Risks:** Avoid imbalanced or intolerable diets. They can cause deficiencies with serious consequences. Children are particularly at risk.
Physical therapies Full immersion baths with whey, milk, tea, or oil additives such as camomile or rosemary, and healing earth wraps are said to stop itchiness. Alternating temperature or cold washing, cold douches (*see* pages 875–6), and exercise therapy (*see* page 868) are said to tone up the system and improve circulation through the skin.	**Useful** as an individually directed, short-term treatment attempt. Some case reports claim efficacy; however, success is probably seen in only a proportion of patients (*see* Placebo, page xxi).	**Suitable for DIY** Qualified guidance is recommended though not essential. These treatments can differ widely in their effects and must be checked for efficacy. **Risks:** Skin damage may be caused to persons with diminished temperature sensation when extreme temperatures are applied.
Probiotics The introduction of certain bacteria into the gut is claimed to bring the intestinal flora back into balance and to have a beneficial effect on the immune system (*see* page 878).	**Of little use** Possibly acceptable as a short-term treatment attempt when more established methods have been unsuccessful. Some case reports claim efficacy; however, success is probably seen in only a proportion of patients (*see* Placebo, page xxi).	**Requires a qualified practitioner** Practitioners should be properly qualified and should propose a treatment plan. Non-prescription formulations are suitable for do-it-yourself. **Risks:** Fairly unlikely provided treatment is carried out competently.

Treatment	*Rating*	*Point of delivery/risks*
Reflex therapies Reflex zone massage (*see* page 883) and reflexology (*see* page 883) are claimed to act via reflex channels (*see* page 881) to ease pain, itchiness, and the tense feeling in the skin.	**Of little use** Acceptable as a short-term, supportive treatment attempt aimed at alleviating symptoms. Some case reports claim efficacy; however, success is probably seen in only a proportion of patients (*see* Placebo, page xxi).	**Suitable for DIY** Qualified guidance is essential. Practitioners should be properly qualified and should propose a treatment plan. **Risks:** Some people find it hard to tolerate manual stimulation or close physical contact.
Relaxation techniques Autogenic training (*see* page 888), muscle relaxation according to Jacobson (*see* page 893), and various biofeedback techniques (*see* page 891) are said to relieve muscle tension and inner unrest, and so might be instrumental in helping the patient come to terms better with his/her condition. These treatments are sometimes used in combination with psycho- and behavioral therapies.	**May be of some use** as a supportive treatment attempt aimed at relaxing the patient and helping him/her come to terms better with his/her condition. Some case reports claim efficacy for these procedures in the treatment of neurodermatitis; however, success is probably seen in only a small proportion of patients (*see* Placebo, page xxi).	**Suitable for DIY** Once a sound understanding of the technique has been acquired from a trainer in groups or through individual tuition, patients can perform exercises themselves. Therapists should propose a treatment plan. **Risks:** Fairly unlikely.
Vitamins and trace elements The antioxidative properties of beta-carotene, vitamins C and E, and selenium are said to exercise a multitude of positive effects and to be capable, *inter alia*, of boosting the immune system (*see* page 900).	**Useful** as an organic diet (*see* page 4) with a high fruit and vegetable content. Of little use when vitamin supplementation is attempted. No definitive recommendations can be made based on present knowledge.	**Suitable for DIY** Qualified guidance is recommended though not essential. **Risks:** Intolerance and overdosage are possible. Recent studies imply that beta-carotene might increase the risk of cancer.

Herbal remedies for neurodermatitis

Active ingredient/preparation	Rating
Borage oil (*Borago officinalis*)	**May be of some use** as a treatment attempt. Borage oil is mostly used as a cheaper alternative to evening primrose oil. **Daily dose:** 4–5g oil. **Individual dose:** Half a teaspoon twice daily. **Risks:** Borage oil can cause allergic reactions, also gastrointestinal problems. The quoted risks associated with pyrrolizidine alkaloids apply to the borage plant, though not to the oil. Borage oil should not be taken with any agent that may induce epilepsy (e.g. certain neuroleptics, including phenothiazines).
Evening primrose oil (*Oenothera biennis*)	**May be of some use** as a supportive treatment attempt, especially for children. Contains unsaturated fatty acids of the linoleic/linolenic acid type, which are thought to have a favorable metabolic action. There have not yet been any controlled long-term studies that would permit a definitive assessment. **Dosage:** As instructed by the manufacturer/prescriber. **Risks:** Evening primrose oil should not be taken with any agent that may induce epilepsy (e.g. certain neuroleptics, including phenothiazines).
Marigold flowers (*Calendula officinalis*)	**May be of some use** as an internal or external treatment attempt for superficial wounds that are slow to heal. Marigold is a vulnerary and anti-inflammatory. Marigold leaves receive a negative assessment due to a lack of efficacy. **Daily dose:** 2–5g herb. **Individual dose:** 1–2g petals infused with 5fl oz of hot water for drinking or as a poultice. Use ready-formulated preparations as instructed by the manufacturer/prescriber. **Risks:** Marigold can cause skin irritation.

Warts

Causes and symptoms

Warts can occur anywhere on the skin. They are caused by viruses which are passed on by direct person-to-person contact or caught in swimming pools, etc. Though painless and harmless, they may become an unsightly problem if they spread over the body.

In many cases warts will disappear spontaneously after a couple of months.

Orthodox treatment

Orthodox treatment usually involves destroying the wart with a proprietary salicylic acid paint or poultice. Low-dose cytostatics may also be injected locally if the problem is persistent. Warts can be removed surgically if other treatments have proved unsuccessful.

Complementary therapies

Complementary therapists see an outbreak of warts as a constitutional problem (see Constitution page 927), the manifestation of a weak immune system, a result of disturbed vital energy (*see* Life force, page 928), or the result of environmental influences and toxic damage. Some procedures aim to deal with warts directly via energy links (*see* page 928).

Treatment plan and limited trial

Before administering a complementary treatment, every therapist should propose a treatment plan (*see* page xxiii) that sets out a clear time frame and defines the goal that the treatment is designed to achieve. Treatment should then be tried for a limited term to test the patient's response.

Caution

A doctor should be seen before any attempt is made to treat a persistent wart problem using a complementary therapy. This is to rule out skin cancer as a possible cause.

Complementary treatments for warts

Treatment	Rating	Point of delivery/risks
Acupuncture Acupuncture in its various forms (*see* page 772) aims either to encourage the flow of energy (*see* page 927) and modulate the immune system (*see* page 10) as a general treatment, or to act directly against warts.	**Of little use** Acceptable as a short-term treatment attempt. Case reports and field studies claim efficacy; however, success is probably seen in only a proportion of patients (*see* Placebo, page xxi).	**Requires a qualified practitioner** Acupuncturists should be properly qualified and should propose a treatment plan. **Risks:** Probably rare provided treatment is carried out competently.
Anthroposophical medicine In the AM interpretation (*see* page 781), warts must be addressed by boosting "creative powers." To achieve this aim, antimony compounds in potentized form and as ointments are used.	**Of little use** Acceptable as a short-term treatment attempt. Case reports claim efficacy; however, success is probably seen in only a proportion of patients (*see* Placebo, page xxi).	**Requires a qualified practitioner** Practitioners should be properly qualified and should propose a treatment plan. **Risks:** Allergies and intolerance are possible.

Treatment	Rating	Point of delivery/risks
Aromatherapy Essential oils (*see* page 786) are used to soothe and relax, and to improve the body's own regulatory systems. The essences may be taken orally, used externally as massage oils or bathing emulsions, or inhaled as vapors.	**Of little use** Possibly acceptable as a supportive treatment attempt aimed at improving the body's own regulatory systems. Some case reports claim efficacy for this procedure in the treatment of warts; however, success is probably seen in only a small proportion of patients (*see* Placebo, page xxi).	**Suitable for DIY** Qualified guidance is recommended. The effects of individual essential oils differ widely. **Risks:** Allergies or intolerance are possible. Some oils are carcinogenic in test systems and possibly in humans.
Bioresonance therapy Bioresonance therapists use electrical devices in an attempt to discover the causes of illness and claim to be able to weaken or turn around pathogenic energies and disease related vibrations (*see* page 794).	**Of little use** Possibly acceptable as a short-term treatment attempt in persistent cases when simpler, more established methods have been unsuccessful. Some case reports claim efficacy; however, success is probably seen in only a small proportion of patients (*see* Placebo, page xxi).	**Requires a qualified practitioner** Practitioners should be properly qualified and should propose a treatment plan. No credence should be given to anyone promising immediate or total success. **Risks:** Fairly unlikely.
Cell therapy Injecting or ingesting products extracted from animal tissues or organs is said to have an immune system modulating effect and to enhance the healing of human tissues and organs (*see* page 796).	**Not advised** Based on present knowledge, there is inadequate evidence of the efficacy and mode of action of these costly and relatively risky procedures.	**Risks:** Injecting foreign proteins into the body can provoke (possibly fatal) allergic reactions. Also, pathogens such as those that cause bovine spongiform encephalopathy (BSE) or other serious infections may be introduced.

Treatment	Rating	Point of delivery/risks
Electroacupuncture according to Voll By taking readings of the electrical conductivity of the skin (*see* page 802), therapists claim to be able to derive an insight into diseased areas of the body, pathogenic foci (*see* page 928), and stress factors (*see* Toxins, page 929). The factors that are presumed to be instrumental in the causation of warts can then be addressed.	**Of little use** Possibly acceptable as a short-term treatment attempt in persistent cases when simpler, more established methods have been unsuccessful. Some case reports claim efficacy; however, success is probably seen in only a small proportion of patients (*see* Placebo, page xxi).	**Requires a qualified practitioner** Practitioners should be properly qualified and should propose a treatment plan. No credence should be given to anyone promising immediate or total success. **Risks:** A second opinion must always be obtained from a qualified physician before any attempt is made to "eliminate foci" (e.g. by surgery).
Electroneural therapy according to Croon According to the theory, readings taken at various reactive sites on the skin highlight diseased areas within the body. Based on these readings, targeted electrostimulative measures can be undertaken to eliminate factors presumed to be instrumental in the causation of warts (*see* page 806).	**Of little use** Possibly acceptable as a short-term treatment attempt in persistent cases when simpler, more established methods have been unsuccessful. Some case reports claim efficacy; however, success is probably seen in only a small proportion of patients (*see* Placebo, page xxi).	**Requires a qualified practitioner** Practitioners should be properly qualified and should propose a treatment plan. No credence should be given to anyone promising immediate or total success. **Risks:** Proponents themselves warn that treatment should not be given in acute inflammatory conditions.
Eliminative methods, bloody Bloody cupping (*see* page 815) is claimed to improve the body's own regulatory systems in severe or recurrent attacks of warts.	**Not advised** The efficacy of this relatively invasive method cannot be fully assessed based on present knowledge.	**Risks:** Bloody cupping can cause infection and scarring. Furthermore, it should not be carried out in persons with bleeding disorders.

Treatment	Rating	Point of delivery/risks
Eliminative methods, unbloody Unbloody cupping (*see* page 817) is supposed to improve the body's own regulatory systems and to energize (*see* page 927) the patient.	**Of little use** The efficacy of unbloody cupping cannot be fully assessed based on present knowledge.	**Suitable for DIY** Qualified guidance is recommended. **Risks:** Unlikely provided treatment is carried out competently.
Enzyme therapy The enzymes used are said to dispel and destroy "immune complexes" (*see* page 824) that course in the blood and that are responsible, for instance, for sustaining inflammatory processes. They are also claimed to boost the immune system.	**Of little use** This relatively costly procedure has been little researched. Some case reports claim efficacy; however, success is probably seen in only a small proportion of patients (*see* Placebo, page xxi).	**Requires a qualified practitioner** Practitioners should propose a treatment plan. Non-prescription preparations are suitable for do-it-yourself. **Risks:** Allergies or intolerance are possible.
Flower remedies Flower remedies (*see* page 828) are said to restore emotional balance and assist the body's psychic ability to heal itself.	**Of little use** Acceptable as a short-term, supportive treatment attempt aimed at soothing and relaxing. Some case reports claim efficacy; however, success is probably seen in only a small proportion of patients (*see* Placebo, page xxi).	**Suitable for DIY** Qualified guidance is recommended. Practitioners should propose a treatment plan. **Risks:** Possible intolerance.

Treatment	Rating	Point of delivery/risks
Homeopathy Highly diluted (potentized) solutions (*see* page 831) are believed to be able to redress vital energy imbalance. Organo- and functiotropic (*see* page 833) homeopathy are claimed to be effective for dealing with warts.	**Of little use** Acceptable as a short-term, supportive treatment attempt for persistent warts. Case reports and field studies claim efficacy; however, success is probably seen in only a proportion of patients (*see* Placebo, page xxi).	**Requires a qualified practitioner** Homeopaths should be properly qualified and should propose a treatment plan. Ready-formulated preparations are suitable for do-it-yourself. **Risks:** Allergies and intolerance are possible.
Hypnosis and self-hypnosis In the relaxed and generally altered state of awareness that is induced in hypnosis or self-hypnosis (*see* page 837), physical conditions can be addressed. Hypnosis is often used in combination with other psycho- and behavioral therapies.	**Of little use** Acceptable as an additional treatment attempt for massive or recurrent wart problems. Case reports show that symptoms can be eased in some patients (*see* Placebo, page xxi).	**Requires a qualified practitioner** Hypnotherapists should be properly qualified and should propose a treatment plan. **Risks:** Unlikely provided treatment is carried out competently.
Magnetic field therapy The use of magnetic field generators, magnetic strips, bracelets, and other objects (*see* page 841) allegedly encourages cell metabolism and helps eliminate warts.	**Of little use** Based on present knowledge, there is inadequate evidence of the efficacy and mode of action of magnetic field therapy in warts.	Operation of magnetic field equipment **requires a qualified practitioner**. **Risks:** Magnetic field equipment can cause implanted cardiac pacemakers to malfunction.

Treatment	Rating	Point of delivery/risks
Nutritional therapies An organic diet (*see* page 4) provides the body with essential and secondary plant nutrients that are believed to boost the immune system.	**Useful** as an individually directed supportive measure for dealing with massive or progressively worsening wart problems. Case reports claim efficacy; however, success is probably seen in only a proportion of patients (*see* Placebo, page xxi).	**Suitable for DIY** Qualified guidance is recommended though not essential. **Risks:** Avoid imbalanced or intolerable diets. They can cause deficiencies with serious consequences. Children are particularly at risk.
Physical therapies Washings and other hydrotherapeutic procedures (*see* pages 871–8) are said to encourage the circulation and to have an immune system modulating effect (*see* page 10).	**Of little use** Some case reports claim efficacy for this procedure; however, success is probably seen in only a small proportion of patients (*see* Placebo, page xxi).	**Suitable for DIY** **Risks:** Skin damage may be caused to persons with diminished temperature sensation when extreme temperatures are applied.
Probiotics The introduction of certain bacteria into the gut is claimed to bring the intestinal flora back into balance and to have a beneficial effect on other parts of the immune system (*see* page 878).	**Of little use** Possibly acceptable as a short-term treatment attempt for massive or recurrent wart problems. Case reports claim efficacy; however, success is probably seen in only a small proportion of patients (*see* Placebo, page xxi).	**Requires a qualified practitioner** Practitioners should be properly qualified and should propose a treatment plan. Non-prescription formulations are suitable for do-it-yourself. **Risks:** Fairly unlikely provided treatment is carried out competently.

Treatment	Rating	Point of delivery/risks
Relaxation techniques Autogenic training (*see* page 888), muscle relaxation according to Jacobson (*see* page 893), and various biofeedback techniques (*see* page 891) are said to relieve muscle tension and inner unrest, and so might be instrumental in helping to reduce psychosomatically induced warts.	**May be of some use** as a supportive treatment attempt aimed at relaxing the patient. Some case reports claim efficacy in the prevention or alleviation of warts; however, success is probably seen in only a small proportion of patients (*see* Placebo, page xxi).	**Suitable for DIY** Once a sound understanding of the technique has been acquired from a trainer, patients can perform exercises themselves. Therapists should propose a treatment plan. **Risks:** Fairly unlikely.
Vitamins and trace elements The antioxidative properties of beta-carotene and vitamins C and E are, it is supposed, instrumental in boosting the body's defence systems. High doses of vitamin B12 are said to help dispel warts (*see* page 900).	**Of little use** The efficacy of vitamins in dealing with wart problems cannot be assessed based on present knowledge.	**Suitable for DIY** Qualified guidance is recommended though not essential. **Risks:** Intolerance and overdosage are possible. Recent studies imply that beta-carotene might increase the risk of cancer.

Herbal remedies for warts

Active ingredient/preparation	Rating
Creeping juniper leaves or tincture (*Juniperus sabina*)	**May be of some use** as a treatment attempt for warts. Used externally, this remedy may cause local irritation, blistering, or skin damage depending on the length of time it is left to act. **Dosage:** As instructed by the manufacturer/prescriber. **Risks:** Not suitable for self-medication; see your doctor. The ingredient podophyllotoxin is a powerful skin irritant. Application of excessive amounts may lead to absorption through the skin, possibly leading to poisoning. Do not use during pregnancy.

Active ingredient/preparation	*Rating*
Greater celandine sap (*Chelidonium majus*)	**May be of some use** as a treatment attempt for warts. Apply fresh sap and allow it to dry. The treatment attempt must be continued for some time. **Risks:** Though not known to have any serious side effects when used externally in therapeutic doses, this plant should be used by trained herbalists only. (The Medicines Act 1968 restricts its sale to pharmacists and medical herbalists in the UK.)
Thuja tincture (*Thuja occidentalis*)	**Of little use** as a treatment attempt for warts. Apply tincture to the warts in the morning and evening, continuing for several weeks. The composition of thuja tincture reveals nothing with regard to a possible therapeutic principle. **Dosage:** Apply 3–4 drops to the wart every two to three hours. **Risks:** Do not use during pregnancy.

Eyes

Conjunctivitis

Causes and symptoms

Conjunctivitis, inflammation of the mucous membrane that forms the outer surface of the eyeball, may be caused by an infection or an allergy, or may be a symptom of another disease. Symptoms of acute conjunctivitis are red, itchy, or swollen eyes, increased lacrimation, and sensitivity to light.

Orthodox treatment

Treatment will include elimination of the causative factors, with antibiotics being prescribed where necessary.

Complementary therapies

Most complementary therapies aim simply to ease the symptoms.

Treatment plan and limited trial

Before administering a complementary treatment, every therapist should propose a treatment plan (*see* page xxiii) that sets out a clear time frame and defines the goal that the treatment is designed to achieve. Treatment should then be tried for a limited term to test the patient's response.

Cautions

Proper assessment by an eye specialist will be necessary if the symptoms are severe or prolonged. Many of the herbal remedies that will be suggested are themselves possibly allergenic.

Complementary treatments for conjunctivitis

Treatment	Rating	Point of delivery/risks
Acupressure This treatment (*see* page 769), otherwise known as pressure-point massage, is claimed to bring relief from conjunctivitis. The pressure points chosen can vary from one practitioner to another.	**Of little use** Possibly acceptable as a short-term, supportive treatment attempt for chronic cases. Some case reports claim efficacy; however, success is probably seen in only a proportion of patients (*see* Placebo, page xxi).	**Suitable for DIY** Qualified guidance is recommended. Therapists should be properly qualified. **Risks:** Unlikely provided treatment is carried out competently.
Acupuncture Acupuncture in its various forms (*see* page 772) aims to encourage the flow of energy (*see* page 927) or to act directly to ease symptoms. The acupuncture points chosen can vary from one practitioner to another.	**Of little use** Possibly acceptable as a short-term, supportive treatment attempt for chronic cases when simpler methods have been unsuccessful. Case reports, field studies, and clinical studies confirm that the procedure has a degree of efficacy.	**Requires a qualified practitioner** Acupuncturists should be properly qualified and should propose a treatment plan. **Risks:** Probably rare provided treatment is carried out competently.

Treatment	Rating	Point of delivery/risks
Anthroposophical medicine In AM (*see* page 781), inflammation can be eliminated through the extremities, it is claimed, by means of foot baths and compresses around the lower legs. Potentized eyedrops are also said to bring additional relief.	**May be of some use** as a short-term treatment attempt in persistent cases when simpler, more established methods have been unsuccessful. Some studies claim efficacy; however, success is probably seen in only a proportion of patients (*see* Placebo, page xxi).	**Requires a qualified practitioner** Practitioners should be properly qualified and should propose a treatment plan. **Risks:** Allergies and intolerance are possible.
Homeopathy Highly diluted (potentized) solutions (*see* page 831) are believed to be able to redress vital energy imbalances. Organo- and functiotropic (*see* page 833) homeopathy is claimed to be effective for dealing with symptoms.	**May be of some use** as a supportive treatment attempt for chronic cases when simpler, more established methods have been unsuccessful. Case reports and field studies claim efficacy; however, success is probably seen in only a proportion of patients (*see* Placebo, page xxi).	**Requires a qualified practitioner** Homeopaths should be properly qualified and should propose a treatment plan. Ready-formulated preparations are suitable for do-it-yourself. **Risks:** Allergies and intolerance are possible.

Herbal remedies for conjunctivitis

Active ingredient/preparation	Rating
Barberry bark (*Berberis vulgaris*)	**Not advised**. There are hygiene issues with this type of plant-based remedy. Self-prepared formulations (infusions, poultices, eyewashes, etc.) may damage the eye. Barberry bark must not be used during pregnancy.

Active ingredient/preparation	Rating
Eyebright (*Euphrasia officinalis*)	**Not advised**. Rigorous studies are lacking; also, there are hygiene issues with this type of plant-based remedy. Nevertheless, preparations containing eyebright continue to be advocated. Self-prepared formulations (infusions, poultices, eyewashes, etc.) may damage the eye.
Fennel water, witch hazel, balm extract, camomile baths	**Not advised**. There are hygiene issues with this type of plant-based remedy. Self-prepared formulations (infusions, poultices, eyewashes, etc.) may damage the eye.

Ears

Middle ear infection and earache

Causes and symptoms

A middle ear infection may manifest itself through a variety of symptoms. Acute middle ear infection (acute otitis media) is caused by a virus or bacterium. It often produces a throbbing pain, a high temperature, hearing difficulty and a "bunged-up" sensation in the ear. In small children vomiting is a frequent symptom. Children under 11 years of age are most likely to suffer from otitis media, and the risk of developing it increases in children with nasal polyps, or those who regularly catch colds or suffer from throat infections; it is often associated, also, with classic childhood diseases such as measles, mumps, and scarlet fever.

The eardrum may perforate after a few days, releasing a yellow/green discharge; pain disappears instantaneously, the high temperature drops, and the eardrum slowly heals. If not properly treated, otitis media can develop into chronic serous otitis, possibly leading to permanent deafness and, occasionally, to irritation (and possibly inflammation) of the meninges, the lining of the brain. Surgery will generally be necessary if infection spreads to the bones behind the ear.

Many conditions that produce symptoms similar to those of classic otitis media are not due to bacteria at all, but rather to viral infection, other diseases, activation of trigger points (*see* page 929), psychosomatic factors, and other causes.

Orthodox treatment

Orthodox treatment usually takes the form of antibiotics to eliminate the causative organism, and an antihistamine preparation and analgesic to deal with the symptoms. Doctors are frequently criticized for all too readily prescribing antibiotics when the infection is not of bacterial origin.

Complementary therapies

Some complementary therapies aim primarily to tackle the symptoms. Other approaches see otitis media as being caused by toxins (*see* page 929) or foci (*see* page 928), as the manifestation of a weakened immune system, as a constitutional problem (*see* Constitution, page 927), or as an expression of a disturbed energy flow (*see* Life force, page 928).

Treatment plan and limited trial

Before administering a complementary treatment, every therapist should propose a treatment plan (*see* page xxiii) that sets out a clear time frame and defines the goal that the treatment is designed to achieve. Treatment should then be tried for a limited term to test the patient's response.

Caution

Complementary therapies have at most a supportive function in the treatment of otitis media with ear discharge: for example, to relieve the symptoms. No complementary therapy is a suitable alternative to a properly prescribed course of antibiotics.

Complementary treatments for middle ear infection and earache

Treatment	Rating	Point of delivery/risks
Acupressure This treatment (*see* page 769), otherwise known as pressure-point massage, is claimed to bring relief to persons with earache, to relieve tension, and to improve general well-being when the appropriate pressure points are stimulated.	**Of little use** Acceptable as a short-term treatment attempt aimed at alleviating earache. Case reports claim efficacy; however, success is probably seen in only a proportion of patients (*see* Placebo, page xxi).	**Suitable for DIY** Qualified guidance is recommended. Therapists should be properly qualified. **Risks:** Unlikely provided treatment is carried out competently.
Acupuncture Acupuncture in its various forms (*see* page 772) aims to encourage the flow of energy (*see* page 927) or to alleviate symptoms directly. The acupuncture points chosen can vary from one practitioner to another.	**Of little use** Acceptable as a short-term treatment attempt aimed at alleviating earache. Case reports, field studies, and clinical studies confirm the procedure that offers a degree of efficacy in some patients.	**Requires a qualified practitioner** Practitioners should be properly qualified and should propose a treatment plan. **Risks:** Probably rare provided treatment is carried out competently.
Anthroposophical medicine In AM (*see* page 781), ear inflammation can be eliminated through the extremities, it is claimed, by means of foot baths, compresses around the lower legs, and sweating. Specially tailored preparations are also given.	**May be of some use** as a short-term treatment attempt. Case reports claim efficacy; however, success is probably seen in only a proportion of patients (*see* Placebo, page xxi).	**Requires a qualified practitioner** Practitioners should be properly qualified and should propose a treatment plan. **Risks:** Allergies and intolerance are possible.

Treatment	Rating	Point of delivery/risks
Aromatherapy Essential oils (*see* page 786) are used to soothe and relax, or to invigorate, thereby possibly leading to an easing of symptoms. The essences may be taken orally, used externally as massage oils or bathing emulsions, or inhaled as vapors.	**Of little use** Acceptable as a short-term treatment attempt aimed at soothing and relaxing. Some case reports claim efficacy; however, success is probably seen in only a small proportion of patients (*see* Placebo, page xxi).	**Suitable for DIY** Qualified guidance is recommended. The effects of individual essential oils differ widely. **Risks:** Allergies or intolerance are possible. Some oils are carcinogenic in test systems and possibly in humans.
Bioresonance therapy Bioresonance therapists use electrical devices in an attempt to discover the causes of illness and claim to be able to weaken or turn around pathogenic energies and disease related vibrations (*see* page 794).	**Of little use** Possibly acceptable as a short-term treatment attempt for chronic symptoms when simpler, more established methods have been unsuccessful. Some case reports claim efficacy; however, success is probably seen, if at all, in only a small proportion of patients (*see* Placebo, page xxi).	**Requires a qualified practitioner** Practitioners should be properly qualified and should propose a treatment plan. No credence should be given to anyone promising immediate or total success. **Risks:** Fairly unlikely.
Cell therapy Injecting or ingesting products extracted from the tissues of newborn animals or animal fetuses is said to have a rejuvenating and revitalizing effect and to enhance the healing of human tissues and organs (*see* page 796).	**Not advised** Based on present knowledge, there is inadequate evidence of the efficacy and mode of action of these costly and relatively risky procedures.	**Risks:** Injecting foreign proteins into the body can provoke (possibly fatal) allergic reactions. Also, pathogens such as those that cause bovine spongiform encephalopathy (BSE) or other serious infections may be introduced.

Treatment	Rating	Point of delivery/risks
Electroacupuncture according to Voll By taking readings of the electrical conductivity of the skin (*see* page 802), therapists claim to be able to derive an insight into diseased areas of the body, pathogenic foci (*see* page 928), and stress factors (*see* Toxins, page 929). The factors presumed to be instrumental in the causation of ear problems can then be addressed.	**Of little use** Possibly acceptable as a short-term, supportive treatment attempt for chronic symptoms when simpler, more established methods have been unsuccessful. Some case reports claim efficacy; however, success is probably seen, if at all, in only a small proportion of patients (*see* Placebo, page xxi).	**Requires a qualified practitioner** Practitioners should be properly qualified and should propose a treatment plan. No credence should be given to anyone promising immediate or total success. **Risks:** A second opinion must always be obtained from a qualified physician before any attempt is made to "eliminate foci" (e.g. by surgery).
Electroneural therapy according to Croon According to the theory, readings taken at various reactive sites on the skin highlight diseased areas within the body. Based on these readings, targeted electrostimulative measures can be undertaken to address the factors presumed to be instrumental in causing symptoms (*see* page 806).	**Of little use** Possibly acceptable as a short-term, supportive treatment attempt for chronic symptoms when simpler, more established methods have been unsuccessful. Some case reports claim efficacy; however, success is probably seen, if at all, in only a small proportion of patients (*see* Placebo, page xxi).	**Requires a qualified practitioner** Practitioners should be properly qualified and should propose a treatment plan. No credence should be given to anyone promising immediate or total success. **Risks:** Proponents themselves warn that treatment should not be given in acute inflammatory conditions.

Treatment	Rating	Point of delivery/risks
Eliminative methods, bloody Leeches (*see* page 822) and bloody cupping (*see* page 815) are said to detoxify patients with otitis media and to improve the body's own regulatory systems.	**Of little use** Possibly acceptable as a short-term treatment attempt for chronic symptoms when more established, less invasive methods have been unsuccessful. Some case reports and field studies claim efficacy; however, success is probably seen in only a proportion of patients (*see* Placebo, page xxi). **Not advised** for children.	**Requires a qualified practitioner** Practitioners should be properly qualified and should propose a treatment plan. **Risks:** Bloody cupping can cause infection and scarring. Furthermore, these procedures should not be carried out in persons with bleeding disorders.
Eliminative methods, unbloody Unbloody cupping (*see* page 817) is supposed to improve the body's own regulatory systems and ease pain in persons with otitis media.	**Of little use** Possibly acceptable as a short-term treatment attempt for chronic symptoms. Some case reports claim efficacy; however, success is probably seen in only a proportion of patients (*see* Placebo, page xxi).	**Suitable for DIY** Qualified guidance is recommended. **Risks:** Unlikely provided treatment is carried out competently.
Enzyme therapy The enzymes used are said to dispel and destroy "immune complexes" (*see* page 824) that course in the blood and that are responsible, for instance, for sustaining inflammatory processes.	**Of little use** Some case reports claim efficacy for this little researched therapy; however, success is probably seen in only a small proportion of patients (*see* Placebo, page xxi).	**Requires a qualified practitioner** Practitioners should propose a treatment plan. Non-prescription preparations are suitable for do-it-yourself. **Risks:** Allergies or intolerance are possible.

Treatment	Rating	Point of delivery/risks
Flower remedies Flower remedies (*see* page 828) are said to restore emotional balance and assist the body's psychic ability to heal itself.	**Of little use** Possibly acceptable as a short-term, supportive treatment attempt aimed at soothing and relaxing. Some case reports claim efficacy; however, success is probably seen in only a small proportion of patients (*see* Placebo, page xxi).	**Suitable for DIY** Qualified guidance is recommended. Practitioners should propose a treatment plan. **Risks:** Possible intolerance.
Homeopathy Highly diluted (potentized) solutions (*see* page 831) are believed to be able to redress vital energy imbalances and strengthen the body's defences. Organo- and functiotropic (*see* page 833) homeopathy is claimed to be effective for dealing with symptoms.	**May be of some use** as a short-term treatment attempt for chronic symptoms. Some case reports claim efficacy; however, success is probably seen in only a proportion of patients (*see* Placebo, page xxi).	**Requires a qualified practitioner** Homeopaths should be properly qualified and should propose a treatment plan. Ready-formulated preparations are suitable for do-it-yourself. **Risks:** Allergies and intolerance are possible.
Nutritional therapies An organic diet (*see* page 4) provides the body with essential and secondary plant nutrients that are believed to exercise a multitude of positive effects and to be capable, *inter alia*, of boosting the immune system (*see* page 10).	**Useful** as an individually directed supportive measure. Whether a change in diet has any effect on the course of these conditions is debatable.	**Suitable for DIY** Qualified guidance is recommended though not essential. **Risks:** Avoid imbalanced or intolerable diets. They can cause deficiencies with serious consequences. Children are particularly at risk.

Treatment	Rating	Point of delivery/risks
Physical therapies Heat and cold treatments, warm packs, inhalation of chamomile or elderflower teas, sitz baths, and sweating are said to ease symptoms (*see* pages 871–8).	**Useful** as a short-term treatment attempt. Case reports and field studies claim efficacy; however, success is probably seen in only a proportion of patients (*see* Placebo, page xxi).	**Suitable for DIY** Qualified guidance is recommended. **Risks:** Skin damage may be caused to persons with diminished temperature sensation when extreme temperatures are applied. Some people find it hard to tolerate heat or cold.
Probiotics The introduction of certain bacteria into the gut is claimed to bring the intestinal flora back into balance and to have a beneficial effect on the immune system (*see* page 878).	**Of little use** Possibly acceptable as a short-term treatment attempt for chronic symptoms when more established methods have been unsuccessful. Some case reports claim efficacy; however, success is probably seen in only a proportion of patients (*see* Placebo, page xxi).	**Requires a qualified practitioner** Practitioners should be properly qualified and should propose a treatment plan. Non-prescription formulations are suitable for do-it-yourself. **Risks:** Fairly unlikely provided treatment is carried out competently.
Reflex therapies Reflex zone massage (*see* page 883), reflexology (*see* page 883), and TENS (*see* page 886) are claimed to act via reflex channels (*see* page 881) to affect physical functions and ease pain.	**May be of some use** as a short-term treatment attempt for acute and chronic symptoms. Case reports claim efficacy; however, success is probably seen in only a proportion of patients (*see* Placebo, page xxi). When compared, the individual techniques seem to be of equal merit, though the benefits they provide vary greatly from person to person.	**Suitable for DIY** Qualified guidance is recommended. **Risks:** Some people are sensitive to electrical stimuli and rubber electrodes; others find it hard to tolerate heat, cold, manual stimulation, or close physical contact.

Treatment	Rating	Point of delivery/risks
Relaxation techniques Autogenic training (*see* page 888), muscle relaxation according to Jacobson (*see* page 893), and various biofeedback techniques (*see* page 891) are said to relieve muscle tension and inner unrest, and so might be instrumental in alleviating symptoms.	**Of little use** Acceptable as a supportive treatment attempt for chronic symptoms. Some case reports claim efficacy; however, success is probably seen in only a proportion of patients (*see* Placebo, page xxi).	**Suitable for DIY** Once a sound understanding of the technique has been acquired from a trainer, patients can perform exercises themselves. Therapists should propose a treatment plan. **Risks:** Fairly unlikely.
Vitamins and trace elements The antioxidative properties of beta-carotene, vitamins C and E, and selenium are, it is supposed, instrumental in boosting the body's defence systems (*see* page 900).	**Of little use**, except in vitamin deficiency. No definitive recommendations can be made based on present knowledge.	**Suitable for DIY** Professional guidance is recommended though not essential. **Risks:** Intolerance and overdosage are possible. Recent studies imply that beta-carotene might increase the risk of cancer.

Herbal remedy for middle ear infection

Active ingredient/preparation	Rating
Onion rings in a linen bag or poultices with healing earth	**May be of limited use** as a traditional, supportive treatment attempt for middle ear infection. Onion bags are placed externally on the ear. Onion is said to have an antibacterial action, though it also probably has an anti-inflammatory action achieved through counterirritation. Healing earth poultices have a soothing effect as they draw heat from the inflamed ear.

Tinnitus

Causes and symptoms

Tinnitus is a continuous or intermittent ringing, whistling, or other noise in the ears. It can have many causes, including the presence of wax or foreign objects in the ear canal, otosclerosis (fusion of the small bones in the ear), damage to the eardrum, circulatory disease, and hyperthyroidism (overfunctioning of the thyroid). Sometimes tinnitus may occur as a drug side effect or be the result of lead, mercury, or carbon monoxide poisoning. Emotional factors are also frequently implicated.

Tinnitus is distressing and debilitating. Symptoms may sometimes disappear spontaneously, or become recurrent and chronic.

Orthodox treatment

The orthodox approach is to examine the possible causes of tinnitus. The doctor will treat any underlying disease he or she discovers. Drugs are available to minimize the effect of tinnitus: for example, by promoting blood circulation. Special tinnitus maskers are also available for tinnitus that does not otherwise respond to treatment. These are small devices about the size of a hearing aid that generate a noise to drown out the tinnitus.

Complementary therapies

Various complementary therapies are claimed to alleviate tinnitus. These include relaxation techniques and variants of reflex therapy that aim to lessen or terminate symptoms by acting on trigger points (*see* page 929).

Treatment plan and limited treatment

Before administering a complementary treatment, every therapist should propose a treatment plan (*see* page xxiii) that sets out a clear time frame and defines the goal that the treatment is designed to achieve. Treatment should then be tried for a limited term to test the patient's response.

Caution

Since tinnitus may be a sign of a serious underlying condition, patients with chronic tinnitus should be examined by an ENT specialist as well as being kept under longer term review by a doctor.

Complementary treatments for tinnitus

Treatment	Rating	Point of delivery/risks
Acupressure This treatment (*see* page 769), otherwise known as pressure-point massage, is claimed to bring relief from tinnitus, ease tension, and improve general well-being.	**May be of some use** as a short-term treatment attempt. Case reports claim efficacy; however, success is probably seen in only a proportion of patients (*see* Placebo, page xxi).	**Suitable for DIY** Qualified guidance is recommended. Therapists should be properly qualified. **Risks:** Unlikely provided treatment is carried out competently.
Acupuncture Acupuncture in its various forms (*see* page 772) aims to encourage the flow of energy (*see* page 927) or to address tinnitus directly.	**May be of some use** as a short-term treatment attempt. Case reports, field studies, and case studies confirm this procedure to be efficacious in some patients.	**Requires a qualified practitioner** Practitioners should be properly qualified and should propose a treatment plan. **Risks:** Probably rare provided treatment is carried out competently.

Treatment	Rating	Point of delivery/risks
Aromatherapy Essential oils (*see* page 786) are used to soothe and relax, or to invigorate, thereby possibly bringing relief from tinnitus. The essences may be taken orally, used externally as massage oils or bathing emulsions, or inhaled as vapors.	**May be of some use** as a short-term, supportive treatment attempt aimed at soothing and relaxing. Some case reports claim efficacy; however, success is probably seen in only a small proportion of patients (*see* Placebo, page xxi).	**Suitable for DIY** Qualified guidance is recommended. The effects of individual essential oils differ widely. **Risks:** Allergies or intolerance are possible. Some oils are carcinogenic in test systems and possibly in humans.
Bioresonance therapy Bioresonance therapists use electrical devices in an attempt to discover the causes of illness and claim to be able to weaken or turn around pathogenic energies and disease related vibrations (*see* page 794).	**Of little use** Possibly acceptable as a short-term treatment attempt in persistent cases when simpler, more established methods have been unsuccessful. Some case reports claim efficacy; however, success is probably seen, if at all, in only a small proportion of patients (*see* Placebo, page xxi).	**Requires a qualified practitioner** Practitioners should be properly qualified and should propose a treatment plan. No credence should be given to anyone promising immediate or total success. **Risks:** Fairly unlikely.
Electroacupuncture according to Voll By taking readings of the electrical conductivity of the skin (*see* page 802), therapists claim to be able to derive an insight into diseased areas of the body, pathogenic foci (*see* page 928), and stress factors (*see* Toxins, page 929). The factors presumed to be instrumental in the causation of tinnitus can then be addressed.	**Of little use** Possibly acceptable as a short-term, supportive treatment attempt in persistent cases when simpler, more established methods have been unsuccessful. Some case reports claim efficacy; however, success is probably seen, if at all, in only a small proportion of patients (*see* Placebo, page xxi).	**Requires a qualified practitioner** Practitioners should be properly qualified and should propose a treatment plan. No credence should be given to anyone promising immediate or total success. **Risks:** A second opinion must always be obtained from a qualified physician before any attempt is made to "eliminate foci" (e.g. by surgery).

Treatment	Rating	Point of delivery/risks
Electroneural therapy according to Croon According to the theory, readings taken at various reactive sites on the skin highlight diseased areas within the body. Based on these readings, targeted electrostimulative measures can be undertaken to address the factors presumed to be instrumental in the causation of tinnitus (*see* page 806).	**Of little use** Possibly acceptable as a short-term, supportive treatment attempt in persistent cases when simpler, more established methods have been unsuccessful. Some case reports claim efficacy; however, success is probably seen, if at all, in only a small proportion of patients (*see* Placebo, page xxi).	**Requires a qualified practitioner** Practitioners should be properly qualified and should propose a treatment plan. No credence should be given to anyone promising immediate or total success. **Risks:** Proponents themselves warn that treatment should not be given in acute inflammatory conditions.
Eliminative methods, bloody Leeches (*see* page 822) and bloodletting (*see* page 810) are holistic procedures (*see* page 928) that are said to improve the body's own regulatory systems.	**Of little use** Possibly acceptable as a short-term treatment attempt in chronic cases when more established, less invasive methods have been unsuccessful. Some case reports claim efficacy; however, success is probably seen in only a small proportion of patients (*see* Placebo, page xxi).	**Requires a qualified practitioner** Practitioners should be properly qualified and should propose a treatment plan. **Risks:** These procedures should not be carried out in persons with bleeding disorders.
Eliminative methods, unbloody Unbloody cupping (*see* page 817) is supposed to energize (*see* page 927) the patient, improve the body's own regulatory systems, and so possibly bring relief from tinnitus.	**May be of some use** as a short-term treatment attempt. Some case reports claim efficacy; however, success is probably seen in only a proportion of patients (*see* Placebo, page xxi).	**Suitable for DIY** Unbloody cupping is best carried out under the guidance of a qualified practitioner. **Risks:** Unlikely provided treatment is carried out competently.

Treatment	Rating	Point of delivery/risks
Flower remedies Flower remedies (*see* page 828) are said to restore emotional balance and assist the body's psychic ability to heal itself.	**May be of some use** as a short-term, supportive treatment attempt aimed at soothing and relaxing. Some case reports claim efficacy; however, success is probably seen in only a small proportion of patients (*see* Placebo, page xxi).	**Suitable for DIY** Qualified guidance is recommended. Practitioners should propose a treatment plan. **Risks:** Possible intolerance.
Homeopathy Highly diluted (potentized) solutions (*see* page 831) are believed to be able to redress vital energy imbalances. Organo- and functiotropic (*see* page 833) homeopathy is claimed to be effective for dealing with symptoms.	**May be of some use** as a short-term treatment attempt. Case reports claim efficacy; however, success is probably seen in only a proportion of patients (*see* Placebo, page xxi).	**Requires a qualified practitioner** Homeopaths should be properly qualified and should propose a treatment plan. Ready-formulated preparations are suitable for do-it-yourself. **Risks:** Allergies and intolerance are possible.
Hypnosis and self-hypnosis In the relaxed and generally altered state of awareness that is induced in hypnosis or self-hypnosis (*see* page 837), physical conditions can, it is said, be addressed. Hypnosis is often used in combination with other psycho- and behavioral therapies.	**May be of some use** as a short-term treatment attempt aimed at relaxing the patient and helping him/her come to terms better with his/her condition. Case reports claim efficacy; however, success is probably seen in only a proportion of patients treated (*see* Placebo, page xxi).	**Requires a qualified practitioner** Hypnotherapists should be properly qualified and should propose a treatment plan. **Risks:** Unlikely provided treatment is carried out competently.

Treatment	Rating	Point of delivery/risks
Manual therapies Chiropractors and osteopaths use a series of manipulations to realign allegedly displaced vertebrae. This is said to eliminate the factors presumed to be instrumental in the causation of tinnitus (*see* page 844).	**May be of some use** as a short-term treatment attempt in persistent cases when less risky, more established methods have been unsuccessful. Case reports and field studies claim efficacy for this potentially risky procedure; however, success is probably seen, if at all, in only a small proportion of patients (*see* Placebo, page xxi).	**Requires a qualified practitioner** Practitioners should be properly qualified and should propose a treatment plan. **Risks:** Manipulation of the head and cervical vertebrae can cause serious injury. Osteoporosis is one of several risk factors.
Massage Local massage (*see* page 847) carried out on the neck and shoulder is said to ease tension, exercise a beneficial effect on trigger points (*see* page 929), and bring relief from tinnitus.	**May be of some use** as a short-term, supportive treatment attempt aimed at relaxing the patient. Case reports and field studies claim efficacy; however, success is probably seen in only a proportion of patients (*see* Placebo, page xxi).	**Requires a qualified practitioner** Masseurs/masseuses should be properly qualified and should propose a treatment plan. **Risks:** Some people are sensitive to manual stimuli; others find it hard to tolerate close physical contact.
Reflex therapies Reflex zone massage (see page 883) is said to ease tension, exercise a beneficial effect on trigger points (*see* page 929), and bring relief from tinnitus.	**May be of some use** as a short-term, supportive treatment attempt aimed at relaxing the patient. Case reports and field studies claim efficacy however success is probably seen in only a proportion of patients (*see* Placebo, page xxi).	**Requires a qualified practitioner** Practitioners should be properly qualified and should propose a proper treatment plan. **Risks:** Some people are sensitive to manual stimuli; others find it hard to tolerate close physical contact.

Treatment	Rating	Point of delivery/risks
Relaxation techniques Autogenic training (*see* page 888), muscle relaxation according to Jacobson (*see* page 893), and various biofeedback techniques (*see* page 891) are said to relieve muscle tension and inner unrest, and might be instrumental in helping the patient become better aware of his/her physical and emotional states.	**Useful** as a short-term treatment attempt. Case studies, field studies, and case reports show that tinnitus was eliminated in a small proportion of patients and that, in a larger proportion, the symptoms were at least alleviated, with patients coming to terms better with their condition.	**Suitable for DIY** Once a sound understanding of the technique has been acquired from a trainer in groups or through individual tuition, patients can perform exercises themselves. Therapists should be properly qualified. **Risks:** Fairly unlikely.
TENS The use of low frequency electrical currents on the surface of the skin is said to act through so-called reflex channels (*see* page 881) to bring relief from tinnitus (*see* page 886).	**May be of some use** as a short-term treatment attempt. Case reports and field studies claim efficacy; however, success is probably seen in only a proportion of patients (*see* Placebo, page xxi).	**Requires a qualified practitioner** Practitioners should be properly qualified and should propose a treatment plan. **Risks:** Some people react sensitively to electrical stimuli or rubber electrodes.

Herbal remedies for tinnitus

Active ingredient/preparation	Rating
Ginkgo extract (extracted from the leaves of *Ginkgo biloba* with acetone/water)	**May be of some use** as a treatment attempt for tinnitus. **Dosage:** 4–8oz extract or as instructed by the manufacturer/prescriber. Use for six to eight weeks, then review treatment. Tinnitus must be investigated conventionally; self-treatment is thus not advised. **Risks:** Headaches, mild gastrointestinal disorders. Not to be taken by persons who are hypersensitive to ginkgo. Ginkgo injections should not be used owing to the allergic reactions they may induce.

Active ingredient/preparation	*Rating*
Ginkgo leaves as an infusion	**Of little use** for treating tinnitus. Infusions prepared from *Ginkgo biloba* leaves cannot be recommended as there is no evidence that they work.

Urinary system

Kidney and urinary tract disease

Causes and symptoms

While "kidney disease" is a catchall term for various inflammatory conditions of metabolic or immunological origin, most urinary tract disease is due to kidney stones or to an infection. Renal colic can be a very painful condition.

Orthodox treatment

In kidney disease the treatment directly addresses the condition as diagnosed. Treatment for urinary tract disease strives more to identify the cause, and will include measures to reduce inflammation and ease pain. Kidney stones can nowadays be broken up *in situ* by means of ultrasound.

Complementary therapies

Kidney disease is seen by many complementary practitioners as a disturbed flow of vital energy (*see* Life force, page 928), as a result of chronic exposure to toxins (*see* page 929), or as the expression of an imbalanced immune system. Treatments are suggested accordingly. Treatments for the urinary tract aim to reduce discomfort and, additionally, to flush out the urinary system.

Treatment plan and limited trial

Before administering a complementary treatment, every therapist should propose a treatment plan (*see* page xxiii) that sets out a clear time frame and defines the goal that the treatment is designed to achieve. Treatment should then be tried for a limited term to test the patient's response.

Caution

Non-orthodox treatments have at most a supportive function in the relief of discomfort and in preventing infection. Claims that some treatments can dissolve larger kidney stones have not been substantiated.

In severe urinary tract infection, especially when there is a high temperature, the complementary remedies on offer are no substitute for a necessary course of antibiotics.

Complementary treatments for kidney and urinary tract infections

Treatment	Rating	Point of delivery/risks
Acupressure This treatment (*see* page 769), otherwise known as pressure-point massage, is claimed to ease pain, to dispel the urge to urinate, and to help stop dribbling. The pressure points chosen may differ from one practitioner to another.	**Of little use** Possibly acceptable as a short-term, supportive treatment attempt and as a preventive measure. Some case reports claim efficacy; however, success is probably seen in only a proportion of patients (*see* Placebo, page xxi).	**Suitable for DIY** Qualified guidance is recommended. Therapists should be properly qualified. **Risks:** Unlikely provided treatment is carried out competently.

Treatment	Rating	Point of delivery/risks
Acupuncture Acupuncture in its various forms (*see* page 772) aims to ease pain, to dispel the urge to urinate, and to help stop dribbling. The acupuncture points chosen can vary from one practitioner to another.	**Of little use** Possibly acceptable as a short-term treatment attempt aimed at easing pain, dispelling the urge to urinate, and helping to stop dribbling. Some case reports claim efficacy; however, success is probably seen in only a proportion of patients (*see* Placebo, page xxi).	**Requires a qualified practitioner** Practitioners should be properly qualified and should propose a treatment plan. **Risks:** Probably rare provided treatment is carried out competently.
Anthroposophical medicine Physicians who practice AM (*see* page 781) apply wraps with horsetail near the kidneys and bladder, and use potentized preparations of horsetail or Spanish fly and herbal teas such as uva-ursi.	**Of little use** Acceptable as a short-term treatment attempt. Case reports claim efficacy; however, success is probably seen in only a proportion of patients (*see* Placebo, page xxi).	**Requires a qualified practitioner** Practitioners should be properly qualified and should propose a treatment plan. **Risks:** Allergies and intolerance are possible.
Bioresonance therapy Bioresonance therapists use electrical devices in an attempt to discover the causes of illness and claim to be able to weaken or turn around pathogenic energies and disease related vibrations (*see* page 794).	**Of little use** Possibly acceptable as a short-term, supportive treatment attempt when simpler, more established methods have been unsuccessful. Some case reports claim efficacy; however, success is probably seen, if at all, in only a small proportion of patients (*see* Placebo, page xxi).	**Requires a qualified practitioner** Practitioners should be properly qualified and should propose a treatment plan. No credence should be given to anyone promising immediate or total success. **Risks:** Fairly unlikely.

Treatment	Rating	Point of delivery/risks
Electroacupuncture according to Voll By taking readings of the electrical conductivity of the skin (*see* page 802), therapists claim to be able to derive an insight into diseased areas of the body, pathogenic foci (*see* page 928), and stress factors (*see* Toxins, page 929). The factors presumed to be instrumental in the causation of the disease can then be addressed.	**Of little use** Possibly acceptable as a short-term, supportive treatment attempt when simpler, more established methods have been unsuccessful. Some case reports claim efficacy; however, success is probably seen, if at all, in only a small proportion of patients (*see* Placebo, page xxi).	**Requires a qualified practitioner** Practitioners should be properly qualified and should propose a treatment plan. No credence should be given to anyone promising immediate or total success. **Risks:** A second opinion must always be obtained from a qualified physician before any attempt is made to "eliminate foci" (e.g. by surgery).
Electroneural therapy according to Croon According to the theory, readings taken at various reactive sites on the skin highlight diseased areas within the body. Based on these readings, targeted electrostimulative measures can be undertaken to address the factors presumed to be instrumental in the causation of the disease (*see* page 806).	**Of little use** Possibly acceptable as a short-term, supportive treatment attempt when simpler, more established methods have been unsuccessful. Some case reports claim efficacy; however, success is probably seen, if at all, in only a small proportion of patients (*see* Placebo, page xxi).	**Requires a qualified practitioner** Practitioners should be properly qualified and should propose a treatment plan. No credence should be given to anyone promising immediate or total success. **Risks:** Proponents themselves warn that treatment should not be given in acute inflammatory conditions.
Eliminative methods, unbloody Unbloody cupping (*see* page 817) is supposed to act via so-called reflex channels (*see* page 881) to ease pain, to suppress the urge to urinate, and to help stop dribbling.	**Of little use** Acceptable as a short-term, supportive treatment attempt. Some case reports claim efficacy; however, success is probably seen in only a small proportion of patients (*see* Placebo, page xxi).	**Suitable for DIY** Unbloody cupping is best carried out under the guidance of a qualified practitioner. **Risks:** Unlikely provided treatment is carried out competently.

Treatment	*Rating*	*Point of delivery/risks*
Enzyme therapy The enzymes used are said to speed up healing, to concentrate antibiotics at the site of infection, and to dispel and destroy "immune complexes" (*see* page 824) that are believed to course in the blood and that are thought responsible, for instance, for sustaining inflammatory processes.	**Of little use** Some case reports claim efficacy for this little researched therapy; however, success is probably seen in only a small proportion of patients (*see* Placebo, page xxi).	**Requires a qualified practitioner** Practitioners should propose a treatment plan. Non-prescription preparations are suitable for do-it-yourself. **Risks:** Allergies or intolerance are possible.
Homeopathy Highly diluted (potentized) solutions (*see* page 831) are believed to be able to redress vital energy imbalances. Organo- and functiotropic (*see* page 833) homeopathy is claimed to be effective for dealing with urinary tract infections.	**Of little use** Acceptable as a short-term, supportive treatment attempt. Some case reports claim efficacy; however, success is probably seen in only a proportion of patients (*see* Placebo, page xxi).	**Requires a qualified practitioner** Homeopaths should be properly qualified and should propose a treatment plan. Ready-formulated preparations are suitable for do-it-yourself. **Risks:** Allergies and intolerance are possible.
Manual therapies Chiropractors and osteopaths (*see* page 844) use a series of manipulations to realign allegedly displaced vertebrae which, it is believed, are associated with urinary tract infection, so alleviating the disease.	**Of little use** Possibly acceptable as a short-term, supportive treatment attempt in particularly persistent cases. Some case reports claim efficacy for these potentially risky procedures; however, success is probably seen, if at all, in only a small proportion of patients (*see* Placebo, page xxi).	**Requires a qualified practitioner** Practitioners should be properly qualified and should propose a treatment plan. **Risks:** Manipulation of the head and cervical vertebrae can cause serious injury. Osteoporosis is one of several risk factors.

Treatment	Rating	Point of delivery/risks
Nutritional therapies An organic diet (*see* page 4) provides the body with essential and secondary plant nutrients that are believed to exercise a multitude of positive effects (*see* pages 858–67).	**May be of some use** as a supportive, general measure.	**Suitable for DIY** Qualified guidance is recommended. Individual diets for persons with kidney stones must be discussed with a qualified physician. **Risks:** Avoid imbalanced or intolerable diets. They can cause deficiencies with serious consequences. Children are particularly at risk.
Physical therapies Lukewarm or hot packs on the abdomen are claimed to ease pain (*see* page 878). Rising temperature foot or sitz baths can be used supportively (*see* page 874).	**May be of some use** as a short-term, supportive treatment attempt. Some case reports claim efficacy; however, success is probably seen in only a proportion of patients (*see* Placebo, page xxi).	**Suitable for DIY** Qualified guidance is recommended though not essential. **Risks:** Skin damage may be caused to persons with diminished temperature sensation when extreme temperatures are applied.
Reflex therapies Reflex zone massage (*see* page 883) and reflexology (*see* page 883) are claimed to act via reflex channels (*see* page 881) to ease pain and inflammation, and speed up healing.	**Of little use** Acceptable as a short-term treatment attempt aimed at alleviating pain. Some case reports claim efficacy; however, success is probably seen in only a proportion of patients (*see* Placebo, page xxi).	**Requires a qualified practitioner** Practitioners should be properly qualified and should propose a treatment plan. **Risks:** Some people are sensitive to pressure or find it hard to tolerate close physical contact.

Treatment	Rating	Point of delivery/risks
TENS The use of low frequency electrical currents on the surface of the skin is said to act through so-called reflex channels (*see* page 886) to reduce pain and speed up healing.	**Of little use** Acceptable as a short-term, supportive treatment attempt aimed at easing pain. Some case reports claim efficacy; however, success is probably seen in only a proportion of patients (*see* Placebo, page xxi).	**Requires a qualified practitioner** Practitioners should be properly qualified and should propose a treatment plan. **Risks:** Some people react sensitively to electrical stimuli or rubber electrodes.

Herbal remedies for urinary tract infections

Active ingredient/preparation	Rating
Asparagus root (*Asparagus officinalis*)	**Only useful** as a supportive treatment attempt to flush the urinary tract in inflammatory conditions of the efferent urinary tract and for prevention of kidney gravel (its own diuretic action has only been demonstrated in animals). **Daily dose:** 1½–2oz root. **Individual dose:** 2 dessertspoons to 1 cup of hot water. Use ready-formulated preparations as instructed by the manufacturer/prescriber. **Risks:** Allergic reactions are possible. Not suitable as a diuretic for persons with edema resulting from impaired cardiac or renal function.
Butterbur root (*Petasites hybridus*)	**Not advised** as a supportive measure in painful spasm of the bladder, especially when calculi are present. **Risks:** The pyrrolizidine alkaloids which butterbur contains are hepatotoxic and potentially carcinogenic. Butterbur can also cause loss of appetite with nausea and diarrhea.

Active ingredient/preparation	Rating

Couch grass root
(*Agropyron repens*)

Only useful as a treatment attempt to flush the urinary tract in inflammatory diseases, and for prevention of kidney gravel. Its essential oil has antibacterial properties.
Daily dose: 6–9g herb. **Individual dose:** 3g to 1 cup of boiling water.
Risks: Not suitable as a diuretic for persons with edema resulting from impaired cardiac or renal function.

Goldenrod
(*Solidago virgaurea*)

Only useful as a supportive treatment attempt to flush the urinary tract in conditions such as kidney stones and gravel, also as a preventive measure. Goldenrod has a mild relaxant and anti-inflammatory action.
Daily dose: 6–12g herb. **Individual dose:** Pour 1 cup of hot water over 3g and infuse. Use ready-formulated preparations as instructed by the manufacturer/prescriber.
Risks: Not suitable as a diuretic for persons with edema resulting from impaired cardiac or renal function.

Horseradish root
(*Armoracia rusticana*)

Only useful for supportive flushing in infections of the efferent urinary tract on account of its mild antibacterial action.
Daily dose: Press 10g of fresh root and swallow the juice twice daily.
Risks: Gastrointestinal problems are possible. Not to be used by persons with ulcers or nephritis. Children under four years of age should not be given horseradish root. It may cause severe allergic reactions. It also tends to depress the function of the thyroid, so should not be used when thyroid levels are low.

Horsetail
(*Equisetum arvense*)

Only useful as a treatment attempt to flush the urinary tract in bacterial and inflammatory disease of the urinary tract and in kidney gravel.
Daily dose: 6g herb. **Individual dose:** 2g to 1 cup of hot water. Use ready-formulated preparations as instructed by the manufacturer/prescriber.
Risks: Not suitable as a diuretic for persons with edema resulting from impaired cardiac and renal function. The plant contains nicotine.

Active ingredient/preparation	Rating
Lovage root (*Levisticum officinale*)	**Only useful** as a treatment attempt to flush the urinary tract in inflammation of the efferent urinary tract, and for prevention of kidney gravel. **Daily dose:** 4–8g herb. **Individual dose:** 1.5g to 1 cup of hot water. Use ready-formulated preparations as instructed by the manufacturer/prescriber. **Risks:** Lovage can render persons with a light complexion more sensitive to light. Not to be used in persons with acute nephritis or impaired renal function. Not suitable as a diuretic for persons with edema resulting from impaired cardiac or renal function.
Nettle (*Urtica dioica*)	**Only useful** as a supportive treatment attempt to flush the urinary tract, and as a prevention against kidney gravel. **Daily dose:** 8–12g herb. **Individual dose:** Pour 1 cup of boiling water over 2–4g of dried herb. Use ready-formulated preparations as instructed by the manufacturer/prescriber. **Risks:** Occasional allergic reactions. Not suitable as a diuretic for persons with oedema resulting from impaired cardiac or renal function.
Orthosiphon leaves (*Orthosiphon spicatus*)	**Only useful** for supportive flushing in bacterial and inflammatory conditions of the efferent urinary tract, and in kidney gravel. Also has a mild relaxant action. **Daily dose:** 6–12g herb. **Individual dose:** 2.5g to 1 cup of boiling water. Use ready-formulated preparations as instructed by the manufacturer/prescriber. **Risks:** Not suitable as a diuretic for persons with edema resulting from impaired cardiac or renal function.

Active ingredient/preparation	Rating

Parsley herb and root
(*Petroselinum crispum*)

Of little use. Perhaps acceptable for flushing the urinary tract as well as for preventing and treating kidney gravel.
Individual dose: 2g root to 1 cup of hot water. Use ready-formulated preparations as instructed by the manufacturer/prescriber.
Risks: The root contains small amounts (0.2–0.3 percent) of oil of parsley. This damages the liver and kidneys as well as being potentially carcinogenic, so should not be used in isolated form. Parsley can cause miscarriages, so should not be used as a diuretic tea during pregnancy. It must not be used as a diuretic by persons with edema resulting from impaired cardiac or renal function.

Purple coneflower
(*Echinacea purpurea*)

May be of some use as a supportive treatment attempt for recurrent urinary tract infection. Possibly improves the body's resistance to disease.
Daily dose: 900mg root or 1–2 teaspoons expressed juice. Fifty drops at the first signs of infection, then 10–20 drops in water every one to two hours for several days, otherwise in infection-free periods take three times a year for a total of three to four weeks. Use ready-formulated preparations as instructed by the manufacturer/prescriber.
Risks: Parenteral administration (injection) is not advised. Possible untoward effects following parenteral administration: poor diabetic control, nausea, shivering attacks, allergic reactions (possibly shock). Echinacea should not be used for diseases such as tuberculosis, rheumatic disease, multiple sclerosis, or if the patient has an allergic tendency, nor during pregnancy.

Restharrow root
(*Ononis spinosa*)

Only useful as a treatment attempt to flush the efferent urinary tract, and for prevention of kidney gravel.
Daily dose: 6–12g herb. Pour 1 cup of hot water over 3g and infuse. Use ready-formulated preparations as instructed by the manufacturer/prescriber.
Risks: Not suitable as a diuretic for persons with edema resulting from impaired cardiac or renal function.

Active ingredient/preparation	Rating
Silver birch leaves (*Betula pendula*)	**Only useful** as a treatment attempt to flush the urinary tract in bacterial and inflammatory disease of the efferent urinary tract and in kidney gravel; can also be drunk as a supportive treatment attempt for rheumatic conditions. **Daily dose:** 6–10g dried leaves. **Individual dose:** Pour hot water over 2–3g of dried leaves and infuse. Use ready-formulated preparations as instructed by the manufacturer/prescriber. **Risks:** Not suitable as a diuretic in persons with edema resulting from impaired cardiac and renal function.
Uva-ursi leaves (*Arctostaphylos uva-ursi*)	**Only useful** as a treatment attempt to flush the urinary tract in inflammation of the efferent urinary tract. Reported to have an antibacterial and antimicrobial action. **Daily dose:** 3g of dried leaves or 400–840mg hydroquinone derivative (arbutin) up to four times a day. **Individual dose:** 3g of dried leaves to 5fl oz hot water or the same quantity prepared with cold water (steep for two to three hours, heat, and drink). Use ready-formulated preparations as instructed by the manufacturer/prescriber. **Risks:** Nausea or vomiting are possible. Very occasionally, respiratory problems and skin eruptions have been noted. Not to be taken with agents that acidify the urine. Not to be used during pregnancy or breastfeeding. Not to be taken by children under 12 years of age. Use for a maximum of one week and not more than five times a year for a total of one to two weeks.
White sandalwood (*Santalum album*)	**Only useful** as a supportive treatment attempt in infections of the efferent urinary tract. White sandalwood has a mild antibacterial and relaxant action. **Daily dose:** As a decoction: 10–20g dried herb. **Individual dose:** 5g to 1 cup of boiling water. **Risks:** Nausea, itching of the skin. Isolated sandalwood oil should be administered in gastric-resistant capsules as it can severely irritate the stomach. Not to be used in persons with conditions affecting the renal parenchyma. Not to be used for longer than six weeks.

Prostate enlargement

Causes and symptoms

Prostate enlargement is due to the overgrowth of glandular tissue in the prostate (benign prostatic hyperplasia or benign prostatic hypertrophy). Symptoms include a need to pass urine more frequently, a reduction in the force of the urine stream, inability to void the bladder fully, and dribbling from the urethra; ultimately there may be urine retention within the bladder. Bedwetting may become a problem and late symptoms may include pointers to renal dysfunction, such as thirst, vomiting, diarrhea, and weight loss. Prostate enlargement generally begins between the ages of 40 and 50 for reasons that are not fully understood. It may be due to cancer; therefore make sure you see your doctor when suffering from the symptoms listed above.

Inability to void the bladder completely leads to cystitis, which cannot heal properly once the normal flushing function of the urine has been lost. Cystitis may progressively worsen and lead to other problems such as pyelitis, glomerulonephritis, renal failure, and toxemia.

Orthodox treatment

Treatment for the initial phase of the condition will include plant-based preparations to reduce the symptoms. Later stages will generally be treated by a surgical procedure known as transurethral resection.

Complementary therapies

Some complementary practitioners claim to be able to influence the prostate directly through energy links (*see* page 928) and so reduce the symptoms. Certain nonorthodox therapists believe prostate enlargement to be caused by foci (*see* page 928), toxins, or a lack of vital energy (*see* Life force, page 928). Treatments are suggested accordingly.

Treatment plan and limited trial

Before administering a complementary treatment, every therapist should propose a treatment plan (*see* page xxiii) that sets out a clear time frame and defines the goal that the treatment is designed to achieve. Treatment should then be tried for a limited term to test the patient's response.

Caution

No complementary treatment is adequate on its own for dealing with conditions caused by enlargement of the prostate gland. In prostate enlargement and its sequelae, complementary therapies may at most be useful in a supportive role: e.g. to provide relief from discomfort.

For any pain, however slight, the advice must be: see a doctor. There is a risk otherwise of inappropriate treatment being given for a possibly serious prostate disease.

Complementary treatments for benign prostate enlargement

Treatment	Rating	Point of delivery/risks
Acupressure This treatment (*see* page 769), otherwise known as pressure-point massage, is claimed to ease pain and improve general well-being.	**May be of some use** as a short-term treatment attempt aimed at alleviating pain. Case reports claim efficacy; however, success is probably seen in only a proportion of patients (*see* Placebo, page xxi).	**Suitable for DIY** Qualified guidance is recommended. Therapists should be properly qualified. **Risks:** Unlikely provided treatment is carried out competently.

Treatment	Rating	Point of delivery/risks
Acupuncture Acupuncture in its various forms (*see* page 772) aims to encourage the flow of energy (*see* page 927) or to act directly to ease pain.	**May be of some use** as a short-term treatment attempt for pain and inflammation. Case reports claim efficacy; however, success is probably seen in only a proportion of patients (*see* Placebo, page xxi).	**Requires a qualified practitioner** Acupuncturists should be properly qualified and should propose a treatment plan. **Risks:** Probably rare provided treatment is carried out competently.
Anthroposophical medicine AM (*see* page 781) uses potentized saw palmetto preparations for pain relief.	**May be of some use** as a short-term, supportive treatment attempt. Some case reports claim efficacy; however, success is probably seen in only a proportion of patients (*see* Placebo, page xxi).	**Requires a qualified practitioner** Practitioners should be properly qualified and should propose a treatment plan. **Risks:** Allergies and intolerance are possible.
Aromatherapy Essential oils (*see* page 786) are used to soothe and relax, or to invigorate, thereby helping to alleviate symptoms. The essences may be taken orally, used externally as massage oils or bathing emulsions, or inhaled as vapors.	**May be of some use** as a short-term, supportive treatment attempt aimed at soothing and relaxing. Some case reports claim efficacy; however, success is probably seen in only a proportion of patients (*see* Placebo, page xxi).	**Suitable for DIY** Qualified guidance is recommended. The effects of individual essential oils differ widely. **Risks:** Allergies or intolerance are possible. Some oils are carcinogenic in test systems and possibly in humans.

Treatment	Rating	Point of delivery/risks
Bioresonance therapy Bioresonance therapists use electrical devices in an attempt to discover the causes of illness and claim to be able to weaken or turn around pathogenic energies and disease related vibrations (*see* page 794).	**Of little use** Possibly acceptable as a short-term treatment attempt when simpler, more established methods have been unsuccessful. Some case reports claim efficacy; however, success is probably seen, if at all, in only a small proportion of patients (*see* Placebo, page xxi).	**Requires a qualified practitioner** Practitioners should be properly qualified and should propose a treatment plan. No credence should be given to anyone promising immediate or total success. **Risks:** Fairly unlikely.
Cell therapy Injecting or ingesting products extracted from the tissues of newborn animals or animal fetuses is said to have a rejuvenating and revitalizing effect and to enhance the healing of human tissues and organs (*see* page 796).	**Not advised** Based on present knowledge, there is inadequate evidence of the efficacy and mode of action of these costly and relatively risky procedures.	**Risks:** Injecting foreign proteins into the body can provoke (possibly fatal) allergic reactions. Also, pathogens such as those that cause bovine spongiform encephalopathy (BSE) or other serious infections may be introduced.
Electroacupuncture according to Voll By taking readings of the electrical conductivity of the skin (*see* page 802), therapists claim to be able to derive an insight into diseased areas of the body, pathogenic foci (*see* page 928), and stress factors (*see* Toxins, page 929). The factors presumed to be instrumental in the causation of prostate enlargement can then be addressed.	**Of little use** Possibly acceptable as a short-term, supportive treatment attempt for severe, chronic conditions when simpler, more established methods have been unsuccessful. Some case reports claim efficacy; however, success is probably seen, if at all, in only a small proportion of patients (*see* Placebo, page xxi).	**Requires a qualified practitioner** Practitioners should be properly qualified and should propose a treatment plan. No credence should be given to anyone promising immediate or total success. **Risks:** A second opinion must always be obtained from a qualified physician before any attempt is made to "eliminate foci" (e.g. by surgery).

Treatment	Rating	Point of delivery/risks
Electroneural therapy according to Croon According to the theory, readings taken at various reactive sites on the skin highlight diseased areas within the body. Based on these readings, targeted electrostimulative measures can be undertaken to address the factors presumed to be instrumental in the causation of prostate enlargement (*see* page 806).	**Of little use** Possibly acceptable as a short-term, supportive treatment attempt for severe symptoms when simpler, more established methods have been unsuccessful. Some case reports claim efficacy; however, success is probably seen, if at all, in only a small proportion of patients (*see* Placebo, page xxi).	**Requires a qualified practitioner** Practitioners should be properly qualified and should propose a treatment plan. No credence should be given to anyone promising immediate or total success. **Risks:** Proponents themselves warn that treatment should not be given in acute inflammatory conditions.
Eliminative methods, bloody Bloody cupping (*see* page 815) is said to ease pain. This procedure is primarily intended as a holistic (*see* page 928) treatment rather than a direct attempt at pain relief.	**Of little use** Possibly acceptable as a short-term, supportive treatment attempt for persistent pain when more established, less invasive methods have been unsuccessful. Some case reports and field studies claim efficacy; however, success is probably seen in only a proportion of patients (*see* Placebo, page xxi).	**Requires a qualified practitioner** Practitioners should be properly qualified and should propose a treatment plan. No credence should be given to anyone promising immediate or total success. **Risks:** Bloody cupping can cause infection and scarring. Furthermore, it should not be carried out in persons with bleeding disorders.

Treatment	Rating	Point of delivery/risks
Eliminative methods, unbloody Unbloody cupping (*see* page 817) or cantharide poultices (*see* page 812) are occasionally used to relieve pain in patients with an enlarged prostate.	Cantharide poultices are **of little use**. Unbloody cupping **may be of some use** as a short-term, supportive treatment attempt aimed at easing persistent pain when more established methods have been unsuccessful. Some case reports claim efficacy; however, success is probably seen in only a small proportion of patients (*see* Placebo, page xxi).	**Suitable for DIY** Unbloody cupping is best carried out under the guidance of a qualified practitioner. Treatment with cantharide poultices requires a qualified practitioner. **Risks:** Cantharide poultices can cause second-degree burns.
Flower remedies Flower remedies (*see* page 828) are said to restore emotional balance and assist the body's psychic ability to heal itself.	**May be of some use** as a short-term, supportive treatment attempt aimed at soothing and relaxing. Some case reports claim efficacy; however, success is probably seen in only a small proportion of patients (*see* Placebo, page xxi).	**Suitable for DIY** Qualified guidance is recommended. Practitioners should propose a treatment plan. **Risks:** Possible intolerance.
Homeopathy The highly diluted (potentized) solutions (*see* page 831) used in organo- and functiotropic (*see* page 833) homeopathy are claimed to be effective in bringing symptomatic relief to prostate disorders.	**May be of some use** as a short-term, supportive treatment attempt. Some case reports claim efficacy; however, success is probably seen in only a proportion of patients (*see* Placebo, page xxi).	**Requires a qualified practitioner** Homeopaths should be properly qualified and should propose a treatment plan. Ready-formulated preparations are suitable for do-it-yourself. **Risks:** Allergies and intolerance are possible.

Treatment	Rating	Point of delivery/risks
Manual therapies Chiropractors and osteopaths (*see* page 844) use a series of manipulations to realign vertebrae allegedly displaced by prostate enlargement. This is said to have a beneficial effect on the prostate and to ease pain.	**Of little use** Possibly acceptable as a short-term treatment attempt for persistent symptoms when less risky, more established methods have been unsuccessful. Some case reports claim efficacy; however, success is probably seen, if at all, in only a small proportion of patients (*see* Placebo, page xxi).	**Requires a qualified practitioner** Practitioners should be properly qualified and should propose a treatment plan. **Risks:** Manipulation of the head and cervical vertebrae can cause serious injury. Osteoporosis is one of several risk factors.
Nutritional therapies An organic diet (*see* page 4) provides the body with essential and secondary plant nutrients that are believed to exercise a multitude of positive effects.	**Useful** as an individually directed supportive measure.	**Suitable for DIY** Qualified guidance is recommended though not essential. **Risks:** Avoid imbalanced or intolerable diets. They can cause deficiencies with serious consequences. Children are particularly at risk.
Physical therapies Rising temperature foot baths, sitz baths, or partial immersion baths, warm packs, mud and thermal baths can, it is claimed, improve the circulation, ease pain, and alleviate other symptoms (*see* pages 871–8).	**May be of some use** as a short-term treatment attempt aimed at alleviating pain. Case reports and field studies claim efficacy; however, success is probably seen in only a proportion of patients (*see* Placebo, page xxi).	**Suitable for DIY** Qualified guidance is recommended though not essential. **Risks:** Skin damage may be caused to persons with diminished temperature sensation when extreme temperatures are applied.

Treatment	Rating	Point of delivery/risks
Reflex therapies Connective tissue massage, reflexology (*see* page 883), and TENS (*see* page 886) are claimed to act via reflex channels (*see* page 881) to encourage bladder function and ease pain and other symptoms.	**May be of some use** as a short-term treatment attempt aimed at alleviating pain. Some case reports claim efficacy; however, success is probably seen in only a proportion of patients (*see* Placebo, page xxi).	**Requires a qualified practitioner** Practitioners should be properly qualified and should propose a treatment plan. **Risks:** Some people are sensitive to electrical stimuli and rubber electrodes; others find it hard to tolerate manual stimulation or close physical contact.
Relaxation techniques Autogenic training (*see* page 888), muscle relaxation according to Jacobson (*see* page 893), and various biofeedback techniques (*see* page 891) are said to relieve muscle tension and inner unrest, to ease pain, and to help the patient become more perceptive toward his physical and emotional states.	**May be of some use** as a short-term, supportive treatment attempt aimed at relaxing the patient and helping him come to terms better with his condition. Some case reports claim efficacy; however, success is probably seen in only a proportion of patients (*see* Placebo, page xxi).	**Suitable for DIY** Once a sound understanding of the technique has been acquired from a trainer in group sessions or through individual tuition, patients can perform exercises themselves. Therapists should be properly qualified **Risks:** Fairly unlikely.

Herbal remedies for prostate enlargement

Active ingredient/preparation	Rating
Nettle root (*Urtica dioica*)	**May be of some use** as a treatment attempt for problems with micturition due to prostate enlargement (stages I–II). Nettle root raises urine volume output and maximum urine flow, while reducing the formation of residual urine in the bladder. **Daily dose:** 4–6g root. **Individual dose:** Pour hot water over 1.5–2g of root and infuse. Use ready-formulated preparations as instructed by the manufacturer/prescriber. **Risks:** Occasional slight gastrointestinal complaints. Allergic skin reactions are possible. Nettle root does not reduce the size of the prostate. Regular medical checks are necessary. Talk to your doctor before taking nettle root.
Pumpkin seeds (*Cucurbita pepo*)	**Useful** as a treatment attempt for problems with micturition due to prostate enlargement (stages I–II). Pumpkin seeds raise urine volume output and maximum urine flow, while reducing the formation of residual urine in the bladder. **Daily dose:** 10g seeds. **Individual dose:** 5g to 1 cup of water; stir and drink. Use ready-formulated preparations as instructed by the manufacturer/prescriber. **Risks:** Pumpkin seeds are not known to have any serious side effects. Talk to your doctor before taking them. Regular medical checks are advised.

Active ingredient/preparation	Rating
Saw palmetto berries (*Serenoa repens*)	**Useful** as a treatment attempt for problems with micturition due to prostate enlargement (stages I–II). Saw palmetto increases volume output and maximum urine flow, while reducing the formation of residual urine in the bladder. Counteracts the male sex hormone and inflammation induced fluid loss from the blood vessels (aqueous extract). Contains beta-sitosterol. **Daily dose:** 1–2g of berries to 1 cup of hot water. Use ready-formulated preparations as instructed by the manufacturer/prescriber. **Risks:** Saw palmetto is not known to have any serious side effects. Consult your doctor before using this remedy.
Seedless green bean (*Phaseolus vulgaris*)	**May be of some use** as a supportive treatment attempt for problems with micturition. Has a mild diuretic action. **Daily dose:** 5–15g pod. **Individual dose:** 3–5g to 1 cup of hot water. **Risks:** Mild, transient gastrointestinal complaints may occasionally occur.
White poplar extract (*Populus tremuloides*) or equivalent non-prostate active combination preparations	**Of little use.** Extract of white poplar is primarily an anti-inflammatory. **Risks:** Gastrointestinal complaints may occasionally occur. Side effects are the same as after taking salicylates.

Prostatitis

Causes and symptoms

Acute bacterial prostatitis is an infection of the prostate that presents as pain or difficulty in passing urine or defecating, with a urethral discharge that is sometimes bloody. There may also be a temperature. Infection is caused by streptococci or by intestinal bacteria that have penetrated via the urethra or through the blood circulation. If not properly treated, acute bacterial prostatitis may become chronic and lead to potency (*see* Sexual problems, page 692) and fertility problems (*see* page 656).

More widespread than bacterial prostatitis, however, is chronic non-bacterial prostatitis, the cause of which is not known.

Orthodox treatment

Bacterial inflammation needs to be treated with antibiotics. Surgery may be required if abscesses or fistulae have developed. Chronic non-bacterial prostatitis is frequently treated with various physical methods of pain relief.

Complementary therapies

Prostatitis is believed by some complementary therapists to be a problem of disturbed life force (*see* page 928); others see it as being caused by foci (*see* page 928), the result of chronic exposure to toxins (*see* page 929), as an energy imbalance (*see* page 927), or as an expression of lowered immunity. Treatments will be suggested accordingly. Some therapists aim to treat symptoms directly through energy links (*see* page 928).

Treatment plan and limited trial

Before administering a complementary treatment, every therapist should propose a treatment plan (*see* page xxiii) that sets out a clear time frame and defines the goal that the treatment is designed to achieve. Treatment should then be tried for a limited term to test the patient's response.

Caution

The various complementary therapies on offer are no substitute for effective modern antibiotics in acute bacterial prostatitis, nor for other orthodox procedures in malignant growth of the prostate.

Complementary treatments for prostatitis

Treatment	Rating	Point of delivery/risks
Acupressure This treatment (*see* page 769), otherwise known as pressure-point massage, is claimed to ease pain and improve general well-being. The pressure points chosen may differ from one practitioner to another.	**May be of some use** as a short-term treatment attempt aimed at alleviating pain. Some case reports claim efficacy; however, success is probably seen in only a proportion of patients (*see* Placebo, page xxi).	**Suitable for DIY** Qualified guidance is recommended. Therapists should be properly qualified. **Risks:** Unlikely provided treatment is carried out competently.
Acupuncture Acupuncture in its various forms (*see* page 772) aims to encourage the flow of energy (*see* page 927) or to act directly to alleviate pain and reduce swelling and inflammation.	**May be of some use** as a short-term treatment attempt aimed at alleviating pain. Case reports and field studies claim efficacy; however, success is probably seen in only a proportion of patients (*see* Placebo, page xxi).	**Requires a qualified practitioner** Acupuncturists should be properly qualified and should propose a treatment plan. **Risks:** Probably rare provided treatment is carried out competently.
Anthroposophical medicine AM (*see* page 781) sees prostatitis as a predominantly psychosomatic condition against which constitutional therapy will generally be attempted.	**May be of some use** as a short-term treatment attempt for chronic symptoms. Some studies claim efficacy; however, success is probably seen in only a proportion of patients (*see* Placebo, page xxi).	**Requires a qualified practitioner** Practitioners should be properly qualified and should propose a treatment plan. **Risks:** Allergies and intolerance are possible.

Treatment	Rating	Point of delivery/risks
Aromatherapy Essential oils (*see* page 786) are used to soothe and relax, or to invigorate, thereby possibly improving general well-being. The essences may be taken orally, used externally as massage oils or bathing emulsions, or inhaled as vapors.	**Of little use** Acceptable as a short-term, supportive treatment attempt aimed at soothing and relaxing. Some case reports claim efficacy; however, success is probably seen in only a proportion of patients (*see* Placebo, page xxi).	**Suitable for DIY** Qualified guidance is recommended. The effects of individual essential oils differ widely. **Risks:** Allergies or intolerance are possible. Some oils are carcinogenic in test systems and possibly in humans.
Bioresonance therapy Bioresonance therapists use electrical devices in an attempt to discover the causes of illness and claim to be able to weaken or turn around pathogenic energies and disease related vibrations (*see* page 794).	**Of little use** Possibly acceptable as a short-term treatment attempt for persistent, chronic prostatitis when simpler, more established methods have been unsuccessful. Some case reports claim efficacy; however, success is probably seen, if at all, in only a small proportion of patients (*see* Placebo, page xxi).	**Requires a qualified practitioner** Practitioners should be properly qualified and should propose a treatment plan. No credence should be given to anyone promising immediate or total success. **Risks:** Fairly unlikely.
Cell therapy Injecting or ingesting products extracted from the tissues of newborn animals or animal fetuses is said to have a rejuvenating and revitalizing effect and to enhance the healing of human tissues and organs (*see* page 796).	**Not advised** Based on present knowledge, there is inadequate evidence of the efficacy and mode of action of these costly and relatively risky procedures.	**Risks:** Injecting foreign proteins into the body can provoke (possibly fatal) allergic reactions. Also, pathogens such as those that cause bovine spongiform encephalopathy (BSE) or other serious infections may be introduced.

Treatment	Rating	Point of delivery/risks
Electroacupuncture according to Voll By taking readings of the electrical conductivity of the skin (*see* page 802), therapists claim to be able to derive an insight into diseased areas of the body, pathogenic foci (*see* page 928), and stress factors (*see* Toxins, page 929). The factors presumed to be instrumental in the causation of prostatitis can then be addressed.	**Of little use** Possibly acceptable as a short-term treatment attempt for persistent, chronic prostatitis when simpler, more established methods have been unsuccessful. Some case reports claim efficacy; however, success is probably seen, if at all, in only a small proportion of patients (*see* Placebo, page xxi).	**Requires a qualified practitioner** Practitioners should be properly qualified and should propose a treatment plan. No credence should be given to anyone promising immediate or total success. **Risks:** A second opinion must always be obtained from a qualified physician before any attempt is made to "eliminate foci" (e.g. by surgery).
Electroneural therapy according to Croon According to the theory, readings taken at various reactive sites on the skin highlight diseased areas within the body. Based on these readings, targeted electrostimulative measures can be undertaken to address the factors presumed to be instrumental in the causation of prostatitis (*see* page 806).	**Of little use** Possibly acceptable as a short-term treatment attempt for persistent, chronic prostatitis when simpler, more established methods have been unsuccessful. Some case reports claim efficacy; however, success is probably seen, if at all, in only a small proportion of patients (*see* Placebo, page xxi).	**Requires a qualified practitioner** Practitioners should be properly qualified and should propose a treatment plan. No credence should be given to anyone promising immediate or total success. **Risks:** Proponents themselves warn that treatment should not be given in acute inflammatory conditions.

Treatment	Rating	Point of delivery/risks
Eliminative methods, bloody Bloody cupping (*see* page 815) is sometimes used in prostatitis to ease pain.	**Of little use** Possibly acceptable as a short-term treatment attempt for chronic, persistent prostatitis when more established, less invasive methods have been unsuccessful. Some case reports and field studies claim efficacy; however, success is probably seen in only a small proportion of patients (*see* Placebo, page xxi).	**Requires a qualified practitioner** Practitioners should be properly qualified and should propose a treatment plan. **Risks:** Bloody cupping can cause infection and scarring. Furthermore, it should not be carried out in persons with bleeding disorders.
Eliminative methods, unbloody Unbloody cupping (*see* page 817) is used as a reflex therapy (*see* page 881) aimed at easing pain, energizing (*see* page 927) the patient and improving the body's own regulatory systems.	**May be of some use** as a short-term, supportive treatment attempt aimed at easing pain. Some case reports claim efficacy; however, success is probably seen in only a proportion of patients (*see* Placebo, page xxi).	**Suitable for DIY** Unbloody cupping is best carried out under the guidance of a qualified practitioner. **Risks:** Unlikely provided treatment is carried out competently.
Enzyme therapy The enzymes used are said to dispel and destroy "immune complexes" (*see* page 824) that course in the blood and that are responsible, for instance, for sustaining inflammatory processes.	**Of little use** Possibly acceptable as a short-term treatment attempt for chronic, non-bacterial prostatitis. Some case reports claim efficacy for this little researched therapy; however, success is probably seen, if at all, in only a small proportion of patients (*see* Placebo, page xxi).	**Requires a qualified practitioner** Practitioners should propose a treatment plan. Non-prescription preparations are suitable for do-it-yourself. **Risks:** Allergies or intolerance are possible.

Treatment	*Rating*	*Point of delivery/risks*
Flower remedies Flower remedies (*see* page 828) are said to restore emotional balance and assist the body's psychic ability to heal itself.	**Of little use** Acceptable as a short-term, supportive treatment attempt aimed at soothing and relaxing. Some case reports claim efficacy; however, success is probably seen in only a proportion of patients (*see* Placebo, page xxi).	**Suitable for DIY** Qualified guidance is recommended. Practitioners should propose a treatment plan. **Risks:** Possible intolerance.
Homeopathy Highly diluted (potentized) solutions (*see* page 831) are believed to be able to redress vital energy imbalances and strengthen the body's defences. Organo- and functiotropic (*see* page 833) homeopathy is claimed to be effective for dealing with symptoms of prostatitis.	**May be of some use** as a supportive treatment attempt for persistent, chronic symptoms. Case reports and field studies claim efficacy; however, success is probably seen in only a proportion of patients (*see* Placebo, page xxi).	**Requires a qualified practitioner** Homeopaths should be properly qualified and should propose a treatment plan. Ready-formulated preparations are suitable for do-it-yourself. **Risks:** Allergies and intolerance are possible.
Manual therapies Chiropractors and osteopaths (*see* page 844) use a series of manipulations to realign vertebrae allegedly displaced by prostatitis. This is said to have a beneficial effect on the prostate and to ease pain.	**Of little use** Possibly acceptable as a short-term treatment attempt for persistent, chronic pain when less risky, more established methods have been unsuccessful. Some case reports claim efficacy; however, success is probably seen, if at all, in only a small proportion of patients (*see* Placebo, page xxi).	**Requires a qualified practitioner** Practitioners should be properly qualified and should propose a treatment plan. **Risks:** Manipulation of the head and cervical vertebrae can cause serious injury. Osteoporosis is one of several risk factors.

Treatment	Rating	Point of delivery/risks
Nutritional therapies An organic diet (*see* page 4) provides the body with essential and secondary plant nutrients that are capable, it is said, of boosting the immune system.	**Useful** in chronic prostatitis as an individually directed supportive measure.	**Suitable for DIY** Qualified guidance is recommended though not essential. **Risks:** Avoid imbalanced or intolerable diets. They can cause deficiencies with serious consequences. Children are particularly at risk.
Physical therapies Warm and hot sitz baths, mud baths, and wraps (*see* pages 871–8) are said to improve the circulation, reduce swelling, and ease pain in patients with prostatitis.	**May be of some use** as a short-term treatment attempt for acute and chronic symptoms. Case reports and field studies claim efficacy; however, success is probably seen in only a proportion of patients (*see* Placebo, page xxi).	**Suitable for DIY** Qualified guidance is recommended though not essential. **Risks:** Skin damage may be caused to persons with diminished temperature sensation when extreme temperatures are applied.
Reflex therapies Connective tissue massage, reflexology (*see* page 883) and TENS (*see* page 886) are claimed to act via reflex channels (*see* page 881) to reduce pain and exercise a beneficial influence on the prostate.	**May be of some use** as a short-term treatment attempt aimed at alleviating pain. Case reports claim efficacy; however, success is probably seen in only a proportion of patients (*see* Placebo, page xxi).	**Requires a qualified practitioner** Practitioners should be properly qualified and should propose a treatment plan. **Risks:** Some people are sensitive to electrical stimuli and rubber electrodes; others find it hard to tolerate manual stimulation or close physical contact.

Treatment	Rating	Point of delivery/risks
Relaxation techniques Autogenic training (*see* page 888), muscle relaxation according to Jacobson (*see* page 893), and various biofeedback techniques (*see* page 891) are said to relieve muscle tension and inner unrest, and might be instrumental in helping the patient to become better aware of his physical and emotional states.	**May be of some use** as a short-term, supportive treatment attempt aimed at relaxing the patient and improving self-awareness. Some case reports claim efficacy; however, success is probably seen in only a proportion of patients (*see* Placebo, page xxi).	**Suitable for DIY** Once a sound understanding of the technique has been acquired from a trainer in group sessions or through individual tuition, patients can perform exercises themselves. Therapists should be properly qualified. **Risks:** Fairly unlikely.

Herbal remedies for prostatitis

See herbal remedies for prostate enlargement and urinary tract infections (*see* pages 386–90, 399–400).

Heart and circulation

Angina pectoris

Causes and symptoms

Angina pectoris is a condition that occurs when the arteries supplying blood to the heart muscle become clogged or constricted. If the coronary blood supply drops below a critical minimum or if the heart momentarily needs more blood than the coronary arteries can supply, the heart muscle cells become underoxygenated. The patient feels a tight, crushing pain in the center of the chest, sometimes radiating to the arms or wrists, the back, the neck, or the jaw. Pain is mostly spasmodic and accompanied by a feeling of severe distress.

Smokers, diabetics, persons with high blood pressure, and those with excessive blood uric acid, fibrinogen, homocystein, or cholesterol levels are more likely to suffer from coronary disease and are thus more prone to angina pectoris. Angina pectoris can be the first sign of a heart attack. Worldwide, it is one of the most common causes of death.

Orthodox treament

Emergency medical treatment will include medication in the form of nitroglycerin capsules and sprays or capsules containing nifedipine. Nitroglycerin frequently causes headaches, however. In the longer term, beta-blockers will be given to reduce the heart's work rate and oxygen demand; organic nitrate preparations will also be prescribed, and calcium antagonists will be used in patients who do not tolerate beta-blockers.

Various possibilities exist for treating patients with coronary heart disease and angina pectoris. Apart from medication, treatments may include coronary dilation (passing a balloon catheter into the coronary arteries and then inflating it to remove constrictions) and coronary artery bypass grafting.

Complementary therapies

Complementary therapies are suitable at best as supportive measures, e.g. for relieving pain or other symptoms. They cannot cure angina pectoris. Advice about lifestyle changes can be useful in preventing further problems.

Treatment plan and limited trial

Before administering a complementary treatment, every therapist should propose a treatment plan (*see* page xxiii) that sets out a clear time frame and defines the goal that the treatment is designed to achieve. Treatment should then be tried for a limited term to test the patient's response.

Caution

Before undergoing any complementary treatment for symptoms that point to angina pectoris, patients must always see a doctor to obtain an orthodox diagnosis; they otherwise risk missing the opportunity of receiving potentially life-saving orthodox medical treatment for their condition. A prolonged episode of angina pectoris may also signal the start of a heart attack.

There is no documented proof to substantiate claims that certain complementary therapies can effectively treat acute attacks.

Complementary treatments for angina pectoris

Treatment	Rating	Point of delivery/risks
Acupressure This treatment (*see* page 769), otherwise known as pressure-point massage, is claimed to alleviate pain when the appropriate pressure points are stimulated. The pressure points chosen may differ from one practitioner to another.	**Inappropriate** as the sole treatment for angina pectoris. **May be of some use** as a short-term, supportive treatment attempt aimed at alleviating pain. Field studies claim efficacy; however, success is probably seen in only a small proportion of patients (*see* Placebo, page xxi).	**Suitable for DIY** Qualified guidance is recommended. Therapists should be properly qualified. **Risks:** Unlikely provided treatment is carried out competently.
Acupuncture Acupuncture in its various forms (*see* page 772) aims to encourage the flow of energy (*see* page 927) or to alleviate pain directly. The acupuncture points chosen can vary from one practitioner to another.	**Inappropriate** as the sole treatment for angina pectoris. **May be of some use** as a short-term, supportive treatment attempt aimed at alleviating pain. Field studies claim efficacy; however, success is probably seen in only a proportion of patients (*see* Placebo, page xxi).	**Requires a qualified practitioner** Practitioners should be properly qualified and should propose a treatment plan. **Risks:** Probably rare provided treatment is carried out competently.
Anthroposophical medicine Doctors who practice AM (*see* page 781) see the heart not as a pump but as an organ that works in association with other organs of the "liquid organism." Curative eurhythmy and preparations that include cactus and potentized gold are used for treating the liver, spleen, and kidneys.	**Inappropriate** as the sole treatment for angina pectoris. **May be of some use** as a preventive measure and as a short-term, supportive treatment attempt. Some case reports claim efficacy; however, success is probably seen in only a proportion of patients (*see* Placebo, page xxi).	**Requires a qualified practitioner** Practitioners should be properly qualified and should propose a treatment plan. No credence should be given to anyone promising immediate or total success. **Risks:** Allergies and intolerance are possible.

Treatment	Rating	Point of delivery/risks
Aromatherapy Essential oils (*see* page 786) are used to soothe and relax, or to invigorate, thereby helping to ease symptoms. The essences may be taken orally, used externally as massage oils or bathing emulsions, or inhaled as vapors.	**Inappropriate** as the sole treatment for angina pectoris. **May be of some use** as a short-term, supportive treatment attempt aimed at soothing and relaxing. Some case reports claim efficacy; however, success is probably seen in only a proportion of patients (*see* Placebo, page xxi).	**Suitable for DIY** Qualified guidance is recommended. The effects of individual essential oils differ widely. **Risks:** Allergies or intolerance are possible. Some oils are carcinogenic in test systems and possibly in humans.
Bioresonance therapy Bioresonance therapists use electrical devices in an attempt to discover the causes of illness and claim to be able to weaken or turn around pathogenic energies and disease related vibrations (*see* page 794).	**Of little use** Possibly acceptable as a short-term, supportive treatment attempt when simpler, more established methods have been unsuccessful. Some case reports claim efficacy; however, success is probably seen, if at all, in only a small proportion of patients (*see* Placebo, page xxi).	**Requires a qualified practitioner** Practitioners should be properly qualified and should propose a treatment plan. No credence should be given to anyone promising immediate or total success. **Risks:** Fairly unlikely.
Cell therapy Injecting or ingesting products extracted from the tissues of newborn animals or animal fetuses is said to have a rejuvenating and revitalizing effect and to enhance the healing of human tissues and organs (*see* page 796).	**Not advised** Based on present knowledge, there is inadequate evidence of the efficacy and mode of action of these costly and relatively risky procedures.	**Risks:** Injecting foreign proteins into the body can provoke (possibly fatal) allergic reactions. Also, pathogens such as those that cause bovine spongiform encephalopathy (BSE) or other serious infections may be introduced.

Treatment	Rating	Point of delivery/risks
Chelation therapy The chelating agent EDTA (*see* page 800) is able, it is claimed, to bind calcareous deposits in the blood vessels. These are subsequently eliminated from the body, so that arteriosclerotic disease can, according to the theory, be reversed.	**Not advised** Evidence of the therapeutic usefulness of this risky procedure is lacking.	**Risks:** EDTA can cause a deficit of calcium and essential heavy metals and, in extreme cases, can lead to cardiac arrhythmia, respiratory failure, cramps, and death.
Electroacupuncture according to Voll By taking readings of the electrical conductivity of the skin (*see* page 802), therapists claim to be able to derive an insight into diseased areas of the body, pathogenic foci (*see* page 928), and stress factors (*see* Toxins, page 929). The factors presumed to be instrumental in the causation of angina pectoris can then be addressed.	**Of little use** Possibly acceptable as a short-term, supportive treatment attempt when simpler, more established methods have been unsuccessful. Some case reports claim efficacy; however, success is probably seen, if at all, in only a small proportion of patients (*see* Placebo, page xxi).	**Requires a qualified practitioner** Practitioners should be properly qualified and should propose a treatment plan. No credence should be given to anyone promising immediate or total success. **Risks:** A second opinion must always be obtained from a qualified physician before any attempt is made to "eliminate foci" (e.g. by surgery).

Treatment	Rating	Point of delivery/risks
Electroneural therapy according to Croon According to the theory, readings taken at various reactive sites on the skin highlight diseased areas within the body. Based on these readings, targeted electrostimulative measures can be undertaken to address the factors presumed to be instrumental in the causation of angina pectoris (*see* page 806).	**Of little use** Possibly acceptable as a short-term, supportive treatment attempt when simpler, more established methods have been unsuccessful. Some case reports claim efficacy; however, success is probably seen, if at all, in only a small proportion of patients (*see* Placebo, page xxi).	**Requires a qualified practitioner** Practitioners should be properly qualified and should propose a treatment plan. No credence should be given to anyone promising immediate or total success. **Risks:** Proponents themselves warn that treatment should not be given in acute inflammatory conditions.
Eliminative methods, bloody Bloody cupping (*see* page 815) is said to improve general well-being and the body's own regulatory systems in patients with angina pectoris.	**Not advised** Evidence of the efficacy of this relatively invasive procedure is lacking.	**Risks:** Bloody cupping can cause infection and scarring. Furthermore, it should not be carried out in persons with bleeding disorders.
Eliminative methods, unbloody Unbloody cupping (*see* page 817) is supposed to energize (*see* page 927) the patient and improve the body's own regulatory systems.	**Inappropriate** as the sole treatment for angina pectoris. **May be of some use** as a short-term, supportive treatment attempt aimed at alleviating pain. Some case reports claim a degree of efficacy; however, success is probably seen in only a small proportion of patients (*see* Placebo, page xxi).	**Suitable for DIY** Qualified guidance is essential. **Risks:** Unlikely provided treatment is carried out competently.

Treatment	Rating	Point of delivery/risks
Enzyme therapy The enzymes used (*see* page 824) can, it is claimed, prevent vascular disease and stop its progression.	**Of little use** Some case reports claim efficacy for this little researched and relatively costly procedure; however, success is probably seen in only a small proportion of patients (*see* Placebo, page xxi).	**Requires a qualified practitioner** Practitioners should propose a treatment plan. Non-prescription preparations are suitable for do-it-yourself. **Risks:** Allergies or intolerance are possible.
Flower remedies Flower remedies (*see* page 828) are said to restore emotional balance and assist the body's psychic ability to heal itself. Bach Rescue Remedy is often used for acute attacks.	**Inappropriate** as the sole treatment for angina pectoris. Possibly acceptable as a short-term treatment attempt aimed at soothing and relaxing. Some case reports claim a degree of efficacy; however, success is probably seen in only a proportion of patients (*see* Placebo, page xxi).	**Suitable for DIY** Qualified guidance is recommended. Practitioners should propose a treatment plan. **Risks:** Possible intolerance.
Homeopathy Highly diluted (potentized) solutions (see page 831) are believed to be able to redress vital energy imbalances and strengthen the body's defences. Organo- and functiotropic (*see* page 833) homeopathy is claimed to be effective for dealing directly with symptoms.	**Inappropriate** as the sole treatment for angina pectoris. **May be of some use** as a supportive treatment attempt and for helping the patient come to terms better with his/her condition. Case reports claim success for homeopathic treatments; however, success is probably seen in only a proportion of patients (*see* Placebo, page xxi).	**Requires a qualified practitioner** Homeopaths should be properly qualified and should propose a treatment plan. Ready-formulated preparations are suitable for do-it-yourself. **Risks:** Allergies and intolerance are possible.

Treatment	Rating	Point of delivery/risks
Hypnosis and self-hypnosis In the relaxed and generally altered state of awareness that is induced in hypnosis or self-hypnosis (*see* page 837), physical and mental conditions can be addressed and pain alleviated. Hypnosis is often used in combination with other psycho- and behavioral therapies.	**Inappropriate** as the sole treatment for angina pectoris. **May be of some use** as a short-term, supportive treatment attempt, as a method of relaxing the patient, and as a way of helping him/her come to terms better with his/her condition. Some case reports claim efficacy; however, success is probably seen in only a proportion of patients treated (*see* Placebo, page xxi).	**Requires a qualified practitioner** Hypnotherapists should be properly qualified and should propose a treatment plan. No credence should be given to anyone promising immediate or total success. **Risks:** Unlikely provided treatment is carried out competently.
Magnetic field therapy The use of magnetic field generators, magnetic strips, bracelets, and other objects (*see* page 841) allegedly encourages cell metabolism and so eases symptoms.	**Of little use** Based on present knowledge, there is inadequate evidence of the efficacy and mode of action of magnetic field therapy in angina pectoris.	Operation of magnetic field equipment **requires a qualified practitioner**. **Risks:** Magnetic field equipment can cause implanted cardiac pacemakers to malfunction.
Manual therapies Chiropractors and osteopaths (*see* page 844) use a series of manipulations to realign allegedly displaced vertebrae. This is said to reduce pain and free energy blockages.	**Inappropriate** as the sole treatment for angina pectoris. Possibly acceptable as a short-term treatment attempt aimed at relieving persistent pain when less risky, more established methods have been unsuccessful. Some case reports claim efficacy for these potentially risky procedures; however, success is probably seen, if at all, in only a small proportion of patients (*see* Placebo, page xxi).	**Requires a qualified practitioner** Practitioners should be properly qualified and should propose a treatment plan. **Risks:** Manipulation of the head and cervical vertebrae can cause serious injury. Osteoporosis is one of several risk factors.

Treatment	Rating	Point of delivery/risks
Massage Classical massage (*see* page 847) can be used to ease muscular and emotional tension.	**Inappropriate** as the sole treatment for angina pectoris. May be of some use as a short-term, supportive treatment attempt aimed at relaxing the patient and improving general well-being. Case reports claim efficacy; however, success is probably seen in only a proportion of patients (*see* Placebo, page xxi).	**Requires a qualified practitioner** Masseurs/masseuses should be properly qualified and should propose a treatment plan. **Risks:** Some people are sensitive to manual stimuli; others find it hard to tolerate close physical contact.
Nutritional therapies An organic diet (*see* page 4) provides the body with essential and secondary plant nutrients (antioxidants), which are believed to exercise a multitude of positive effects and to be capable, *inter alia*, of preventing vascular disease.	**Inappropriate** as the sole treatment for angina pectoris. **Useful** as an individually directed supportive measure. Studies ascribe a degree of efficacy in the treatment of arteriosclerosis, in the prevention of infarction, and in the prevention of further problems if infarction has already occurred.	**Suitable for DIY** Qualified guidance is recommended though not essential. **Risks:** Avoid imbalanced or intolerable diets. They can cause deficiencies with serious consequences. Children are particularly at risk.
Physical therapies Hot arm washes and compresses, hot mustard poultices, and brush massaging are said to improve the circulation (*see* pages 871–8). Exercise therapy (*see* page 868), as a supportive measure, is supposed to prevent infarction.	**Inappropriate** as the sole treatment for angina pectoris. **Useful** as a longer-term, preventive measure. Case reports and field studies claim efficacy; however, success is probably seen in only a proportion of patients (*see* Placebo, page xxi).	**Suitable for DIY** Qualified guidance is recommended. An individual plan of treatment should be defined in association with the treating physician. **Risks:** Skin damage may be caused to persons with diminished temperature sensation when extreme temperatures are applied.

Treatment	Rating	Point of delivery/risks
Probiotics The introduction of certain bacteria into the gut is claimed to bring the intestinal flora back into balance and to have a beneficial effect on vascular processes and arteriosclerosis (*see* page 878).	**Inappropriate** as the sole treatment for angina pectoris. Possibly acceptable as a short-term, supportive treatment attempt when more established methods have been unsuccessful. Some case reports claim efficacy; however, success is probably seen in only a small proportion of patients (*see* Placebo, page xxi).	**Requires a qualified practitioner** Practitioners should be properly qualified and should propose a treatment plan. Non-prescription formulations are suitable for do-it-yourself. **Risks:** Fairly unlikely provided treatment is carried out competently.
Reflex therapies Reflex zone massage (*see* page 883), reflexology (*see* page 883), and TENS (*see* page 886) are claimed to act via reflex channels (*see* page 881) to ease pain.	**Inappropriate** as the sole treatment for angina pectoris. **May be of some use** as a short-term, supportive treatment attempt aimed at alleviating acute pain. Field studies claim efficacy; however, success is probably seen in only a proportion of patients (*see* Placebo, page xxi).	**Suitable for DIY** Qualified guidance is essential. Therapists should propose a treatment plan. **Risks:** Some people are sensitive to electrical stimuli and rubber electrodes; others find it hard to tolerate manual stimulation or close physical contact.
Relaxation techniques Autogenic training (*see* page 880), muscle relaxation according to Jacobson (*see* page 893), and various biofeedback techniques (*see* page 891) are said to relieve tension and inner unrest and so might be instrumental in helping the patient achieve a change of lifestyle.	**Inappropriate** as the sole treatment for angina pectoris. **Useful** as a supportive measure aimed at relaxing the patient and encouraging a change of lifestyle. Some case reports claim efficacy; however, success is probably seen in only a proportion of patients (*see* Placebo, page xxi).	**Suitable for DIY** Once a sound understanding of the technique has been acquired from a trainer, patients can perform exercises themselves. Therapists should propose a treatment plan. **Risks:** Fairly unlikely.

Treatment	Rating	Point of delivery/risks
Vitamins and trace elements The antioxidative properties of beta-carotene, vitamins C and E, and selenium are, it is supposed, instrumental in countering the formation of free radicals and in boosting the body's antioxidative defence systems (*see* page 900).	**Inappropriate** as the sole treatment for angina pectoris. **May be of some use** as a preventive measure. Studies ascribe a degree of success to this treatment. No definitive recommendations can be made based on present knowledge. In the elderly, in particular, there may be some benefit in taking certain vitamins.	**Suitable for DIY** Qualified guidance is recommended though not essential. **Risks:** Intolerance and overdosage are possible. Recent studies imply that beta-carotene might increase the risk of cancer.

Herbal remedy for angina pectoris

Active ingredient/preparation	Rating
Hawthorn leaves and blossom (*Crataegus monogyna* and *Crataegus laevigata*)	**May be of some use** as a supportive treatment attempt for mild and stable forms of angina pectoris. Hawthorn is a coronary vasodilator that helps guard against oxygen deficit. Talk to your doctor before taking hawthorn. **Daily dose:** 1g herb. **Individual dose:** Pour hot water over 0.2–0.3g of herb and infuse, three to four times a day. Use ready-formulated preparations as instructed by the manufacturer/prescriber. **Risks:** Hawthorn may in some cases cause nausea, headaches and vertigo. Remedies containing hawthorn may possibly potentiate the action and thus the toxicity of digitalis. It must not be used, therefore, with cardiac tonics that contain digitalis. It is not suitable for self-medication.

Atherosclerosis

Causes and symptoms

Atherosclerosis is a gradual clogging or hardening of the arteries, leading to poor circulation. It ranges in severity from slightly reduced bloodflow to partial or complete arterial blockage. Common early symptoms of atherosclerosis include angina pectoris, pain felt while walking, and leg cramps (intermittent claudication); as the disease progresses, leg pains are experienced at rest, the skin becomes sensitive, and the legs may become ulcerated.

Orthodox treatment

Orthodox treatment will vary depending on the part of the body affected and how advanced the disease is. Doctors will usually advise patients to avoid risk factors such as smoking. Modern treatments include expansion of the blood vessels with a balloon catheter and various other surgical procedures.

Complementary therapies

There is no evidence to suggest that any complementary therapy can improve blood circulation in relatively advanced atherosclerosis. The majority of available therapies are suitable at best for prevention or for alleviating symptoms.

Treatment plan and limited trial

Before administering a complementary treatment, every therapist should propose a treatment plan (*see* page xxiii) that sets out a clear time frame and defines the goal that the treatment is designed to achieve. Treatment should then be tried for a limited term to test the patient's response.

Caution

Complementary medicine can offer no substitute for surgical procedures designed to expand and unblock arteries.

Complementary treatments for atherosclerosis

Treatment	Rating	Point of delivery/risks
Acupressure This treatment (*see* page 769), otherwise known as pressure-point massage, is claimed to alleviate pain when the appropriate pressure points are stimulated. The pressure points chosen may differ from one practitioner to another.	**Inappropriate** as a treatment for atherosclerosis. **May be of some use** as a short-term, supportive treatment attempt aimed at alleviating pain. Case reports ascribe a degree of efficacy to this procedure; however, success is probably seen in only a proportion of patients (*see* Placebo, page xxi).	**Suitable for DIY** Qualified guidance is recommended. Therapists should be properly qualified. **Risks:** Unlikely provided treatment is carried out competently.
Acupuncture Acupuncture in its various forms (*see* page 772) aims to encourage the flow of energy (*see* page 927) or to act directly to alleviate pain and improve the circulation. The acupuncture points chosen can vary from one practitioner to another.	**Inappropriate** as a treatment for atherosclerosis. **May be of some use** as a short-term, supportive treatment attempt aimed at alleviating pain and improving the circulation. Case reports and field studies claim efficacy; however, success is probably seen in only a proportion of patients (*see* Placebo, page xxi).	**Requires a qualified practitioner** Practitioners should be properly qualified and should propose a treatment plan. **Risks:** Probably rare provided treatment is carried out competently.

Treatment	Rating	Point of delivery/risks
Anthroposophical medicine As a preventive measure, doctors who practice AM (*see* page 781) prescribe potentized "compositions" of lead compounds. Art therapy used supportively is claimed to improve intellectual activity and *joie de vivre*, and so to contribute to a healthier style of life.	**Inappropriate** as a treatment for atherosclerosis. Possibly acceptable as a preventive measure and as a supportive treatment attempt in advanced stages of the disease, in which conventional treatments have in the past usually been found to be ineffective. Case reports claim efficacy; however, success is probably seen in only a proportion of patients (*see* Placebo, page xxi).	**Requires a qualified practitioner** Practitioners should be properly qualified and should propose a treatment plan. No credence should be given to anyone promising immediate or total success. **Risks:** Allergies and intolerance are possible.
Aromatherapy Essential oils (*see* page 786) are used to soothe and relax, or to invigorate, thereby possibly leading to an easing of symptoms. The essences may be taken orally, used externally as massage oils or bathing emulsions, or inhaled as vapors.	**Inappropriate** as a treatment for atherosclerosis. Possibly acceptable as a short-term, supportive treatment attempt aimed at soothing and relaxing. Some case reports claim efficacy; however, success is probably seen in only a small proportion of patients (*see* Placebo, page xxi).	**Suitable for DIY** Qualified guidance is recommended. The effects of individual essential oils differ widely. **Risks:** Allergies or intolerance are possible. Some oils are carcinogenic in test systems and possibly in humans.

Treatment	Rating	Point of delivery/risks
Bioresonance therapy Bioresonance therapists use electrical devices in an attempt to discover the causes of illness and claim to be able to weaken or turn around pathogenic energies and disease related vibrations (*see* page 794).	**Inappropriate** as a treatment for atherosclerosis. **Of little use** Possibly acceptable as a short-term, supportive treatment attempt when simpler, more established methods have been unsuccessful. Some case reports claim efficacy; however, success is probably seen, if at all, in only a small proportion of patients (*see* Placebo, page xxi).	**Requires a qualified practitioner** Practitioners should be properly qualified and should propose a treatment plan. No credence should be given to anyone promising immediate or total success. **Risks:** Fairly unlikely.
Cell therapy Products extracted from the tissues of newborn animals or animal fetuses are said to have a rejuvenating and revitalizing effect and to enhance the healing of human tissues and organs (*see* page 796).	**Not advised** Based on present knowledge, there is inadequate evidence of the efficacy and mode of action of these costly and relatively risky procedures.	**Risks:** Injecting foreign proteins into the body can provoke (possibly fatal) allergic reactions. Also, pathogens such as those that cause bovine spongiform encephalopathy (BSE) or other serious infections may be introduced.
Chelation therapy The chelating agent EDTA (*see* page 800) is able, it is claimed, to bind calcareous deposits and heavy metals in the blood vessels. These are subsequently eliminated from the body.	**Not advised** Controlled clinical studies have confirmed the worthlessness of this risky procedure.	**Risks:** EDTA can cause a deficit of calcium and essential heavy metals and, in extreme cases, can lead to cardiac arrhythmia, respiratory failure, cramps, and death.

Treatment	*Rating*	*Point of delivery/risks*
Electroacupuncture according to Voll By taking readings of the electrical conductivity of the skin (*see* page 802), therapists claim to be able to derive an insight into diseased areas of the body, pathogenic foci (*see* page 928), and stress factors (*see* Toxins, page 929). The factors presumed to be instrumental in the causation of atherosclerosis can then be addressed.	**Inappropriate** as a treatment for atherosclerosis. Possibly acceptable as a short-term, supportive treatment attempt when simpler, more established methods have been unsuccessful. Some case reports claim efficacy; however, success is probably seen, if at all, in only a small proportion of patients (*see* Placebo, page xxi).	**Requires a qualified practitioner** Practitioners should be properly qualified and should propose a treatment plan. No credence should be given to anyone promising immediate or total success. **Risks:** A second opinion must always be obtained from a qualified physician before any attempt is made to "eliminate foci" (e.g. by surgery).
Electroneural therapy according to Croon According to the theory, readings taken at various reactive sites on the skin highlight diseased areas within the body. Based on these readings, targeted electrostimulative measures can be undertaken to address factors presumed to be instrumental in the causation of atherosclerosis (*see* page 806).	**Inappropriate** as a treatment for atherosclerosis. Possibly acceptable as a short-term, supportive treatment attempt when simpler, more established methods have been unsuccessful. Some case reports claim efficacy; however, success is probably seen, if at all, in only a small proportion of patients (*see* Placebo, page xxi).	**Requires a qualified practitioner** Practitioners should be properly qualified and should propose a treatment plan. No credence should be given to anyone promising immediate or total success. **Risks:** Proponents themselves warn that treatment should not be given in acute inflammatory conditions.

Treatment	Rating	Point of delivery/risks
Eliminative methods, bloody Bloody cupping (*see* page 815) is said to encourage the circulation and improve the body's own regulatory systems.	**Not advised** There is insufficient documentary evidence of the efficacy and mode of action of this invasive and sometimes risky procedure.	**Risks:** Bloody cupping can cause infection and scarring. Furthermore, it should not be carried out in persons with bleeding disorders.
Eliminative methods, unbloody Unbloody cupping (*see* page 817) is supposed to ease pain in persons with atherosclerosis, energize (*see* page 927) the patient, and improve the body's own regulatory systems.	**Inappropriate** as a treatment for atherosclerosis. Acceptable as a short-term, supportive treatment attempt aimed at easing pain. Case reports claim efficacy; however, success is probably seen in only a proportion of patients (*see* Placebo, page xxi).	**Suitable for DIY** Unbloody cupping is best carried out under the guidance of a qualified practitioner. **Risks:** Unlikely provided treatment is carried out competently.
Enzyme therapy The enzymes used (*see* page 824) are said to dispel and destroy "immune complexes" that course in the blood and that are responsible, for instance, for sustaining inflammatory processes that might be responsible for vascular damage and arteriosclerosis.	**Of little use** Some case reports claim efficacy for this little researched therapy; however, success is probably seen in only a small proportion of patients (*see* Placebo, page xxi).	**Requires a qualified practitioner** Practitioners should propose a treatment plan. Non-prescription preparations are suitable for do-it-yourself. **Risks:** Allergies or intolerance are possible.

Treatment	Rating	Point of delivery/risks
Flower remedies Flower remedies (*see* page 828) are said to restore emotional balance and assist the body's psychic ability to heal itself.	**Inappropriate** as a treatment for atherosclerosis. Possibly acceptable as a short-term treatment attempt aimed at soothing and relaxing. Some case reports claim efficacy; however, success is probably seen in only a small proportion of patients (*see* Placebo, page xxi).	**Suitable for DIY** Qualified guidance is recommended. Practitioners should propose a treatment plan. **Risks:** Possible intolerance.
Homeopathy Highly diluted (potentized) solutions (*see* page 831) are believed to be able to redress vital energy imbalances. Organo- and functiotropic (*see* page 833) homeopathy is claimed to be effective for dealing with symptoms.	**Inappropriate** as a treatment for atherosclerosis. Possibly acceptable as a supportive treatment attempt. Case reports claim efficacy; however, success is probably seen in only a small proportion of patients (*see* Placebo, page xxi).	**Requires a qualified practitioner** Homeopaths should be properly qualified and should propose a treatment plan. Ready-formulated preparations are suitable for do-it-yourself. **Risks:** Allergies and intolerance are possible.
Magnetic field therapy The use of magnetic field generators, magnetic strips, bracelets, and other objects (*see* page 841) allegedly encourages cell metabolism and eases symptoms.	**Of little use** Based on present knowledge, there is inadequate evidence of the efficacy and mode of action of magnetic field therapy in atherosclerosis.	Operation of magnetic field equipment **requires a qualified practitioner**. **Risks:** Magnetic field equipment can cause implanted cardiac pacemakers to malfunction.

Treatment	Rating	Point of delivery/risks
Manual therapies Chiropractors and osteopaths (*see* page 844) use a series of manipulations to realign allegedly displaced vertebrae. This is said to reduce pain and release energy blockages (*see* page 927).	**Inappropriate** as a treatment for atherosclerosis. Possibly acceptable as a short-term treatment attempt aimed at alleviating pain. Some case reports claim efficacy for this potentially risky procedure; however, success is probably seen, if at all, in only a small proportion of patients (*see* Placebo, page xxi).	**Requires a qualified practitioner** Practitioners should be properly qualified and should propose a treatment plan. **Risks:** Manipulation of the head and cervical vertebrae can cause serious injury. Osteoporosis is one of several risk factors.
Massage Classical massage (*see* page 847) is said to ease muscular and emotional tension.	**Inappropriate** as a treatment for atherosclerosis. **May be of some use** as a supportive measure aimed at relaxing the patient. Case reports claim efficacy; however, success is probably seen in only a proportion of patients (*see* Placebo, page xxi).	**Suitable for DIY** Qualified guidance is recommended. Masseurs/masseuses should be properly qualified. **Risks:** Some people are sensitive to pressure; others find it hard to tolerate close physical contact.
Nutritional therapies Organic and vegetarian diets (*see* page 4) provide the body with essential and secondary plant nutrients, dietary fibers, antioxidants, etc., and may achieve a reduction in cholesterol levels. Therapeutic fasting (*see* page 864) is also often recommended for initiating a change of diet.	**Inappropriate** as a treatment for atherosclerosis. **Useful** as an individually directed supportive measure. Various controversial reports and studies ascribe major significance to a change-over to organic or vegetarian diets.	**Suitable for DIY** Qualified guidance is recommended though not essential. Food low in salt and protein but rich in potassium and magnesium is sometimes recommended. These recommendations are controversial, however. **Risks:** Avoid imbalanced or intolerable diets. They can cause deficiencies with serious consequences. Children are particularly at risk.

Treatment	Rating	Point of delivery/risks
Physical therapies Exercise therapy (*see* page 868) is said to improve the circulation and increase perfusion of the legs. Various hydrotherapeutic techniques are also said to improve the circulation (*see* pages 871–8).	**Useful** as an individually directed, supportive treatment attempt. Field studies, case reports, and initial clinical studies (carbon dioxide baths) ascribe a degree of efficacy to this treatment in some patients, especially in the initial stages of the disease.	**Suitable for DIY** Qualified guidance is recommended. An individual plan of treatment should be defined in association with the treating physician. **Risks:** In stage III, exercise therapy should be used in moderation and to suit the individual.
Reflex therapies Reflex zone massage (*see* page 883), reflexology (*see* page 883), and TENS (*see* page 886) are claimed to act via reflex channels (*see* page 881) to ease pain, to relax the patient, and to improve his/her circulation.	**Inappropriate** as a treatment for atherosclerosis. **May be of some use** as a short-term treatment attempt aimed at alleviating pain and improving the circulation. Field studies claim efficacy; however, success is probably seen in only a proportion of patients (*see* Placebo, page xxi).	**Suitable for DIY** Qualified guidance is essential. **Risks:** Some people are sensitive to electrical stimuli and rubber electrodes; others find it hard to tolerate manual stimulation or close physical contact.
Relaxation techniques Autogenic training (*see* page 888), muscle relaxation according to Jacobson (*see* page 893), and various biofeedback techniques (*see* page 891) are said to relieve muscle tension and inner unrest.	**Inappropriate** as a treatment for atherosclerosis. **Useful** as a supportive measure aimed at soothing and relaxing. Some case reports claim efficacy; however, success is probably seen in only a proportion of patients (*see* Placebo, page xxi).	**Suitable for DIY** Once a sound understanding of the technique has been acquired from a trainer, patients can perform exercises themselves. Therapists should be properly qualified. **Risks:** Fairly unlikely.

Treatment	Rating	Point of delivery/risks
Vitamins and trace elements The antioxidative properties of beta-carotene, vitamins C and E, and selenium are, it is supposed, instrumental in countering the formation of free radicals and in boosting the body's antioxidative defence systems (*see* page 900).	**Inappropriate** as a treatment for atherosclerosis. **May be of some use** as a short-term treatment attempt aimed at generally strengthening the body and trying to prevent high blood pressure and arteriosclerosis. No definitive recommendations can be made based on present knowledge. High vitamin C doses do appear to offer some benefits.	**Suitable for DIY** Qualified guidance is recommended though not essential. **Risks:** Intolerance and overdosage are possible. Recent studies imply that beta-carotene might increase the risk of cancer.

Herbal remedies for atherosclerosis

Active ingredient/preparation	Rating
Garlic corms (*Allium sativum*)	**Only useful** as a supportive treatment (with diet) for raised blood fat values and as a preventive measure against age-related vascular changes. Thins the blood and thus possibly also improves its flow properties. **Dosage:** As instructed by the manufacturer/prescriber (600–1200mg dry powder or 4g fresh corms [2–4 small cloves]). **Risks:** Gastric problems and asthma are possible. Garlic may prolong natural wound closure after accidental incisions owing to its blood-thinning properties. Consult your doctor before using garlic for this indication.

Active ingredient/preparation	Rating
Garlic oil maceration products	**Of little use**, as the chemical compostions of the preparations differ widely and no general daily dosage recommendations can be given. **Dosage:** As instructed by the manufacturer/prescriber. **Risks:** Gastric problems and asthma are possible in rare cases. Consult your doctor before using garlic for this indication.
Ginkgo leaves	**Of little use**. Teas prepared from ginkgo leaves have no proven efficacy. **Daily dose:** 4–8oz leaves. **Individual dose:** Pour 1 cup of hot water over 0.1g of leaves and infuse. **Risks:** Allergic reactions are possible.
Ginkgo extract (*Ginkgo biloba*)	**Useful** as a treatment attempt for circulatory problems in the legs resulting from vascular changes in conjunction with exercise designed to improve walking distances. **Dosage:** As instructed by the manufacturer/prescriber. **Risks:** Mild gastrointestinal problems, headaches and allergic skin reactions are possible. Not to be taken by persons who are hypersensitive to ginkgo. Injectable ginkgo preparations have been withdrawn owing to hypersensitivity reactions.
Soy lecithin (*Glycine max*)	**Of little use**. This is a rarely used and (at most) supportive treatment for mild disorders of fat metabolism, such as hypercholesteremia, in association with (or after) dietary measures to prevent hardening of the arteries. Soy lecithin reportedly changes the LDL/HDL ratio and so possibly has blood fat-lowering properties. **Dosage:** As instructed by the manufacturer/prescriber. **Risks:** Soy lecithin is not known to have any serious side effects.

High blood pressure (hypertension)

Causes and symptoms

Hypertension is a persistent rise in systolic blood pressure (the peak pressure when the heart contracts) above the normal limit of 140mm Hg, and in diastolic blood pressure (the lower pressure between heartbeats) above the normal limit of 90mm Hg (mm Hg or millimetres of mercury is the unit used to denote the displacement that occurs in a column of mercury when a given pressure is applied to it). Hypertension is further classified by degree, based principally on diastolic pressure. Values of between 90 and 95, for instance, are often referred to as "borderline hypertension." In the elderly, the limits at which medication becomes essential are generally set higher.

There are many causes of high blood pressure. The form most frequently diagnosed is primary or essential hypertension, the specific cause of which is not known. Some hypertension is the result of kidney disease or hormonal dysfunction. Other causes are: drugs, diet, cardiovascular disease, pregnancy, or damage to the central nervous system. Persistent hypertension is one of the risk factors for arterioclerosis and it may also damage structures such as the eyes, heart, kidneys, and brain. Symptoms associated with high blood pressure are giddiness, headaches and visual disturbance. These are not necessarily felt unless the pressure is elevated to extreme values.

Orthodox treatment

Disease-induced hypertension will be treated by addressing the underlying cause. Essential hypertension caused by other factors can be treated with exercise, by a change of diet, or through weight reduction. Where medication is required, this will be prescribed in the form of diuretics (to reduce the fluid status of the body), beta-blockers, calcium antagonists, and ACE inhibitors, either alone or in combination. Such treatments have been shown to reduce blood pressure, and subsequently organ damage, thus increasing life expectancy.

Complementary therapies

Exercise and nutritional therapies are the first line of defence in the complementary treatment of high blood pressure. Other complementary therapies are claimed to be able to reduce high blood pressure, though there have not as yet been any systematic long-term studies into these.

Treatment plan and limited trial

Before administering a complementary treatment, every therapist should propose a treatment plan (*see* page xxiii) that sets out a clear time frame and defines the goal that the treatment is designed to achieve. Treatment should then be tried for a limited term to test the patient's response.

Caution

Conventional and complementary therapies can be combined in an effective long-term treatment program. However, in high blood pressure crises involving sudden high rises in blood pressure, complementary medicine has nothing to match modern orthodox treatments.

Complementary treatments for high blood pressure

Treatment	Rating	Point of delivery/risks
Acupressure This treatment (*see* page 769), otherwise known as pressure-point massage, is used to energize (*see* page 927) the patient and to stimulate points associated with blood pressure.	**May be of some use** as a supportive treatment attempt. Case reports claim efficacy; however, success is probably seen in only a proportion of patients (*see* Placebo, page xxi).	**Suitable for DIY** Qualified guidance is recommended. Therapists should be properly qualified. **Risks:** Unlikely provided treatment is carried out competently.

Treatment	Rating	Point of delivery/risks
Acupuncture Acupuncture in its various forms (*see* page 772) aims to encourage the flow of energy (*see* page 927) or to act directly to influence blood pressure.	**May be of some use** as a supportive treatment attempt. Case reports and field studies claim efficacy; however, success is probably seen in only a proportion of patients (*see* Placebo, page xxi).	**Requires a qualified practitioner** Practitioners should be properly qualified and should propose a treatment plan. **Risks:** Probably rare provided treatment is carried out competently.
Anthroposophical medicine For prevention and as a supportive measure, AM (*see* page 781) uses constitutional therapy with measures aimed at relaxing the patient and restoring a correct rhythm, as well as a special diet and potentized gold.	**May be of some use** as a supportive treatment attempt when simpler, more established methods have been unsuccessful. Some studies claim efficacy; however, success is probably seen in only a proportion of patients (*see* Placebo, page xxi).	**Requires a qualified practitioner** Practitioners should be properly qualified and should propose a treatment plan. **Risks:** Allergies and intolerance are possible.
Aromatherapy Essential oils (*see* page 786) are used to soothe and relax, and to help improve general well-being. The essences may be taken orally, used externally as massage oils or bathing emulsions, or inhaled as vapors.	**May be of some use** as a supportive measure aimed at soothing and relaxing. Case reports claim efficacy for this procedure in the treatment of high blood pressure; however, success is probably seen in only a proportion of patients (*see* Placebo, page xxi).	**Suitable for DIY** Qualified guidance is recommended. The effects of individual essential oils differ widely. **Risks:** Allergies or intolerance are possible. Some oils are carcinogenic in test systems and possibly in humans.

Treatment	Rating	Point of delivery/risks
Bioresonance therapy Bioresonance therapists use electrical devices in an attempt to discover the causes of illness and claim to be able to weaken or turn around pathogenic energies and disease related vibrations (*see* page 794).	**Of little use** Possibly acceptable as a short-term, supportive treatment attempt when simpler, more established methods have been unsuccessful. Some case reports claim efficacy; however, success is probably seen, if at all, in only a small proportion of patients (*see* Placebo, page xxi).	**Requires a qualified practitioner** Practitioners should be properly qualified and should propose a treatment plan. No credence should be given to anyone promising immediate or total success. **Risks:** Fairly unlikely.
Cell therapy Injecting or ingesting products extracted from animal tissues or organs is said to have a rejuvenating effect and to enhance the healing of human tissues and organs (*see* page 796).	**Not advised** Based on present knowledge, there is inadequate evidence of the efficacy and mode of action of these costly and relatively risky procedures.	**Risks:** Injecting foreign proteins into the body can provoke (possibly fatal) allergic reactions. Also, pathogens such as those that cause bovine spongiform encephalopathy (BSE) or other serious infections may be introduced.
Chelation therapy The chelating agent EDTA (*see* page 800) is able, it is claimed, to cure high blood pressure by binding calcareous deposits and heavy metals in the blood vessels. These are subsequently eliminated from the body.	**Not advised** Evidence of the therapeutic usefulness of this risky procedure is lacking.	**Risks:** EDTA can cause a deficit of calcium and essential heavy metals and, in extreme cases, can lead to cardiac arrhythmia, respiratory failure, cramps, and death.

Treatment	Rating	Point of delivery/risks
Electroacupuncture according to Voll By taking readings of the electrical conductivity of the skin (*see* page 802), therapists claim to be able to derive an insight into diseased areas of the body, pathogenic foci (*see* page 928), and stress factors (*see* Toxins, page 929). The factors presumed to be instrumental in the causation of high blood pressure can then be addressed.	**Of little use** Possibly acceptable as a short-term, supportive treatment attempt when simpler, more established methods have been unsuccessful. Some case reports claim efficacy; however, success is probably seen, if at all, in only a small proportion of patients (*see* Placebo, page xxi).	**Requires a qualified practitioner** Practitioners should be properly qualified and should propose a treatment plan. No credence should be given to anyone promising immediate or total success. **Risks:** A second opinion must always be obtained from a qualified physician before any attempt is made to "eliminate foci" (e.g. by surgery).
Electroneural therapy according to Croon According to the theory, readings taken at various reactive sites on the skin highlight diseased areas within the body. Based on these readings, targeted electrostimulative measures can be undertaken to address the factors presumed to be instrumental in the causation of high blood pressure (*see* page 806).	**Of little use** Possibly acceptable as a short-term, supportive treatment attempt when simpler, more established methods have been unsuccessful. Some case reports claim efficacy; however, success is probably seen, if at all, in only a small proportion of patients (*see* Placebo, page xxi).	**Requires a qualified practitioner** Practitioners should be properly qualified and should propose a treatment plan. No credence should be given to anyone promising immediate or total success. **Risks:** Proponents themselves warn that treatment should not be given in acute inflammatory conditions.

Treatment	*Rating*	*Point of delivery/risks*
Eliminative methods, bloody Bloodletting (*see* page 810) is sometimes attempted in patients with high blood pressure. This technique is often used as part of a holistic (*see* page 928) approach rather than directly against high blood pressure.	**Of little use** Possibly acceptable as a short-term, supportive treatment attempt when more established, less invasive methods have been unsuccessful. Some case reports claim efficacy; however, success is probably seen in only a small proportion of patients (*see* Placebo, page xxi).	**Requires a qualified practitioner** Practitioners should be properly qualified and should propose a treatment plan. No credence should be given to anyone promising immediate or total success. **Risks:** Bloodletting should not be carried out in persons with bleeding disorders.
Eliminative methods, unbloody Unbloody cupping (*see* page 817) is said to energize (*see* page 927) the patient and improve the body's own regulatory systems.	**May be of some use** as a short-term, supportive treatment attempt. Some case reports claim efficacy; however, success is probably seen in only a small proportion of patients (*see* Placebo, page xxi).	**Suitable for DIY** Unbloody cupping is best carried out under the guidance of a qualified practitioner. **Risks:** Fairly unlikely provided treatment is carried out competently.
Enzyme therapy The enzymes used are said to dispel and destroy "immune complexes" (*see* page 826) that course in the blood and that are responsible, for instance, for causing arteriosclerotic changes in the body (*see* pages 824–6).	**Of little use** Some case reports claim efficacy for this little researched and relatively costly therapy; however, success is probably seen in only a small proportion of patients (*see* Placebo, page xxi).	**Requires a qualified practitioner** Practitioners should propose a treatment plan. Non-prescription preparations are suitable for do-it-yourself. **Risks:** Allergies or intolerance are possible.

Treatment	Rating	Point of delivery/risks
Flower remedies To the flower therapist high blood pressure can be an expression of psychological problems. Flower remedies (*see* page 828) are said to restore emotional balance and assist the body's psychic ability to heal itself.	**May be of some use** as a supportive treatment attempt aimed at soothing and relaxing the patient and at helping him/her come to terms better with his/her condition. Some case reports claim efficacy for this procedure in the treatment of high blood pressure; however, success is probably seen in only a proportion of patients (*see* Placebo, page xxi).	**Suitable for DIY** Qualified guidance is recommended. Therapists should propose a treatment plan. **Risks:** Possible intolerance.
Homeopathy Highly diluted (potentized) solutions (*see* page 831) are believed to be able to redress vital energy imbalances. Organo- and functiotropic (*see* page 833) homeopathy is claimed to be effective for reducing high blood pressure directly.	**May be of some use** as a supportive treatment attempt. Case studies suggest that an unknown number of patients might profit from supportive homeopathic treatments (*see* Placebo, page xxi).	**Requires a qualified practitioner** Homeopaths should be properly qualified and should propose a treatment plan. Ready-formulated preparations are suitable for do-it-yourself. **Risks:** Allergies and intolerance are possible.
Hypnosis and self-hypnosis In the relaxed and generally altered state of awareness that is induced in hypnosis or self-hypnosis (*see* page 837), physical and mental conditions can be addressed. Hypnosis is often used in combination with other psycho- and behavioral therapies.	**May be of some use** as a short-term, supportive treatment attempt when simpler, more established methods of treating high blood pressure have been unsuccessful. Case reports claim efficacy; however, success is probably seen in only a proportion of patients treated (*see* Placebo, page xxi).	**Requires a qualified practitioner** Hypnotherapists should be properly qualified and should propose a treatment plan. No credence should be given to anyone promising immediate or total success. **Risks:** Unlikely provided treatment is carried out competently.

Treatment	*Rating*	*Point of delivery/risks*
Magnetic field therapy The use of magnetic field generators, magnetic strips, bracelets, and other objects (*see* page 841) allegedly encourages cell metabolism and so alleviates symptoms.	**Of little use** Based on present knowledge, there is inadequate evidence of the efficacy and mode of action of magnetic field therapy in high blood pressure.	Operation of magnetic field equipment **requires a qualified practitioner**. **Risks:** Magnetic field equipment can cause implanted cardiac pacemakers to malfunction.
Manual therapies Chiropractors and osteopaths (*see* page 844) use a series of manipulations to realign allegedly displaced vertebrae and joints which, it is believed, irritate the nerves and may thus be co-responsible for high blood pressure.	**Of little use** Possibly acceptable as a short-term, supportive treatment attempt when less risky, more established methods of treating high blood pressure have been unsuccessful. Some case reports claim efficacy for this potentially risky procedure; however, success is probably seen, if at all, in only a small proportion of patients (*see* Placebo, page xxi).	**Requires a qualified practitioner** Practitioners should be properly qualified and should propose a treatment plan. **Risks:** Manipulation of the head and cervical vertebrae can cause serious injury. Osteoporosis is one of several risk factors.
Massage Classical massage (*see* page 847) can, it is claimed, ease muscular and emotional tension and improve general well-being.	**May be of some use** as a supportive measure aimed at relaxing the patient. Some case reports claim efficacy for this procedure in the treatment of high blood pressure; however, success is probably seen in only a proportion of patients (*see* Placebo, page xxi).	**Suitable for DIY** Qualified guidance is essential. **Risks:** Some people are sensitive to manual stimuli; others find it hard to tolerate close physical contact.

Treatment	Rating	Point of delivery/risks
Nutritional therapies An organic diet (*see* page 4) provides the body with essential and secondary plant nutrients (dietary fiber, antioxidants, etc.), which are believed to be instrumental in the prevention and treatment of high blood pressure.	**Useful** as a preventive measure and as a supportive treatment attempt aimed at lowering high blood pressure. Studies ascribe a degree of efficacy to this procedure. In addition, salt intake should be moderated; there is at present no consensus regarding maximum daily intake.	**Suitable for DIY** Qualified guidance is recommended though not essential. **Risks:** Avoid imbalanced or intolerable diets. They can cause deficiencies with serious consequences. Children are particularly at risk.
Physical therapies Exercise therapies (*see* page 868) and various hydro- and hydrothermal therapies (*see* pages 871–8) are said to improve the circulation and lower blood pressure.	**Useful** as a treatment attempt. Studies suggest that exercise therapy is efficacious. Based on present knowledge, moderate, sustained exercise (e.g. walking, running, cycling) for about 30 minutes three times a week is considered beneficial. Some case reports, field studies, and case studies claim efficacy for bathing and saunas; however, success is probably seen in only a proportion of patients (*see* Placebo, page xxi).	**Suitable for DIY** Qualified guidance is recommended though not essential. Practitioners should be properly qualified and should propose a treatment plan. **Risks:** Skin damage may be caused to persons with diminished temperature sensation when extreme temperatures are applied.

Treatment	Rating	Point of delivery/risks
Probiotics The introduction of certain bacteria into the gut is claimed to bring the intestinal flora back into balance and to have a beneficial effect on vascular reactions and arteriosclerotic processes (*see* page 878).	**Of little use** Evidence of the efficacy and mode of action of this procedure in the treatment of high blood pressure is lacking. Some case reports claim efficacy; however, success is probably seen in only a small proportion of patients (*see* Placebo, page xxi).	**Suitable for DIY** Practitioners should be properly qualified and should propose a treatment plan. Non-prescription formulations are suitable for do-it-yourself. **Risks:** Fairly unlikely provided treatment is carried out competently.
Reflex therapies Reflex zone massage (*see* page 883), reflexology (*see* page 883), and TENS (*see* page 886) are claimed to act via reflex channels (*see* page 881) to relax the patient and exert a number of physical effects, including the lowering of blood pressure.	**May be of some use** as a short-term, supportive treatment attempt. Some case reports claim efficacy for these procedures in the treatment of high blood pressure; however, success is probably seen in only a proportion of patients (*see* Placebo, page xxi).	**Requires a qualified practitioner** Practitioners should be properly qualified and should propose a treatment plan. **Risks:** Some people are sensitive to electrical stimuli and rubber electrodes; others find it hard to tolerate manual stimulation or close physical contact.
Relaxation techniques Autogenic training (*see* page 888), muscle relaxation according to Jacobson (*see* page 893), and various biofeedback techniques (*see* page 891) are able, it is claimed, to help reduce muscle tension, inner unrest, and stress.	**Useful** as a treatment attempt aimed at relaxing the patient. Case reports, field studies, and case studies claim efficacy for these procedures in the treatment of high blood pressure; however, success is probably seen in only a proportion of patients (*see* Placebo, page xxi).	**Suitable for DIY** Once a sound understanding of the technique has been acquired from a trainer, patients can perform exercises themselves. Therapists should be properly qualified. **Risks:** Fairly unlikely.

Treatment	Rating	Point of delivery/risks
Vitamins and trace elements The antioxidative properties of beta-carotene, vitamins C and E, and selenium are, it is supposed, able to exert a favorable influence on arteriosclerotic processes (*see* page 900).	**May be of some use** Studies into the relationships between beta-carotene, vitamins C and E, and arteriosclerosis produced variable results. No definitive recommendations can be made.	**Suitable for DIY** Medical supervision is recommended though not essential. **Risks:** Intolerance and overdosage are possible. Recent studies imply that beta-carotene might increase the risk of cancer.

Herbal remedies for high blood pressure

Active ingredient/preparation	Rating
Garlic corms (*Allium sativum*)	**May be of some use** as a treatment attempt for lowering slightly raised blood pressure values. **Dosage:** 4g fresh garlic corms (2–4 small cloves) or 600–1200g dried powder, or as instructed by the manufacturer/prescriber. **Risks:** Gastric complaints and asthma are possible in rare cases. External use of garlic may cause skin irritation. Consult your doctor before using garlic for this indication.
Hawthorn leaves and blossom (*Crataegus monogyna* and *Crataegus laevigata*)	**May be of some use** as a supportive treatment attempt for lowering high blood pressure. **Daily dose:** 1g herb. **Individual dose:** Pour hot water over 0.2–0.3g of herb and infuse, three to four times a day. Use ready-formulated preparations as instructed by the manufacturer/prescriber. **Risks:** Hawthorn may in some cases cause nausea, headaches and vertigo. Remedies containing hawthorn may possibly potentiate the action and thus the toxicity of digitalis. It must not be used, therefore, with cardiac tonics that contain digitalis. Hawthorn is not suitable for unsupervised self-medication.

Active ingredient/preparation	Rating

Mistletoe stem and leaves
(*Viscum album*)

Of little use. Despite traditional beliefs, mistletoe stem and leaves are not effective against high blood pressure. The same applies to their use for heart conditions, headaches, tinnitus, vertigo, irritability, forgetfulness, and blood pressure fluctuations.
Dosage: As instructed by the manufacturer/prescriber.
Risks: Allergic reactions may occur in rare cases. Severe allergies or circulatory problems may occur following an injection of mistletoe. The berries must not be used.

Rauwolfia root
(*Rauwolfia serpentina*)

May be of some use as a treatment attempt for mild essential hypertension, especially in raised excitability with sinus tachycardia (racing heart), anxiety, nervous tension, and psychomotor unrest, in cases where dietary measures have not been adequate. Rauwolfia is available by prescription only, so is not suitable for self-treatment.
Daily dose: Initially, 100–200mg powdered whole root twice daily. **Maintenance dose** 50–300mg daily depending on response; or as instructed by the manufacturer/prescriber.
Risks: Rauwolfia may cause depression, tiredness, cold symptoms, and problems of sexual potency. Even at recommended dosages, it may affect a person's ability to drive and operate machinery. Caution should be exercised by persons also taking cardiac stimulants, antipsychotic drugs, barbiturates, or levodopa. Not to be taken if the patient suffers from depression, a gastric ulcer, or disease of the adrenal medulla; nor during pregnancy or lactation.

Rhododendron leaves
(*Rhododendri folium*)

Not advised. Rhododendron leaves are not advised for treating high blood pressure because of the risk of side effects and overdosage (the plant is toxic), and because no efficacy has so far been demonstrated.

Low blood pressure (hypotension)

Causes and symptoms

Hypotension is when the blood pressure is lower than it should be. It is said to exist when the systolic (peak) pressure falls in men to below 110mm Hg (millimetres of mercury), and in women to below 100mm Hg, or when in both sexes the diastolic value (the lower pressure measured between two heartbeats) falls below 60mm Hg. These arbitrary limits are not universally recognized, however.

Hypotension may be further classified as follows:

- secondary hypotension resulting from a variety of diseases, some serious, e.g. heart failure, heart valve defects, pericarditis, myocardial infarction, hormonal disturbance, and low fluid status
- constitutional hypotension—this is not universally recognized as a valid medical condition, nor is there any precise definition; common symptoms are fainting, perspiration, giddiness, and (sometimes) depressive moods
- orthostatic hypotension, with low resting blood pressure values and frequent blackouts and giddiness upon standing upright.

Having low blood pressure can adversely affect a person's performance and *joie de vivre*.

Orthodox treatment

The principal approach will be to treat any underlying disease. For hypotension resulting from other causes, the most commonly advocated treatments include various physical therapies and regular sustained exercise. Tablets will sometimes be prescribed in an attempt to raise the person's blood pressure. However, there is no evidence that the most commonly prescribed medications have any long-term beneficial effect.

Complementary therapies

Complementary therapies are tried mostly in patients with constitutional or orthostatic hypotension. Depending on their particular approach, therapists will attempt either to remove symptoms directly, to raise the blood pressure, or to restore balance to the circulation.

Treatment plan and limited trial

Before administering a complementary treatment, every therapist should propose a treatment plan (*see* page xxiii) that sets out a clear time frame and defines the goal that the treatment is designed to achieve. Treatment should then be tried for a limited term to test the patient's response.

Caution

In low blood pressure resulting from a serious medical condition such as cardiovascular disease, the procedures used by complementary therapists are no match for modern orthodox treatments.

Complementary treatments for low blood pressure

Treatment	Rating	Point of delivery/risks
Acupressure This treatment (*see* page 769), otherwise known as pressure-point massage, is used to energize (*see* page 927) the patient and to stimulate points associated with blood pressure.	**May be of some use** as a short-term, supportive treatment attempt. Some case reports claim efficacy; however, success is probably seen in only a proportion of patients (*see* Placebo, page xxi).	**Suitable for DIY** Qualified guidance is recommended. Therapists should be properly qualified. **Risks:** Unlikely provided treatment is carried out competently.

Treatment	Rating	Point of delivery/risks
Acupuncture Acupuncture in its various forms (*see* page 772) aims to encourage the flow of energy (*see* page 927) or to act directly to influence blood pressure.	**May be of some use** as a short-term, supportive treatment attempt. Some case reports and field studies claim efficacy; however, success is probably seen in only a proportion of patients (*see* Placebo, page xxi).	**Requires a qualified practitioner** Acupuncturists should be properly qualified and should propose a treatment plan. **Risks:** Probably rare provided treatment is carried out competently.
Anthroposophical medicine As a preventive measure and a supportive therapy, AM uses constitutional therapy (*see* page 781) in association with restorative measures, curative eurhythmy, and potentized iron preparations.	**May be of some use** as a short-term, supportive treatment attempt when simpler, more established methods have been unsuccessful. Case reports claim efficacy; however, success is probably seen in only a proportion of patients (*see* Placebo, page xxi).	**Requires a qualified practitioner** Practitioners should be properly qualified and should propose a treatment plan. **Risks:** Allergies and intolerance are possible.
Aromatherapy Essential oils (*see* page 786) are used to soothe and relax, or to invigorate, thereby helping to produce an improvement in general well-being. The essences may be taken orally, used externally as massage oils or bathing emulsions, or inhaled as vapors.	**Of little use** Acceptable as a supportive measure aimed at improving general well-being. Some case reports claim efficacy; however, success is probably seen in only a proportion of patients (*see* Placebo, page xxi).	**Suitable for DIY** Qualified guidance is recommended. The effects of individual essential oils differ widely. **Risks:** Allergies or intolerance are possible. Some oils are carcinogenic in test systems and possibly in humans.

Treatment	Rating	Point of delivery/risks
Bioresonance therapy Bioresonance therapists use electrical devices in an attempt to discover the causes of illness and claim to be able to weaken or turn around pathogenic energies and disease related vibrations (*see* page 794).	**Of little use** Possibly acceptable as a short-term, supportive treatment attempt when simpler, more established methods have been unsuccessful. Some case reports claim efficacy; however, success is probably seen, if at all, in only a small proportion of patients (*see* Placebo, page xxi).	**Requires a qualified practitioner** Practitioners should be properly qualified and should propose a treatment plan. No credence should be given to anyone promising immediate or total success. **Risks:** Fairly unlikely.
Cell therapy Injecting or ingesting products extracted from animal tissues or organs is said to have a rejuvenating and invigorating effect and to enhance the healing of human tissues and organs (*see* page 796).	**Not advised** Based on present knowledge, there is inadequate evidence of the efficacy and mode of action of these costly and relatively risky procedures.	**Risks:** Injecting foreign proteins into the body can provoke (possibly fatal) allergic reactions. Also, pathogens such as those that cause bovine spongiform encephalopathy (BSE) or other serious infections may be introduced.
Chelation therapy The chelating agent EDTA (*see* page 800) is able, it is claimed, to bind calcareous deposits and heavy metals in the blood vessels. These are subsequently eliminated from the body.	**Not advised** Evidence of the therapeutic usefulness of this risky procedure is lacking.	**Risks:** EDTA can cause a deficit of calcium and essential heavy metals and, in extreme cases, can lead to cardiac arrhythmia, respiratory failure, cramps, and death.

Treatment	Rating	Point of delivery/risks
Electroacupuncture according to Voll By taking readings of the electrical conductivity of the skin (*see* page 802), therapists claim to be able to derive an insight into diseased areas of the body, pathogenic foci (*see* page 928), and stress factors (*see* Toxins, page 929). The factors presumed to be instrumental in the causation of low blood pressure can then be addressed.	**Of little use** Possibly acceptable as a short-term, supportive treatment attempt when simpler, more established methods have been unsuccessful. Some case reports claim efficacy; however, success is probably seen, if at all, in only a small proportion of patients (*see* Placebo, page xxi).	**Requires a qualified practitioner** Practitioners should be properly qualified and should propose a treatment plan. No credence should be given to anyone promising immediate or total success. **Risks:** A second opinion must always be obtained from a qualified physician before any attempt is made to "eliminate foci" (e.g. by surgery).
Electroneural therapy according to Croon According to the theory, readings taken at various reactive sites on the skin highlight diseased areas within the body. Based on these readings, targeted electrostimulative measures can be undertaken to address the factors presumed to be instrumental in the causation of low blood pressure (*see* page 806).	**Of little use** Possibly acceptable as a short-term, supportive treatment attempt when simpler, more established methods have been unsuccessful. Some case reports claim efficacy; however, success is probably seen, if at all, in only a small proportion of patients (*see* Placebo, page xxi).	**Requires a qualified practitioner** Practitioners should be properly qualified and should propose a treatment plan. No credence should be given to anyone promising immediate or total success. **Risks:** Proponents themselves warn that treatment should not be given in acute inflammatory conditions.

Treatment	*Rating*	*Point of delivery/risks*
Eliminative methods, bloody Bloody cupping (*see* page 815) is said to invigorate patients with low blood pressure and to help improve the body's own regulatory systems.	**Not advised** Evidence of the efficacy of this relatively invasive treatment is lacking.	**Risks:** Bloody cupping can cause infection and scarring. Furthermore, it should not be carried out in persons with bleeding disorders.
Eliminative methods, unbloody Unbloody cupping (*see* page 817) is supposed to energize (*see* page 927) patients with low blood pressure and improve the body's own regulatory systems.	**May be of some use** as a short-term, supportive treatment attempt. Some case reports claim efficacy; however, success is probably seen in only a proportion of patients (*see* Placebo, page xxi).	**Suitable for DIY** Unbloody cupping is best carried out under the guidance of a qualified practitioner. **Risks:** Unlikely provided treatment is carried out competently.
Flower remedies Flower remedies (*see* page 824) are said to restore emotional balance and assist the body's psychic ability to heal itself.	**May be of some use** as a treatment attempt aimed at helping patients come to terms emotionally with their condition. Some case reports claim efficacy for flower remedies in the treatment of low blood pressure; however, success is probably seen in only a proportion of patients (*see* Placebo, page xxi).	**Suitable for DIY** Qualified guidance is recommended. Practitioners should propose a treatment plan. **Risks:** Possible intolerance.

Treatment	Rating	Point of delivery/risks
Homeopathy Highly diluted (potentized) solutions (*see* page 831) are believed to be able to redress vital energy imbalances. Organo- and functiotropic (*see* page 833) homeopathy is claimed to be effective for treating low blood pressure.	**May be of some use** as a treatment attempt and as additional motivation for the patient to come to terms with his/her condition and to change his/her lifestyle. Case studies and reports claim efficacy for homeopathic treatments; however, success is probably seen in only a proportion of patients (*see* Placebo, page xxi).	**Requires a qualified practitioner** Homeopaths should be properly qualified and should propose a treatment plan. Ready-formulated preparations are suitable for do-it-yourself. **Risks:** Allergies and intolerance are possible.
Hypnosis and self-hypnosis In the relaxed and generally altered state of awareness that is induced in hypnosis or self-hypnosis (*see* page 837), physical and mental conditions can be addressed. Hypnosis is often used in combination with other psycho- and behavioral therapies.	**Of little use** Acceptable as a short-term, supportive treatment attempt when simpler methods of raising blood pressure have been unsuccessful. Case reports claim efficacy in the treatment of low blood pressure; however, success is probably seen in only a proportion of patients treated (*see* Placebo, page xxi).	**Requires a qualified practitioner** Hypnotherapists should be properly qualified and should propose a treatment plan. **Risks:** Unlikely provided treatment is carried out competently.
Magnetic field therapy The use of magnetic field generators, magnetic strips, bracelets, and other objects (*see* page 841) is allegedly able to encourage cell metabolism and so raise blood pressure.	**Of little use** Based on present knowledge, there is inadequate evidence of the efficacy and mode of action of magnetic field therapy in low blood pressure.	Operation of magnetic field equipment **requires a qualified practitioner**. **Risks:** Magnetic field equipment can cause implanted cardiac pacemakers to malfunction.

Treatment	Rating	Point of delivery/risks
Manual therapies Chiropractors and osteopaths (*see* page 844) use a series of manipulations to realign allegedly displaced vertebrae and joints which, it is believed, irritate the nerves and may thus be co-responsible for low blood pressure.	**Of little use** Possibly acceptable as a short-term, supportive treatment attempt when less risky, more established methods of treating high blood pressure have been unsuccessful. Some case reports claim efficacy for this potentially risky procedure; however, success is probably seen, if at all, in only a small proportion of patients (*see* Placebo, page xxi).	**Requires a qualified practitioner** Practitioners should be properly qualified and should propose a treatment plan. **Risks:** Manipulation of the head and cervical vertebrae can cause serious injury. Osteoporosis is one of several risk factors.
Massage Classical massage (*see* page 847) is said to have a relaxing and restorative effect. Ice massage (*see* page 878) is claimed to improve a number of physical functions, to invigorate the patient, and to raise his/her blood pressure.	**Useful** as a supportive treatment attempt. Case reports claim efficacy in the treatment of low blood pressure; however, success is probably seen in only a small proportion of patients (*see* Placebo, page xxi).	**Suitable for DIY** Qualified guidance is essential. Masseurs/masseuses should be properly qualified. **Risks:** Some people are sensitive to manual stimuli; others find it hard to tolerate close physical contact.
Nutritional therapies An organic diet (*see* page 4) provides the body with essential and secondary plant nutrients, dietary fiber, antioxidants, etc., which are believed to exercise a multitude of positive effects and to be capable, *inter alia*, of giving the patient more energy.	**Useful** as an individually directed supportive measure.	**Suitable for DIY** Qualified guidance is recommended though not essential. **Risks:** Avoid imbalanced or intolerable diets. They can cause deficiencies with serious consequences. Children are particularly at risk.

Treatment	Rating	Point of delivery/risks

Physical therapies
Exercise therapy (*see* page 868) and various forms of hydrotherapy (*see* pages 871–8), saunas, and climatic cures are able, it is claimed, to improve the circulation and raise blood pressure. These procedures are often used in combination.

Useful as a treatment attempt. These therapies can differ widely in their effects. Case reports, case studies, and field studies claim efficacy; however, success is probably seen in only a proportion of patients (*see* Placebo, page xxi).

Suitable for DIY
Qualified guidance is recommended though not essential. Therapists should propose a treatment plan.
Risks: Skin damage may be caused to persons with diminished temperature sensation when extreme temperatures are applied.

Probiotics
The introduction of certain bacteria into the gut is claimed to bring the intestinal flora back into balance and to have a beneficial effect on vascular reactions and blood pressure (*see* page 878).

Of little use
Possibly acceptable as a short-term, supportive treatment attempt when more established methods have been unsuccessful. Case reports claim efficacy; however, success is probably seen in only a proportion of patients (*see* Placebo, page xxi).

Requires a qualified practitioner
Practitioners should be properly qualified and should propose a treatment plan. Non-prescription formulations are suitable for do-it-yourself.
Risks: Fairly unlikely provided treatment is carried out competently.

Reflex therapies
Reflex zone massage (*see* page 883), reflexology (*see* page 883), TENS (*see* page 886), cooling sprays, and electroacupuncture are claimed to act via reflex channels (*see* page 881) to improve a number of physical functions, to invigorate the patient, and to raise his/her blood pressure.

May be of some use as a short-term, supportive treatment attempt. These therapies can differ widely in their effects. Some case reports claim efficacy; however, success is probably seen in only a proportion of patients (*see* Placebo, page xxi).

Suitable for DIY
Qualified guidance is essential. Therapists should propose a treatment plan.
Risks: Some people are sensitive to electrical stimuli and rubber electrodes; others find it hard to tolerate manual stimulation or close physical contact.

Treatment	Rating	Point of delivery/risks
Relaxation techniques Autogenic training (*see* page 888), muscle relaxation according to Jacobson (*see* page 893), and various biofeedback techniques (*see* page 891) are said to relax the patient physically and emotionally and to have a beneficial effect on low blood pressure.	**May be of some use** as a supportive treatment attempt aimed at providing physical and emotional relaxation. Some case reports claim efficacy for these treatments in raising blood pressure; however, success is probably seen in only a proportion of patients (*see* Placebo, page xxi).	**Suitable for DIY** Once a sound understanding of the technique has been acquired from a trainer in group sessions or through individual tuition, patients can perform exercises themselves. Therapists should propose a treatment plan. **Risks:** Fairly unlikely.
Vitamins and trace elements The antioxidative properties of beta-carotene and vitamins C and E are, it is supposed, instrumental in reducing the formation of free radicals and individual lipids, thereby exercising a generally restorative function (*see* page 900).	**Useful** in vitamin deficiency. **May be of some use** as a supportive treatment attempt aimed at generally strengthening the system. No definitive recommendations can be given based on present knowledge.	**Suitable for DIY** Qualified guidance is recommended though not essential. **Risks:** Intolerance and overdosage are possible. Recent studies imply that beta-carotene might increase the risk of cancer.

Herbal remedies for low blood pressure

Active ingredient/preparation	Rating
Caffeine from coffee beans, kola nuts, or leaf tea	**Only useful** as a short-term attempt to raise blood pressure. Its action is only weak. **Daily dose:** maximum 0.6g. **Individual dose:** 0.1g on average (the amount contained in a large cup of coffee). **Risks:** Sleeplessness, inner unrest, tachycardia, and gastrointestinal problems are possible.

Active ingredient/preparation	Rating

Camphor
(*Cinnamomum camphora*)

Only useful as "smelling salts" in cardiovascular conditions such as low blood pressure.
Dosage: For external application or as "smelling salts", use in a maximum 11 percent alcoholic solution.
Risks: Camphor can cause contact eczema. Do not use on damaged skin. Do not apply to the nose and face of infants and young children, as collapse has occurred.

Ephedra
(*Ephedra sinica*)

Of little use. The active constituent, ephedrin, may have a transitory anti-hypotensive action. In animal experiments ephedrin has been shown to be an effective antitussive.
Dosage: As instructed by the manufacturer/prescriber.
Risks: Sleeplessness, nausea, vomiting, problems with micturition, cardiac arrhythmia, and dependence at high dosages. Ephedra is controlled under the Medicines Act 1968 in the UK. It must not be used by persons with high blood pressure, anxiety or unrest, glaucoma, circulatory problems, a prostate adenoma with formation of residual urine in the bladder, an adrenomedulla tumor, or an overactive thyroid.

Hawthorn leaves and blossom
(*Crataegus monogyna* and *Crataegus laevigata*)

May be of some use as a supportive treatment attempt for low blood pressure.
Daily dose: 1g herb. **Individual dose:** Pour hot water over 0.2–0.3g of herb and infuse, three to four times a day. Use ready-formulated preparations as instructed by the manufacturer/prescriber.
Risks: Remedies containing hawthorn may possibly potentiate the effect and thus the toxicity of digitalis. It must not be used, therefore, with cardiac tonics that contain digitalis. Hawthorn is not suitable for self-medication.

Active ingredient/preparation	Rating
Lavender flowers (*Lavandula angustifolia*)	**May be of some use** as a supportive treatment attempt for low blood pressure or as a bath to assist the blood circulation. **Dosage:** 20–100g herb to 20 litres of bathwater, then made up to a full immersion bath. **Risks:** Lavender flowers are not known to have any serious side effects.
Rosemary leaves (*Rosmarinus officinalis*)	**May be of some use** as a supportive treatment attempt for poor circulation and low blood pressure (as an addition to bathwater or an embrocation). Acts as a skin and circulatory stimulant. **Dosage:** 10–20 drops of essential oil or 50–100g of herb to a full immersion bath. **Risks:** Large amounts of rosemary oil may inflame the lining of the gut and the kidneys. Preparations containing rosemary (including teas) should not be taken during pregnancy. Rosemary oil may cause skin reactions in hypersensitive individuals.

Cardiac arrhythmia

Causes and symptoms

Situated in the right auricle of the heart are so-called sino-atrial nodes that give the heart muscle the instruction to pump—about 70 times a minute at precisely defined intervals. Doctors talk of cardiac arrhythmia when the normal rhythm of heartbeats is disturbed.

Arrhythmias can have a number of causes, including psychological problems, stress, excessive alcohol, coffee or nicotine, and certain drugs. In addition, cardiac arrhythmia can be a symptom of cardiovascular disease or of some other serious disease. The most common forms of arrhythmia are occasional extra heartbeats (extrasystoles) and atrial flutter, when the atrial contractions are regular but too frequent.

Orthodox treatment

Any disease that is causing the arrhythmia will need to be treated. As cardiac arrhythmia may have a significant psychological cause, relaxation exercises, psychotherapy, and counselling will generally be advised. In many cases a pacemaker, an artificial device to control the heartbeat, can be the solution.

Complementary therapies

Various complementary procedures are used in the belief that patients with cardiac arrhythmia can be relaxed or that energy links (*see* page 928) can be used to influence the action of the heart directly. Often, symptoms are interpreted as pointing to a constitutional problem (*see* Constitution, page 927) or to a deficient flow of vital energy (*see* Life force, page 928).

Treatment plan and limited trial

Before administering a complementary treatment, every therapist should propose a treatment plan (*see* page xxiii) that sets out a clear time frame and defines the goal that the treatment is designed to achieve. Treatment should then be tried for a limited term to test the patient's response.

Cautions

Before starting any treatment, the patient should consult a qualified physician to discover whether the rhythm disturbance has a medically treatable cause. Cardiac arrhythmias can be life threatening.

Complementary procedures are no substitute for a proper diagnosis and treatment by a mainstream doctor.

Complementary treatments for cardiac arrhythmia

Treatment	Rating	Point of delivery/risks
Acupressure This treatment (*see* page 769), otherwise known as pressure-point massage, is claimed to reduce atrial tachycardia when pressure is applied to the appropriate points. The pressure points chosen may differ from one practitioner to another.	**Of little use** Acceptable as a short-term treatment attempt for atrial tachycardia. Some case reports claim efficacy; however, success is probably seen in only a proportion of patients (*see* Placebo, page xxi). This treatment is no substitute for a visit to your doctor.	**Suitable for DIY** Qualified guidance is recommended. Therapists should be properly qualified. **Risks:** Unlikely provided treatment is carried out competently.
Acupuncture Acupuncture in its various forms (*see* page 772) aims to encourage the flow of energy (*see* page 927) or to act directly to reduce atrial tachycardia. The acupuncture points chosen can vary from one practitioner to another.	**Of little use** Acceptable as a short-term treatment attempt for atrial tachycardia. Some case reports claim efficacy; however, success is probably seen in only a small proportion of patients (*see* Placebo, page xxi).	**Requires a qualified practitioner** Practitioners should be properly qualified and should propose a treatment plan. **Risks:** Probably rare provided treatment is carried out competently.
Anthroposophical medicine Doctors who practice AM (*see* page 781) look for the causes of arrhythmia and treat these through constitutional therapy. The composition Cardiodoron is one of the principal preparations used.	**May be of some use** as a short-term treatment attempt. Case studies claim efficacy; however, success is probably seen in only a proportion of patients (*see* Placebo, page xxi).	**Requires a qualified practitioner** Practitioners should be properly qualified and should propose a treatment plan. **Risks:** Allergies and intolerance are possible.

Treatment	Rating	Point of delivery/risks
Aromatherapy Essential oils (*see* page 786) are used to soothe and relax, or to invigorate, so contributing to an easing of symptoms. The essences may be taken orally, used externally as massage oils or bathing emulsions, or inhaled as vapors.	**Of little use** Acceptable as a short-term, supportive treatment attempt aimed at soothing and relaxing patients with atrial tachycardia. Case reports claim efficacy; however, success is probably seen in only a small proportion of patients (*see* Placebo, page xxi).	**Suitable for DIY** Qualified guidance is recommended. The effects of individual essential oils differ widely. **Risks:** Allergies or intolerance are possible. Some oils are carcinogenic in test systems and possibly in humans.
Bioresonance therapy Bioresonance therapists use electrical devices in an attempt to discover the causes of illness and claim to be able to weaken or turn around pathogenic energies and disease related vibrations (*see* page 794).	**Of little use** Possibly acceptable as a short-term, supportive treatment attempt when simpler, more established methods have been unsuccessful. Some case reports claim efficacy; however, success is probably seen, if at all, in only a small proportion of patients (*see* Placebo, page xxi).	**Requires a qualified practitioner** Practitioners should be properly qualified and should propose a treatment plan. No credence should be given to anyone promising immediate or total success. **Risks:** Fairly unlikely.
Cell therapy Injecting or ingesting products extracted from the tissues of newborn animals or animal fetuses is said to have a rejuvenating and revitalizing effect and to enhance the healing of human tissues and organs (*see* page 796).	**Not advised** Based on present knowledge, there is inadequate evidence of the efficacy and mode of action of these costly and relatively risky procedures.	**Risks:** Injecting foreign proteins into the body can provoke (possibly fatal) allergic reactions. Also, pathogens such as those that cause bovine spongiform encephalopathy (BSE) or other serious infections may be introduced.

Treatment	Rating	Point of delivery/risks
Chelation therapy The chelating agent EDTA (*see* page 800) is able, it is claimed, to bind calcareous deposits in the blood vessels. These are subsequently eliminated from the body, so that arteriosclerotic disease can, according to the theory, be reversed.	**Not advised** Evidence of the therapeutic usefulness of this risky procedure is lacking.	**Risks:** EDTA can cause a deficit of calcium and essential heavy metals and, in extreme cases, can lead to cardiac arrhythmia, respiratory failure, cramps, and death.
Electroacupuncture according to Voll By taking readings of the electrical conductivity of the skin (*see* page 802), therapists claim to be able to derive an insight into diseased areas of the body, pathogenic foci (*see* page 928), and stress factors (*see* Toxins, page 929). The factors presumed to be instrumental in the causation of cardiac arrhythmia can then be addressed.	**Of little use** Possibly acceptable as a short-term, supportive treatment attempt when simpler, more established methods have been unsuccessful. Some case reports claim efficacy; however, success is probably seen, if at all, in only a small proportion of patients (*see* Placebo, page xxi).	**Requires a qualified practitioner** Practitioners should be properly qualified and should propose a treatment plan. No credence should be given to anyone promising immediate or total success. **Risks:** A second opinion must always be obtained from a qualified physician before any attempt is made to "eliminate foci" (e.g. by surgery).

Treatment	Rating	Point of delivery/risks
Electroneural therapy according to Croon According to the theory, readings taken at various reactive sites on the skin highlight diseased areas within the body. Based on these readings, targeted electrostimulative measures can be undertaken to address the factors presumed to be instrumental in the causation of cardiac arrhythmia (*see* page 806).	**Of little use** Possibly acceptable as a short-term, supportive treatment attempt when simpler, more established methods have been unsuccessful. Some case reports claim efficacy; however, success is probably seen, if at all, in only a small proportion of patients (*see* Placebo, page xxi).	**Requires a qualified practitioner** Practitioners should be properly qualified and should propose a treatment plan. No credence should be given to anyone promising immediate or total success. **Risks:** Proponents themselves warn that treatment should not be given in acute inflammatory conditions.
Eliminative methods, bloody Bloody cupping (*see* page 815) is said to alleviate pain, to improve the body's own regulatory systems, and to ease symptoms.	**Not advised** Proof of the efficacy and mode of action of this invasive and sometimes risky procedure is lacking.	**Risks:** Bloody cupping can cause infection and scarring. Furthermore, it should not be carried out in persons with bleeding disorders.
Eliminative methods, unbloody Unbloody cupping (*see* page 817) is supposed to soothe and energize (*see* page 927) patients with cardiac arrhythmia, to ease symptoms, and to improve the body's own regulatory systems.	**Of little use** Acceptable as a short-term, supportive treatment attempt aimed at alleviating persistent symptoms. Some case reports claim efficacy; however, success is probably seen in only a proportion of patients (*see* Placebo, page xxi).	**Requires a qualified practitioner** Practitioners should be properly qualified and should propose a treatment plan. **Risks:** Unlikely provided treatment is carried out competently.

Treatment	*Rating*	*Point of delivery/risks*
Enzyme therapy The enzymes used (*see* page 824) are said, *inter alia*, to have a beneficial effect on the blood vessels.	**Of little use** Some case reports claim efficacy for this little researched therapy; however, success is probably seen in only a small proportion of patients (*see* Placebo, page xxi).	**Requires a qualified practitioner** Practitioners should propose a treatment plan. Non-prescription preparations are suitable for do-it-yourself. **Risks:** Allergies or intolerance are possible.
Flower remedies Flower remedies (*see* page 828) are said to restore emotional balance and assist the body's psychic ability to heal itself.	**Of little use** Acceptable as a short-term, supportive treatment attempt aimed at soothing and relaxing. Some case reports claim efficacy; however, success is probably seen in only a small proportion of patients (*see* Placebo, page xxi).	**Suitable for DIY** Qualified guidance is recommended. Practitioners should propose a treatment plan. **Risks:** Possible intolerance.
Homeopathy Highly diluted (potentized) solutions (*see* page 831) are believed to be able to redress vital energy imbalances. Organo- and functiotropic (*see* page 833) homeopathy is claimed to be effective for dealing with cardiac arrhythmia.	**Of little use** Acceptable as a supportive treatment attempt. Case reports claim efficacy; however, success is probably seen in only a proportion of patients (*see* Placebo, page xxi).	**Requires a qualified practitioner** Homeopaths should be properly qualified and should propose a treatment plan. Ready-formulated preparations are suitable for do-it-yourself. **Risks:** Allergies and intolerance are possible.

Treatment	Rating	Point of delivery/risks
Hypnosis and self-hypnosis In the relaxed and generally altered state of awareness that is induced in hypnosis or self-hypnosis (*see* page 837), physical and mental conditions can be addressed.	**Of little use** Acceptable as a short-term, supportive treatment attempt for paroxysmal atrial tachycardia when more established methods have been unsuccessful. Some case reports claim efficacy; however, success is probably seen in only a proportion of patients treated (*see* Placebo, page xxi).	**Requires a qualified practitioner** Hypnotherapists should be properly qualified and should propose a treatment plan. **Risks:** Unlikely provided treatment is carried out competently.
Magnetic field therapy The use of magnetic field generators, magnetic strips, bracelets, and other objects (*see* page 841) allegedly eases symptoms.	**Inappropriate** Based on present knowledge, there is inadequate evidence of the efficacy and mode of action of magnetic field therapy in cardiac arrhythmia.	Operation of magnetic field equipment **requires a qualified practitioner**. **Risks:** Magnetic field equipment can cause implanted cardiac pacemakers to malfunction.
Manual therapies Chiropractors and osteopaths (*see* page 844) use a series of manipulations to realign allegedly displaced vertebrae. This is said to release energy blockages (*see* page 927) and address factors that may be at the root of cardiac arrhythmia.	**Of little use** Possibly acceptable as a short-term, supportive treatment attempt when less risky, more established methods have been unsuccessful. Some case reports claim efficacy for these potentially risky procedures; however, success is probably seen, if at all, in only a small proportion of patients (*see* Placebo, page xxi).	**Requires a qualified practitioner** Practitioners should be properly qualified and should propose a treatment plan. **Risks:** Manipulation of the head and cervical vertebrae can cause serious injury. Osteoporosis is one of several risk factors.

Treatment	Rating	Point of delivery/risks
Massage Classical massage (*see* page 847) can soothe the patient, as well as ease muscular and emotional tension.	**May be of some use** as a short-term, supportive treatment and as a means of relaxing the patient. Case reports claim efficacy; however, success is probably seen in only a proportion of patients (*see* Placebo, page xxi).	**Suitable for DIY** Qualified guidance is recommended. Masseurs/masseuses should be properly qualified. **Risks:** Some people are sensitive to manual stimuli; others find it hard to tolerate close physical contact.
Nutritional therapies An organic diet (*see* page 4) provides the body with essential and secondary plant nutrients, dietary fiber, antioxidants, etc., which are believed to exercise a multitude of positive effects.	**Useful** as an individually directed preventive measure in persons with obesity, metabolic disorders, diabetes, or vascular disease. Case reports claim efficacy in the treatment of cardiac arrhythmia; however, success is probably seen in only a small proportion of patients (*see* Placebo, page xxi).	**Suitable for DIY** Qualified guidance is recommended though not essential. **Risks:** Avoid imbalanced or intolerable diets. They can cause deficiencies with serious consequences. Children are particularly at risk.
Physical therapies Cold washings, cold compresses applied to the neck, cold thyroid wraps (*see* pages 871–8), breathing exercises, and exercise therapy (*see* page 868) are supposed to relax and invigorate the patient and ease symptoms.	**Useful** as a short-term treatment attempt for tachycardia. Some case reports and field studies claim efficacy; however, success is probably seen in only a proportion of patients (*see* Placebo, page xxi).	**Suitable for DIY** Qualified guidance is recommended. **Risks:** Skin damage may be caused to persons with diminished temperature sensation when extreme temperatures are applied.

Treatment	Rating	Point of delivery/risks
Reflex therapies Reflex zone massage (*see* page 883), reflexology (*see* page 883), and TENS (*see* page 886) are claimed to act via reflex channels (*see* page 881) to soothe and relax, or to invigorate.	**Of little use** Acceptable as a short-term treatment attempt for tachycardia. Case reports and field studies claim efficacy; however, success is probably seen in only a proportion of patients (*see* Placebo, page xxi).	**Suitable for DIY** Qualified guidance is essential. **Risks:** Some people are sensitive to electrical stimuli and rubber electrodes; others find it hard to tolerate manual stimulation or close physical contact.
Relaxation techniques Autogenic training (*see* page 888), muscle relaxation according to Jacobson (*see* page 893), and various biofeedback techniques (*see* page 891) are said to relieve tension and inner unrest, and so might be instrumental in helping the patient change his/her lifestyle.	**Useful** as a supportive treatment attempt aimed at relaxing the patient. Some case reports claim efficacy; however, success is probably seen in only a proportion of patients (*see* Placebo, page xxi).	**Suitable for DIY** Once a sound understanding of the technique has been acquired from a trainer, patients can perform exercises themselves. Therapists should propose a treatment plan. **Risks:** Fairly unlikely.
Vitamins and trace elements The antioxidative properties of beta-carotene, vitamins C and E, and selenium are, it is supposed, instrumental in countering the formation of free radicals and in boosting the body's antioxidative defence systems (*see* page 900).	**Of little use** No definitive dosage recommendations can be made based on present knowledge, as they vary widely and are probably set to rise. Slightly higher intake is probably beneficial to the elderly.	**Suitable for DIY** Qualified guidance is recommended though not essential. **Risks:** Intolerance and overdosage are possible. Recent studies imply that beta-carotene might increase the risk of cancer.

Herbal remedies for cardiac arrhythmia

There are no recommended herbal remedies for use in this indication.

Heart attack

Causes and symptoms

A lowering of coronary perfusion below a critical cut-off deprives the heart muscle of oxygen, leading to pain or permanent, irreversible damage. We speak of a myocardial infarction (MI) when the heart muscle cells actually die. The most common cause of MI is arteriosclerosis, a thickening of the arterial walls, with acute blockage usually being caused by a clot, or thrombus, that develops at an already constricted site. Smoking (*see* page 66), high blood pressure (*see* page 431), diabetes (*see* page 627), a surfeit of LDL cholesterol in the blood, gout (*see* page 180) and also—it is assumed—obesity (*see* page 6), stress, and other emotional factors all increase the infarction risk.

There are various ways to guard against heart attack. The most important of these are: stopping smoking, normalizing weight, reducing the LDL component of blood fats, obtaining treatment for high blood pressure, regular sustained exercise, and stress reduction.

Orthodox treatment

Attempts will be made in the first hour after a heart attack to dissolve (lyse) the blood clot that is blocking the artery, using drugs. Heparin, an anticoagulant, will be given to persons confined to bed for long periods, to prevent a pulmonary embolism.

After being hospitalized, heart-attack patients will often receive rehabilitation treatment, in order to increase their physical performance.

Depending on the state of the coronary arteries, life expectancy may be raised by a bypass operation.

One frequently recommended method of preventing further heart attacks is to take a low daily dose of aspirin (e.g. 100mg), though this may cause gastric irritation. There is disagreement as to the benefit of taking other anticoagulant drugs, which can provoke hemorrhaging. Controlled clinical studies show that beta-blockers can increase the life expectancy of infarction patients.

Complementary therapies

Apart from nutritional and some physical therapies that are also used by mainstream medicine to treat heart attack patients, complementary methods have at most a supportive role in relieving pain or stress following an attack. Present findings show there to be no satisfactory alternative to orthodox diagnosis and treatment.

Treatment plan and limited trial

Before administering a complementary treatment, every therapist should propose a treatment plan (*see* page xxiii) that sets out a clear time frame and defines the goal that the treatment is designed to achieve. Treatment should then be tried for a limited term to test the patient's response.

Caution

Patients contemplating receiving only a complementary therapy for heart attack are exposing themselves to an unacceptably high risk and will almost certainly miss out on life-saving orthodox treatment.

Complementary treatments following a heart attack

Treatment	Rating	Point of delivery/risks
Acupressure This treatment (*see* page 769), otherwise known as pressure-point massage, is claimed to stimulate and activate patients and to reduce pain and depression. Some of the proponents of acupressure see it as an energizing (*see* page 927) treatment.	**May be of some use** as a short-term, supportive treatment attempt aimed at reducing pain and depression and at stimulating and activating the patient. Some case reports claim efficacy; however, success is probably seen in only a proportion of patients (*see* Placebo, page xxi).	**Suitable for DIY** Qualified guidance is recommended. Therapists should be properly qualified. **Risks:** Unlikely provided treatment is carried out competently.

Treatment	Rating	Point of delivery/risks
Acupuncture Acupuncture in its various forms (*see* page 772) aims to stimulate and activate patients following a heart attack and to reduce pain and depression. The acupuncture points chosen can vary from one practitioner to another.	**May be of some use** as a short-term, supportive treatment attempt aimed at alleviating pain and depression and stimulating and activating the patient. Case reports claim efficacy; however, success is probably seen in only a proportion of patients (*see* Placebo, page xxi).	**Requires a qualified practitioner** Practitioners should be properly qualified and should propose a treatment plan. Acupuncture should not be carried out on patients on oral anticoagulants. **Risks:** Probably rare provided treatment is carried out competently.
Anthroposophical medicine Measures used following a heart attack include rhythmic massage, curative eurhythmy, and various compositions to speed up rehabilitation (*see* page 781).	**May be of some use** as a supportive measure. Some case reports claim efficacy; however, success is probably seen in only a proportion of patients (*see* Placebo, page xxi).	**Requires a qualified practitioner** Practitioners should be properly qualified and should propose a treatment plan. **Risks:** Allergies and intolerance are possible.
Aromatherapy Essential oils (*see* page 786) are said to have a relaxing or invigorating effect. The essences may be taken orally, used externally as massage oils or bathing emulsions, or inhaled as vapors.	**May be of some use** as a supportive measure aimed at relaxing the patient and improving his/her general well-being. Some case reports claim efficacy; however, success is probably seen in only a proportion of patients (*see* Placebo, page xxi).	**Suitable for DIY** Qualified guidance is recommended. The effects of individual essential oils differ widely. **Risks:** Allergies or intolerance are possible. Some oils are carcinogenic in test systems and possibly in humans.

Treatment	Rating	Point of delivery/risks
Bioresonance therapy Bioresonance therapists use electrical devices in an attempt to discover the causes of illness and claim to be able to weaken or turn around pathogenic energies and disease related vibrations (*see* page 794).	**Of little use** There is little evidence of the efficacy of this relatively involved procedure.	**Requires a qualified practitioner** Practitioners should be properly qualified and should propose a treatment plan. No credence should be given to anyone promising immediate or total success. **Risks:** Fairly unlikely.
Cell therapy Products extracted from the tissues or organs of animals are said to have a rejuvenating effect and to enhance the healing of human tissues and organs (*see* page 796).	**Not advised** Based on present knowledge, there is inadequate evidence of the efficacy and mode of action of these costly and relatively risky procedures.	**Risks:** Injecting foreign proteins into the body can provoke (possibly fatal) allergic reactions. Also, pathogens such as those that cause bovine spongiform encephalopathy (BSE) or other serious infections may be introduced.
Chelation therapy The chelating agent EDTA (*see* page 800) is able, it is claimed, to bind calcareous deposits in the blood vessels. These are subsequently eliminated from the body, so that arteriosclerotic disease and its sequelae can, it is claimed, be prevented.	**Not advised** Evidence of the efficacy of this risky procedure is lacking.	**Risks:** EDTA can cause a deficit of calcium and essential heavy metals and, in extreme cases, can lead to cardiac arrhythmia, respiratory failure, cramps, and death.

Treatment	Rating	Point of delivery/risks
Electroacupuncture according to Voll By taking readings of the electrical conductivity of the skin, therapists claim to be able to address factors presumed to be associated with infarction (*see* page 802).	**Of little use** Evidence of the efficacy of this relatively involved procedure is lacking.	**Requires a qualified practitioner** Practitioners should be properly qualified and should propose a treatment plan. No credence should be given to anyone promising immediate or total success. **Risks:** A second opinion must always be obtained from a qualified physician before any attempt is made to "eliminate foci" (e.g. by surgery).
Electroneural therapy according to Croon According to the theory, readings taken at various reactive sites on the skin enable measures to be taken against factors associated with infarction (*see* page 806).	**Of little use** Evidence of the efficacy of this relatively involved procedure is lacking.	**Requires a qualified practitioner** Practitioners should be properly qualified and should propose a treatment plan. No credence should be given to anyone promising immediate or total success. **Risks:** Proponents themselves warn that treatment should not be given in acute inflammatory conditions.
Eliminative methods, bloody Bloody cupping (*see* page 815) is said to have a restorative effect following heart attack, to improve the body's own regulatory systems, and to release energy blockages (*see* page 927).	**Not advised** Evidence of the efficacy of this invasive and relatively risky procedure is lacking.	**Risks:** Bloody cupping can cause infection and scarring. Furthermore, it should not be carried out on persons with bleeding disorders, nor on patients on oral anticoagulants.

Treatment	Rating	Point of delivery/risks
Eliminative methods, unbloody Unbloody cupping (*see* page 817) is used following heart attack with the aim of stimulating and activating patients and reducing pain and depression.	**May be of some use** as a short-term, supportive treatment attempt aimed at reducing pain and depression. Some case reports claim efficacy; however, success is probably seen in only a proportion of patients (*see* Placebo, page xxi).	**Suitable for DIY** Unbloody cupping is best carried out under the guidance of a qualified practitioner. **Risks:** This treatment should not be carried out on patients on oral anticoaguants.
Enzyme therapy Enzymes (*see* page 824) obtained from plant or animal tissues are claimed to have a restorative effect following heart attack, as well as an anti-inflammatory and immune system modulating effect (*see* page 10). They are also said to hasten recovery.	**Of little use** Some case reports claim efficacy for this little researched therapy; however, success is probably seen in only a small proportion of patients (*see* Placebo, page xxi).	**Requires a qualified practitioner** Practitioners should propose a treatment plan. Non-prescription preparations are suitable for do-it-yourself. **Risks:** Allergies or intolerance are possible.
Flower remedies Flower remedies (*see* page 828) are said to restore emotional balance and assist the body's psychic ability to heal itself.	**May be of some use** as a short-term, supportive treatment attempt aimed at relieving anxiety and feelings of hopelessness. Some case reports claim efficacy; however, success is probably seen in only a proportion of patients (*see* Placebo, page xxi).	**Requires a qualified practitioner** Qualified guidance is recommended. Practitioners should propose a treatment plan. **Risks:** Possible intolerance.

Treatment	Rating	Point of delivery/risks
Homeopathy Highly diluted (potentized) solutions (*see* page 831) are believed to be able to redress vital energy imbalances and strengthen the body's defences. Organo- and functiotropic (*see* page 833) homeopathy is claimed to be effective for dealing with symptoms.	**Of little use** Acceptable as a supportive measure and as an additional motivation for the person to come to terms better with his/her condition. Some case reports claim success for homeopathic treatments; however, success is probably seen in only a proportion of patients (*see* Placebo, page xxi).	**Requires a qualified practitioner** Homeopaths should be properly qualified and should propose a treatment plan. Ready-formulated preparations are suitable for do-it-yourself. **Risks:** Allergies and intolerance are possible.
Hypnosis and self-hypnosis In the relaxed and generally altered state of awareness that is induced in hypnosis or self-hypnosis (*see* page 837), anxiety can be reduced and the patient can be helped to come to terms better with his/her condition. These treatments are frequently used in combination with psycho- or behavioral therapy.	**Of little use** Acceptable as a short-term, supportive treatment attempt aimed at relieving anxiety and helping the patient come to terms better with his/her condition and to bring about a change of lifestyle. Some case reports claim efficacy; however, success is probably seen in only a proportion of patients (*see* Placebo, page xxi).	**Requires a qualified practitioner** Hypnotherapists should be properly qualified and should propose a treatment plan. **Risks:** Unlikely provided treatment is carried out competently.
Magnetic field therapy The use of magnetic field generators, magnetic strips, bracelets, and other objects (*see* page 841) allegedly encourages cell metabolism.	**Inappropriate** Based on present knowledge, there is inadequate evidence of the efficacy and mode of action of magnetic field therapy following heart attack.	Operation of magnetic field equipment **requires a qualified practitioner**. **Risks:** Magnetic field equipment can cause implanted cardiac pacemakers to malfunction.

Treatment	Rating	Point of delivery/risks
Manual therapies Chiropractors and osteopaths use a series of manipulations to realign allegedly displaced vertebrae. This is said to release energy blockages (*see* page 927), ease pain, improve the body's own regulatory systems, and hasten recovery (*see* page 844).	**Of little use** Possibly acceptable as a short-term, supportive treatment attempt aimed at alleviating tension and pain in the skeletomuscular system. Case reports claim efficacy; however, success is probably seen, if at all, in only a proportion of patients (*see* Placebo, page xxi).	**Requires a qualified practitioner** Practitioners should be properly qualified and should propose a treatment plan. **Risks:** Manipulation of the head and cervical vertebrae can cause serious injury. Osteoporosis is one of several risk factors.
Massage Classical massage (*see* page 847) is claimed to invigorate the patient, relieve muscular and emotional tension, and ease pain.	**Useful** as a short-term treatment attempt aimed at relaxing the patient and easing muscular pain. Some case reports claim efficacy; however, success is probably seen in only a proportion of patients (*see* Placebo, page xxi).	**Suitable for DIY** Qualified guidance is recommended. **Risks:** Some people are sensitive to manual stimuli; others find it hard to tolerate close physical contact.
Nutritional therapies An organic diet (*see* page 4) can influence possible risk factors, such as obesity and blood fat levels, as well as improve general performance and well-being.	**Useful** as an individually directed supportive and preventive measure. Controlled studies suggest that this procedure is clearly efficacious in the prevention of heart attack.	**Suitable for DIY** Qualified guidance is recommended though not essential. **Risks:** Avoid imbalanced or intolerable diets. They can cause deficiencies with serious consequences.

Treatment	Rating	Point of delivery/risks
Physical therapies Following a heart attack, patients are sometimes treated through exercise therapy (*see* page 868), ascending temperature arm baths, hot mustard arm wraps, brush massage, or bathing cures (*see* pages 871–8).	**Useful** as an attempted treatment aimed at rehabilitating the patient. Controlled clinical studies confirm the efficacy of specially tailored treatment packages, especially physiotherapy, during rehabilitation.	**Requires a qualified practitioner** Practitioners should be properly qualified and should propose a treatment plan. **Risks:** Skin damage may be caused to persons with diminished temperature sensation when extreme temperatures are applied.
Probiotics The introduction of certain bacteria into the gut is claimed to bring the intestinal flora back into balance and to reduce risk factors such as arteriosclerosis (*see* page 878).	**Of little use** Possibly acceptable as a short-term treatment attempt when more established methods have been unsuccessful. Some case reports claim efficacy; however, success is probably seen in only a small proportion of patients (*see* Placebo, page xxi).	**Requires a qualified practitioner** Practitioners should be properly qualified and should propose a treatment plan. Non-prescription formulations are suitable for do-it-yourself. **Risks:** Fairly unlikely provided treatment is carried out competently.
Reflex therapies Reflex zone massage (*see* page 883), reflexology (*see* page 883), and TENS (*see* page 886) are claimed to act via reflex channels (*see* page 881) to ease pain, relax the patient, reduce tiredness and lassitude, and possibly influence the patient's blood pressure and heartbeat.	**Useful** as an individually directed, supportive treatment attempt provided the treatment is perceived to be pleasant and relaxing and to bring relief from pain. Some case reports claim efficacy; however, success is probably seen in only a proportion of patients (*see* Placebo, page xxi).	**Requires a qualified practitioner** Practitioners should be properly qualified and should propose a treatment plan. **Risks:** Some people are sensitive to electrical stimuli and rubber electrodes; others find it hard to tolerate manual stimulation or close physical contact.

Treatment	Rating	Point of delivery/risks
Relaxation techniques Autogenic training (*see* page 888), muscle relaxation according to Jacobson (*see* page 893), and various biofeedback techniques (*see* page 891) are said to relieve muscle tension and inner unrest, and to reduce stress and feelings of hopelessness. These procedures are frequently combined with psycho- or behavioral therapy.	**Useful** as a short-term, supportive treatment attempt for tension and feelings of hopelessness, provided the patient is fit enough to receive treatment and the treatment he or she has chosen is perceived to be pleasant and efficacious. Case reports claim efficacy; however, success is probably seen in only a proportion of patients (*see* Placebo, page xxi).	**Suitable for DIY** Once a sound understanding of the technique has been acquired from a trainer in group sessions or through individual tuition, patients can perform exercises themselves. Therapists should propose a treatment plan. **Risks:** Fairly unlikely.
Vitamins and trace elements The antioxidative properties of so-called "free radical interceptors" are thought to be instrumental in the prevention of arteriosclerosis (*see* page 900).	**May be of some use** High-dosed vitamins (vitamins E, C, and beta-carotene) may be useful in the prevention of arteriosclerosis. The results of some studies are contradictory in nature.	**Suitable for DIY** Qualified guidance is recommended though not essential. Risks: Intolerance and overdosage are possible. Recent studies imply that beta-carotene might increase the risk of cancer.

Herbal remedies for use after a heart attack

Active ingredient/preparation	Rating
Garlic corms (*Allium sativum*)	**May be of some use** as a supportive treatment (with diet) for thinning the blood after a heart attack (garlic promotes the flow properties of blood) and for preventing age-related vascular changes. **Dosage:** As instructed by the manufacturer/ prescriber (600–1200mg dry extract or 4g fresh corms—2–4 small cloves). **Risks:** Gastric problems and asthma are possible in rare cases. Skin irritation is possible when garlic is applied externally. Consult your doctor before using garlic for this indication.

Active ingredient/preparation	Rating
Garlic in combination with other herbal constituents	**Of little use**. These preparations frequently contain mistletoe, wheatgerm oil, ginseng, hawthorn, St. John's wort, etc. In all of the common combination preparations, however, both garlic and allicin are underdosed. Also, the efficacy of many of the other herbal constituents is in doubt (e.g. mistletoe). Suitably dosed pure garlic preparations should therefore be used in preference. **Dosage:** As instructed by the manufacturer/prescriber. **Risks:** Gastric problems and asthma are possible in rare cases. Skin irritation is possible when garlic is applied externally. Consult your doctor before using garlic for this indication.
Garlic oil maceration products	**Of little use**, as the chemical compositions of the preparations differ widely and no general daily dosage recommendations can be given. **Dosage:** As instructed by the manufacturer/prescriber. **Risks:** Gastric problems and asthma are possible in rare cases. Skin irritation is possible when garlic is applied externally. Consult your doctor before using garlic for this indication.

Heart failure (cardiac insufficiency)

Causes and symptoms

Heart failure (cardiac insufficiency) is when the heart is unable to keep the blood circulating as it should. As the heart's pumping efficiency diminishes, blood begins to collect in the veins, leading to a surfeit of fluid, and swelling, in the tissues. Heart failure is mostly a condition of the elderly.

There are numerous causes of heart failure, including coronary heart disease and its possible sequelae, such as angina pectoris (*see* page 409), myocardial infarction (*see* Heart attack, page 464), carditis and heart valve disease, as well as high blood pressure (*see* page 431) and pulmonary embolisms.

Symptoms vary depending on which side of the heart is affected. Failure of the left heart is marked by breathlessness and rapid palpitations, while insufficiency of the right heart is associated with such symptoms as swollen ankles, a feeling of fullness, and fatigue. Without proper treatment heart failure can lead to cardiac arrhythmia (*see* page 454). Failure of the left heart may result in the life-threatening accumulation of fluid in the lungs (pulmonary edema). Edematous swelling when the right heart fails can damage the skin and underlying tissues in the legs, the gastric mucosa, the liver, and the kidneys.

Heart failure is one of the most common diagnoses by doctors. For practical reasons, it is classified by degree, with distinct treatments being offered for each level of severity.

Orthodox treatment

An orthodox doctor will treat heart failure with digoxin (to strengthen the heart), diuretics (to increase fluid output), angiotensin-converting enzyme (ACE) inhibitors, or other medications. In very severe cases a heart transplant operation may be advised where medication has failed to improve the heart's efficiency. In less severe cases exercise may be prescribed.

Complementary therapies

There are complementary therapists who claim to be able to treat, or even cure, heart failure by addressing the symptoms or by allegedly increasing cardiac output by exploiting energy links (*see* page 928). In some complementary philosophies, heart failure is deemed to be a constitutional problem (*see* Constitution, page 927) or to be caused by toxins (*see* page 929). The majority of treatments are useful at best as an adjunct to orthodox treatment, but are able to assist in nothing more than the mildest degrees of heart failure.

Treatment plan and limited trial

Before administering a complementary treatment, every therapist should propose a treatment plan (*see* page xxiii) that sets out a clear time frame and defines the goal that the treatment is designed to achieve. Treatment should then be tried for a limited term to test the patient's response.

Caution

It is important for patients to be examined by a physician in case their cardiac insufficiency is treatable by conventional means.

In advanced heart failure, complementary medicine can offer no substitute for modern orthodox methods.

Complementary treatments for heart failure

Treatment	*Rating*	*Point of delivery/risks*
Acupressure This treatment (*see* page 769), otherwise known as pressure-point massage, is used to stimulate points associated with the heart, to energize (*see* page 927) the patient, and generally to raise his/her performance.	**Of little use** Acceptable as a short-term, supportive treatment attempt in the initial stages of heart failure. Some case reports and field studies claim efficacy; however, success is probably seen in only a proportion of patients (*see* Placebo, page xxi).	**Suitable for DIY** Qualified guidance is recommended. Therapists should be properly qualified and should propose a treatment plan. **Risks:** Unlikely provided treatment is carried out competently.

Treatment	*Rating*	*Point of delivery/risks*
Acupuncture Acupuncture in its various forms (*see* page 772) is used to stimulate points associated with the heart, to energize (*see* page 927) the patient, and generally to raise his/her performance.	**Of little use** Acceptable as a short-term, supportive treatment attempt when simpler, more established methods have been unsuccessful. Case reports claim efficacy; however, success is probably seen in only a proportion of patients (*see* Placebo, page xxi).	**Requires a qualified practitioner** Practitioners should be properly qualified and should propose a treatment plan. **Risks:** Probably rare provided treatment is carried out competently.
Anthroposophical medicine AM (*see* page 781) interprets heart failure as an expression of a weak liver that is no longer able to sustain the movement of fluids through the body. Therapy is based on herbal remedies such as Crataegus and potentized drugs containing Crataegus, adonis, or squill.	**May be of some use** as a short-term, supportive treatment attempt when simpler, more established methods have been unsuccessful. Some studies claim efficacy; however, success is probably seen in only a small proportion of patients (*see* Placebo, page xxi).	**Requires a qualified practitioner** Practitioners should be properly qualified and should propose a treatment plan. **Risks:** Allergies and intolerance are possible.
Aromatherapy Essential oils (*see* page 786) are used to soothe and relax, or to invigorate, thereby increasing general well-being. The essences may be taken orally, used externally as massage oils or bathing emulsions, or inhaled as vapors.	**Of little use** Acceptable as a short-term, supportive treatment attempt aimed at invigorating the patient and improving his/her general well-being. Some case reports claim efficacy; however, success is probably seen in only a small proportion of patients (*see* Placebo, page xxi).	**Suitable for DIY** Qualified guidance is recommended. The effects of individual essential oils differ widely. **Risks:** Allergies or intolerance are possible. Some oils are carcinogenic in test systems and possibly in humans.

Treatment	Rating	Point of delivery/risks
Bioresonance therapy Bioresonance therapists use electrical devices in an attempt to discover the causes of illness and claim to be able to weaken or turn around pathogenic energies and disease related vibrations (*see* page 794).	**Of little use** Possibly acceptable as a short-term, supportive treatment attempt in the early stages of heart failure when simpler, more established methods have been unsuccessful. Some case reports claim efficacy; however, success is probably seen, if at all, in only a small proportion of patients (*see* Placebo, page xxi).	**Requires a qualified practitioner** Practitioners should be properly qualified and should propose a treatment plan. No credence should be given to anyone promising immediate or total success. **Risks:** Fairly unlikely.
Cell therapy Injecting or ingesting products extracted from the tissues and organs of animals is said to have a rejuvenating and revitalizing effect and to enhance the healing of human tissues and organs (*see* page 796).	**Not advised** Based on present knowledge, there is inadequate evidence of the efficacy and mode of action of these costly and relatively risky procedures.	**Risks:** Injecting foreign proteins into the body can provoke (possibly fatal) allergic reactions. Also, pathogens such as those that cause bovine spongiform encephalopathy (BSE) or other serious infections may be introduced.
Chelation therapy The chelating agent EDTA (*see* page 800) is able, it is claimed, to bind calcareous deposits and heavy metals in the blood vessels. These are then supposedly eliminated from the body, enabling arteriosclerotic disease to be cured.	**Not advised** Evidence of the therapeutic usefulness of this risky procedure is lacking.	**Risks:** EDTA can cause a deficit of calcium and essential heavy metals and, in extreme cases, can lead to cardiac arrhythmia, respiratory failure, cramps, and death.

Treatment	Rating	Point of delivery/risks
Electroacupuncture according to Voll By taking readings of the electrical conductivity of the skin (*see* page 802), therapists claim to be able to derive an insight into diseased areas of the body, pathogenic foci (*see* page 928), and stress factors (*see* Toxins, page 929). The factors presumed to be instrumental in the causation of heart failure can then be addressed.	**Of little use** Possibly acceptable as a short-term, supportive treatment attempt when simpler, more established methods have been unsuccessful. Some case reports claim efficacy; however, success is probably seen, if at all, in only a small proportion of patients (*see* Placebo, page xxi).	**Requires a qualified practitioner** Practitioners should be properly qualified and should propose a treatment plan. No credence should be given to anyone promising immediate or total success. **Risks:** A second opinion must always be obtained from a qualified physician before any attempt is made to "eliminate foci" (e.g. by surgery).
Electroneural therapy according to Croon According to the theory, readings taken at various reactive sites on the skin highlight diseased areas within the body. Based on these readings, targeted electrostimulative measures can be undertaken to address the factors presumed to be instrumental in the causation of heart failure (*see* page 806).	**Of little use** Possibly acceptable as a short-term, supportive treatment attempt when simpler, more established methods have been unsuccessful. Some case reports claim efficacy; however, success is probably seen, if at all, in only a small proportion of patients (*see* Placebo, page xxi).	**Requires a qualified practitioner** Practitioners should be properly qualified and should propose a treatment plan. No credence should be given to anyone promising immediate or total success. **Risks:** Proponents themselves warn that treatment should not be given in acute inflammatory conditions.

Treatment	Rating	Point of delivery/risks
Eliminative methods, bloody Bloody cupping (*see* page 815) and bloodletting (*see* page 810) are said to give the patient strength and to improve the body's own regulatory systems.	**Of little use** Possibly acceptable as a short-term treatment attempt when more established, less invasive methods have been unsuccessful. Some case reports claim efficacy for this invasive and little researched method; however, success is probably seen, if at all, in only a proportion of patients (*see* Placebo, page xxi).	**Requires a qualified practitioner** Practitioners should be properly qualified and should propose a treatment plan. No credence should be given to anyone promising immediate or total success. **Risks:** Bloody cupping can cause infection and scarring. Neither procedure should be carried out on persons with bleeding disorders.
Eliminative methods, unbloody Unbloody cupping (*see* page 817) is supposed to energize (*see* page 927) the patient and improve the body's own regulatory systems in persons with a weak heart.	**May be of some use** as a short-term, supportive treatment attempt. Some case reports claim efficacy; however, success is probably seen in only a small proportion of patients (*see* Placebo, page xxi).	**Suitable for DIY** Unbloody cupping is best carried out under the guidance of a qualified practitioner. **Risks:** Fairly unlikely provided treatment is carried out competently.
Enzyme therapy Enzymes obtained from plant and animal tissues are claimed to have a restorative effect, as well as inhibiting inflammation, modulating the immune system (*see* page 824), having a general strengthening effect, and improving well-being.	**Of little use** Some case reports claim efficacy for this little researched method; however, success is probably seen in only a small proportion of patients (*see* Placebo, page xxi).	**Requires a qualified practitioner** Practitioners should propose a treatment plan. Non-prescription preparations are suitable for do-it-yourself. **Risks:** Allergies or intolerance are possible.

Treatment	Rating	Point of delivery/risks
Flower remedies Flower remedies (*see* page 828) are said to restore emotional balance and assist the body's psychic ability to heal itself.	**Of little use** Acceptable as a short-term treatment attempt aimed at helping the patient come to terms emotionally with his/her condition. Some case reports claim efficacy; however, success is probably seen in only a small proportion of patients (*see* Placebo, page xxi).	**Suitable for DIY** Qualified guidance is recommended. Practitioners should propose a treatment plan. **Risks:** Possible intolerance.
Homeopathy Highly diluted (potentized) solutions (*see* page 831) are believed to be able to redress vital energy imbalances and strengthen the body's defences. Organo- and functiotropic (*see* page 833) homeopathy is claimed to be effective for dealing with heart failure.	**Of little use** Acceptable as a supportive treatment attempt and as an additional motivation for the patient to come to terms with his/her condition. Some case reports claim that homeopathic treatments can be used to strengthen the heart; however, success is probably seen in only a proportion of patients (*see* Placebo, page xxi).	**Requires a qualified practitioner** Homeopaths should be properly qualified and should propose a treatment plan. Ready-formulated preparations are suitable for do-it-yourself. **Risks:** Allergies and intolerance are possible.
Hypnosis and self-hypnosis In the relaxed and generally altered state of awareness that is induced in hypnosis or self-hypnosis (*see* page 837), physical conditions can be addressed. Hypnosis is often used in combination with other psycho- and behavioral therapies.	**Of little use** Acceptable as a short-term, supportive treatment attempt when simpler, more established methods have been unsuccessful. Some case reports claim that these procedures can be used to strengthen the heart; however, success is probably seen in only a small proportion of patients (*see* Placebo, page xxi).	**Requires a qualified practitioner** Hypnotherapists should be properly qualified and should propose a treatment plan. No credence should be given to anyone promising immediate or total success. **Risks:** Unlikely provided treatment is carried out competently.

Treatment	*Rating*	*Point of delivery/risks*
Magnetic field therapy The use of magnetic field generators, magnetic strips, bracelets, and other objects (*see* page 841) allegedly encourages cell metabolism and has a general restorative and invigorating effect.	**Inappropriate** Based on present knowledge, there is inadequate evidence of the efficacy and mode of action of magnetic field therapy in heart failure.	Operation of magnetic field equipment **requires a qualified practitioner**. **Risks:** Magnetic field equipment can cause implanted cardiac pacemakers to malfunction.
Manual therapies Chiropractors and osteopaths (*see* page 844) use a series of manipulations to realign allegedly displaced vertebrae. This is said to reduce nerve blockages and irritation thought to be co-responsible for heart failure.	**Of little use** Possibly acceptable as a short-term treatment attempt when less risky, more established methods have been unsuccessful. Some case reports claim efficacy for these potentially risky procedures; however, success is probably seen, if at all, in only a small proportion of patients (*see* Placebo, page xxi).	**Requires a qualified practitioner** Practitioners should be properly qualified and should propose a treatment plan. **Risks:** Manipulation of the head and cervical vertebrae can cause serious injury. Osteoporosis is one of several risk factors.
Massage Classical massage (*see* page 847) is said to ease muscular and emotional tension, to have a restorative effect, and to improve general well-being.	**Of little use** Acceptable as a supportive treatment attempt aimed at relaxing the patient. Some case reports claim efficacy for this treatment of heart failure; however, success is probably seen in only a proportion of patients (*see* Placebo, page xxi).	**Suitable for DIY** Qualified guidance is recommended. Masseurs/masseuses should be properly qualified and should propose a treatment plan. **Risks:** Some people are sensitive to manual stimuli; others find it hard to tolerate close physical contact.

Treatment	Rating	Point of delivery/risks
Nutritional therapies An organic diet (*see* page 4) provides the body with essential and secondary plant nutrients, dietary fiber, antioxidants, etc., which are believed to exercise a multitude of positive effects.	**Useful** as an individually directed supportive measure. Some case reports claim efficacy for this type of treatment in strengthening the heart; however, success is probably seen in only a proportion of patients (*see* Placebo, page xxi).	**Suitable for DIY** Qualified guidance is recommended though not essential. **Risks:** Avoid imbalanced or intolerable diets. They can cause deficiencies with serious consequences. Children are particularly at risk.
Physical therapies Exercise therapy (*see* page 868), cold washings, various forms of hydrotherapy (*see* pages 871–8), and climatic cures supposedly stimulate the circulation. These procedures are often used in combination.	**Useful** as a supportive treatment attempt, mainly in the initial stages of heart failure. The results achieved may differ widely from one person to another. Case reports and field studies claim efficacy; however, success is probably seen in only a proportion of patients (*see* Placebo, page xxi).	**Suitable for DIY** Qualified guidance is recommended though not essential. **Risks:** Insufficient as the sole measure in advanced stages of heart failure. Skin damage may be caused to persons with diminished temperature sensation when extreme temperatures are applied.
Reflex therapies Reflex zone massage (*see* page 883), reflexology (*see* page 883), and TENS (*see* page 886) are claimed to act via reflex channels (*see* page 881) to invigorate and stimulate.	**May be of some use** as a short-term supportive treatment attempt aimed at generally strengthening the heart. Case reports claim efficacy; however, success is probably seen in only a proportion of patients (*see* Placebo, page xxi).	**Suitable for DIY** Qualified guidance is recommended. **Risks:** Some people are sensitive to electrical stimuli and rubber electrodes; others find it hard to tolerate manual stimulation or close physical contact.

Treatment	*Rating*	*Point of delivery/risks*
Relaxation techniques Autogenic training (*see* page 888), muscle relaxation according to Jacobson (*see* page 893), and various biofeedback techniques (*see* page 891) are said to relieve physical and emotional tension and lessen anxiety and overexcitability.	**May be of some use** as a supportive treatment attempt aimed at physical and emotional relaxation. Some case reports claim efficacy; however, success is probably seen in only a proportion of patients (*see* Placebo, page xxi).	**Suitable for DIY** Once a sound understanding of the technique has been acquired from a trainer in group sessions or through individual tuition, patients can perform exercises themselves. Therapists should propose a treatment plan. **Risks:** Fairly unlikely.
Vitamins and trace elements The antioxidative properties of beta-carotene, and of vitamins C and E, are supposed to reduce levels of individual lipids, to have a general restorative effect, and to prevent high blood pressure and arteriosclerosis (*see* page 900).	**May be of some use** as a supportive measure aimed at generally building up strength and as an attempt to prevent high blood pressure and arteriosclerosis. Based on present knowledge, no definitive recommendations can be given; however, high vitamin C doses do appear to provide some benefits.	**Suitable for DIY** Qualified guidance is recommended though not essential. **Risks:** Intolerance and overdosage are possible. Recent studies suggest that beta-carotene might increase the risk of cancer.

Herbal remedies for heart failure

Active ingredient/preparation	Rating
Hawthorn leaves and blossom (*Crataegus monogyna* and *Crataegus laevigata*)	**Useful** as a treatment attempt for stage I and II heart failure when there is not yet a need for digitalis preparations or ACE inhibitors. **Daily dose:** 1g herb. **Individual dose:** Pour hot water over 0.2–0.3g of herb and infuse, three to four times a day. Use ready-formulated preparations as instructed by the manufacturer/prescriber. **Risks:** Consult a doctor if heart failure and water retention in the legs have not cleared up after six weeks. A doctor must be consulted if there are severe symptoms (pain near the heart, in the arms, upper abdomen, or neck). Hawthorn may in some cases cause nausea, headaches, and vertigo. Remedies containing hawthorn may possibly potentiate the action and thus the toxicity of digitalis. Hawthorn must not be used, therefore, with cardiac tonics that contain digitalis. It is not suitable for self-medication.
Hawthorn in combination with other ingredients	**Of little use**, as only hawthorn itself is described as having a cardioactive action, so appropriately dosed pure hawthorn preparations should be used in preference. **Dosage:** As instructed by the manufacturer/prescriber. Not suitable for self-medication. **Risks:** As for hawthorn. See the package insert for details of other constituents.

Active ingredient/preparation	Rating

Lily of the valley
(*Convallaria majalis*)

May be of some use as a treatment attempt for mild heart weakness under load and senile heart.
Daily dose: 0.6g powder or as instructed by the manufacturer/prescriber. Not suitable for self-medication.
Risks: Nausea, vomiting, cardiac arrhythmia. Drug interactions: augments the action of saluretics (agents that promote the excretion of sodium and chloride ions in the urine, e.g. in hypertension), high doses of laxatives, and cortisone preparations. Not to be taken with cardiac tonics that contain digitalis, as it can raise digitalis toxicity. Not to be taken by persons with digitalis intoxication or potassium deficiency.
Caution: Lily of the valley is controlled by the Medicines Act 1968 in the UK. Persons using it must be kept under medical supervision.

Lily of the valley in combination with other constituents

Of little use. Cardioactive agents should be individually dosed. This cannot be optimally achieved in combination preparations. Also, not all constituents in such combinations (e.g. oleander) have been tested for cardiac activity or been shown to be efficacious enough in the case of heart failure.
Dosage: As instructed by the manufacturer/prescriber. Not suitable for self-medication.
Risks: As for lily of the valley. See the package insert for details of other constitutents.

Active ingredient/preparation	*Rating*

Spring adonis
(*Adonis vernalis*)

May be of some use as a treatment attempt for slight cardiac weakness under load, senile heart, and nervous heart conditions. Not suitable for self-medication.
Daily dose: 0.6g powdered adonis, maximum 3g. **Individual dose:** 1g, two to three times a day as a tea drink. Use ready-formulated preparations as instructed by the manufacturer/prescriber. Not suitable for self-medication.
Risks: Overdosage can cause nausea, vomiting, and cardiac arrhythmia. Drug interactions: augments the action of saluretics (agents that promote the excretion of sodium and chloride ions in the urine, e.g. in hypertension), high doses of laxatives, and cortisone preparations. Not to be taken by persons with digitalis intoxication or potassium deficiency.

Adonis fluid extract in combination preparations

Of little use. Cardioactive agents should be individually dosed. This cannot be optimally achieved in combination preparations. Also, not all combination partners (e.g. oleander) have been shown to be efficacious enough in the case of heart failure.
Dosage: As instructed by the manufacturer/prescriber. Not suitable for self-medication.
Risks: Not to be taken with cardiac tonics that contain digitalis, as it can raise digitalis toxicity.

Active ingredient/preparation	Rating
Squill (*Urginea maritima*)	**May be of some use** as a treatment attempt for mild heart failure, also in impaired renal function. **Dosage:** As instructed by the manufacturer/prescriber. Not suitable for self-medication. **Risks:** Nausea, vomiting, gastric problems, diarrhea, irregular pulse. Squill interacts with substances such as quinidine, calcium, laxatives, saluretics, etc. Do not take when calcium levels are too high or too low, or in cases of tachycardia, extreme bradycardia, or digitalis intoxication. Care is needed for persons with problems of cardiac stimulus conduction or receiving intravenous calcium. Not to be taken with cardiac tonics that contain digitalis, as it can raise digitalis toxicity.
Squill in combination with other constituents	**Of little use**. Powdered squill must be individually dosed. This cannot be optimally achieved in combination preparations. Also, not all constituents in such combinations (e.g. oleander) have been tested or been shown to be efficacious enough in cases of heart failure. **Dosage:** As instructed by the manufacturer/prescriber. Not suitable for self-medication. **Risks:** As for squill. See the package insert for details of other constituents.

Stroke

Causes and symptoms

A stroke is the result of damage to blood vessels supplying the brain. When the cerebral arteries become blocked or sclerotic, the supply of oxygen and nutrients to the brain is reduced or cut off. A stroke is most commonly caused by a clot (thrombus) in one of the cerebral arteries. In other instances a cerebral blood vessel may burst. In both scenarios this leads to loss of consciousness and cerebral functions, and possibly to paralysis. Partial or complete recovery is possible, although approximately every third patient will suffer lasting effects.

Orthodox treatment

Persons suspected of having a stroke should immediately be admitted to a hospital, where their circulation, respiration, and blood pressure can be monitored. After a stroke, support will generally be provided through various forms of physiotherapy plus speech and other appropriate supportive therapies to improve recovery. Anti-hypertensive drugs and anticoagulation therapy will be prescribed where needed.

Following a stroke, patients will usually be given help to improve their physical and intellectual performance.

Complementary therapies

Apart from exercise (which is also used in the mainstream treatment of a stroke) and possibly acupuncture, complementary procedures have little to offer except pain relief. As things stand at present, they are no substitute for diagnosis and therapy by a qualified physician.

Treatment plan and limited trial

Before administering a complementary treatment, every therapist should propose a treatment plan (*see* page xxiii) that sets out a clear time frame and defines the goal that the treatment is designed to achieve. Treatment should then be tried for a limited term to test the patient's response.

Caution

Patients receiving just a complementary treatment following a stroke will miss out on essential orthodox treatment.

Complementary treatments following a stroke

Treatment	Rating	Point of delivery/risks
Acupressure This treatment (*see* page 769), otherwise known as pressure-point massage, is used after a stroke as a means of stimulating and activating the patient, and of hastening and improving recovery.	**Useful** as a supportive treatment attempt aimed at stimulating and activating the patient and for hastening rehabilitation. Some case reports claim efficacy; however, success is probably seen in only a proportion of patients (*see* Placebo, page xxi).	**Suitable for DIY** Qualified guidance is recommended. Therapists should be properly qualified. **Risks:** Unlikely provided treatment is carried out competently.
Acupuncture Acupuncture in its various forms (*see* page 772) is used with the aim of stimulating and activating patients following a stroke, and of hastening and improving recovery. The acupuncture points chosen can vary from one practitioner to another.	**Useful** as a supportive treatment attempt aimed at stimulating and activating the patient and for hastening rehabilitation. Case reports, field studies, and one controlled clinical study suggest that at present an incalculable number of patients profits from acupuncture as a supportive measure.	**Requires a qualified practitioner** Practitioners should be properly qualified and should propose a treatment plan. **Risks:** Probably rare provided treatment is carried out competently. Acupuncture should not be carried out on patients taking oral anticoagulants.
Anthroposophical medicine Supportive measures used following a stroke include rhythmic massage, curative eurhythmy, and potentized arnica, lead, and organ preparations (*see* page 781).	**May be of some use** as a supportive treatment attempt aimed at rehabilitating the patient. Numerous case reports claim efficacy; however, success is probably seen in only a proportion of patients (*see* Placebo, page xxi).	**Requires a qualified practitioner** Practitioners should be properly qualified and should propose a treatment plan. **Risks:** Allergies and intolerance are possible.

Treatment	Rating	Point of delivery/risks
Aromatherapy Essential oils (*see* page 786) are used to invigorate and relax the patient. The essences may be taken orally, used externally as massage oils or bathing emulsions, or inhaled as vapors.	**May be of some use** as a supportive treatment attempt aimed at relaxing the patient and improving his/her general well-being. Some case reports claim efficacy; however, success is probably seen in only a small proportion of patients (*see* Placebo, page xxi).	**Suitable for DIY** Qualified guidance is recommended. The effects of individual essential oils differ widely. **Risks:** Allergies or intolerance are possible. Some oils are carcinogenic in test systems and possibly in humans.
Bioresonance therapy Bioresonance therapists use electrical devices in an attempt to discover the causes of illness and claim to be able to weaken or turn around pathogenic energies and disease related vibrations (*see* page 794).	**Of little use** Evidence of the efficacy of this relatively involved procedure is lacking.	**Requires a qualified practitioner** Practitioners should be properly qualified and should propose a treatment plan. No credence should be given to anyone promising immediate or total success. **Risks:** Fairly unlikely.
Cell therapy Injecting or ingesting products extracted from the tissues and organs of animals is said to have a rejuvenating and revitalizing effect and to enhance the healing of human tissues and organs (*see* page 796).	**Not advised** Based on present knowledge, there is inadequate evidence of the efficacy and mode of action of these costly and relatively risky procedures.	**Risks:** Injecting foreign proteins into the body can provoke (possibly fatal) allergic reactions. Also, pathogens such as those that cause bovine spongiform encephalopathy (BSE) or other serious infections may be introduced.

Treatment	Rating	Point of delivery/risks
Electroacupuncture according to Voll By taking readings of the electrical conductivity of the skin, therapists claim to be able to address symptoms (*see* page 802).	**Of little use** Evidence of the efficacy of this relatively involved procedure is lacking.	**Requires a qualified practitioner** Practitioners should be properly qualified and should propose a treatment plan. No credence should be given to anyone promising immediate or total success. **Risks:** A second opinion must always be obtained from a qualified physician before any attempt is made to "eliminate foci" (e.g. by surgery).
Electroneural therapy according to Croon According to the theory, readings taken at various reactive sites on the skin enable measures to be taken against symptoms (*see* page 806).	**Of little use** Evidence of the efficacy of this relatively involved procedure is lacking.	**Requires a qualified practitioner** Practitioners should be properly qualified and should propose a treatment plan. No credence should be given to anyone promising immediate or total success. **Risks:** Proponents themselves warn that treatment should not be given in acute inflammatory conditions.
Eliminative methods, bloody Bloody cupping (*see* page 815) is said to have a restorative effect following a stroke and to release blocked energy (*see* page 927).	**Not advised** Evidence of the efficacy of this invasive and relatively risky procedure is lacking.	**Risks:** Bloody cupping can cause infection and scarring. Furthermore, it should not be carried out on persons with bleeding disorders or those taking oral anticoagulants.

Treatment	*Rating*	*Point of delivery/risks*
Eliminative methods, unbloody Unbloody cupping (*see* page 817) is said to have an analgesic, muscle-relaxing and energizing (*see* page 927) effect in patients who have had a stroke, and also to improve the prospects of recovery.	**May be of some use** as a supportive treatment attempt aimed at pain relief and muscle relaxation. Field studies and case reports claim efficacy; however, success is probably seen in only a proportion of patients (*see* Placebo, page xxi).	**Suitable for DIY** Qualified guidance is recommended. **Risks:** Unlikely provided treatment is carried out competently.
Enzyme therapy Enzymes (*see* page 824) obtained from plant and animal tissues are claimed to have a restorative effect following a stroke and to hasten recovery.	**Of little use** Some case reports claim efficacy for this little researched therapy; however, success is probably seen in only a small proportion of patients (*see* Placebo, page xxi).	**Requires a qualified practitioner** Practitioners should propose a treatment plan. Non-prescription preparations are suitable for do-it-yourself. **Risks:** Allergies or intolerance are possible.
Flower remedies Flower remedies (*see* page 828) are said to restore emotional balance and assist the body's psychic ability to heal itself.	**May be of some use** as a short-term, supportive treatment attempt aimed at countering anxiety and feelings of hopelessness. Some case reports claim efficacy; however, success is probably seen in only a proportion of patients (*see* Placebo, page xxi).	**Suitable for DIY** Qualified guidance is recommended. Practitioners should propose a treatment plan. **Risks:** Possible intolerance.

Treatment	Rating	Point of delivery/risks
Homeopathy Highly diluted (potentized) solutions (*see* page 831) are believed to be able to redress vital energy imbalances and strengthen the body's defences. Organo- and functiotropic (*see* page 833) homeopathy is claimed to be effective for dealing with the aftermath of a stroke.	**Of little use** Acceptable as a treatment attempt and for helping the patient come to terms better with his/her condition. Case reports claim success for homeopathic treatments; however, success is probably seen in only a proportion of patients (*see* Placebo, page xxi).	**Requires a qualified practitioner** Homeopaths should be properly qualified and should propose a treatment plan. Ready-formulated preparations are suitable for do-it-yourself. **Risks:** Allergies and intolerance are possible.
Hypnosis and self-hypnosis In the relaxed and generally altered state of awareness that is induced in hypnosis or self-hypnosis (*see* page 837), anxiety can be reduced and the patient can be helped to come to terms better with his/her condition.	**May be of some use** as a short-term supportive treatment attempt aimed at relieving anxiety and at helping the patient come to terms better with his/her condition. Some case reports claim efficacy; however, success is probably seen in only a proportion of patients treated (*see* Placebo, page xxi).	**Requires a qualified practitioner** Hypnotherapists should be properly qualified and should propose a treatment plan. No credence should be given to anyone promising immediate or total success. **Risks:** Unlikely provided treatment is carried out competently.
Magnetic field therapy The use of magnetic field generators, magnetic strips, bracelets, and other objects (*see* page 841) allegedly encourages cell metabolism and so has an invigorating effect.	**Inappropriate** Based on present knowledge, there is inadequate evidence of the efficacy and mode of action of magnetic field therapy following a stroke.	Operation of magnetic field equipment **requires a qualified practitioner**. **Risks:** Magnetic field equipment can cause implanted cardiac pacemakers to malfunction.

Treatment	Rating	Point of delivery/risks
Manual therapies Chiropractors and osteopaths (*see* page 844) use a series of manipulations to realign allegedly displaced vertebrae. This is said to reduce pain, improve the body's own regulatory systems, and hasten rehabilitation. Sometimes these procedures are used to release blocked energy (*see* page 927).	**Of little use** Possibly acceptable as a short-term treatment attempt aimed at alleviating pain in the locomotor system. Some case reports claim efficacy for these potentially risky procedures; however, success is probably seen, if at all, in only a small proportion of patients (*see* Placebo, page xxi).	**Requires a qualified practitioner** Practitioners should be properly qualified and should propose a treatment plan. **Risks:** Manipulation of the head and cervical vertebrae can cause serious injury. Osteoporosis is one of several risk factors.
Massage Classical massage (*see* page 847) is claimed to invigorate the patient, as well as ease muscular and emotional tension and alleviate muscular pain.	**Useful** as a supportive treatment attempt aimed at relaxing the patient and easing muscular pain. Case reports claim efficacy; however, success is probably seen in only a proportion of patients (*see* Placebo, page xxi).	**Suitable for DIY** Qualified guidance is recommended. Masseurs/masseuses should be properly qualified. **Risks:** Some people are sensitive to manual stimuli; others find it hard to tolerate close physical contact.
Nutritional therapies An organic diet (*see* page 4) can influence possible risk factors such as obesity and blood fat levels, as well as improve general performance and well-being.	**Useful** as a supportive and preventive measure provided that the diet is tolerated.	**Suitable for DIY** Qualified guidance is recommended though not essential. **Risks:** Avoid imbalanced or intolerable diets. They can cause deficiencies with serious consequences. Children are particularly at risk.

Treatment	Rating	Point of delivery/risks
Physical therapies Individually directed treatment packages with various activating concepts, exercise therapies (*see* page 868) are used for rehabilitation, sometimes in combination with psycho- or behavioral therapy.	**Useful** as a treatment attempt during rehabilitation. Controlled clinical studies confirm the efficacy of individually tailored treatment packages, especially physiotherapy.	**Requires a qualified practitioner** Practitioners should be properly qualified. **Risks:** Unlikely provided treatment is carried out competently. Expert guidance should be sought if the rehabilitation program is continued at home.
Probiotics The introduction of certain bacteria into the gut is claimed to bring the intestinal flora back into balance and to lessen risk factors such as arteriosclerosis (*see* page 878).	**Of little use** Acceptable as a treatment attempt when the intestinal flora has been damaged by a poor diet. Case reports claim efficacy; however, success is probably seen in only a small proportion of patients (*see* Placebo, page xxi).	**Requires a qualified practitioner** Practitioners should be properly qualified and should propose a treatment plan. Non-prescription formulations are suitable for do-it-yourself. **Risks:** Fairly unlikely provided treatment is carried out competently.
Reflex therapies Reflex zone massage (*see* page 883), reflexology (*see* page 883), and TENS (*see* page 886) are claimed to act via reflex channels (*see* page 881) to ease pain and help rehabilitate the patient.	**Useful** as an individually directed supportive measure aimed at pain relief. Case reports claim efficacy; however, success is probably seen in only a proportion of patients (*see* Placebo, page xxi).	**Requires a qualified practitioner** Practitioners should be properly qualified and should propose a treatment plan. **Risks:** Some people are sensitive to electrical stimuli and rubber electrodes; others find it hard to tolerate manual stimulation or close physical contact.

Treatment	Rating	Point of delivery/risks
Relaxation techniques Autogenic training (*see* page 888), muscle relaxation according to Jacobson (*see* page 893), and various biofeedback techniques (*see* page 891) are said to relieve muscle tension and inner unrest, and to reduce stress and feelings of hopelessness.	**May be of some use** as a short-term, supportive treatment attempt aimed at relieving tension and feelings of hopelessness, provided the patient is fit enough to receive treatment. Case reports claim efficacy; however, success is probably seen in only a proportion of patients (*see* Placebo, page xxi).	**Suitable for DIY** Once a sound understanding of the technique has been acquired from a trainer, patients can perform exercises themselves. Therapists should be properly qualified. **Risks:** Patients are frequently unable to practice autogenic training or muscle relaxation according to Jacobson.
Vitamins The antioxidative properties of so-called radical interceptors are said to play a beneficial role in the prevention of arteriosclerosis (*see* page 900).	High vitamin doses (vitamins E, C, and beta-carotene) **may be of some use** for preventing arteriosclerosis and further strokes. The findings of various studies sometimes contradict one another.	**Suitable for DIY** Qualified guidance is recommended though not essential. **Risks:** Intolerance and overdosage are possible. Recent studies imply that beta-carotene might increase the risk of cancer.

Herbal remedies for use after a stroke

Active ingredient/preparation	Rating
Garlic corms (*Allium sativum*)	**May be of some use** as a supportive treatment (with diet) for thinning the blood and preventing age-related vascular changes. As garlic thins the blood, it possibly also improves its flow properties. **Dosage:** As instructed by the manufacturer/prescriber (600–1200mg dry extract or 4g fresh corms—2–4 small cloves). **Risks:** Gastric problems and asthma are possible in rare cases. Consult your doctor before using garlic for this indication.

Active ingredient/preparation	Rating
Garlic in combination with other herbal constituents	**Of little use**. These preparations frequently contain mistletoe, wheatgerm oil, ginseng, hawthorn, St. John's wort, etc. In all of the common combination preparations, however, both garlic and allicin are underdosed. Also, the efficacy of many of the other herbal constituents is in doubt (e.g. mistletoe). Suitably dosed pure garlic preparations should therefore be used in preference. **Dosage:** As instructed by the manufacturer/prescriber. **Risks:** Gastric problems and asthma are possible in rare cases. Consult your doctor before using garlic for this indication.
Garlic oil maceration products	**Of little use**, as the chemical compositions of the preparations differ widely and no general daily dosage recommendations can be given. **Dosage:** As instructed by the manufacturer/prescriber. **Risks:** Gastric problems and asthma are possible in rare cases. Consult your doctor before using garlic for this indication.
Ginkgo biloba **leaves**	**Of little use**. Teas prepared from ginkgo leaves have no proven efficacy. **Daily dose:** 0.5g leaves. **Individual dose:** Pour 1 cup of hot water over 0.1g of leaves and infuse. **Risks:** Allergic reactions are possible.
Ginkgo extract (*Ginkgo biloba*)	**May be of some use** as a supportive treatment attempt. Ginkgo can improve the flow properties of the blood and so improve cerebral circulation following a stroke. **Dosage:** As instructed by the manufacturer/prescriber. **Risks:** Mild gastrointestinal problems, headaches and allergic skin reactions are possible. Consult a doctor before taking it. Not to be taken by persons who are hypersensitive to ginkgo. Injectable ginkgo preparations have been withdrawn owing to hypersensitivity reactions.

Varicose veins, phlebitis, and chronic venous insufficiency

Causes and symptoms

Varicose veins is a condition in which the veins, usually those in the legs, become distended and swollen with blood pooled in the area. Phlebitis is a superficial inflammation that often accompanies varicose veins. Chronic venous insufficiency is suffered by a large number of people, involves a general weakening of the venous circulation, and is often associated with one or both of the other two conditions. Typical symptoms of all three conditions include tired, heavy legs, tenderness, pain, and swelling.

Genetic factors may be significant in the causation of these conditions, as well as workplace conditions, frequent or prolonged standing, pregnancy, obesity, and psychological stress.

Orthodox treatment

The basis of any treatment for varicose veins and chronic venous insufficiency will be physiotherapeutic measures and compression therapy (with support stockings, etc.). Varicose veins may also be removed surgically. Chronic venous insufficiency can be treated with (herbal) drugs, too, though assessments of the efficacy of these differ.

Complementary therapies

Many complementary procedures are based on the same principles as orthodox treatments, though some complementary therapists use methods that are constitution oriented (*see* Constitution, page 927) or that will allegedly invigorate the veins and, indeed, the entire vascular system. Many of the medicines used are botanicals.

Treatment plan and limited trial

Before administering a complementary treatment, every therapist should propose a treatment plan (*see* page xxiii) that sets out a clear time frame and defines the goal that the treatment is designed to achieve. Treatment should then be tried for a limited term to test the patient's response.

Cautions

In the treatment of deep vein thrombosis, a potentially life-threatening condition, none of the complementary remedies on offer will be an adequate substitute for the methods of modern mainstream medicine.

Complementary treatments for varicose veins, phlebitis, and chronic venous insufficiency

Treatment	Rating	Point of delivery/risks
Acupressure This treatment (*see* page 769), otherwise known as pressure-point massage, is claimed to ease pain, alleviate heaviness of the legs, and relieve feelings of fullness and itchiness when pressure is applied to the appropriate points. The pressure points chosen may differ from one practitioner to another.	**Inappropriate** as the sole treatment for varicose veins, phlebitis, and chronic venous insufficiency. **May be of some use** as a short-term, supportive treatment attempt aimed at easing pain, heaviness of the legs, and itchiness. Initial studies, case reports, and observational studies ascribe a degree of efficacy to this treatment in some patients (*see* Placebo, page xxi).	**Suitable for DIY** Qualified guidance is recommended. Therapists should be properly qualified. **Risks:** Unlikely provided treatment is carried out competently.

Treatment	Rating	Point of delivery/risks
Acupuncture Acupuncture in its various forms (*see* page 772) aims to encourage the flow of energy (*see* page 927) or to act directly to ease pain and improve the circulation. The acupuncture points chosen can vary from one practitioner to another.	**Inappropriate** as the sole treatment for varicose veins, phlebitis, and chronic venous insufficiency. **May be of some use** as a short-term, supportive treatment attempt aimed at easing pain and improving the circulation. Case reports claim efficacy; however, success is probably seen in only a proportion of patients (*see* Placebo, page xxi).	**Requires a qualified practitioner** Acupuncturists should be properly qualified and should propose a treatment plan. **Risks:** Probably rare provided treatment is carried out competently.
Anthroposophical medicine For the treatment of varicose veins and edema, doctors who practice AM (*see* page 781) advise the use of curative eurhythmy and various compositions to stimulate the flow of fluids within the body.	**Inappropriate** as the sole treatment for varicose veins, phlebitis, and chronic venous insufficiency. **May be of some use** as a preventive measure and as a short-term treatment. Case reports claim efficacy; however, success is probably seen in only a proportion of patients (*see* Placebo, page xxi).	**Requires a qualified practitioner** Practitioners should be properly qualified and should propose a treatment plan. **Risks:** Allergies and intolerance are possible.
Aromatherapy Essential oils (*see* page 786) are used to soothe and relax, or to invigorate, so possibly easing symptoms. The essences may be taken orally, used externally as massage oils or bathing emulsions, or inhaled as vapors.	**Inappropriate** as the sole treatment for varicose veins, phlebitis, and chronic venous insufficiency. **May be of some use** as a short-term, supportive treatment attempt aimed at soothing and relaxing. Some case reports claim efficacy; however, success is probably seen in only a small proportion of patients (*see* Placebo, page xxi).	**Suitable for DIY** Qualified guidance is recommended. The effects of individual essential oils differ widely. **Risks:** Allergies or intolerance are possible. Some oils are carcinogenic in test systems and possibly in humans.

Treatment	Rating	Point of delivery/risks
Bioresonance therapy Bioresonance therapists use electrical devices in an attempt to discover the causes of illness and claim to be able to weaken or turn around pathogenic energies and disease related vibrations (*see* page 794).	**Inappropriate** as the sole treatment for varicose veins, phlebitis, and chronic venous insufficiency. **Of little use** Possibly acceptable as a short-term, supportive treatment attempt in persistent cases when simpler, more established methods have been unsuccessful. Some case reports claim efficacy; however, success is probably seen, if at all, in only a small proportion of patients (*see* Placebo, page xxi).	**Requires a qualified practitioner** Practitioners should be properly qualified and should propose a treatment plan. No credence should be given to anyone promising immediate or total success. **Risks:** Fairly unlikely.
Cell therapy Injecting or ingesting products extracted from the tissues of newborn animals or animal fetuses is said to have a rejuvenating and revitalizing effect and to enhance the healing of human tissues and organs (*see* page 796).	**Not advised** Based on present knowledge, there is inadequate evidence of the efficacy and mode of action of these costly and relatively risky procedures.	**Risks:** Injecting foreign proteins into the body can provoke (possibly fatal) allergic reactions. Also, pathogens such as those that cause bovine spongiform encephalopathy (BSE) or other serious infections may be introduced.

Treatment	Rating	Point of delivery/risks
Electroacupuncture according to Voll By taking readings of the electrical conductivity of the skin (*see* page 802), therapists claim to be able to derive an insight into diseased areas of the body, pathogenic foci (*see* page 928), and stress factors (*see* Toxins, page 929). The factors presumed to be instrumental in the causation of varicose veins, phlebitis, and chronic venous insufficiency can then be addressed.	**Inappropriate** as the sole treatment for varicose veins, phlebitis, and chronic venous insufficiency. Possibly acceptable as a short-term, supportive treatment attempt in persistent cases when simpler, more established methods have been unsuccessful. Some case reports claim efficacy; however, success is probably seen, if at all, in only a small proportion of patients (*see* Placebo, page xxi).	**Requires a qualified practitioner** Practitioners should be properly qualified and should propose a treatment plan. No credence should be given to anyone promising immediate or total success. **Risks:** A second opinion must always be obtained from a qualified physician before any attempt is made to "eliminate foci" (e.g. by surgery).
Electroneural therapy according to Croon According to the theory, readings taken at various reactive sites on the skin highlight diseased areas within the body. Based on these readings, targeted electrostimulative measures can be undertaken to address the factors presumed to be instrumental in the causation of varicose veins, phlebitis, and chronic venous insufficiency (*see* page 806).	**Inappropriate** as the sole treatment for varicose veins, phlebitis, and chronic venous insufficiency. Possibly acceptable as a short-term, supportive treatment attempt in persistent cases when simpler, more established methods have been unsuccessful. Some case reports claim efficacy; however, success is probably seen, if at all, in only a small proportion of patients (*see* Placebo, page xxi).	**Requires a qualified practitioner** Practitioners should be properly qualified and should propose a treatment plan. No credence should be given to anyone promising immediate or total success. **Risks:** Proponents themselves warn that treatment should not be given in acute inflammatory conditions.

Treatment	Rating	Point of delivery/risks
Eliminative methods, bloody Leeches (*see* page 822) are used to inhibit inflammation and to "thin" the blood.	**Inappropriate** as the sole treatment for varicose veins, phlebitis, and chronic venous insufficiency. Possibly acceptable as a short-term, supportive treatment attempt. Case reports and field studies claim efficacy; however, success is probably seen in only a small proportion of patients (*see* Placebo, page xxi).	**Suitable for DIY** Qualified guidance is essential. **Risks:** Leeches should not be used in persons with bleeding disorders. They should be used once only owing to the risk of infection.
Eliminative methods, unbloody Unbloody cupping (*see* page 817) is supposed to ease pain, tension, and feelings of having heavy legs, as well as improving the body's own regulatory systems.	**Inappropriate** as the sole treatment for varicose veins, phlebitis, and chronic venous insufficiency. **May be of some use** as a short-term, supportive treatment attempt aimed at alleviating pain. Some case reports claim efficacy; however, success is probably seen in only a proportion of patients (*see* Placebo, page xxi).	**Suitable for DIY** Unbloody cupping is best carried out under the guidance of a qualified practitioner. **Risks:** Unlikely provided treatment is carried out competently.
Enzyme therapy The enzymes used (*see* page 824) are said to dispel and destroy "immune complexes" that course in the blood and that are responsible, for instance, for sustaining inflammatory processes.	**Of little use** Some case reports claim efficacy for this little researched therapy; however, success is probably seen in only a small proportion of patients (*see* Placebo, page xxi).	**Requires a qualified practitioner** Practitioners should propose a treatment plan. Non-prescription preparations are suitable for do-it-yourself. **Risks:** Allergies or intolerance are possible.

Treatment	Rating	Point of delivery/risks
Flower remedies Flower remedies (*see* page 828) are said to restore emotional balance and assist the body's psychic ability to heal itself.	**Inappropriate** as the sole treatment for varicose veins, phlebitis, and chronic venous insufficiency. **May be of some use** as a short-term, supportive treatment attempt aimed at soothing and relaxing. Some case reports claim efficacy; however, success is probably seen in only a small proportion of patients (*see* Placebo, page xxi).	**Suitable for DIY** Qualified guidance is recommended. Practitioners should propose a treatment plan. **Risks:** Possible intolerance.
Homeopathy Highly diluted (potentized) solutions (*see* page 831) are believed to be able to redress vital energy imbalances and strengthen the body's defences. Organo- and functiotropic (*see* page 833) homeopathy is claimed to be effective for dealing with symptoms.	**Inappropriate** as the sole treatment for varicose veins, phlebitis, and chronic venous insufficiency. **May be of some use** as a supportive treatment attempt aimed at easing symptoms. Case reports claim success for organotropic preparations; however, success is probably seen in only a small proportion of patients (*see* Placebo, page xxi).	**Requires a qualified practitioner** Homeopaths should be properly qualified and should propose a treatment plan. Ready-formulated preparations are suitable for do-it-yourself. **Risks:** Allergies and intolerance are possible.
Magnetic field therapy The use of magnetic field generators, magnetic strips, bracelets, and other objects (*see* page 841) allegedly encourages cell metabolism and so eases symptoms.	**Inappropriate** Based on present knowledge, there is inadequate evidence of the efficacy and mode of action of magnetic field therapy in varicose veins, phlebitis, and chronic venous insufficiency.	Operation of magnetic field equipment **requires a qualified practitioner**. **Risks:** Magnetic field equipment can cause implanted cardiac pacemakers to malfunction.

Treatment	Rating	Point of delivery/risks
Massage Classical massage (*see* page 847) is said to invigorate the patient, as well as ease muscular and emotional tension. Lymphatic drainage (*see* page 850) is claimed to ease symptoms in persons with chronic venous insufficiency.	**Inappropriate** as the sole treatment for varicose veins, phlebitis, and chronic venous insufficiency. **May be of some use** as a supportive measure provided the treatment is perceived as being pleasant and soothing. Some case reports claim efficacy; however, success is probably seen in only a proportion of patients (*see* Placebo, page xxi).	**Suitable for DIY** Qualified guidance is recommended. Masseurs/masseuses should be properly qualified. **Risks:** Parts of the body affected by thrombosis must not be massaged.
Nutritional therapies An organic diet (*see* page 4) provides the body with essential and secondary plant nutrients, dietary fiber, antioxidants, etc., which are believed to exercise a multitude of positive effects (*see* pages 858–67).	**Inappropriate** as the sole treatment for varicose veins, phlebitis, and chronic venous insufficiency. **Useful** as an individually tailored supportive measure. The concrete effects of numerous recommended diets for preventing and treating varicose veins, phlebitis, and chronic venous insufficiency have not been fully documented.	**Suitable for DIY** Qualified guidance is recommended though not essential. **Risks:** Avoid imbalanced or intolerable diets. They can cause deficiencies with serious consequences. Children are particularly at risk.

Treatment	*Rating*	*Point of delivery/risks*
Physical therapies Various hydrotherapeutic measures (*see* pages 871–8) are claimed to ease symptoms of chronic venous insufficiency. Raising the legs and carrying out breathing exercises is claimed to improve the circulation; leg exercises and walking are said to stimulate the pumping action of the muscles. If sores are present, cold to warm wraps with various additives and bathing of the lower legs are said to have a disinfecting effect; alternating temperature knee and thigh douches are said to ease symptoms (*see* page 875).	**Useful** as an individually directed treatment attempt. Observational studies, case reports, and initial clinical studies (on carbon dioxide and Kneipp treatments) ascribe a degree of efficacy to these treatments in some patients.	**Suitable for DIY** Qualified guidance is recommended. Practitioners should be properly qualified and should propose a treatment plan. An individual plan of treatment should be defined in association with the treating physician. **Risks:** Skin damage may be caused to persons with diminished temperature sensation when extreme temperatures are applied.
Reflex therapies Reflex zone massage (*see* page 883), reflexology (*see* page 883), and TENS (*see* page 886) are claimed to act via reflex channels (*see* page 881) to ease pain, to relax the patient, and to improve his/her circulation.	**Inappropriate** as the sole treatment for varicose veins, phlebitis, and chronic venous insufficiency. **May be of some use** as a short-term, supportive treatment attempt aimed at alleviating pain and improving the circulation. Observational studies claim efficacy; however, success is probably seen in only a proportion of patients (*see* Placebo, page xxi).	**Suitable for DIY** Qualified guidance is essential. Therapists should propose a treatment plan. **Risks:** Some people are sensitive to electrical stimuli and rubber electrodes; others find it hard to tolerate manual stimulation or close physical contact.

Treatment	Rating	Point of delivery/risks
Relaxation techniques Autogenic training (*see* page 888), muscle relaxation according to Jacobson (*see* page 893), and various biofeedback techniques (*see* page 891) are said to relieve muscle tension and inner unrest.	**Inappropriate** as the sole treatment for varicose veins, phlebitis, and chronic venous insufficiency. **May be of some use** as a supportive treatment attempt aimed at soothing and relaxing. Case reports claim efficacy; however, success is probably seen in only a proportion of patients (*see* Placebo, page xxi).	**Suitable for DIY** Once a sound understanding of the technique has been acquired from a trainer, patients can perform exercises themselves. Therapists should be properly qualified. **Risks:** Fairly unlikely.
Vitamins and trace elements The antioxidative properties of beta-carotene, vitamins C and E, and selenium are, it is supposed, instrumental in countering the formation of free radicals and in boosting the body's antioxidative defence systems (*see* page 900).	**Inappropriate** as the sole treatment for varicose veins, phlebitis, and chronic venous insufficiency. **May be of some use** as a supportive measure. No definitive recommendations can be made based on present knowledge. Case reports claim efficacy; however, success is probably seen in only a small proportion of patients (*see* Placebo, page xxi).	**Suitable for DIY** Qualified guidance is recommended though not essential. **Risks:** Intolerance and overdosage are possible. Recent studies imply that beta-carotene might increase the risk of cancer.

Herbal remedies for varicose veins, phlebitis, and chronic venous insufficiency

Active ingredient/preparation	Rating
Arnica flowers (*Arnica montana*)	**Of little use** for external application in venous disease and superficial phlebitis. There is some doubt as to whether externally applied preparations for varicose veins have any efficacy. **Dosage:** As an embrocation, 2g to 4fl oz of water for rubbing onto the legs; for compresses use tincture diluted three- to tenfold; ointments should contain 20–25 percent tincture or maximum 15 percent oil. To apply, rub a few drops several times daily onto the area causing pain. Use ready-formulated preparations as instructed by the manufacturer/prescriber. **Risks:** Do not use internally. Do not use on broken skin. Arnica can damage skin and cause blistering.
Horse chestnut extract (*Aesculus hippocastanum*)	Taken internally, horse chestnut extract is **useful** for chronic venous insufficiency, soft tissue swellings, and swollen ankles. Used externally, it is **of little use**. There is some doubt as to whether externally applied preparations for varicose veins have any efficacy. **Daily dose:** 500–625mg extract or as instructed by the manufacturer/prescriber. **Risks:** Horse chestnut may cause gastric irritation, nausea, and itchiness. In injectables, aescin (the active principle in horse chestnut extract) may cause renal failure and kidney damage. Be sure to persist with other medically prescribed measures such as pressure dressings, support hosiery, and bathing with cold water.

Active ingredient/preparation	*Rating*
Horse chestnut extract in combination preparations	**Of little use**. In these combinations, horse chestnut extract is mixed with cardioactive herbal ingredients, vitamins, diuretics, and other preparations for varicose veins. Such combinations do not increase the efficacy of the product, but may produce a wide variety of side effects. **Dosage:** As instructed by the manufacturer/ prescriber. **Risks:** Horse chestnut may cause gastric irritation, nausea, and itchiness. In injectables, aescin (the active principle in horse chestnut extract) may cause renal failure and kidney damage. Be sure to persist with other medically prescribed measures such as pressure dressings, support hosiery, and bathing with cold water.
Shepherd's myrtle root (*Ruscus aculeatus*)	**May be of some use** (e.g. as a supportive measure alongside other physical therapies such as massage, support hosiery, etc.) in chronic venous insufficiency, also in muscular cramp in the calf, pruritus, swellings, and burns. In animal experiments, shepherd's myrtle has been seen to increase the tonus of the venous system. **Of little use** used externally. There is some doubt as to whether externally applied preparations for varicose veins have any efficacy. **Dosage:** As instructed by the manufacturer/ prescriber. **Risks:** Gastric problems and nausea may occur.
Sweet clover (*Melilotus officinalis*)	Taken orally, sweet clover is **useful** in chronic venous insufficiency and as a supportive measure in the treatment of superficial phlebitis. Applied externally, it is **of little use**. There is some doubt as to whether externally applied preparations for varicose veins have any efficacy. **Dosage:** As instructed by the manufacturer/ prescriber. **Risks:** May cause headaches when taken internally.

Active ingredient/preparation	Rating
Witch hazel leaves and bark (*Hamamelis virginiana*)	**Of little use** in venous disease and varicose veins. There is some doubt as to whether externally applied preparations for varicose veins have any efficacy. **Dosage:** for externally applied infusions: 0.1–1g herb one to three times daily; alternatively, add to bath water or use as an embrocation (ointment, gel, etc.). Use ready-formulated preparations as instructed by the manufacturer/prescriber. **Risks:** Witch hazel is not known to have any serious side effects.

Stomach, intestine, digestive system

Constipation

Causes and symptoms

Constipation, the difficult or infrequent passing of stools, can have a variety of causes, including acute or chronic emotional problems, stress, a poor diet, and jetlag; it may also be the result of toxins, bowel disease, or a neurological disorder, and can occur temporarily during pregnancy, after surgery, or as a side effect of certain drugs. Chronic constipation can lead to diverticulosis, the formation of small sacs (diverticulae) in the walls of the large intestine. Serious complications, including peritonitis, may set in if the diverticulae become chronically inflamed (diverticulitis). Chronic digestive problems are frequently equated with an increased risk of bowel cancer.

Constipation is probably less common than many people think. Having a motion only three times a week is normal and not a cause for alarm; though subjective feelings should be the final arbiter, measures need only be taken when there has not been a bowel movement for more than three days.

Orthodox treatment

Modern nutritionists recommend a high-fiber diet with plenty of fruit, vegetables, and cereals, as well as an adequate intake of fluids. This provides bulk and stimulates bowel movements. Counselling or psychotherapy may be recommended if chronic constipation is the result of stress or emotional problems.

For chronic constipation it is usual to prescribe laxatives; however, taken in the long term, they upset the body's fluid balance, lead to a loss of electrolytes (causing potassium and magnesium deficiency), and reduce the tone of the bowel muscles. Even natural plant-based laxatives can elicit these effects.

Complementary therapies

Various complementary therapies are claimed to relieve constipation. As in mainstream medicine, the emphasis will be on a high-fiber diet to stop constipation from occurring in the first place. Natural laxatives are used to encourage bowel movements.

Reflexologists claim to be able to relax body and mind and to directly influence bowel activity through energy links (*see* page 928). Some therapists see constipation as a constitutional problem (*see* Constitution, page 927) or as being caused by toxins (see page 929).

Treatment plan and limited trial

Before administering a complementary treatment, every therapist should propose a treatment plan (*see* page xxiii) that sets out a clear time frame and defines the goal that the treatment is designed to achieve. Treatment should then be tried for a limited term to test the patient's response.

Caution

You must consult a qualified physician if you notice any sudden change in your bowel activity that is not simply attributable to a change of diet or to taking prescribed medications.

Complementary treatments for constipation

Treatment	Rating	Point of delivery/risks
Acupressure This treatment (*see* page 769), otherwise known as pressure-point massage, is claimed to encourage bowel movements and improve general well-being when pressure is applied to the appropriate points.	**May be of some use** as a short-term treatment attempt. Case reports claim efficacy; however, success is probably seen in only a proportion of patients (*see* Placebo, page xxi).	**Suitable for DIY** Qualified guidance is recommended. Therapists should be properly qualified. **Risks:** Unlikely provided treatment is carried out competently.
Acupuncture Acupuncture in its various forms (*see* page 772) aims to encourage the flow of energy (*see* page 927) or to act directly to activate the digestive processes. The acupuncture points chosen can vary from one practitioner to another.	**May be of some use** as a short-term treatment attempt for chronic constipation. Some case reports claim efficacy; however, success is probably seen in only a proportion of patients (*see* Placebo, page xxi).	**Requires a qualified practitioner** Acupuncturists should be properly qualified and should propose a treatment plan. **Risks:** Probably rare provided treatment is carried out competently.
Anthroposophical medicine AM (*see* page 781) interprets constipation as sluggishness of the astral body, and treats it through dietary measures, with bitters, and with the preparation Digestodoron.	**May be of some use** as a short-term treatment attempt for chronic constipation. Case reports claim efficacy; however, success is probably seen in only a proportion of patients (*see* Placebo, page xxi).	**Requires a qualified practitioner** Practitioners should be properly qualified and should propose a treatment plan. **Risks:** Allergies and intolerance are possible.

Treatment	Rating	Point of delivery/risks
Aromatherapy Essential oils (*see* page 786) are used to soothe and relax, or to invigorate, thereby encouraging bowel movement and contributing to an easing of symptoms. The essences may be taken orally, used externally as massage oils or bathing emulsions, or inhaled as vapors.	**Of little use** Possibly acceptable as a short-term, supportive treatment attempt aimed at soothing and relaxing the gut. Some case reports claim efficacy; however, success is probably seen in only a small proportion of patients (*see* Placebo, page xxi).	**Suitable for DIY** Qualified guidance is recommended. The effects of individual essential oils differ widely. **Risks:** Allergies or intolerance are possible. Some oils are carcinogenic in test systems and possibly in humans.
Bioresonance therapy Bioresonance therapists use electrical devices in an attempt to discover the causes of illness and claim to be able to weaken or turn around pathogenic energies and disease related vibrations (*see* page 794).	**Of little use** Possibly acceptable in chronic constipation as a short-term treatment attempt when simpler, more established methods have been unsuccessful. Some case reports claim efficacy; however, success is probably seen, if at all, in only a small proportion of patients (*see* Placebo, page xxi).	**Requires a qualified practitioner** Practitioners should be properly qualified and should propose a treatment plan. No credence should be given to anyone promising immediate or total success. **Risks:** Fairly unlikely.
Cell therapy Injecting or ingesting products extracted from the tissues of newborn animals or animal fetuses is said to have a rejuvenating and revitalizing effect and to enhance the healing of human tissues and organs (*see* page 796).	**Not advised** Based on present knowledge, there is inadequate evidence of the efficacy and mode of action of these costly and relatively risky procedures.	**Risks:** Injecting foreign proteins into the body can provoke (possibly fatal) allergic reactions. Also, pathogens such as those that cause bovine spongiform encephalopathy (BSE) or other serious infections may be introduced.

Treatment	Rating	Point of delivery/risks
Electroacupuncture according to Voll By taking readings of the electrical conductivity of the skin (*see* page 802), therapists claim to be able to derive an insight into diseased areas of the body, pathogenic foci (*see* page 928), and stress factors (*see* Toxins, page 929). The factors presumed to be instrumental in the causation of constipation can then be addressed.	**Of little use** Possibly acceptable as a short-term treatment attempt for chronic constipation when simpler, more established methods have been unsuccessful. Some case reports claim efficacy; however, success is probably seen, if at all, in only a small proportion of patients (*see* Placebo, page xxi).	**Requires a qualified practitioner** Practitioners should be properly qualified and should propose a treatment plan. No credence should be given to anyone promising immediate or total success. **Risks:** A second opinion must always be obtained from a qualified physician before any attempt is made to "eliminate foci" (e.g. by surgery).
Electroneural therapy according to Croon According to the theory, readings taken at various reactive sites on the skin highlight diseased areas within the body. Based on these readings, targeted electrostimulative measures can be undertaken to address factors presumed to be instrumental in the causation of constipation (*see* page 806).	**Of little use** Possibly acceptable as a short-term, supportive treatment attempt for chronic constipation when simpler, more established methods have been unsuccessful. Some case reports claim efficacy; however, success is probably seen, if at all, in only a small proportion of patients (*see* Placebo, page xxi).	**Requires a qualified practitioner** Practitioners should be properly qualified and should propose a treatment plan. No credence should be given to anyone promising immediate or total success. **Risks:** Proponents themselves warn that treatment should not be given in acute inflammatory conditions.

Treatment	*Rating*	*Point of delivery/risks*
Eliminative methods, unbloody Enemas (*see* page 819) can provide relief from acute constipation. Unbloody cupping (*see* page 817) is said to ease symptoms and improve the body's own regulatory systems in chronic constipation.	Enemas are possibly **useful** in chronic constipation. Unbloody cupping **may be of some use** as a short-term treatment attempt for chronic constipation. Some case reports claim efficacy; however, success is probably seen in only a proportion of patients (*see* Placebo, page xxi).	**Suitable for DIY** Unbloody cupping is best carried out under the guidance of a qualified practitioner. **Risks:** Unlikely provided treatment is carried out competently.
Enzyme therapy The enzymes used (*see* page 824) are said to dispel and destroy "immune complexes" that course in the blood and that are responsible, for instance, for affecting digestion.	**Of little use** Some case reports claim efficacy for this little researched therapy; however, success is probably seen in only a small proportion of patients (*see* Placebo, page xxi).	**Requires a qualified practitioner** Practitioners should propose a treatment plan. Non-prescription preparations are suitable for do-it-yourself. **Risks:** Allergies or intolerance are possible.
Flower remedies Flower remedies (*see* page 828) are said to restore emotional balance and assist the body's psychic ability to heal itself.	**Of little use** Acceptable in chronic constipation as a short-term, supportive treatment attempt aimed at soothing and relaxing. Some case reports claim efficacy; however, success is probably seen in only a small proportion of patients (*see* Placebo, page xxi).	**Suitable for DIY** Qualified guidance is recommended. **Risks:** Possible intolerance.

Treatment	*Rating*	*Point of delivery/risks*
Homeopathy Highly diluted (potentized) solutions (*see* page 831) are believed to be able to redress vital energy imbalances and strengthen the body's defences. Organo- and functiotropic (*see* page 833) homeopathy is claimed to be effective for dealing directly with constipation.	**May be of some use** as a supportive treatment attempt for chronic constipation. Observational studies claim success for homeopathic treatments; however, success is probably seen in only a small proportion of patients (*see* Placebo, page xxi).	**Requires a qualified practitioner** Homeopaths should be properly qualified and should propose a treatment plan. Ready-formulated preparations are suitable for do-it-yourself. **Risks:** Allergies and intolerance are possible.
Hypnosis and self-hypnosis In the relaxed and generally altered state of awareness that is induced in hypnosis or self-hypnosis (*see* page 837), physical conditions can be addressed. Some professionally organized courses in self-hypnosis are now available. Hypnosis is sometimes used in combination with other psycho- and behavioral therapies.	**Of little use** Acceptable in chronic constipation as a short-term, supportive treatment attempt. Some case reports claim efficacy; however, success is probably seen in only a small proportion of patients (*see* Placebo, page xxi).	**Requires a qualified practitioner** Hypnotherapists should be properly qualified and should propose a treatment plan. **Risks:** Unlikely provided treatment is carried out competently.
Manual therapies Chiropractors and osteopaths (*see* page 844) use a series of manipulations to realign allegedly displaced vertebrae. This is said to ease tension, release energy blockages (*see* page 927), and address factors that may be at the root of constipation.	**Of little use** Possibly acceptable as a short-term treatment attempt for chronic constipation when more established methods have been unsuccessful. Some case reports claim efficacy; however, success is probably seen in only a proportion of patients (*see* Placebo, page xxi).	**Requires a qualified practitioner** Practitioners should be properly qualified and should propose a treatment plan. **Risks:** Manipulation of the head and cervical vertebrae can cause serious injury. Osteoporosis is one of several risk factors.

Treatment	Rating	Point of delivery/risks
Massage Classical massage (*see* page 847) is said to have an invigorating effect and to ease muscular and emotional tension, thereby possibly improving bowel movements. Colonic massage is said to be beneficial in chronic constipation.	**Of little use** Acceptable as a short-term treatment attempt for chronic constipation. Some case reports claim efficacy; however, success is probably seen in only a proportion of patients (*see* Placebo, page xxi).	**Requires a qualified practitioner** Masseurs/masseuses should be properly qualified and should propose a treatment plan. **Risks:** Some people are sensitive to manual stimuli; others find it hard to tolerate close physical contact.
Nutritional therapies An organic diet (*see* page 4) provides the body with essential and secondary plant nutrients that are believed to exercise a multitude of positive effects and to be capable, *inter alia*, of improving digestion (*see* pages 858–67).	**Useful** and recommended as an individually directed supportive measure. Observational studies, case reports, case studies, etc. confirm the efficacy of nutritional therapies for constipation.	**Suitable for DIY** Qualified guidance is recommended. Brief curative fasting can be a prelude to a change of diet. **Risks:** Avoid imbalanced or intolerable diets. They can cause deficiencies with serious consequences. Children are particularly at risk.
Physical therapies Cold treatments such as baths, foot baths, body wraps, knee douches, or cold abdominal washings are said to encourage digestion in persons with a sluggish bowel. Alternating temperature treatments, it is claimed, can give the body extra strength. Heat treatments such as ascending temperature sitz baths, wraps, or hot water bottles are said to ease a spastic colon (*see* pages 871–8).	**Useful** as a short-term treatment attempt for chronic constipation. Some case reports claim efficacy; however, success is probably seen in only a proportion of patients (*see* Placebo, page xxi).	**Suitable for DIY** Qualified guidance is recommended. Practitioners should be properly qualified and should propose a treatment plan. These treatments should be given in association with a nutritional therapy and an exercise therapy. **Risks:** Skin damage may be caused to persons with diminished temperature sensation when extreme temperatures are applied.

Treatment	Rating	Point of delivery/risks
Probiotics The introduction of certain bacteria into the gut is claimed to bring the intestinal flora back into balance and to improve digestion (*see* page 878).	**May be of some use** in persons with persistent symptoms, as a short-term treatment attempt aimed at rapid reinstatement of the intestinal flora after successful treatment for constipation. Some case reports claim efficacy; however, success is probably seen in only a proportion of patients (*see* Placebo, page xxi).	**Requires a qualified practitioner** Practitioners should be properly qualified and should propose a treatment plan. Non-prescription formulations are suitable for do-it-yourself. **Risks:** Fairly unlikely provided treatment is carried out competently.
Reflex therapies Reflex zone massage (*see* page 883), reflexology (*see* page 883), and TENS (*see* page 886) are claimed to act via reflex channels (*see* page 881) to relax the patient, ease symptoms, and improve digestion.	**May be of some use** as a short-term treatment attempt for chronic constipation. Some case reports claim efficacy; however, success is probably seen in only a small proportion of patients (*see* Placebo, page xxi). Comparison has shown all of these procedures to be of roughly equal merit, although their effects differ widely from one patient to another.	**Requires a qualified practitioner** Practitioners should be properly qualified and should propose a treatment plan. **Risks:** Some people are sensitive to electrical stimuli and rubber electrodes; others find it hard to tolerate manual stimulation or close physical contact.
Relaxation techniques Autogenic training (*see* page 888), muscle relaxation according to Jacobson (*see* page 893), and various biofeedback techniques (*see* page 891) are said to relieve muscle tension and inner unrest. These procedures are sometimes used in association with psycho- or behavioral therapies.	**Useful** as a short-term treatment attempt for chronic constipation. Some case reports and field studies claim efficacy; however, success is probably seen in only a proportion of patients (*see* Placebo, page xxi).	**Suitable for DIY** Once a sound understanding of the technique has been acquired from a trainer in group sessions or through individual tuition, patients can perform exercises themselves. Therapists should be properly qualified. **Risks:** Fairly unlikely.

Treatment	Rating	Point of delivery/risks
Vitamins and trace elements The antioxidative properties of beta-carotene, vitamins C and E, and selenium are, it is supposed, instrumental in countering the formation of free radicals, in boosting the body's own antioxidative defence systems, and in exercising a multitude of other beneficial effects (*see* page 900).	**Only useful** as a supportive treatment attempt in vitamin deficiency associated with the misuse of laxatives. There is no evidence to suggest that vitamins are efficacious in the treatment of constipation.	**Suitable for DIY** Qualified guidance is recommended though not essential. **Risks:** Intolerance and overdosage are possible. Recent studies imply that beta-carotene might increase the risk of cancer.

Herbal remedies for constipation

Active ingredient/preparation	Rating
Alder buckthorn (*Rhamnus frangula*)	**Of little use**. Taken orally, alder buckthorn is possibly acceptable as a treatment attempt for constipation or for conditions requiring a looser stool. Only to be used when the desired effect has not already been achieved by changing to a diet with a high fiber content. **Daily dose:** As a tea drink, 2g of bark to 1 cup of boiling water, taken in the evening. Use ready-formulated preparations as instructed by the manufacturer/prescriber. **Risks:** Contains anthraquinone alkaloids, which are suspected of causing gene mutations. Not to be used by persons with intestinal occlusion, acute inflammation of the bowel, hemorrhoids, or potassium deficiency, nor by children under 12 years old. Do not use during pregnancy, breastfeeding, or menstruation. Following prolonged use of alder buckthorn (longer than one to two weeks), the bowel may become more sluggish. Its use may also result in hypokalemia (increased digitalis sensitivity), pigmentary infiltration, and reddening of the urine.

Active ingredient/preparation	*Rating*
Aloes (sap from the leaves) (*Aloe barbadensis* and *ferox*)	**Of little use.** Taken orally, aloe sap is possibly acceptable as a treatment attempt for constipation or for conditions requiring a looser stool. Only to be used when the desired effect has not already been achieved by changing to a diet with a high fiber content. **Dosage:** As instructed by the manufacturer/prescriber. **Risks:** Contains anthraquinone alkaloids, which are suspected of causing gene mutations. May color the urine red. Not to be used by persons with intestinal occlusion or hemorrhoids, during menstruation, in acute inflammatory bowel disease, in children under 12 years old, during pregnancy (as it stimulates uterine contractions), and during breastfeeding. Following protracted use (longer than one to two weeks), it can make the bowel more sluggish. Also its use may result in loss of electrolytes, hypokalemia (increased digitalis sensitivity), and pigmentary infiltration of the intestine.
Cascara sagrada (*Rhamnus purshiana*)	**Of little use.** Taken orally, cascara sagrada is possibly acceptable as a treatment attempt for constipation or for conditions requiring a looser stool. **Daily dose:** In the evening as a decoction, 0.3–2.4g of bark to 1 cup of boiling water. **Risks:** Contains anthraquinone alkaloids, which are suspected of causing gene mutations. Do not use for long periods (maximum one to two weeks). Its use may result in pigmentary infiltration of the wall of the intestine and upset the electrolyte balance. The action of cardiac glycosides may be intensified. Not to be used by persons with intestinal occlusion, inflammation of the bowel, hemorrhoids, or potassium deficiency; nor during pregnancy and breastfeeding.

Active ingredient/preparation	Rating

Flea seeds (dark psyllium)
(*Plantago psyllium* and *indica*)

Taken orally, flea seeds **may be of some use** as a treatment attempt for constipation caused, for example, by prolonged sitting, by ignoring the defecation stimulus, or by an irritable bowel. They help regulate the bowel muscles. Take with plenty of fluid.
Daily dose: 10–30g seeds. **Individual dose:** 10–15g powder to be taken with 1 glass of cold water. Use ready-formulated preparations as instructed by the manufacturer/prescriber.
Risks: Flea seeds can cause allergic reactions. Not to be taken by persons with narrowing of the esophagus or of the gastrointestinal tract.

Linseed
(*Linum usitatissimum*)

Taken orally, linseed **may be of some use** as a treatment attempt for constipation and inflammation of the colon. It is also a demulcent.
Daily dose: 3 tablespoons (45g). **Individual dose:** Drink 1 tablespoon with 1 glass of cold water. Use ready-formulated preparations as instructed by the manufacturer/prescriber.
Risks: May cause other drugs taken simultaneously to be absorbed more slowly. Not to be taken by persons with any form of intestinal obstruction or occlusion.

Manna
(dried exudate from *Fraxinus ornus*)

Taken orally, manna **may be of some use** as a treatment attempt for constipation or for conditions requiring a looser stool.
Daily dose: 20–30g dried exudate (for children 2–16g). **Individual dose:** Take 10g dried exudate (for children 1–5g) with 1 glass of cold water. Use ready-formulated preparations as instructed by the manufacturer/prescriber.
Risks: Nausea and flatulence are possible. Not to be taken by persons with intestinal occlusion. Do not use for any length of time without speaking to your doctor.

Active ingredient/preparation	*Rating*
Pale psyllium (*Plantago ovata* and *ispaghula*)	Taken orally, pale psyllium **may be of some use** as a treatment attempt for habit-related constipation and conditions requiring a looser stool; as a supportive measure in diarrhea and irritable bowel syndrome. As well as being a laxative, pale psyllium reduces cholesterol levels. **Daily dose:** Seeds up to 15g. **Pale psyllium seeds, individual dose:** Take 3–5g dried seeds with 5fl oz of water. **Pale psyllium seed cases, individual dose:** Take 10g with 1 glass of water, maximum two to three times per day. Use ready-formulated preparations as instructed by the manufacturer/prescriber. **Risks:** Can lead to hypersensitivities and may slow down absorption of various drugs (take half to one hour apart). Not to be used in persons with intestinal occlusion, poor diabetic control, or pathological narrowing of the gastrointestinal tract. Insulin-dependent diabetics should consider reducing their insulin dose (ask your doctor first). Consult a doctor if symptoms persist (for more than three to four days).
Rhubarb root (*Rheum palmatum* or *officinale*)	**Of little use**. Taken orally, rhubarb root may be acceptable as a treatment attempt for constipation or for conditions requiring a looser stool. **Daily dose:** rhizome/root 0.2–1.0g. **Individual dose:** To prepare a decoction, cover 1g of root with 1 cup of boiling water, bring to the boil, simmer for ten minutes, strain, and drink, preferably in the evening. Use ready-formulated preparations as instructed by the manufacturer/prescriber. **Risks:** Contains anthraquinone alkaloids, which are suspected of causing gene mutations. Do not use for long periods (maximum one to two weeks). Its use may result in pigmentary infiltration of the wall of the intestine and upset the electrolyte balance. Not to be used by persons with intestinal occlusion, inflammation of the bowel, hemorrhoids, or potassium deficiency; nor during pregnancy, breastfeeding, or menstruation.

Active ingredient/preparation	Rating
Senna fruits (pods) and leaves (*Cassia senna* and *angustifolia*)	Taken orally, senna **may be of some use** as a treatment attempt for constipation or for conditions requiring a looser stool, e.g. in patients having to take strong painkillers such as morphine. The leaves contain a higher concentration of active principle than the pods. **Daily dose:** 0.5–1.5g dried pods or leaves. **Individual dose:** 2 teaspoons of leaves or pods. Cover leaves with cold or lukewarm water, allow to steep for one to two hours, strain, and drink in the evening. Alternatively, cover fruits with 1 cup of hot water, allow to steep for five minutes, strain, and drink. Use ready-formulated preparations as instructed by the manufacturer/prescriber. **Risks:** Contains anthraquinone alkaloids, which are suspected of causing gene mutations. Its use may result in pigmentary infiltration of the wall of the intestine and upset the electrolyte balance. Senna may also intensify the action of cardiac glycosides, cause protein and red blood cells to be excreted in the urine, and damage the plexus myentericus (ganglion cells in the gastrointestinal tract). Not to be used by persons with intestinal occlusion, inflammation of the bowel, hemorrhoids or potassium deficiency; nor during pregnancy, breastfeeding, and menstruation. Do not use for long periods (maximum one to two weeks).

Diarrhea

Causes and symptoms

Diarrhea may accompany a number of infectious and non-infectious diseases. Various psychological factors, or a serious physical ailment, can cause chronic diarrhea.

Orthodox treatment

Replacement of fluid and electrolytes (oral rehydration) is the mainstay of orthodox treatment. As well as treating the disease, if any, thought to be causing the problem, doctors will frequently prescribe a medication to make stools less watery.

Complementary therapies

The most common treatments in complementary medicine center around nutritional therapy, reflexology, and herbalism.

Treatment plan and limited trial

Before administering a complementary treatment, every therapist should propose a treatment plan (*see* page xxiii) that sets out a clear time frame and defines the goal that the treatment is designed to achieve. Treatment should then be tried for a limited term to test the patient's response.

Caution

Always consult a physician if diarrhea is recurrent or persistent, as the symptoms may point to something more serious.

Complementary treatments for diarrhea

Treatment	Rating	Point of delivery/risks
Acupressure This treatment (*see* page 769), otherwise known as pressure-point massage, is claimed to influence bowel function when pressure is applied to the appropriate points.	**Of little use** Acceptable as a short-term treatment attempt. Some case reports claim efficacy; however, success is probably seen in only a proportion of patients (*see* Placebo, page xxi).	**Suitable for DIY** Qualified guidance is recommended. Therapists should be properly qualified. **Risks:** Unlikely provided treatment is carried out competently.

Treatment	*Rating*	*Point of delivery/risks*
Acupuncture Acupuncture in its various forms (*see* page 772) aims to encourage the flow of energy (*see* page 927) or to act directly to strengthen the bowel. The acupuncture points chosen can vary from one practitioner to another.	**Of little use** Acceptable as a short-term treatment attempt in persistent cases. Some case reports claim efficacy; however, success is probably seen in only a proportion of patients (*see* Placebo, page xxi).	**Requires a qualified practitioner** Practitioners should be properly qualified and should propose a treatment plan. **Risks:** Probably rare provided treatment is carried out competently.
Anthroposophical medicine For chronic diarrhea, doctors who practice AM (*see* page 781) carry out a constitutional treatment based on psychosomatic considerations, and prescribe individual compositions.	**May be of some use** as a short-term treatment attempt for chronic diarrhea when simpler methods have been unsuccessful. Case reports claim efficacy; however, success is probably seen in only a proportion of patients (*see* Placebo, page xxi).	**Requires a qualified practitioner** Practitioners should be properly qualified and should propose a treatment plan. **Risks:** Allergies and intolerance are possible.
Aromatherapy Essential oils (*see* page 786) are used to soothe and relax, or to invigorate, and so contribute to an easing of symptoms. The essences may be taken orally, used externally as massage oils or bathing emulsions, or inhaled as vapors.	**Of little use** Acceptable as a short-term treatment attempt aimed at soothing and relaxing the patient and improving mental outlook. Some case reports claim efficacy; however, success is probably seen, if at all, in only a small proportion of patients (*see* Placebo, page xxi).	**Suitable for DIY** Qualified guidance is recommended. The effects of individual essential oils differ widely. **Risks:** Allergies or intolerance are possible. Some oils are carcinogenic in test systems and possibly in humans.

Treatment	*Rating*	*Point of delivery/risks*
Bioresonance therapy Bioresonance therapists use electrical devices in an attempt to discover the causes of illness and claim to be able to weaken or turn around pathogenic energies and disease related vibrations (*see* page 794).	**Of little use** Possibly acceptable as a short-term, supportive treatment attempt for chronic diarrhea when simpler, more established methods have been unsuccessful. Some case reports claim efficacy; however, success is probably seen, if at all, in only a small proportion of patients (*see* Placebo, page xxi).	**Requires a qualified practitioner** Practitioners should be properly qualified and should propose a treatment plan. No credence should be given to anyone promising immediate or total success. **Risks:** Fairly unlikely.
Cell therapy Injecting or ingesting products extracted from the tissues of newborn animals or animal fetuses is said to have a rejuvenating and revitalizing effect and to enhance the healing of human tissues and organs (*see* page 796).	**Not advised** Based on present knowledge, there is inadequate evidence of the efficacy and mode of action of these costly and relatively risky procedures.	**Risks:** Injecting foreign proteins into the body can provoke (possibly fatal) allergic reactions. Also, pathogens such as those that cause bovine spongiform encephalopathy (BSE) or other serious infections may be introduced.
Electroacupuncture according to Voll By taking readings of the electrical conductivity of the skin (*see* page 802), therapists claim to be able to derive an insight into diseased areas of the body, pathogenic foci (*see* page 928), and stress factors (*see* Toxins, page 929). The factors presumed to be instrumental in the causation of diarrhea can then be addressed.	**Of little use** Possibly acceptable as a short-term, supportive treatment attempt for chronic diarrhea when simpler, more established methods have been unsuccessful. Some case reports claim efficacy; however, success is probably seen, if at all, in only a small proportion of patients (*see* Placebo, page xxi).	**Requires a qualified practitioner** Practitioners should be properly qualified and should propose a treatment plan. No credence should be given to anyone promising immediate or total success. **Risks:** A second opinion must always be obtained from a qualified physician before any attempt is made to "eliminate foci" (e.g. by surgery).

Treatment	Rating	Point of delivery/risks
Electroneural therapy according to Croon According to the theory, readings taken at various reactive sites on the skin highlight diseased areas within the body. Based on these readings, targeted electrostimulative measures can be undertaken to address factors presumed to be instrumental in the causation of diarrhea (*see* page 806).	**Of little use** Possibly acceptable as a short-term, supportive treatment attempt for persistent diarrhea when simpler, more established methods have been unsuccessful. Some case reports claim efficacy; however, success is probably seen, if at all, in only a small proportion of patients (*see* Placebo, page xxi).	**Requires a qualified practitioner** Practitioners should be properly qualified and should propose a treatment plan. No credence should be given to anyone promising immediate or total success. **Risks:** Proponents themselves warn that treatment should not be given in acute inflammatory conditions.
Enzyme therapy The enzymes used (*see* page 824) are said to dispel and destroy "immune complexes" that course in the blood and that are responsible, for instance, for sustaining inflammatory processes.	**Of little use** Some case reports claim efficacy for this little researched therapy; however, success is probably seen in only a small proportion of patients (*see* Placebo, page xxi).	**Requires a qualified practitioner** Practitioners should propose a treatment plan. Non-prescription preparations are suitable for do-it-yourself. **Risks:** Allergies or intolerance are possible.
Flower remedies For many flower therapists, diarrhea is an expression of emotional disharmony. Flower remedies (*see* page 828) are said to restore emotional balance and assist the body's psychic ability to heal itself.	**Of little use** Acceptable as a short-term, supportive treatment attempt aimed at soothing and relaxing. Some case reports claim efficacy; however, success is probably seen in only a small proportion of patients (*see* Placebo, page xxi).	**Suitable for DIY** Qualified guidance is recommended. Practitioners should propose a treatment plan. **Risks:** Possible intolerance.

Treatment	Rating	Point of delivery/risks
Homeopathy Highly diluted (potentized) solutions (*see* page 831) are believed to be able to redress vital energy imbalances. Organo- and functiotropic (*see* page 833) homeopathy is claimed to be effective for dealing with diarrhea.	**May be of some use** in chronic diarrhea as a supportive treatment attempt. Case reports and initial studies claim success for homeopathic treatments for diarrhea; however, success is probably seen in only a proportion of patients (*see* Placebo, page xxi).	**Requires a qualified practitioner** Homeopaths should be properly qualified and should propose a treatment plan. Ready-formulated preparations are suitable for do-it-yourself. **Risks:** Allergies and intolerance are possible.
Hypnosis and self-hypnosis In the relaxed and generally altered state of awareness that is induced in hypnosis or self-hypnosis (*see* page 837), physical and mental conditions can be addressed. Professionally organized courses in self-hypnosis are occasionally available.	**Of little use** Acceptable in persistent cases as a short-term treatment attempt aimed at relaxing the patient. Case reports claim efficacy; however, success is probably seen in only a proportion of patients (*see* Placebo, page xxi).	**Requires a qualified practitioner** Hypnotherapists should be properly qualified and should propose a treatment plan. **Risks:** Unlikely provided treatment is carried out competently.
Manual therapies Chiropractors and osteopaths (*see* page 844) use a series of manipulations to realign allegedly displaced vertebrae. This is said to overcome dysfunctions, release energy blockages (*see* page 927), and ease symptoms.	**Of little use** Possibly acceptable in persistent cases as a short-term, supportive treatment attempt when less risky, more established methods have been unsuccessful. Case reports claim efficacy; however, success is probably seen, if at all, in only a proportion of patients (*see* Placebo, page xxi).	**Requires a qualified practitioner** Practitioners should be properly qualified and should propose a treatment plan. **Risks:** Manipulation of the head and cervical vertebrae can cause serious injury. Osteoporosis is one of several risk factors.

Treatment	Rating	Point of delivery/risks
Massage Classical massage (*see* page 847) can, it is said, soothe the bowel and ease muscular and emotional tension.	**Of little use** Acceptable in persistent cases as a treatment attempt aimed at relaxing the patient. Some case reports claim efficacy; however, success is probably seen, if at all, in only a small proportion of patients (*see* Placebo, page xxi).	**Requires a qualified practitioner** Masseurs/masseuses should be properly qualified and should propose a treatment plan. **Risks:** Some people are sensitive to manual stimuli; others find it hard to tolerate close physical contact.
Nutritional therapies Brief therapeutic fasting (*see* page 864) is said to be good for the treatment of acute diarrhea. The fluids and minerals lost should be replenished by drinking herbal teas and freshly boiled non-fatty vegetable broths.	**Useful** as an individually directed short-term treatment attempt for acute diarrhea (*see* Placebo, page xxi).	**Suitable for DIY** Qualified guidance is recommended. **Risks:** Avoid imbalanced or intolerable diets. They can cause deficiencies with serious consequences. Children are particularly at risk.
Physical therapies Moist wraps and packs (*see* pages 877–8) or a hayseed pillow are said to soothe and relax persons with acute diarrhea.	**Of little use** Acceptable as a short-term, supportive treatment attempt. Some case reports claim efficacy; however, success is probably seen in only a small proportion of patients (*see* Placebo, page xxi).	**Suitable for DIY** Qualified guidance is recommended though not essential. **Risks:** Unlikely provided treatment is carried out competently.

Treatment	Rating	Point of delivery/risks
Probiotics The introduction of certain bacteria into the gut is claimed to bring the intestinal flora back into balance and to have a beneficial effect in the treatment of diarrhea (*see* page 878).	**Of little use** Acceptable as a short-term treatment attempt for chronic diarrhea when more established methods have been unsuccessful. Some case reports claim efficacy; however, success is probably seen in only a proportion of patients (*see* Placebo, page xxi).	**Requires a qualified practitioner** Practitioners should be properly qualified and should propose a treatment plan. Non-prescription formulations are suitable for do-it-yourself. **Risks:** Fairly unlikely provided treatment is carried out competently.
Reflex therapies Reflex zone massage (*see* page 883) and reflexology (*see* page 883) are claimed to act via reflex channels (*see* page 881) to alleviate symptoms.	**Of little use** Acceptable as a short-term, supportive treatment attempt. Some case reports and field studies claim efficacy; however, success is probably seen in only a proportion of patients (*see* Placebo, page xxi).	**Suitable for DIY** Qualified guidance is essential. **Risks:** Some people are sensitive to electrical stimuli and rubber electrodes; others find it hard to tolerate manual stimulation or close physical contact.
Relaxation techniques Autogenic training (*see* page 888), muscle relaxation according to Jacobson (*see* page 893), and various biofeedback techniques (*see* page 891) are said to relieve muscle tension and inner unrest, and might be instrumental in bringing relief from chronic diarrhea.	**Of little use** Acceptable as a treatment attempt for relaxing patients with chronic diarrhea. Some case reports claim efficacy; however, success is probably seen in only a small proportion of patients (*see* Placebo, page xxi).	**Suitable for DIY** Once a sound understanding of the technique has been acquired from a trainer in group sessions or through individual tuition, patients can perform exercises themselves. Therapists should propose a treatment plan **Risks:** Fairly unlikely.

Herbal remedies for diarrhea

Active ingredient/preparation	Rating
Agrimony (*Agrimonia eupatoria*)	Taken orally, agrimony **may be of some use** as a treatment attempt for mild acute diarrhea. **Daily dose:** 3–6g dried herb. **Individual dose:** Pour 1 cup of hot water over 1.5g of herb and infuse. Drink before meals. Use ready-formulated preparations as instructed by the manufacturer/prescriber. **Risks:** Agrimony is not known to have any serious side effects.
Bilberries (*Vaccinium myrtillus*)	Taken orally, bilberries **may be of some use** as a treatment attempt for acute diarrhea. **Mean daily dose:** 20–60g berries. **Individual dose:** Pour 1 cup of water over 10g of berries, bring to a boil and simmer for 30 minutes, strain, and drink; alternatively, chew 1 tablespoon of bilberries several times a day. Be sure to see your doctor if the diarrhea persists (for longer than three to four days). **Risks:** Bilberries are not known to have any serious side effects.
Carbo coffea (*Coffea arabica*)	Taken orally, this remedy **may be of some use** as a treatment attempt for acute diarrhea. It has an astringent action and binds organisms that cause diarrhea. **Daily dose:** 9g. **Individual dose:** Stir 3g in cold water or juice and drink. Use ready-formulated preparations as instructed by the manufacturer/prescriber. **Risks:** Carbo coffea is not known to have any serious side effects.
Jambul (*Syzygium cumini*)	Taken orally, jambul **may be of some use** as a treatment attempt for acute diarrhea. It has an astringent action. **Daily dose:** 3–6g dried fruit. **Individual dose:** Pour 1 cup of hot water over 1–2g of dried fruit and infuse. Be sure to see your doctor if the diarrhea persists (for longer than three to four days). **Risks:** Possible gastric complaints.

Active ingredient/preparation	Rating

Lady's mantle
(*Alchemilla vulgaris*)

Taken orally, lady's mantle **may be of some use** as a treatment attempt for mild bouts of diarrhea. It has an astringent action.
Daily dose: 5–10g herb. **Individual dose:** Pour 1 cup of boiling water over 2.5g of dried herb and infuse. Be sure to see your doctor if the diarrhea persists (for longer than three to four days).
Risks: Lady's mantle is not known to have any serious side effects.

Oak bark
(*Quercus robur* and *petraea*)

Taken orally, oak bark **may be of some use** as a treatment attempt for acute diarrhea.
Daily dose: 3g bark.
Individual dose: For a decoction: 1g of bark to 1 cup of cold water, bring to the boil, and simmer briefly. Drink several times daily half an hour before meals. Be sure to see your doctor if the diarrhea persists (for longer than three to four days).
Risks: Drinking oak bark tea can reduce the uptake of alkaline and alkaloid-containing drugs.

Opium tincture
(*Papaver somniferum*)

Only useful as an oral treatment attempt for severe diarrhea that has not responded to other measures (for example, it may be tried in elderly persons with uncontrolled bowel movements or in patients with bowel cancer).
Dosage: The maximum prescribed amount of tincture per day is 20g. Opium tincture is a controlled substance.
Risks: Sedation, nausea, lethargy, respiratory depression. Quickly leads to drug dependency.

Pectin

Of little use. Pectin is said to be able to bind bacteria. There is no definitive evidence that it works, however. Pectin is found, for instance, in apple peel, which is why grated apple mixed with banana and rusks is a recommended remedy for diarrhea.
Dosage: As instructed by the manufacturer/ prescriber.
Risks: Pectin is not known to have any serious side effects.

Active ingredient/preparation	Rating
Silverweed (*Potentilla anserina*)	Taken orally, silverweed **may be of some use** as a treatment attempt for acute diarrhea (mild forms). **Daily dose:** 4–6g herb. **Individual dose:** Pour 1 cup of boiling water over 2g of dried herb and infuse. Drink several times daily. Use ready-formulated preparations as instructed by the manufacturer/prescriber. **Risks:** Stomach irritation may occur. Silverweed can also cause the uterine muscle to contract.
Tormentil root (*Potentilla erecta*)	Taken orally, tormentil **may be of some use** as a treatment attempt for acute diarrhea. It has an astringent action. **Daily dose:** 4–6g dried root. **Individual dose:** For a decoction, place 2g in cold water, bring to a boil, simmer, and strain; alternatively, 10–20 drops of tincture to 1 cup of water, or on sugar. Use capsules as instructed by the manufacturer/prescriber. **Risks:** Possible gastric complaints.
Uzara root (*Xysmalobium undulatum*)	Taken orally, uzara root **may be of some use** as a treatment attempt for acute diarrhea. **Daily dose:** Up to 1.2g root. **Individual dose:** Pour hot water over 0.5–1g of root. Use ready-formulated preparations as instructed by the manufacturer/prescriber. Be sure to see your doctor if the diarrhea persists (for longer than three to four days). **Risks:** Not to be taken with digitalis glycosides, as the root itself contains digitalis and may increase the risk of digitalis intoxication.

Active ingredient/preparation	*Rating*
Dried yeast (*Saccharomyces cerevisiae*)	**May be of some use** in acute diarrhea and for preventing "travel tummy" and diarrhea often associated with tube feeding. **Dosage:** For children over two years and adults five days before departure, 250–500mg daily (prophylaxis), 250–500mg daily (therapy). The preparations are for oral use. For diarrhea from tube feeding: 500mg per quart nutrient solution. Use ready-formulated preparations as instructed by the manufacturer/prescriber. **Risks:** Occasionally there will be hypersensitivity with itchiness, rarely even Quincke's edema. Has a hypertensive action when taken together with MAO inhibitors (a type of antidepressant drug). Not to be taken by persons known to be hypersensitive to yeast. It can cause flatulence.

Gall bladder disease

Causes and symptoms

"Gall bladder disease" is a term covering a number of inflammatory and non-inflammatory diseases of the gall bladder and bile ducts. It presents in a variety of ways, ranging from nausea and vomiting to colicky pains in the upper right abdomen.

Orthodox treatment

Depending on its etiology and symptoms, gall bladder disease will be treated with drugs, by endoscopy, or by surgery.

Complementary therapies

Complementary practitioners generally take a symptom oriented approach to the treatment of gall bladder disease.

Treatment plan and limited trial

Before administering a complementary treatment, every therapist should propose a treatment plan (*see* page xxiii) that sets out a clear time frame and defines the goal that the treatment is designed to achieve. Treatment should then be tried for a limited term to test the patient's response.

Caution

When the disease is associated with acute, severe, or febrile symptoms, complementary medicine has no effective alternative to modern antibiotics and state of the art surgical techniques.

Complementary treatments for gallbladder disease

Treatment	Rating	Point of delivery/risks
Acupressure This treatment (*see* page 769), otherwise known as pressure-point massage, is used to relieve pain in the upper right abdomen, to ease tension, and to improve general well-being. Acupressure is also used as a restorative measure designed to impart vital energy (*see* Life force, page 928).	**May be of some use** as a short-term, supportive treatment attempt aimed at alleviating pain, e.g. in the upper right abdomen. Case reports ascribe a degree of efficacy to this treatment; however, success is probably seen in only a proportion of patients (*see* Placebo, page xxi).	**Suitable for DIY** Qualified guidance is essential. Therapists should be properly qualified and should propose a treatment plan. **Risks:** Unlikely provided treatment is carried out competently.
Acupuncture Acupuncture in its various forms (*see* page 772) aims to encourage the flow of energy (*see* page 927) or to act directly to ease pain in the upper right abdomen. The acupuncture points chosen can vary from one practitioner to another.	**May be of some use** as a short-term, supportive treatment attempt aimed at alleviating pain, e.g. in the upper right abdomen. Case reports and field studies claim efficacy; however, success is probably seen in only a proportion of patients (*see* Placebo, page xxi).	**Requires a qualified practitioner** Acupuncturists should be properly qualified and should propose a treatment plan. **Risks:** Probably rare provided treatment is carried out competently.

Treatment	Rating	Point of delivery/risks
Anthroposophical medicine AM (*see* page 781) interprets gall bladder disease as an expression of excessive hardening in metabolic reactions. The preparation Choleodoron is used to encourage the flow of bile, while in attacks of colic the potentized preparation Oxalis Compositum is used.	**May be of some use** as a short-term, supportive treatment attempt. Case reports claim efficacy; however, success is probably seen in only a proportion of patients (*see* Placebo, page xxi).	**Requires a qualified practitioner** Practitioners should be properly qualified and should propose a treatment plan. **Risks:** Allergies and intolerance are possible.
Aromatherapy Essential oils (*see* page 786) are used to soothe and relax, or to invigorate, contributing to pain relief. The essences may be taken orally, used externally as massage oils or bathing emulsions, or inhaled as vapors.	**Of little use** Acceptable as a short-term, supportive treatment attempt aimed at soothing and relaxing, or invigorating. Some case reports ascribe a degree of efficacy to this treatment in the relief of pain; however, success is probably seen in only a small proportion of patients (*see* Placebo, page xxi).	**Suitable for DIY** Qualified guidance is recommended. The effects of individual essential oils differ widely. **Risks:** Allergies or intolerance are possible. Some oils are carcinogenic in test systems and possibly in humans.
Bioresonance therapy Bioresonance therapists use electrical devices in an attempt to discover the causes of illness and claim to be able to weaken or turn around pathogenic energies and disease related vibrations (*see* page 794).	**Of little use** Possibly acceptable as a short-term, supportive treatment attempt when simpler, more established methods have been unsuccessful. Some case reports claim efficacy; however, success is probably seen, if at all, in only a small proportion of patients (*see* Placebo, page xxi).	**Requires a qualified practitioner** Practitioners should be properly qualified and should propose a treatment plan. No credence should be given to anyone promising immediate or total success. **Risks:** Fairly unlikely.

Treatment	Rating	Point of delivery/risks
Cell therapy Injecting or ingesting products extracted from animal tissues or organs is said to have a rejuvenating and revitalizing effect and to enhance the healing of human tissues and organs (*see* page 796).	**Not advised** Based on present knowledge, there is inadequate evidence of the efficacy and mode of action of these costly and relatively risky procedures.	**Risks:** Injecting foreign proteins into the body can provoke (possibly fatal) allergic reactions. Also, pathogens such as those that cause bovine spongiform encephalopathy (BSE) or other serious infections may be introduced.
Chelation therapy The chelating agent EDTA (*see* page 800) is able, it is claimed, to bind calcareous deposits. These are subsequently eliminated from the body. It is also reputed to be able to dissolve gall stones.	**Not advised** Evidence of the therapeutic usefulness of this risky procedure is lacking.	**Risks:** EDTA can cause a deficit of calcium and essential heavy metals and, in extreme cases, can lead to cardiac arrhythmia, respiratory failure, cramps, and death.
Electroacupuncture according to Voll By taking readings of the electrical conductivity of the skin (*see* page 802), therapists claim to be able to derive an insight into diseased areas of the body, pathogenic foci (*see* page 928), and stress factors (*see* Toxins, page 929). The factors presumed to be instrumental in the causation of gall bladder disease can then be addressed.	**Of little use** Possibly acceptable as a short-term, supportive treatment attempt when simpler, more established methods have been unsuccessful. Some case reports claim a degree of efficacy in the treatment of gall bladder disease; however, success is probably seen, if at all, in only a small proportion of patients (*see* Placebo, page xxi).	**Requires a qualified practitioner** Practitioners should be properly qualified and should propose a treatment plan. No credence should be given to anyone promising immediate or total success. **Risks:** A second opinion must always be obtained from a qualified physician before any attempt is made to "eliminate foci" (e.g. by surgery).

Treatment	Rating	Point of delivery/risks
Electroneural therapy according to Croon According to the theory, readings taken at various reactive sites on the skin highlight diseased areas within the body. Based on these readings, targeted electrostimulative measures can be undertaken to address factors presumed to be instrumental in the causation of gall bladder disease (*see* page 806).	**Of little use** Possibly acceptable as a short-term, supportive treatment attempt when simpler, more established methods have been unsuccessful. Some case reports claim efficacy; however, success is probably seen, if at all, in only a small proportion of patients (*see* Placebo, page xxi).	**Requires a qualified practitioner** Practitioners should be properly qualified and should propose a treatment plan. No credence should be given to anyone promising immediate or total success. **Risks:** Proponents themselves warn that treatment should not be given in acute inflammatory conditions.
Eliminative methods, bloody Bloody cupping (*see* page 815) is occasionally used in patients with persistent pain in the upper right abdomen, as a means of improving the body's own regulatory systems.	**Of little use** Possibly acceptable as a short-term, supportive treatment attempt in persistent cases when more established, less invasive methods have been unsuccessful. Some case reports ascribe a degree of efficacy to this treatment; however, success is probably seen in only a small proportion of patients (*see* Placebo, page xxi).	**Requires a qualified practitioner** Practitioners should be properly qualified and should propose a treatment plan. **Risks:** Bloody cupping can cause infection and scarring. Furthermore, it should not be carried out in persons with bleeding disorders.
Eliminative methods, unbloody Unbloody cupping (*see* page 817) is occasionally used in patients with pain in the upper right abdomen, as a means of easing pain, improving the body's own regulatory systems, and energizing (*see* page 927) the patient.	**May be of some use** as a short-term, supportive treatment attempt aimed at alleviating pain. Some case reports and field studies claim efficacy; however, success is probably seen in only a proportion of patients (*see* Placebo, page xxi).	**Suitable for DIY** Unbloody cupping is best carried out under the guidance of a qualified practitioner. **Risks:** Unlikely provided treatment is carried out competently.

Treatment	Rating	Point of delivery/risks
Enzyme therapy The enzymes used (*see* page 824) are said to dispel and destroy "immune complexes" that course in the blood and that are responsible, for instance, for sustaining inflammatory processes.	**Of little use** Some case reports claim efficacy for this little researched therapy; however, success is probably seen in only a small proportion of patients (*see* Placebo, page xxi).	**Requires a qualified practitioner** Practitioners should propose a treatment plan. Non-prescription preparations are suitable for do-it-yourself. **Risks:** Allergies or intolerance are possible.
Flower remedies Flower remedies (*see* page 828) are said to restore emotional balance and assist the body's psychic ability to heal itself.	**Of little use** Acceptable as a short-term, supportive treatment attempt aimed at soothing and relaxing. Case reports claim a degree of efficacy in the treatment of gall bladder disease; however, success is probably seen in only a small proportion of patients (*see* Placebo, page xxi).	**Suitable for DIY** Qualified guidance is recommended. Practitioners should propose a treatment plan. **Risks:** Possible intolerance.
Homeopathy Highly diluted (potentized) solutions (*see* page 831) are believed to be able to redress vital energy imbalances. Organo- and functiotropic (*see* page 833) homeopathy is claimed to be effective for dealing with gall bladder disease.	**May be of some use** as a supportive treatment attempt. Case reports and field studies claim efficacy; however, success is probably seen in only a proportion of patients (*see* Placebo, page xxi).	**Requires a qualified practitioner** Homeopaths should be properly qualified and should propose a treatment plan. Ready-formulated preparations are suitable for do-it-yourself. **Risks:** Allergies and intolerance are possible.

Treatment	Rating	Point of delivery/risks
Hypnosis and self-hypnosis In the relaxed and generally altered state of awareness that is induced in hypnosis or self-hypnosis (*see* page 837), physical and mental conditions can be addressed. Hypnosis is often used in combination with other psycho- and behavioral therapies to help the patient change his/her lifestyle.	**Of little use** Acceptable as a short-term, supportive treatment attempt aimed at relaxing the patient and helping to bring about a change in his/her lifestyle when simpler, more established methods have been unsuccessful. Some case reports claim efficacy; however, success is probably seen in only a proportion of patients (*see* Placebo, page xxi).	**Requires a qualified practitioner** Hypnotherapists should be properly qualified and should propose a treatment plan. **Risks:** Unlikely provided treatment is carried out competently.
Manual therapies Chiropractors and osteopaths (*see* page 844) use a series of manipulations to realign allegedly displaced vertebrae. This is said to reduce pain and release energy blockages (*see* page 927).	**Of little use** Acceptable as a short-term, supportive treatment attempt in persistent cases when less risky, more established methods have been unsuccessful. Some case reports claim efficacy for these potentially risky procedures; however, success is probably seen, if at all, in only a small proportion of patients (*see* Placebo, page xxi).	**Requires a qualified practitioner** Practitioners should be properly qualified and should propose a treatment plan. **Risks:** Manipulation of the head and cervical vertebrae can cause serious injury. Osteoporosis is one of several risk factors.
Massage Classical massage (*see* page 847) can soothe or invigorate the patient, as well as relieve pain and ease muscular and emotional tension.	**Of little use** Acceptable as a short-term, supportive treatment attempt aimed at relaxing the patient. Case reports and field studies claim efficacy; however, success is probably seen in only a proportion of patients (*see* Placebo, page xxi).	**Suitable for DIY** Qualified guidance is recommended. Masseurs/masseuses should propose a treatment plan. **Risks:** Some people are sensitive to manual stimuli; others find it hard to tolerate close physical contact.

Treatment	Rating	Point of delivery/risks
Nutritional therapies An organic diet (*see* page 4) provides the body with essential and secondary plant nutrients that are believed to exercise a multitude of positive effects.	**Useful** as an individually directed general measure aimed at prevention and lessening the tendency to relapse.	**Suitable for DIY** Qualified guidance is recommended though not essential. **Risks:** Avoid imbalanced or intolerable diets. They can cause deficiencies with serious consequences. Children are particularly at risk.
Physical therapies Ascending temperature foot baths, sitz baths, hot vapor compresses, hot packs (*see* pages 871–8), etc. are claimed to relax the patient and alleviate pain. An individual plan of treatment should be defined in association with the treating physician.	**May be of some use** as a short-term, supportive treatment attempt aimed at alleviating pain and easing cramps. Case reports and field studies claim efficacy; however, success is probably seen in only a proportion of patients (*see* Placebo, page xxi).	**Suitable for DIY** Qualified guidance is recommended though not essential. Therapists should propose a treatment plan. **Risks:** Skin damage may be caused in persons with diminished temperature sensation when extreme temperatures are applied.
Reflex therapies Reflex zone massage (*see* page 883), reflexology (*see* page 883), and TENS (*see* page 886) are claimed to act via reflex channels (*see* page 881) to ease pain and relax the patient.	**May be of some use** as a short-term, supportive treatment attempt aimed at easing cramps and alleviating pain in acute colicky attacks. Case reports and field studies claim efficacy; however, success is probably seen in only a proportion of patients (*see* Placebo, page xxi).	**Suitable for DIY** Qualified guidance is essential. The effects of the various therapies can differ significantly from one person to another. **Risks:** Some people are sensitive to electrical stimuli and rubber electrodes; others find it hard to tolerate manual stimulation or close physical contact.

Treatment	Rating	Point of delivery/risks
Relaxation techniques Autogenic training (*see* page 888), muscle relaxation according to Jacobson (*see* page 893), and various biofeedback techniques (*see* page 891) are said to relieve muscle tension and inner unrest, and might be instrumental in easing pain.	**Useful** only as a short-term, supportive treatment attempt aimed at relaxing the patient. Some case reports and field studies claim efficacy; however, success is probably seen in only a proportion of patients (*see* Placebo, page xxi).	**Suitable for DIY** Once a sound understanding of the technique has been acquired from a trainer, patients can perform exercises themselves. Therapists should propose a treatment plan. **Risks:** Fairly unlikely.
Vitamins and trace elements The antioxidative properties of beta-carotene, vitamins C and E, and selenium are, it is supposed, instrumental in countering the formation of free radicals and boosting the body's own antioxidative defence systems (*see* page 900).	**Useful** in vitamin deficiency, e.g. when too little bile flows into the intestine. Based on present knowledge, no definitive recommendations can be given with regard to dosages of vitamins with anti-oxidative properties.	**Suitable for DIY** Qualified guidance is recommended though not essential. **Risks:** Intolerance and overdosage are possible. Recent studies imply that beta-carotene might increase the risk of cancer.

Herbal remedies for gallbladder disease

Active ingredient/preparation	Rating
Dandelion root and leaves (*Taraxacum officinale*)	Taken orally, dandelion root and leaves **may be of some use** as a treatment attempt for problems with bile flow. Dandelion is a cholagog and diuretic. **Daily dose:** As a tincture, 10–15 drops three times a day; to prepare a decoction, add 1 cup of hot water to 3–4g of herb, bring to a boil, simmer, and strain. Use ready-formulated preparations as instructed by the manufacturer/prescriber. **Risks:** If you have gall stones, ask your doctor before taking dandelion. Not to be taken by persons with occlusion of the bile duct, gall bladder empyema, or intestinal occlusion. Risk of stomach disorders through an excess of gastric acid.
Fumitory (*Fumaria officinalis*)	Taken orally, fumitory **may be of some use** as a treatment attempt for gall bladder disease and gastrointestinal spasms. It relieves spasms in the upper part of the alimentary canal. **Daily dose:** 6g herb. **Individual dose:** Pour 1 cup of hot water over 2g of herb and infuse. Use ready-formulated preparations as instructed by the manufacturer/prescriber. **Risks:** The alkaloid fumarin contained in fumitory may be responsible for the development of an edema and increased intra-ocular pressure. This theory is still to be proven, however.
Globe artichoke leaves (*Cynara scolymus*)	**May be of some use** as a treatment attempt for gall bladder disease. **Daily dose:** 1–4g dried leaves. **Individual dose:** Pour 1 cup of hot water over 1–2g of dried leaves and infuse. For the extract (depending on how prepared), 200–600mg. Use ready-formulated preparations as instructed by the manufacturer/prescriber. **Risks:** contact allergies are possible. Not to be taken by persons with occlusion of the bile duct or gall stones. If you are pregnant or breastfeeding, ask your doctor before taking globe artichoke leaves.

Active ingredient/preparation	Rating

Greater celandine
(*Chelidonium majus*)

Taken orally, greater celandine **may be of some use** as a treatment attempt for painful spasms of the gall bladder and gastrointestinal tract. Its action is antispasmodic.

Daily dose: 2–5g. **Individual dose:** As an infusion, 1.0g to 1 cup of hot water.

Use ready-formulated preparations as instructed by the manufacturer/prescriber.

Risks: Do not use in children, as there have been reports of intoxication following consumption of this plant. Greater celandine is controlled by the Medicines Act 1968 in the UK. Its sale is restricted to medical herbalists and pharmacists. It should be used with care as it has been known to cause anemia.

Peppermint leaves
(*Mentha piperita*)

Taken orally, peppermint leaves **may be of some use** as a treatment attempt for painful spasm of the gall bladder and biliary tract. Peppermint is a cholagogue and carminative and has an antispasmodic action on the smooth musculature.

Daily dose: 3–6g herb. **Individual dose:** Pour 1 cup of boiling water over 1.5g of dried herb and infuse. Alternatively, 1 teaspoon of tincture in water, several times daily.

Risks: If you have gall stones, ask your doctor before taking peppermint leaves. The volatile oil contained in peppermint may cause allergic reactions.

Active ingredient/preparation	*Rating*
Peppermint oil (*Mentha piperita*)	Taken orally, peppermint oil **may be of some use** as a treatment attempt for spasms of the biliary tract. Peppermint oil is an antispasmodic, carminative, and antibacterial. **Daily dose:** For internal use: 6–12 drops (when inhaled, 3–4 drops in water). **Individual dose:** 2–4 drops, e.g. on sugar. Use ready-formulated preparations as instructed by the manufacturer/prescriber. **Risks:** Gastric problems. On contact with the skin, peppermint oil causes local irritation. If you have gall stones, ask your doctor before taking peppermint oil. Not to be taken by persons with occlusion of the bile duct, gall bladder inflammation, or severe liver damage. Do not apply to the nose and face of infants and young children.
Radish root (*Raphanus sativus* var. *niger*)	Taken orally, radish root **may be of some use** as a treatment attempt for functional problems with the gall bladder. It is a choleretic and antimicrobial which stimulates gastrointestinal motoricity. **Dosage:** Take 1–2 teaspoons of freshly expressed juice several times daily. Use ready-formulated preparations as instructed by the manufacturer/prescriber. **Risks:** Retching, contraction of the pupils, drowsiness, and proteinuria are possible. Not to be taken by persons with gallstones.
Wormwood (*Artemisia absinthium*)	Taken orally, wormwood **may be of some use** as a treatment attempt for painful spasm of the biliary tract. Contains bitter principles and volatile oil. **Daily dose:** 3–5g herb. **Individual dose:** As an infusion, 1g of dried herb to 1 cup of hot water. Take 2 cups morning and noon each day. Use ready-formulated preparations as instructed by the manufacturer/prescriber. **Risks:** Do not use oil of wormwood. The isolated essential oil can damage the nervous system and impair intellectual faculties. Many countries therefore forbid alcoholic solutions and the pure oil.

Gastritis, heartburn, gastric ulcers, and duodenal ulcers

Causes and symptoms

Gastritis is a collective term for various forms of gastric inflammation, the causes of which are manifold. Symptoms differ widely depending on their cause and may be associated with other organ disease affecting, for instance, the heart, liver, bowel, kidneys, and pancreas. Gastritis and gastric ulcers often present with a feeling of fullness, lack of appetite, nausea, vomiting, heartburn, stomach ache, and abdominal pain. Occasionally, patients may show no symptoms.

Gastric and duodenal ulcers are frequently characterized by the same sets of symptoms. However, duodenal ulcers are associated additionally with hunger pains.

The conditions listed in this section may be caused by emotional and social factors, diet, and the consumption of coffee, tea, and alcohol; more recent research has shown that *Helicobacter pylori*, a bacterium often found in the stomach, is also implicated in their causation.

Orthodox treatment

Orthodox treatment will mostly involve endoscopic examination and analysis of bioptic specimens. Attempts are sometimes made to eliminate the *Helicobacter pylori* bacterium through a combination of treatments. A new class of drugs called H_2 antagonists may be prescribed. Surgery is now seldom carried out.

When symptoms are chronic or recurrent, gastroscopy or duodenoscopy is generally carried out to achieve a diagnosis.

Complementary therapies

Various complementary procedures aim to calm and relax the patient and reduce pain and nausea. Sometimes the practitioner takes a constitutional approach (*see* Constitution, page 927). Great emphasis is placed on a healthy, organic diet and on eating little and often.

Treatment plan and limited trial

Before administering a complementary treatment, every therapist should propose a treatment plan (*see* page xxiii) that sets out a clear time frame and defines the goal that the treatment is designed to achieve. Treatment should then be tried for a limited term to test the patient's response.

Caution

Malignant tumors may present with symptoms similar to those seen in gastritis or in a gastric or duodenal ulcer. It is thus vital that you see your doctor.

Complementary treatments for gastritis, heartburn, gastric ulcers, and duodenal ulcers

Treatment	Rating	Point of delivery/risks
Acupressure This treatment (*see* page 769), otherwise known as pressure-point massage, is claimed to reduce pain, wind, and nausea when pressure is applied to the appropriate points. The pressure points chosen may differ from one practitioner to another.	**May be of some use** as a short-term, supportive treatment attempt, especially for easing pain. Some case reports claim efficacy; however, success is probably seen in only a proportion of patients (*see* Placebo, page xxi).	**Suitable for DIY** Qualified guidance is recommended. Therapists should be properly qualified. **Risks:** Unlikely provided treatment is carried out competently.

Treatment	Rating	Point of delivery/risks
Acupuncture Acupuncture in its various forms (*see* page 772) aims to encourage the flow of energy (*see* page 927) or to act directly to ease pain, nausea, and retching, to influence the production of gastric acid, and to eliminate the disease.	**Useful** as a short-term, supportive treatment attempt for easing pain. Case reports and field studies show that symptoms were indeed alleviated in some patients, and that the production of gastric acid was influenced. The efficacy described is probably seen in only a proportion of patients (*see* Placebo, page xxi).	**Requires a qualified practitioner** Acupuncturists should be properly qualified and should propose a treatment plan. No credence should be given to anyone promising immediate or total success. **Risks:** Probably rare provided treatment is carried out competently.
Anthroposophical medicine For gastritis and duodenal ulcers, doctors who practice AM (*see* page 781) prescribe potentized antimony compounds, dialog therapy, eurhythmy, and individually tailored diets.	**May be of some use** as a short-term treatment attempt. Case reports claim efficacy; however, success is probably seen in only a proportion of patients (*see* Placebo, page xxi).	**Requires a qualified practitioner** Practitioners should be properly qualified and should propose a treatment plan. **Risks:** Allergies and intolerance are possible.
Aromatherapy Essential oils (*see* page 786) are used to soothe and relax, or to invigorate, thereby contributing to pain relief. The essences may be taken orally, used externally as massage oils or bathing emulsions, or inhaled as vapors.	**Of little use** Acceptable as a short-term treatment attempt aimed at soothing and relaxing. Some case reports claim efficacy; however, success is probably seen in only a proportion of patients (*see* Placebo, page xxi).	**Suitable for DIY** Qualified guidance is recommended. The effects of individual essential oils differ widely. **Risks:** Allergies or intolerance are possible. Some oils are carcinogenic in test systems and possibly in humans.

Treatment	Rating	Point of delivery/risks
Bioresonance therapy Bioresonance therapists use electrical devices in an attempt to discover the causes of illness and claim to be able to weaken or turn around pathogenic energies and disease related vibrations (*see* page 794).	**Of little use** Possibly acceptable as a short-term treatment attempt in persistent cases when simpler, more established methods have been unsuccessful. Some case reports claim efficacy; however, success is probably seen, if at all, in only a small proportion of patients (*see* Placebo, page xxi).	**Requires a qualified practitioner** Practitioners should be properly qualified and should propose a treatment plan. No credence should be given to anyone promising immediate or total success. **Risks:** Fairly unlikely.
Cell therapy Injecting or ingesting products extracted from the tissues of newborn animals or animal fetuses is said to have a rejuvenating and revitalizing effect and to enhance the healing of human tissues and organs (*see* page 796).	**Not advised** Based on present knowledge, there is inadequate evidence of the efficacy and mode of action of these costly and relatively risky procedures.	**Risks:** Injecting foreign proteins into the body can provoke (possibly fatal) allergic reactions. Also, pathogens such as those that cause bovine spongiform encephalopathy (BSE) or other serious infections may be introduced.
Electroacupuncture according to Voll By taking readings of the electrical conductivity of the skin (*see* page 802), therapists claim to be able to derive an insight into diseased areas of the body, pathogenic foci (*see* page 928), and stress factors (*see* Toxins, page 929). The factors presumed to be instrumental in the causation of these disorders can then be addressed.	**Of little use** Possibly acceptable as a short-term, supportive treatment attempt in persistent cases when simpler, more established methods have been unsuccessful. Some case reports claim a degree of efficacy; however, success is probably seen, if at all, in only a small proportion of patients (*see* Placebo, page xxi).	**Requires a qualified practitioner** Practitioners should be properly qualified and should propose a treatment plan. No credence should be given to anyone promising immediate or total success. **Risks:** A second opinion must always be obtained from a qualified physician before any attempt is made to "eliminate foci" (e.g. by surgery).

Treatment	Rating	Point of delivery/risks
Electroneural therapy according to Croon According to the theory, readings taken at various reactive sites on the skin highlight diseased areas within the body. Based on these readings, targeted electrostimulative measures can be undertaken to address factors presumed to be instrumental in the causation of these disorders (*see* page 806).	**Of little use** Possibly acceptable as a short-term, supportive treatment attempt in persistent cases when simpler, more established methods have been unsuccessful. Some case reports claim a degree of efficacy; however, success is probably seen, if at all, in only a small proportion of patients (*see* Placebo, page xxi).	**Requires a qualified practitioner** Practitioners should be properly qualified and should propose a treatment plan. No credence should be given to anyone promising immediate or total success. **Risks:** Proponents themselves warn that treatment should not be given in acute inflammatory conditions.
Eliminative methods, bloody Bloody cupping (*see* page 815) of areas of the body associated with the gut (*see* Reflex therapies, page 881) is said to act on gastritis and a duodenal ulcer by improving the body's own regulatory systems and by easing symptoms.	**Of little use** Possibly acceptable as a short-term treatment attempt in persistent cases when more established, less invasive methods have been unsuccessful. Some case reports claim efficacy; however, success is probably seen in only a proportion of patients (*see* Placebo, page xxi).	**Requires a qualified practitioner** Practitioners should be properly qualified and should propose a treatment plan. **Risks:** Bloody cupping can cause infection and scarring. Furthermore, it should not be carried out in persons with bleeding disorders.
Eliminative methods, unbloody Unbloody cupping (*see* page 817) of areas of the body associated with the gut (*see* Reflex therapies, page 881) is said to ease symptoms and improve the body's own regulatory systems.	**May be of some use** in persistent cases as a short-term treatment attempt. Some case reports claim efficacy; however, success is probably seen in only a proportion of patients (*see* Placebo, page xxi).	**Suitable for DIY** Unbloody cupping is best carried out under the guidance of a qualified practitioner. **Risks:** Unlikely provided treatment is carried out competently.

Treatment	Rating	Point of delivery/risks
Enzyme therapy The enzymes used (*see* page 824) are said to dispel and destroy "immune complexes" that course in the blood and that are responsible, for instance, for sustaining inflammatory processes.	**Of little use** Some case reports claim efficacy for this little researched therapy; however, success is probably seen in only a small proportion of patients (*see* Placebo, page xxi).	**Requires a qualified practitioner** Practitioners should propose a treatment plan. Non-prescription preparations are suitable for do-it-yourself. **Risks:** Allergies or intolerance are possible.
Flower remedies Flower remedies (*see* page 828) are said to restore emotional balance and assist the body's psychic ability to heal itself.	**Of little use** Acceptable as a short-term, supportive treatment attempt aimed at soothing and relaxing. Some case reports claim a degree of efficacy; however, success is probably seen in only a small proportion of patients (*see* Placebo, page xxi).	**Suitable for DIY** Qualified guidance is recommended. Practitioners should propose a treatment plan. **Risks:** Possible intolerance.
Homeopathy Highly diluted (potentized) solutions (*see* page 831) are believed to be able to redress vital energy imbalances and strengthen the body's defences. Organo- and functiotropic (*see* page 833) homeopathy is claimed to be effective for dealing with symptoms.	**Of little use** Acceptable as a supportive treatment attempt in persistent cases and for helping the patient come to terms emotionally with his/her condition. Case reports claim success for homeopathic treatments; however, success is probably seen in only a proportion of patients (*see* Placebo, page xxi).	**Requires a qualified practitioner** Homeopaths should be properly qualified and should propose a treatment plan. Ready-formulated preparations are suitable for do-it-yourself. **Risks:** Allergies and intolerance are possible.

Treatment	Rating	Point of delivery/risks
Hypnosis and self-hypnosis In the relaxed and generally altered state of awareness that is induced in hypnosis or self-hypnosis (*see* page 837), physical and mental conditions can be addressed and pain relieved. Hypnosis is often used in combination with other psycho- and behavioral therapies in order to help the patient to change his/her lifestyle.	**Of little use** Acceptable in persistent cases as a short-term, supportive treatment attempt aimed at relaxing the patient and at helping him/her come to terms better with his/her condition. Some case reports claim efficacy; however, success is probably seen in only a proportion of patients treated (*see* Placebo, page xxi).	**Requires a qualified practitioner** Hypnotherapists should be properly qualified and should propose a treatment plan. **Risks:** Unlikely provided treatment is carried out competently.
Manual therapies Chiropractors and osteopaths (*see* page 844) use a series of manipulations to realign allegedly displaced vertebrae said to be associated with the patient's condition. This procedure, it is claimed, eases symptoms and addresses factors that are presumed to be instrumental in the causation of these disorders.	**Of little use** Acceptable as a short-term, supportive treatment attempt when less risky, more established methods have been unsuccessful. Some case reports claim efficacy; however, success is probably seen, if at all, in only a small proportion of patients (*see* Placebo, page xxi).	**Requires a qualified practitioner** Practitioners should be properly qualified and should propose a treatment plan. **Risks:** Manipulation of the head and cervical vertebrae can cause serious injury. Osteoporosis is one of several risk factors.
Massage Classical massage (*see* page 847) can invigorate the patient, as well as ease muscular and emotional tension.	**May be of some use** as a supportive treatment attempt provided it is perceived as being pleasant and relaxing. Some case reports claim a degree of efficacy; however, success is probably seen in only a proportion of patients (*see* Placebo, page xxi).	**Suitable for DIY** Qualified guidance is recommended. Masseurs/masseuses should propose a treatment plan. **Risks:** Some people are sensitive to manual stimuli; others find it hard to tolerate close physical contact.

Treatment	Rating	Point of delivery/risks
Physical therapies Local heat treatments, e.g. torso wraps or ascending temperature foot baths, are said to ease acute pain. Warm foot baths or sitz baths (*see* pages 871–8) are said to have a relaxing effect.	**May be of some use** as a treatment attempt. Observational studies claim efficacy; however, success is probably seen in only a proportion of patients (*see* Placebo, page xxi).	**Suitable for DIY** Qualified guidance is recommended though not essential. Therapists should propose a treatment plan. **Risks:** Unlikely provided treatment is carried out competently.
Probiotics The introduction of certain bacteria into the gut is claimed to bring the intestinal flora back into balance and to have a beneficial effect on the gut (*see* page 878).	**May be of some use** as a short-term treatment attempt when more established methods have been unsuccessful. Case reports claim efficacy; however, success is probably seen in only a proportion of patients (*see* Placebo, page xxi).	**Requires a qualified practitioner** Practitioners should be properly qualified and should propose a treatment plan. Non-prescription formulations are suitable for do-it-yourself. **Risks:** Fairly unlikely provided treatment is carried out competently.
Reflex therapies Connective tissue massage, periosteal massage, reflexology (*see* page 883), and TENS (*see* page 886) are claimed to act via reflex channels (*see* page 881) to ease symptoms.	**May be of some use** as a short-term treatment attempt aimed at alleviating pain. Observational studies claim efficacy; however, success is probably seen in only a proportion of patients (*see* Placebo, page xxi).	**Suitable for DIY** Qualified guidance is recommended. **Risks:** Some people are sensitive to electrical stimuli and rubber electrodes; others find it hard to tolerate manual stimulation or close physical contact.

Treatment	Rating	Point of delivery/risks
Relaxation techniques Autogenic training (*see* page 888), muscle relaxation according to Jacobson (*see* page 893), and various biofeedback techniques (*see* page 891) are said to relieve muscle tension and inner unrest, and might be instrumental in easing symptoms.	**Useful** as a short-term, supportive treatment attempt. Case reports, case studies, and field studies claim a degree of efficacy in some patients (*see* Placebo, page xxi).	**Suitable for DIY** Once a sound understanding of the technique has been acquired from a trainer, patients can perform exercises themselves. Therapists should propose a treatment plan. **Risks:** Fairly unlikely.
Vitamins and trace elements The antioxidative properties of beta-carotene, vitamins C and E, and selenium are, it is supposed, instrumental in countering the formation of free radicals, in boosting the body's own antioxidative defence systems, and in suppressing inflammation (*see* page 900).	**Of little use** Acceptable as a short-term, supportive treatment attempt. No definitive dosage recommendations can be given based on present knowledge.	**Suitable for DIY** Qualified guidance is recommended though not essential. **Risks:** Intolerance and overdosage are possible. Recent studies imply that beta-carotene might increase the risk of cancer.

Herbal remedies for indigestion

Herbal remedies are altogether of little use for indigestion, as they have hardly any acid-binding capacity. *See also* Lack of appetite, page 592, Wind, page 620, and below.

Herbal remedies for gastritis

Active ingredient/preparation	Rating
Angelica root (*Angelica archangelica*)	Taken orally, angelica root **may be of some use** as a treatment attempt for digestive disorders, lack of appetite, and flatulence. It is an antispasmodic agent and cholagog, and promotes the secretion of gastric fluid. **Daily dose:** As a decoction, 4.5g of herb. **Individual dose:** Pour boiling water over 1.5g of herb. Drink unsweetened half an hour before meals; 20–40 drops of tincture on sugar. **Risks:** Photosensitization (persons should avoid direct sunlight after taking angelica root, or they may suffer allergic skin irritation).
Blessed thistle (*Cnicus benedictus*)	Taken orally, blessed thistle **may be of some use** as a treatment attempt for digestive disorders. It promotes the formation of saliva and gastric fluid. **Daily dose:** 4–6g herb. **Individual dose:** Pour 1 cup of hot water over 2g of herb and infuse. **Risks:** Blessed thistle may cause allergies, so do not if use if you are allergic to blessed thistle or compositae.
Buck bean leaves (*Menyanthes trifoliata*)	Taken orally, buck bean leaves **may be of some use** as a treatment attempt for digestive disorders. It promotes the secretion of saliva and gastric fluid. **Daily dose:** 4.5g herb. **Individual dose:** Pour 1 cup of hot water over 1.5g of leaves and infuse. **Risks:** Buck bean is not known to have any serious side effects.

Active ingredient/preparation	Rating
Centaury (*Centaurium minus*)	Taken orally, centaury **may be of some use** as a treatment attempt for digestive disorders. It is a digestive stimulant. **Daily dose:** 6g herb. **Individual dose:** 1–2g of herb with approximately 5oz of boiling water before meals. Use ready-formulated preparations as instructed by the manufacturer/prescriber. **Risks:** Centaury is not known to have any serious side effects.
Chicory leaves and root (*Cichorium intybus* var. *intybus*)	Taken orally, chicory leaves and root **may be of some use** as a treatment attempt for digestive disorders. **Daily dose:** 3g herb. **Individual dose:** Pour boiling water over 1g, infuse for five minutes, and strain. **Risks:** Allergic reactions are possible. Not to be taken by persons who are allergic to chicory and compositae. If you have gallstones, ask your doctor before taking chicory.
Chinese cinnamon bark (*Cinnamomum aromaticum*)	Taken orally, Chinese cinnamon bark **may be of some use** as a treatment attempt for lack of appetite, digestive disorders, and flatulence. Encourages bowel activity. **Daily dose:** 2–4g herb. **Individual dose:** Pour 1 cup of boiling water over 1g of dried inner bark and infuse; 2–8 drops of essential oil on sugar. **Risks:** Allergic skin and mucosal reactions are common. Not to be used during pregnancy or by persons who are to cinnamon or balsam of Tolu.

Active ingredient/preparation	Rating

Cinchona bark
(*Cinchona succirubra/pubescens*)

Taken orally, cinchona bark **may be of some use** as a treatment attempt for digestive problems and flatulence. It encourages the secretion of digestive juices and saliva.
Daily dose: 1–3g of bark. **Individual dose:** Pour boiling water over 1g of bark, infuse for 10 minutes, strain, and drink half an hour before meals; 20–40 drops of tincture on sugar.
Risks: Increased bleeding and hypersensitive reactions are possible. Cinchona bark should not be used during pregnancy, nor by individuals suffering from an allergy. Cinchona bark intensifies the action of anticoagulants. It should not be taken for long periods of time, as it may give rise to symptoms of cinchonism (characterized by tinnitus, headaches, visual disturbances, nausea). In the UK it may only be sold to practitioners.

Cinnamon bark
(*Cinnamomum verum*)

Taken orally, cinnamon bark **may be of some use** as a treatment attempt for digestive disorders and flatulence. It is a gentle digestive tonic with an antibacterial and antifungal action.
Daily dose: 2–4g dried inner bark.
Individual dose: Pour 1 cup of hot water over 1g of dried inner bark and infuse.
Risks: Allergic skin and mucosal reactions are common. Not to be used during pregnancy or by persons who are allergic to cinnamon or balsam of Tolú.

Coriander seeds
(*Coriandrum sativum* var. *vulgare*)

Taken orally, coriander seeds **may be of some use** as a treatment attempt for digestive disorders and lack of appetite.
Daily dose: 3g seeds. **Individual dose:** To prepare an infusion drunk several times a day between meals, bruise 1g of seeds with the back of a knife, pour on 1 cup of boiling water, and infuse. Use ready-formulated preparations as instructed by the manufacturer/prescriber.
Risks: Coriander seeds are not known to have any serious side effects.

Active ingredient/preparation	Rating
Dandelion (*Taraxacum officinale*)	Taken orally, dandelion **may be of some use** as a treatment attempt for digestive disorders and a feeling of fullness. **Daily dose:** 10g herb. **Individual dose:** Pour 1 cup of hot water over 2–3g of herb and infuse. Use ready-formulated preparations as instructed by the manufacturer/prescriber. **Risks:** Contact allergies can occur (rarely). Not to be taken by persons with occlusion of the bile duct, gall bladder empyema, or intestinal occlusion. If you have gall stones, ask your doctor before taking dandelion.
Galangal root (*Alpinia officinarum*)	Taken orally, galangal **may be of some use** as a treatment attempt for digestive disorders and lack of appetite. Its action is antispasmodic, anti-inflammatory, and antibacterial. **Daily dose:** 2–4g of herb or 2–4g of tincture. **Individual dose:** Pour 1 cup of boiling water over 1g of dried rhizome and infuse. Use ready-formulated preparations as instructed by the manufacturer/prescriber. **Risks:** Galangal is not known to have any serious side effects.
German camomile flowers (*Chamomilla recutita*)	Taken orally, German camomile flowers **may be of some use** as a treatment attempt for spasm and inflammation of the gastrointestinal tract. Its action is anti-inflammatory, antispasmodic, vulnerary, and antibacterial. **Daily dose:** 12g flowers. **Individual dose:** As a tea drink taken several times a day between meals, 3g herb to 1 cup of boiling water. Use ready-formulated preparations as instructed by the manufacturer/prescriber. **Risks:** Severe allergic (anaphylactic) reactions in rare cases.

Active ingredient/preparation	Rating
Iceland moss (*Cetraria islandica, Lichen islandicus*)	Taken orally, Iceland moss **may be of some use** as a treatment attempt for lack of appetite. **Daily dose:** 4–6g lichen. **Individual dose:** Pour 1 cup of boiling water over 2g of shredded moss and infuse. Drink several times a day. **Risks:** Iceland moss is not known to have any serious side effects.
Lemon balm leaves (*Melissa officinalis*)	Taken orally, lemon balm **may be of some use** as a treatment attempt for functional gastric disorders. It has a relaxing effect and relieves flatulence. **Daily dose:** 8–10g leaves. **Individual dose:** Pour 1 cup of hot water over 1.5–4.5g of leaves and infuse. Use ready-formulated preparations as instructed by the manufacturer/prescriber. **Risks:** The ethereal oil in lemon balm may cause allergic reactions.
Orange peel (*Citrus sinensis*)	Taken orally, orange peel **may be of some use** as a treatment attempt for lack of appetite. **Daily dose:** 10–15g peel. **Individual dose:** Pour 1 cup of hot water over 5g and infuse. Take half an hour before meals. **Risks:** Orange peel is not known to have any serious side effects.
Peppermint leaves (*Mentha piperita*)	Taken orally, peppermint leaves **may be of some use** as a treatment attempt for painful spasm of the gastrointestinal tract. Peppermint is a cholagogue and has an antispasmodic action on the smooth muscles as well as relieving flatulence. **Daily dose:** 3–6g leaves. **Individual dose:** Pour 1 cup of boiling water over 1.5g of leaves and infuse. 1 teaspoon of tincture in water. Use ready-formulated preparations as instructed by the manufacturer/prescriber. **Risks:** If you have gall stones, ask your doctor before taking peppermint.

Active ingredient/preparation	Rating
Peppermint oil (*Mentha piperita*)	Taken orally, peppermint oil **may be of some use** as a treatment attempt for spasm of the upper gastrointestinal tract, for gall bladder problems and an irritable bowel. It has an antispasmodic, antibacterial, and cooling action; it also relieves flatulence. **Daily dose:** 6–12 drops (for an inhalation, 3–4 drops in water). **Individual dose:** 0.1ml (approx. 3–4 drops). **Individual dose for an irritable bowel:** 0.2ml (approx. 6–8 drops). Use ready-formulated preparations as instructed by the manufacturer/prescriber. **Risks:** Gastric problems are possible. If you have gall stones, ask your doctor before taking peppermint oil. Not to be taken by persons with biliary tract occlusion, gall bladder inflammation, or severe liver damage. Do not apply to the nose and face of infants and young children.
Sour orange peel (*Citrus aurantium* ssp. *aurantium*)	Taken orally, the peel of sour (Seville) oranges **may be of some use** as a treatment attempt for digestive disorders. **Daily dose:** 4–6g peel, 2–3g tincture. To prepare a tea drink, pour boiling water over 1–2g of peel; 2–3g of tincture on sugar. Use ready-formulated preparations as instructed by the manufacturer/prescriber. **Risks:** Photosensitization (persons with a light complexion should avoid direct sunlight after taking sour orange peel, or they may suffer allergic skin reactions).
White horehound (*Marrubium vulgare*)	Taken orally, white horehound **may be of some use** as a treatment attempt for digestive disorders and a feeling of fullness. The constituent marrubic acid is a cholagogue. **Daily dose:** 4.5g herb. **Individual dose:** Pour 1 cup of boiling water over 1.5g of herb and infuse. **Risks:** White horehound is not known to have any serious side effects.

Active ingredient/preparation	Rating

Wormwood
(*Artemisia absinthium*)

Taken orally, wormwood **may be of some use** as a treatment attempt for digestive disorders. Contains bitter principles and volatile oil.
Daily dose: 3–5g herb. **Individual dose:** Pour 1 cup of hot water over 1.5–2g of dried herb and infuse. Use ready-formulated preparations as instructed by the manufacturer/prescriber.
Risks: Do not use oil of wormwood. The isolated essential oil can damage the nervous system and impair intellectual faculties. Many countries therefore forbid alcoholic solutions and the pure oil.

Yarrow shoot and flowers
(*Achillea millefolium*)

Taken orally, yarrow **may be of some use** as a treatment attempt for digestive disorders. Yarrow is a cholagogue and antispasmodic.
Daily dose: 4.5g aerial parts, 3g yarrow flowers. To prepare a tea drink, pour hot water over 1–1.5g of aerial parts or 1g of flowers. Use ready-formulated preparations as instructed by the manufacturer/prescriber.
Risks: Contact skin allergies are possible. Not to be taken by persons who are allergic to compositae.

Herbal remedy for gastric and duodenal ulcers

Active ingredient/preparation	Rating
Licorice root (*Glycyrrhiza glabra*)	Taken orally, licorice root **may be of some use** as a treatment attempt for gastric and duodenal ulcers. **Daily dose:** 5–15g root. **Individual dose:** To prepare a tea drink, pour 1 cup of boiling water over 1–2g of root, allow to infuse for 15 minutes, and strain. Drink 1 cup several times daily; 1.5–3g of juice per day in water. Use ready-formulated preparations as instructed by the manufacturer/prescriber. **Risks:** Prolonged use and high dosages may lead to edema, potassium deficiency, and high blood pressure. These effects are amplified by simultaneous administration of thiazide and loop diuretics. Not to be taken during pregnancy or by persons with liver disease, hypertension, or potassium deficiency. Do not take for longer than four to six weeks without consulting a doctor. Caution: Licorice increases sensitivity to digitalis. Digitalis intoxication can occur more rapidly.

Hemorrhoids

Causes and symptoms

Hemorrhoids are small varicosities or swellings in the veins in and around the anus. It is not fully understood what causes them. Their chief symptoms are itching, a pressing sensation, a burning or pain around the anus, mucous discharge, inflammation, eczema, bleeding (bright red blood), and prolapse of the rectum. There may occasionally be fecal incontinence.

Orthodox treatment

Good anal hygiene is the cornerstone of effective treatment. Occasionally laxatives will be prescribed to prevent constipation, together with ointments and suppositories. Surgical intervention is sometimes required to freeze or remove hemorrhoids.

Complementary therapies

Complementary treatments, being symptom oriented, are merely palliative.

Treatment plan and limited trial

Before administering a complementary treatment, every therapist should propose a treatment plan (*see* page xxiii) that sets out a clear time frame and defines the goal that the treatment is designed to achieve. Treatment should then be tried for a limited term to test the patient's response.

Caution

Signs of blood in the feces should always be a cue for examination by a qualified physician in case it signals something more serious, such as bowel cancer.

Complementary treatments for hemorrhoids

Treatment	Rating	Point of delivery/risks
Acupressure This treatment (*see* page 769), otherwise known as pressure-point massage, is claimed to ease hemorrhoids when pressure is applied to the appropriate points.	**Of little use** Acceptable as a short-term treatment attempt aimed at alleviating pain. Some case reports claim efficacy; however, success is probably seen in only a proportion of patients (*see* Placebo, page xxi).	**Suitable for DIY** Qualified guidance is recommended. Therapists should be properly qualified. **Risks:** Unlikely provided treatment is carried out competently.

Treatment	*Rating*	*Point of delivery/risks*
Acupuncture Acupuncture in its various forms (*see* page 772) aims to encourage the flow of energy (*see* page 927) or to act directly to relieve symptoms.	**Of little use** Acceptable as a short-term treatment attempt aimed at alleviating pain. Some case reports claim efficacy; however, success is probably seen in only a proportion of patients (*see* Placebo, page xxi).	**Requires a qualified practitioner** Practitioners should be properly qualified and should propose a treatment plan. **Risks:** Probably rare provided treatment is carried out competently.
Anthroposophical medicine Doctors who practice AM (*see* page 781) see hemorrhoids as an expression of a blockage in the bloodstream which is beyond the capabilities of the liver. Liver therapy is combined with analgesic suppositories.	**Of little use** Acceptable as a longer-term treatment attempt when simpler, more established methods have been unsuccessful. Some studies claim efficacy; however, success is probably seen in only a proportion of patients (*see* Placebo, page xxi).	**Requires a qualified practitioner** Practitioners should be properly qualified and should propose a treatment plan. **Risks:** Allergies and intolerance are possible.
Aromatherapy Essential oils (*see* page 786) are used to soothe and relax, or to invigorate, thereby contributing to an easing of symptoms. The essences may be taken orally, used externally as massage oils or bathing emulsions, or inhaled as vapors.	**Of little use** Possibly acceptable as a short-term, supportive treatment attempt aimed at soothing and relaxing. Some case reports claim efficacy; however, success is probably seen in only a proportion of patients (*see* Placebo, page xxi).	**Suitable for DIY** Qualified guidance is recommended. The effects of individual essential oils differ widely. **Risks:** Allergies or intolerance are possible. Some oils are carcinogenic in test systems and possibly in humans.

Treatment	Rating	Point of delivery/risks
Bioresonance therapy Bioresonance therapists use electrical devices in an attempt to discover the causes of illness and claim to be able to weaken or turn around pathogenic energies and disease related vibrations (*see* page 794).	**Of little use** Possibly acceptable as a short-term, supportive treatment attempt in persistent cases when simpler, more established methods have been unsuccessful. Some case reports claim efficacy; however, success is probably seen, if at all, in only a small proportion of patients (*see* Placebo, page xxi).	**Requires a qualified practitioner** Practitioners should be properly qualified and should propose a treatment plan. No credence should be given to anyone promising immediate or total success. **Risks:** Fairly unlikely.
Electroacupuncture according to Voll By taking readings of the electrical conductivity of the skin (*see* page 802), therapists claim to be able to derive an insight into diseased areas of the body, pathogenic foci (*see* page 928), and stress factors (*see* Toxins, page 929). The factors presumed to be instrumental in the causation of hemorrhoids can then be addressed.	**Of little use** Possibly acceptable as a short-term, supportive treatment attempt in persistent cases when simpler, more established methods have been unsuccessful. Some case reports claim efficacy; however, success is probably seen, if at all, in only a small proportion of patients (*see* Placebo, page xxi).	**Requires a qualified practitioner** Practitioners should be properly qualified and should propose a treatment plan. No credence should be given to anyone promising immediate or total success. **Risks:** A second opinion must always be obtained from a qualified physician before any attempt is made to "eliminate foci" (e.g. by surgery).

Treatment	Rating	Point of delivery/risks
Electroneural therapy according to Croon According to the theory, readings taken at various reactive sites on the skin highlight diseased areas within the body. Based on these readings, targeted electrostimulative measures can be undertaken to address factors presumed to be instrumental in the causation of hemorrhoids (*see* page 806).	**Of little use** Possibly acceptable as a short-term treatment attempt in persistent cases when simpler, more established methods have been unsuccessful. Some case reports claim efficacy; however, success is probably seen, if at all, in only a small proportion of patients (*see* Placebo, page xxi).	**Requires a qualified practitioner** Practitioners should be properly qualified and should propose a treatment plan. No credence should be given to anyone promising immediate or total success. **Risks:** Proponents themselves warn that treatment should not be given in acute inflammatory conditions.
Eliminative methods, bloody Leeches (*see* page 822) and bloody cupping (*see* page 815) around the rectum are said to eliminate circulatory blockage and to ease symptoms.	**Of little use** Possibly acceptable as a short-term treatment attempt in persistent cases. Some case reports claim efficacy; however, success is probably seen in only a proportion of patients (*see* Placebo, page xxi).	**Requires a qualified practitioner** Practitioners should be properly qualified and should propose a treatment plan. **Risks:** Bloody cupping can cause infection and scarring. Furthermore, it should not be carried out in persons with bleeding disorders.
Eliminative methods, unbloody Unbloody cupping (*see* page 817) is supposed to alleviate pain and complications, and to improve the body's own regulatory systems.	**Of little use** Acceptable as a short-term, supportive treatment attempt aimed at alleviating pain. Some case reports claim efficacy; however, success is probably seen in only a small proportion of patients (*see* Placebo, page xxi).	**Suitable for DIY** Unbloody cupping is best carried out under the guidance of a qualified practitioner. **Risks:** Unlikely provided treatment is carried out competently.

Treatment	*Rating*	*Point of delivery/risks*
Enzyme therapy The enzymes used (*see* page 824) are said to dispel and destroy "immune complexes" that course in the blood and that are responsible, for instance, for sustaining inflammatory processes.	**Of little use** Some case reports claim efficacy for this little researched therapy; however, success is probably seen in only a small proportion of patients (*see* Placebo, page xxi).	**Requires a qualified practitioner** Practitioners should propose a treatment plan. Non-prescription preparations are suitable for do-it-yourself. **Risks:** Allergies or intolerance are possible.
Flower remedies Some flower therapists see hemorrhoids as an expression of emotional disharmony. Flower remedies (*see* page 828) are said to restore emotional balance and assist the body's psychic ability to heal itself.	**Of little use** Possibly acceptable as a short-term, supportive treatment attempt aimed at soothing and relaxing. Some case reports claim efficacy; however, success is probably seen in only a small proportion of patients (*see* Placebo, page xxi).	**Suitable for DIY** Qualified guidance is recommended. Practitioners should propose a treatment plan. **Risks:** Possible intolerance.
Homeopathy Highly diluted (potentized) solutions (*see* page 831) are believed to be able to redress vital energy imbalances. Organo- and functiotropic (*see* page 833) homeopathy is claimed to be effective for dealing directly with symptoms.	**Of little use** Acceptable as a treatment attempt aimed at easing symptoms. Case reports, case studies, and field studies claim efficacy; however, success is probably seen in only a proportion of patients (*see* Placebo, page xxi).	**Requires a qualified practitioner** Homeopaths should be properly qualified and should propose a treatment plan. Ready-formulated preparations are suitable for do-it-yourself. **Risks:** Allergies and intolerance are possible.

Treatment	*Rating*	*Point of delivery/risks*
Nutritional therapies An organic diet (*see* page 4) provides the body with essential and secondary plant nutrients that are believed to exercise a multitude of positive effects and to be capable, *inter alia*, of softening stools.	**Useful** as an individually directed supportive measure.	**Suitable for DIY** Qualified guidance is recommended though not essential. **Risks:** Avoid imbalanced or intolerable diets. They can cause deficiencies with serious consequences. Children are particularly at risk.
Physical therapies Ascending temperature sitz baths, cold washings, baths or wraps (*see* pages 871–8) with oak bark or horse-chestnut, exercise therapy (*see* page 868), and swimming are said to improve the circulation, inhibit inflammation, ease itching, and alleviate pain.	**Useful** as a short-term, symptomatic treatment attempt. Some case reports claim efficacy; however, success is probably seen in only a proportion of patients (*see* Placebo, page xxi).	**Suitable for DIY** Qualified guidance is recommended though not essential. Practitioners should be properly qualified. **Risks:** Unlikely provided treatment is carried out competently. Hemorrhoids may become more distended when hot water is applied.
Probiotics The introduction of certain bacteria into the gut is claimed to bring the intestinal flora back into balance and to have a beneficial effect on hemorrhoids (*see* page 878).	**Of little use** Possibly acceptable as a short-term treatment attempt aimed at softening stools when more established methods have been unsuccessful. Some case reports claim efficacy; however, success is probably seen in only a proportion of patients (*see* Placebo, page xxi).	**Requires a qualified practitioner** Practitioners should be properly qualified and should propose a treatment plan. Non-prescription formulations are suitable for do-it-yourself. **Risks:** Fairly unlikely provided treatment is carried out competently.

Treatment	Rating	Point of delivery/risks
Reflex therapies Reflex zone massage (*see* page 883), reflexology (*see* page 883), and TENS (*see* page 886) are claimed to act via reflex channels (*see* page 881) to ease symptoms.	**Of little use** Acceptable as a short-term, symptomatic treatment attempt. Some case reports claim efficacy; however, success is probably seen in only a proportion of patients (*see* Placebo, page xxi).	**Suitable for DIY** Qualified guidance is essential. **Risks:** Some people are sensitive to electrical stimuli and rubber electrodes; others find it hard to tolerate manual stimulation or close physical contact.
Relaxation techniques Autogenic training (*see* page 888), muscle relaxation according to Jacobson (*see* page 893), and various biofeedback techniques (*see* page 891) are said to relieve muscle tension and inner unrest, and might be instrumental in easing symptoms.	**Of little use** Acceptable as a supportive treatment attempt aimed at easing symptoms. Some case reports claim efficacy; however, success is probably seen in only a proportion of patients (*see* Placebo, page xxi).	**Suitable for DIY** Once a sound understanding of the technique has been acquired from a trainer, patients can perform exercises themselves. Therapists should be properly qualified. **Risks:** Fairly unlikely.

Herbal remedies for hemorrhoids

Active ingredient/preparation	Rating
Balsam of Tolú (*Myroxylon balsamum* var. *pereira*)	**Not advised**. Reported as being used for hemorrhoids, but not advised owing to its allergizing action. **Dosage:** As instructed by the manufacturer/prescriber. Do not use for longer than 1 week. **Risks:** Not to be used by highly allergic persons.
German camomile flowers (*Chamomilla recutita*)	**Only useful** as an external treatment attempt for slight inflammation in the anal/genital region. **Dosage:** 20g to 1 quart of bath preparation, then make up to a full bath. Use ready-formulated preparations as instructed by the manufacturer/prescriber. **Risks:** Allergic reactions are possible in isolated cases.

Active ingredient/preparation	*Rating*
Oak bark (*Quercus robur*)	**Only useful** as an addition to bathwater for the treatment of slight inflammation in the anal/genital region. It has a strongly astringent action and is said to stop the replication of viruses. **Dosage:** For rinses (moist wipes): 20g bark per quart of bath-warm water; for partial immersion baths: 5g bark per quart of warm water. **Risks:** Not to be used by persons with extensive skin damage. No full immersion baths for persons with suppurating eczema, broken skin, febrile or infectious conditions, severe heart failure, or high blood pressure.
Poplar buds of various species (*Populi gema*)	**May be of some use** as an external treatment attempt. It also has a slight antibacterial action. **Dosage:** As instructed by the manufacturer/prescriber, or 5g per quart for bathing. **Risks:** Allergies. Not to be used by persons who are allergic to poplar buds, propolis, balsam of Tolú, and salicylates.
Shepherd's myrtle root (*Ruscus aculeatus*)	**May be of some use** as a bath or embrocation for itching or burning hemorrhoids. There is no evidence to suggest that its use internally is beneficial. Use ready-formulated preparations as instructed by the manufacturer/prescriber. **Risks:** Gastric problems in isolated cases, nausea when used internally; it may occasionally provoke allergic reactions when used externally.

Active ingredient/preparation	*Rating*
Sweet clover (*Melilotus officinalis*)	Taken orally, sweet clover is **of little use** as a treatment attempt for hemorrhoids. **May be of some use** as an external treatment attempt for hemorroids. **Daily dose:** 3–30mg of the principal constituent, coumarin. **Individual dose:** Use 10g to a pint as addition to bathwater. Use ready-formulated preparations as instructed by the manufacturer/prescriber. **Risks:** Headaches are possible when sweet clover is used internally; allergic reactions can occur when it is used externally. Suggestions that it adversely affects the liver when taken internally have not been confirmed.
Walnut leaves (*Juglans regia*)	**May be of some use** as an external treatment attempt for slight superficial inflammation such as in external hemorrhoids. Walnut leaves have an astringent action. **Individual dose:** Soak 2–3g of leaves in 1 cup of cold water, bring to a boil, simmer, strain, and use for wraps and partial immersion baths. **Risks:** Walnut leaves are not known to have any serious adverse effects.
Witch hazel leaves (*Hamamelis virginiana*)	**Only useful** as an internal or external treatment attempt for hemorrhoids or varicose veins. Witch hazel is an astringent and anti-inflammatory. **Dosage:** One to three times daily, 0.1–1g of herb to a cup of hot water as an infusion for drinking or as a local moist wipe or for tea bathing. Use ready-formulated preparations as instructed by the manufacturer/prescriber. **Risks:** Witch hazel is not known to have any serious side effects.

Irritable bowel syndrome

Causes and symptoms

Irritable bowel syndrome (IBS) is often considered to be a psychosomatic illness. Symptoms range from frequent spasmodic pain, with bouts of diarrhea and constipation (often alternating), to a feeling of fullness and excessive wind. IBS is sometimes a physical response to stress. An irritable stomach may also feature among the functional and/or psychosomatic symptoms.

Orthodox treatment

Various medications are used to treat irritable bowel syndrome. Relaxation exercises, psychotherapy, or counselling may also be prescribed.

Complementary therapies

Herbal treatments and homeopathic remedies play a significant role in the complementary treatment of irritable bowel syndrome. Therapies to alleviate symptoms may be supported additionally by other measures. IBS is sometimes seen as a constitutional problem (*see* Constitution, page 927), a result of the influence of toxins or foci (*see* pages 928–9), or the consequence of one's vital energy being out of balance (*see* Energy imbalance, page 927); complementary treatments are offered accordingly.

Treatment plan and limited trial

Before administering a complementary treatment, every therapist should propose a treatment plan (*see* page xxiii) that sets out a clear time frame and defines the goal that the treatment is designed to achieve. Treatment should then be tried for a limited term to test the patient's response.

Caution

Irritable bowel syndrome is mostly diagnosed by excluding other possible diagnoses, some of which are serious. It is thus important that you see your doctor.

Complementary treatments for irritable bowel syndrome

Treatment	Rating	Point of delivery/risks
Acupressure This treatment (*see* page 769), otherwise known as pressure-point massage, is claimed to ease flatulence, feelings of fullness, constipation, and colicky pains.	**May be of some use** as a short-term, supportive treatment attempt for various symptoms, e.g. pain. Case reports and field studies claim efficacy; however, success is probably seen in only a proportion of patients (*see* Placebo, page xxi).	**Suitable for DIY** Qualified guidance is recommended. Therapists should be properly qualified. **Risks:** Unlikely provided treatment is carried out competently.
Acupuncture Acupuncture in its various forms (*see* page 772) aims to encourage the flow of energy (*see* page 927) or to act directly to ease pain, nausea, and vomiting. The acupuncture points chosen can vary from one practitioner to another.	**May be of some use** as a short-term treatment attempt for various symptoms, e.g. pain. Case reports and field studies claim efficacy; however, success is probably seen in only a proportion of patients (*see* Placebo, page xxi).	**Requires a qualified practitioner** Acupuncturists should be properly qualified and should propose a treatment plan. **Risks:** Probably rare provided treatment is carried out competently.
Anthroposophical medicine In chronic irritable bowel syndrome, doctors who practice AM (*see* page 781) carry out a constitutional treatment based on psychosomatic considerations, and prescribe individual compositions.	**May be of some use** as a short-term treatment attempt for chronic irritable bowel syndrome when simpler methods have been unsuccessful. Case reports claim efficacy; however, success is probably seen in only a proportion of patients (*see* Placebo, page xxi).	**Requires a qualified practitioner** Practitioners should be properly qualified and should propose a treatment plan. **Risks:** Allergies and intolerance are possible.

Treatment	Rating	Point of delivery/risks
Aromatherapy Essential oils (*see* page 786) are used to soothe and relax, or to invigorate, thereby contributing to an easing of symptoms. The essences may be taken orally, used externally as massage oils or bathing emulsions, or inhaled as vapors.	**Of little use** Acceptable as a short-term, supportive treatment attempt aimed at soothing and relaxing. Some case reports claim a degree of efficacy; however, success is probably seen in only a proportion of patients (*see* Placebo, page xxi).	**Suitable for DIY** Qualified guidance is recommended. The effects of individual essential oils differ widely. **Risks:** Allergies or intolerance are possible. Some oils are carcinogenic in test systems and possibly in humans.
Bioresonance therapy Bioresonance therapists use electrical devices in an attempt to discover the causes of illness and claim to be able to weaken or turn around pathogenic energies and disease related vibrations (*see* page 794).	**Of little use** Possibly acceptable as a short-term treatment attempt for persistent symptoms when simpler, more established methods have been unsuccessful. Some case reports claim efficacy; however, success is probably seen, if at all, in only a small proportion of patients (*see* Placebo, page xxi).	**Requires a qualified practitioner** Practitioners should be properly qualified and should propose a treatment plan. No credence should be given to anyone promising immediate or total success. **Risks:** Fairly unlikely.
Cell therapy Injecting or ingesting products extracted from the tissues of newborn animals or animal fetuses is said to have a rejuvenating and revitalizing effect and to enhance the healing of human tissues and organs (*see* page 796).	**Not advised** Based on present knowledge, there is inadequate evidence of the efficacy and mode of action of these costly and relatively risky procedures.	**Risks:** Injecting foreign proteins into the body can provoke (possibly fatal) allergic reactions. Also, pathogens such as those that cause bovine spongiform encephalopathy (BSE) or other serious infections may be introduced.

Treatment	Rating	Point of delivery/risks
Electroacupuncture according to Voll By taking readings of the electrical conductivity of the skin (*see* page 802), therapists claim to be able to derive an insight into diseased areas of the body, pathogenic foci (*see* page 928), and stress factors (*see* Toxins, page 929). The factors presumed to be instrumental in the causation of irritable bowel syndrome can then be addressed.	**Of little use** Possibly acceptable as a short-term, supportive treatment attempt when simpler, more established methods have been unsuccessful. Some case reports claim efficacy; however, success is probably seen, if at all, in only a small proportion of patients (*see* Placebo, page xxi).	**Requires a qualified practitioner** Practitioners should be properly qualified and should propose a treatment plan. No credence should be given to anyone promising immediate or total success. **Risks:** A second opinion must always be obtained from a qualified physician before any attempt is made to "eliminate foci" (e.g. by surgery).
Electroneural therapy according to Croon According to the theory, readings taken at various reactive sites on the skin highlight diseased areas within the body. Based on these readings, targeted electrostimulative measures can be undertaken to address factors presumed to be instrumental in the causation of irritable bowel syndrome (*see* page 806).	**Of little use** Possibly acceptable as a short-term, supportive treatment attempt when simpler, more established methods have been unsuccessful. Some case reports claim efficacy; however, success is probably seen, if at all, in only a small proportion of patients (*see* Placebo, page xxi).	**Requires a qualified practitioner** Practitioners should be properly qualified and should propose a treatment plan. No credence should be given to anyone promising immediate or total success. **Risks:** Proponents themselves warn that treatment should not be given in acute inflammatory conditions.

Treatment	Rating	Point of delivery/risks
Eliminative methods, bloody Bloody cupping (*see* page 815) of zones associated with the gut (*see* Reflex therapies, page 881) is claimed to ease symptoms of irritable bowel syndrome and improve the body's own regulatory systems.	**Of little use** Possibly acceptable as a short-term treatment attempt in extremely persistent cases when more established, less invasive methods have been unsuccessful. Some case reports and field studies claim efficacy; however, success is probably seen in only a proportion of patients (*see* Placebo, page xxi).	**Requires a qualified practitioner** Practitioners should be properly qualified and should propose a treatment plan. **Risks:** Bloody cupping can cause infection and scarring. Furthermore, it should not be carried out in persons with bleeding disorders.
Eliminative methods, unbloody Unbloody cupping (*see* page 817) of zones associated with the gut (*see* Reflex therapies, page 881) is claimed to ease symptoms of irritable bowel and improve the body's own regulatory systems.	**May be of some use** as a short-term treatment attempt aimed at easing pain. Some case reports claim efficacy; however, success is probably seen in only a small proportion of patients (*see* Placebo, page xxi).	**Suitable for DIY** Unbloody cupping is best carried out under the guidance of a qualified practitioner. **Risks:** Unlikely provided treatment is carried out competently.
Enzyme therapy The enzymes used (*see* page 824) are said to dispel and destroy "immune complexes" that course in the blood and that are responsible, for instance, for sustaining inflammatory processes.	**Of little use** Some case reports claim efficacy for this little researched therapy; however, success is probably seen in only a small proportion of patients (*see* Placebo, page xxi).	**Requires a qualified practitioner** Practitioners should propose a treatment plan. Non-prescription preparations are suitable for do-it-yourself. **Risks:** Allergies or intolerance are possible.

Treatment	Rating	Point of delivery/risks
Flower remedies Flower remedies (*see* page 828) are said to restore emotional balance and assist the body's psychic ability to heal itself.	**May be of some use** as a short-term, supportive treatment attempt aimed at soothing and relaxing. Case reports claim efficacy; however, success is probably seen in only a proportion of patients (*see* Placebo, page xxi).	**Suitable for DIY** Qualified guidance is recommended. Practitioners should propose a treatment plan. **Risks:** Possible intolerance.
Homeopathy Highly diluted (potentized) solutions (*see* page 831) are believed to be able to redress vital energy imbalances and strengthen the body's defences. Organo- and functiotropic (*see* page 883) homeopathy is claimed to be effective for dealing with symptoms.	**May be of some use** as a supportive treatment attempt. Case reports claim success for homeopathic treatments; however, success is probably seen in only a proportion of patients (*see* Placebo, page xxi).	**Requires a qualified practitioner** Homeopaths should be properly qualified and should propose a treatment plan. Ready-formulated preparations are suitable for do-it-yourself. **Risks:** Allergies and intolerance are possible.
Manual therapies Chiropractors and osteopaths (*see* page 844) use a series of manipulations to realign allegedly displaced vertebrae. This is said to reduce pain, release energy blockages (*see* page 927), and address factors that may be at the root of irritable bowel syndrome.	**Of little use** Possibly acceptable as a short-term, supportive treatment attempt when less risky, more established methods have been unsuccessful. Some case reports claim efficacy; however, success is probably seen, if at all, in only a small proportion of patients (*see* Placebo, page xxi).	**Requires a qualified practitioner** Practitioners should be properly qualified and should propose a treatment plan. **Risks:** Manipulation of the head and cervical vertebrae can cause serious injury. Osteoporosis is one of several risk factors.

Treatment	Rating	Point of delivery/risks
Massage Classical massage (*see* page 847) can ease muscular and emotional tension.	**May be of some use** as a supportive treatment attempt aimed at relaxing the patient and improving his/her general well-being. Case reports claim efficacy; however, success is probably seen in only a proportion of patients (*see* Placebo, page xxi).	**Suitable for DIY** Qualified guidance is recommended. Masseurs/masseuses should propose a treatment plan. **Risks:** Some people are sensitive to manual stimuli; others find it hard to tolerate close physical contact.
Physical therapies Local heat treatments, e.g. torso wraps and baths, are claimed to ease colicky pains. Warm foot baths or sitz baths are said to relax the patient. Kneipp treatments, it is said, invigorate the patient and improve his/her feeling of general well-being (*see* pages 871–8).	**May be of some use** as a treatment attempt. Some case reports claim efficacy; however, success is probably seen in only a proportion of patients (*see* Placebo, page xxi).	**Suitable for DIY** Qualified guidance is recommended though not essential. **Risks:** Skin damage may be caused in persons with diminished temperature sensation when extreme temperatures are applied.
Probiotics The introduction of certain bacteria into the gut is claimed to bring the intestinal flora back into balance and to have a beneficial effect on the gut (*see* page 878).	**Of little use** Acceptable as a short-term treatment attempt for persistent symptoms when simpler, more established methods have been unsuccessful. Some case reports claim efficacy; however, success is probably seen in only a proportion of patients (*see* Placebo, page xxi).	**Requires a qualified practitioner** Practitioners should be properly qualified and should propose a treatment plan. Non-prescription formulations are suitable for do-it-yourself. **Risks:** Fairly unlikely provided treatment is carried out competently.

Treatment	Rating	Point of delivery/risks
Reflex therapies Connective tissue massage, periosteal massage, reflexology (*see* page 883), and TENS (*see* page 886) are claimed to act via reflex channels (*see* page 881) to ease symptoms.	**May be of some use** as a short-term treatment attempt aimed at alleviating pain. Some case reports claim efficacy; however, success is probably seen in only a proportion of patients (*see* Placebo, page xxi).	**Suitable for DIY** Qualified guidance is recommended. **Risks:** Some people are sensitive to electrical stimuli and rubber electrodes; others find it hard to tolerate manual stimulation or close physical contact.
Relaxation techniques Autogenic training (*see* page 888), muscle relaxation according to Jacobson (*see* page 893), and various biofeedback techniques (*see* page 891) are said to relieve muscle tension and inner unrest, and might be instrumental in easing symptoms.	**Useful** as a short-term treatment attempt. Case studies, observational studies, and case reports ascribe a degree of efficacy to these treatments in a proportion of patients.	**Suitable for DIY** Once a sound understanding of the technique has been acquired from a trainer, patients can perform exercises themselves. Therapists should be properly qualified. **Risks:** Fairly unlikely.

Herbal remedies for irritable bowel syndrome

Active ingredient/preparation	Rating
German camomile flowers (*Chamomilla recutita*)	Taken orally, German camomile **may be of some use** as a treatment attempt for gastrointestinal spasm and inflammation of the lining of the gut. German camomile is an anti-inflammatory, antispasmodic, vulnerary, and antibacterial. **Dosage:** As a tea drink, 3g of dried flowers to 5oz of hot water, three to four times daily. Use ready-formulated preparations as instructed by the manufacturer/prescriber. **Risks:** German camomile may provoke allergies (even anaphylaxis) in rare instances.

Active ingredient/preparation	*Rating*
Linseed (*Linum usitatissimum*)	Taken orally, linseed **may be of some use** as a treatment attempt for irritable bowel syndrome and inflamed colon. It has a demulcent action. **Daily dose:** Take 1 tablespoon with 1 cup of cold liquid two to three times daily. Use ready-formulated preparations as instructed by the manufacturer/prescriber. **Risks:** May cause other drugs taken simultaneously to be absorbed more slowly. Not to be taken by persons with any form of intestinal obstruction or occlusion.
Pale psyllium (*Plantago ovata* and *ispaghula*)	Taken orally, pale psyllium **may be of some use** as a treatment attempt for irritable bowel syndrome. **Daily dose:** Seeds up to 15g. **Pale psyllium seeds, individual dose:** Take 3–5g dried seeds with 5fl oz of water. **Pale psyllium seed cases, individual dose:** Take 10g with 1 glass of water, no more than two to three times per day. Use ready-formulated preparations as instructed by the manufacturer/prescriber. **Risks:** Can lead to hypersensitivities and may slow down absorption of various drugs (take half to one hour apart). Not to be used in persons with intestinal occlusion, poor diabetic control, or pathological narrowing of the gastrointestinal tract. Insulin-dependent diabetics should consider reducing their insulin dose (ask your doctor first). Consult a doctor if diarrhea persists (for more than three to four days).

Active ingredient/preparation	Rating
Peppermint oil (*Mentha piperita*)	**Useful** as a treatment attempt for irritable bowel syndrome. It has an antispasmodic, antibacterial, and carminative action. **Daily dose:** For internal use, 6–12 drops (for an inhalation, 3–4 drops in water). **Individual dose:** 0.2ml (approximately 8 drops) swallowed or diluted in water. Use ready-formulated preparations as instructed by the manufacturer/prescriber. **Risks:** Gastric problems are possible. Peppermint oil occasionally causes severe skin irritation. If you have gall stones, ask your doctor before taking peppermint oil. Not to be taken by persons with biliary tract occlusion, gall bladder inflammation, or severe liver damage. Do not apply to the nose and face of infants and young children.
Yarrow shoot and flowers (*Achillea millefolium*)	Taken orally, yarrow **may be of some use** as a treatment attempt for irritable bowel syndrome. Yarrow is a cholagogue, astringent, and antispasmodic. **Daily dose:** 4.5g aerial parts or 3g yarrow flowers. To prepare a tea drink, pour 1 cup of hot water over 1–1.5g of aerial parts or 1g of flowers, infuse for five minutes, and strain. Drink 1 cup several times a day. Use ready-formulated preparations as instructed by the manufacturer/prescriber. **Risks:** Contact skin allergies are possible. Not to be taken by persons who are allergic to compositae

Lack of appetite

Causes and symptoms

Poor appetite, or a diminished or absent hunger stimulus, can have a diversity of causes and occur as a result of a number of diseases and other disturbances, ranging from the simple common cold to depression and malignant tumors. Everyday stresses and worries can also lead to a lack of appetite.

Orthodox treatment

The condition is mostly treated by addressing the underlying problem. Nevertheless, certain oral appetite stimulants, usually "amara" or bitters, may be given additionally, though their effectiveness has not been substantiated scientifically.

Complementary therapies

Remedies that are commonly recommended include herbals containing amaroids or spices to stimulate the appetite. Some complementary practitioners interpret poor appetite as the result of environmental poisons or poor balance of energies.

Treatment plan and limited trial

Before administering a complementary treatment, every therapist should propose a treatment plan (*see* page xxiii) that sets out a clear time frame and defines the goal that the treatment is designed to achieve. Treatment should then be tried for a limited term to test the patient's response.

Caution

A persistent lack of appetite may be caused by a medically treatable disease.

Complementary treatments for a lack of appetite

Treatment	Rating	Point of delivery/risks
Acupressure This treatment (*see* page 769), otherwise known as pressure-point massage, is used to counter lack of appetite and nausea, which is sometimes associated with it. Some proponents of acupressure see it as an energizing (*see* page 927) treatment.	**Useful** as a short-term treatment attempt aimed at reducing nausea. Some case reports claim efficacy; however, success is probably seen in only a proportion of patients (*see* Placebo, page xxi).	**Suitable for DIY** Qualified guidance is recommended. Therapists should be properly qualified and should propose a treatment plan. **Risks:** Unlikely provided treatment is carried out competently.
Acupuncture Acupuncture in its various forms (*see* page 772) aims to encourage the flow of energy (*see* page 927) or to act directly to rectify lack of appetite.	**Useful** as a short-term treatment attempt aimed at reducing nausea. Some case reports claim efficacy; however, success is probably seen in only a proportion of patients (*see* Placebo, page xxi).	**Requires a qualified practitioner** Practitioners should be properly qualified and should propose a treatment plan. **Risks:** Probably rare provided treatment is carried out competently.
Anthroposophical medicine In the AM (*see* page 781) interpretation, the higher constituent elements are too little involved in the digestive organism. Appetite stimulants, such as amara bitters, may be given.	**May be of some use** as a short-term treatment attempt. Case reports claim efficacy; however, success is probably seen in only a proportion of patients (*see* Placebo, page xxi).	**Requires a qualified practitioner** Practitioners should be properly qualified and should propose a treatment plan. **Risks:** Allergies and intolerance are possible.

Treatment	Rating	Point of delivery/risks
Aromatherapy Essential oils (*see* page 786) are used to soothe and relax, or to invigorate, thereby stimulating the patient's appetite. The essences may be taken orally, used externally as massage oils or bathing emulsions, or inhaled as vapors. Spices are also claimed to be effective.	**May be of some use** as a short-term, supportive treatment attempt aimed at soothing and relaxing the patient and at stimulating his/her appetite. Some case reports claim efficacy; however, success is probably seen in only a proportion of patients (*see* Placebo, page xxi).	**Suitable for DIY** Qualified guidance is recommended. The effects of individual essential oils differ widely. **Risks:** Allergies or intolerance are possible. Some oils are carcinogenic in test systems and possibly in humans.
Bioresonance therapy Bioresonance therapists use electrical devices in an attempt to discover the causes of illness and claim to be able to weaken or turn around pathogenic energies and disease related vibrations (*see* page 794).	**Of little use** Possibly acceptable as a short-term, supportive treatment attempt in persistent cases when simpler, more established methods have been unsuccessful. Some case reports claim efficacy; however, success is probably seen, if at all, in only a small proportion of patients (*see* Placebo, page xxi).	**Requires a qualified practitioner** Practitioners should be properly qualified and should propose a treatment plan. No credence should be given to anyone promising immediate or total success. **Risks:** Fairly unlikely.
Cell therapy Injecting or ingesting products extracted from the tissues or organs of animals is said to have a rejuvenating and revitalizing effect and to restore appetite in sick persons (*see* page 796).	**Not advised** Based on present knowledge, there is inadequate evidence of the efficacy and mode of action of these costly and relatively risky procedures.	**Risks:** Injecting foreign proteins into the body can provoke (possibly fatal) allergic reactions. Also, pathogens such as those that cause bovine spongiform encephalopathy (BSE) or other serious infections may be introduced.

Treatment	Rating	Point of delivery/risks
Electroacupuncture according to Voll By taking readings of the electrical conductivity of the skin (*see* page 802), therapists claim to be able to derive an insight into diseased areas of the body, pathogenic foci (*see* page 928), and stress factors (*see* Toxins, page 929). The factors presumed to be instrumental in the causation of a lack of appetite can then be addressed.	**Of little use** Possibly acceptable as a short-term, supportive treatment attempt in persistent cases when simpler, more established methods have been unsuccessful. Some case reports claim efficacy; however, success is probably seen, if at all, in only a small proportion of patients (*see* Placebo, page xxi).	**Requires a qualified practitioner** Practitioners should be properly qualified and should propose a treatment plan. No credence should be given to anyone promising immediate or total success. **Risks:** A second opinion must always be obtained from a qualified physician before any attempt is made to "eliminate foci" (e.g. by surgery).
Electroneural therapy according to Croon According to the theory, readings taken at various reactive sites on the skin highlight diseased areas within the body. Based on these readings, targeted electrostimulative measures can be undertaken to address the factors presumed to be instrumental in the causation of a lack of appetite (*see* page 806).	**Of little use** Possibly acceptable as a short-term, supportive treatment attempt in persistent cases when simpler, more established methods have been unsuccessful. Some case reports claim efficacy; however, success is probably seen, if at all, in only a small proportion of patients (*see* Placebo, page xxi).	**Requires a qualified practitioner** Practitioners should be properly qualified and should propose a treatment plan. No credence should be given to anyone promising immediate or total success. **Risks:** Proponents themselves warn that treatment should not be given in acute inflammatory conditions.

Treatment	Rating	Point of delivery/risks
Eliminative methods, bloody Bloody cupping (*see* page 815) can, it is claimed, improve the body's own regulatory systems and so stimulate the appetite.	**Not advised** Conclusive proof of the efficacy of this invasive and sometimes risky procedure is lacking. Some case reports claim efficacy; however, success is probably seen, if at all, in only a small proportion of patients (*see* Placebo, page xxi).	**Risks:** Bloody cupping can cause infection and scarring. Furthermore, it should not be carried out in persons with bleeding disorders.
Enzyme therapy Enzymes (*see* page 824) obtained from plant and animal tissues are able, it is claimed, to exert a restorative effect and improve general well-being and appetite.	**Of little use** Some case reports claim efficacy for this little researched therapy; however, success is probably seen in only a small proportion of patients (*see* Placebo, page xxi).	**Requires a qualified practitioner** Practitioners should propose a treatment plan. Non-prescription preparations are suitable for do-it-yourself. **Risks:** Allergies or intolerance are possible.
Flower remedies Flower remedies (*see* page 828) are said to restore emotional balance and assist the body's psychic ability to heal itself.	**May be of some use** as a short-term, supportive treatment attempt aimed at soothing and relaxing. Some case reports claim efficacy; however, success is probably seen in only a proportion of patients (*see* Placebo, page xxi).	**Suitable for DIY** Qualified guidance is recommended. Practitioners should propose a treatment plan. **Risks:** Possible intolerance.

Treatment	Rating	Point of delivery/risks
Homeopathy Highly diluted (potentized) solutions (*see* page 831) are believed to be able to redress vital energy imbalances. Organo- and functiotropic (*see* page 833) homeopathy is claimed to be effective for dealing directly with a lack of appetite.	**May be of some use** as a supportive treatment attempt and as an additional motivation for the patient to face up to his/her condition and to perhaps change his/her lifestyle. Case reports and field studies claim efficacy; however, success is probably seen in only a proportion of patients (*see* Placebo, page xxi).	**Requires a qualified practitioner** Homeopaths should be properly qualified and should propose a treatment plan. Ready-formulated preparations are suitable for do-it-yourself. **Risks:** Allergies and intolerance are possible.
Hypnosis and self-hypnosis In the relaxed and generally altered state of awareness that is induced in hypnosis or self-hypnosis (*see* page 837), physical and mental conditions can be addressed. Hypnosis is often used in combination with other psycho- and behavioral therapies.	**Of little use** Acceptable as a short-term, supportive treatment attempt in persistent cases when simpler methods have been unsuccessful. Case reports claim efficacy; however, success is probably seen in only a proportion of patients (*see* Placebo, page xxi).	**Requires a qualified practitioner** Hypnotherapists should be properly qualified and should propose a treatment plan. **Risks:** Unlikely provided treatment is carried out competently.
Massage Classical massage (*see* page 847) is said to have a relaxing and restorative effect and to improve general well-being.	**Of little use** Acceptable as a short-term, supportive treatment attempt aimed at relaxing the patient and imparting a feeling of improved well-being. Some case reports claim efficacy for this treatment in dealing with a lack of appetite; however, success is probably seen in only a proportion of patients (*see* Placebo, page xxi).	**Suitable for DIY** Qualified guidance is recommended. Masseurs/masseuses should propose a treatment plan. **Risks:** Some people are sensitive to manual stimuli; others find it hard to tolerate close physical contact.

Treatment	Rating	Point of delivery/risks
Nutritional therapies Tasty, fragrant, and appropriately spiced foods are said to stimulate the appetite.	**Useful** as an individually directed supportive measure.	**Suitable for DIY** Qualified guidance is recommended though not essential. **Risks:** Avoid excessively spicy foods; also avoid imbalanced or intolerable diets, which can cause deficiencies with serious consequences, especially in children.
Physical therapies Exercise therapies (*see* page 868), cold washing, bathing and douches (*see* pages 875–6), and saunas (*see* page 876) are claimed to be able to improve the body's own regulatory systems, to improve the feeling of general well-being and to stimulate the appetite. These treatments are often used in combination.	**May be of some use** as a short-term treatment attempt. The effects of these procedures may differ from person to person. Some case reports claim efficacy; however, success is probably seen in only a small proportion of patients (*see* Placebo, page xxi).	**Suitable for DIY** Qualified guidance is recommended though not essential. Therapists should propose a treatment plan. **Risks:** Skin damage may be caused to persons with diminished temperature sensation when extreme temperatures are applied.
Probiotics The introduction of certain bacteria into the gut is claimed to bring the intestinal flora back into balance and to have a beneficial effect on the appetite (*see* page 878).	**Of little use** Possibly acceptable as a short-term treatment attempt in persistent cases when more established methods have been unsuccessful. Case reports claim efficacy; however, success is probably seen in only a proportion of patients (*see* Placebo, page xxi).	**Requires a qualified practitioner** Practitioners should be properly qualified and should propose a treatment plan. Non-prescription formulations are suitable for do-it-yourself. **Risks:** Fairly unlikely provided treatment is carried out competently.

Treatment	Rating	Point of delivery/risks
Reflex therapies Reflex zone massage (*see* page 883), reflexology (*see* page 883), and TENS (*see* page 886) are claimed to act via reflex channels (*see* page 881) to relax or invigorate the patient and so encourage his/her appetite.	**May be of some use** as a short-term treatment attempt. The effects of these procedures may differ widely from person to person. Some case reports claim efficacy; however, success is probably seen in only a proportion of patients (*see* Placebo, page xxi).	**Suitable for DIY** Qualified guidance is essential. **Risks:** Some people are sensitive to electrical stimuli and rubber electrodes; others find it hard to tolerate manual stimulation or close physical contact.
Relaxation techniques Autogenic training (*see* page 888), muscle relaxation according to Jacobson (*see* page 893), and various biofeedback techniques (*see* page 891) are said to relieve physical and emotional tension and so might be instrumental in addressing a lack of appetite associated with stress and tension.	**May be of some use** as a supportive treatment attempt for a lack of appetite associated with stress. Some case reports claim efficacy; however, success is probably seen in only a small proportion of patients (*see* Placebo, page xxi).	**Suitable for DIY** Once a sound understanding of the technique has been acquired from a trainer, patients can perform exercises themselves. Therapists should propose a treatment plan. **Risks:** Fairly unlikely.
Vitamins and trace elements The antioxidative properties of beta-carotene, vitamins C and E, and selenium are, it is supposed, instrumental in the reduction of individual blood fat levels, and so exercise a generally strengthening and possibly appetite stimulating effect (*see* page 900).	**Useful** in vitamin deficiency. **May be of some use** as a supportive treatment attempt aimed at generally strengthening the patient. No definitive recommendations can be made based on present knowledge. However, it would appear to be beneficial for the elderly to increase their intake of vitamins and certain trace elements.	**Suitable for DIY** Medical supervision is recommended though not essential. **Risks:** Intolerance and overdosage are possible. Recent studies imply that beta-carotene might increase the risk of cancer.

Herbal remedies for a lack of appetite

Active ingredient/preparation	*Rating*
Angelica root (*Angelica archangelica*)	**May be of some use** as a treatment attempt for digestive disorders, a lack of appetite, and flatulence. It is an antispasmodic agent and cholagogue, and promotes secretion of gastric fluid. **Daily dose:** As a decoction, 4.5g of herb. **Individual dose:** Pour boiling water over 1.5g of herb. Drink unsweetened half an hour before meals; 1.5–3g fluid extract, 1.5g tincture or 10–20 drops essential oil. Use ready-formulated preparations as instructed by the manufacturer/prescriber. **Risks:** Photosensitization (persons should avoid direct sunlight after taking angelica root, or they may suffer allergic skin irritation. The use of angelica in amounts exceeding those normally used in food should be avoided during pregnancy and breastfeeding.
Blessed thistle (*Cnicus benedictus*)	**May be of some use** as a treatment attempt for a lack of appetite and digestive disorders. It promotes the formation of saliva and gastric fluid. **Daily dose:** 4–6g herb. **Individual dose:** Pour 1 cup of hot water over 2g of herb and infuse. **Risks:** Blessed thistle may cause allergies, so do not use if you are allergic to blessed thistle or compositae.
Buck bean leaves (*Menyanthes trifoliata*)	**May be of some use** as a treatment attempt for a lack of appetite. It promotes the secretion of saliva and gastric fluid. **Daily dose:** 1.5–3g herb. **Individual dose:** Pour 1 cup of hot water over 1g of leaves and infuse. **Risks:** Buck bean is not known to have any serious side effects.

Active ingredient/preparation	*Rating*

Centaury
(*Centaurium minus*)

Taken orally, centaury **may be of some use** as a treatment attempt for a lack of appetite and digestive disorders. It is a digestive stimulant.
Daily dose: 6g herb.
Individual dose: 1–2g of herb with approximately 5oz of boiling water, or 1–2g of extract. Use ready-formulated preparations as instructed by the manufacturer/prescriber.
Risks: Centaury is not known to have any serious side effects.

Chicory leaves and root
(*Cichorium intybus* var. *intybus*)

Taken orally, chicory leaves and root **may be of some use** as a treatment attempt for digestive disorders and a lack of appetite. Chicory is a cholagogue.
Daily dose: 3g herb. **Individual dose:** Pour boiling water over 1g, infuse for five minutes, and strain. Use ready-formulated preparations as instructed by the manufacturer/prescriber.
Risks: Allergic reactions are possible. Not to be taken by persons who are allergic to chicory and compositae. If you have gall stones, ask your doctor before taking chicory.

Cinchona bark
(*Cinchona succirubra/pubescens*)

Taken orally, cinchona bark **may be of some use** as a treatment attempt for a lack of appetite, digestive problems, and flatulence. It encourages the secretion of digestive juices and saliva.
Dosage: Pour boiling water over 1g of bark, infuse for ten minutes, strain, and drink half an hour before meals. Use ready-formulated preparations as instructed by the manufacturer/prescriber.
Risks: Raised hemorrhagic tendency and hypersensitive reactions are possible. Not to be used during pregnancy or if suffering from an allergy. Cinchona bark intensifies the action of anticoagulants. In the UK it may only be sold to practitioners.

Active ingredient/preparation	*Rating*
Cinnamon bark (*Cinnamomum verum*)	Taken orally, cinnamon bark **may be of some use** as a treatment attempt for a lack of appetite, digestive disorders, and flatulence. It is a gentle digestive tonic. **Daily dose:** 2–4g dried inner bark. **Individual dose:** Pour 1 cup of hot water over 1g of dried inner bark and infuse; alternatively, 0.05–0.2g (2–8 drops) of ethereal oil on sugar. **Risks:** Allergic skin and mucosal reactions are common. Not to be used during pregnancy or by persons who are allergic to cinnamon or balsam of Tolú.
Condurango bark (*Marsdenia cundurango*)	**May be of some use** for a lack of appetite. It encourages the secretion of saliva and digestive juices. **Daily dose:** 3–5g herb. **Individual dose:** Pour 1 cup of boiling water over 1.5–2g of dried bark and infuse. Tincture: take 1 teaspoon before meals. Use ready-formulated preparations as instructed by the manufacturer/prescriber. **Risks:** Condurango is not known to have any serious side effects.
Coriander seeds (*Coriandrum sativum* var. *vulgare*)	Taken orally, coriander seeds **may be of some use** as a treatment attempt for digestive disorders and a lack of appetite. **Daily dose:** 3g seeds. **Individual dose:** To prepare an infusion for drinking several times a day between meals, bruise 1g of seeds with the back of a knife, pour on 1 cup of boiling water and infuse for five to ten minutes. Use ready-formulated preparations as instructed by the manufacturer/prescriber. **Risks:** Coriander seeds are not known to have any serious side effects.

Active ingredient/preparation	Rating

Dandelion
(*Taraxacum officinale*)

Taken orally, dandelion **may be of some use** as a treatment attempt for a lack of appetite, digestive disorders, and a feeling of fullness.
Dosage: Three times daily pour hot water over 2–3g of herb and infuse for five to ten minutes. Use ready-formulated preparations as instructed by the manufacturer/prescriber.
Risks: Contact allergies can occur (rarely). Not to be taken by persons with occlusion of the bile duct, gall bladder empyema, or intestinal occlusion. If you have gall stones, ask your doctor before taking dandelion.

Fenugreek seeds
(*Trigonella foenum-graecum*)

May be of some use for a lack of appetite.
Daily dose: 6g.
Individual dose: Allow 1.5–2.0g of seeds to steep in cold water for three hours, then drink.
Risks: May cause unpleasant skin reactions.

Galangal root
(*Alpinia officinarum*)

Taken orally, galangal **may be of some use** as a treatment attempt for digestive disorders and a lack of appetite. Its action is antispasmodic, anti-inflammatory, and antibacterial.
Daily dose: 2–4g of herb or 2–4g of tincture.
Individual dose: Pour 1 cup of boiling water over 1g of dried rhizome and infuse for five to ten minutes. Drink several times a day. Tincture on 1 spoon of sugar. Use ready-formulated preparations as instructed by the manufacturer/prescriber.
Risks: Galangal is not known to have any serious side effects.

Gentian root
(*Gentiana lutea*)

Taken orally, gentian **may be of some use** as a treatment attempt for a lack of appetite, a feeling of fullness, and flatulence. It encourages the secretion of saliva and gastric juices.
Daily dose: 2–4g herb or 1–3g tincture.
Individual dose: As a decoction, 1g of root to 1 cup of boiling water, leave to steep for five to ten minutes, and drink half an hour before meals.
Risks: May cause headaches. Not to be taken by persons with a gastric or duodenal ulcer.

Active ingredient/preparation	Rating
Iceland moss (*Cetraria islandica, Lichen islandicus*)	Taken orally, Iceland moss **may be of some use** as a treatment attempt for a lack of appetite. **Daily dose:** 4–6g lichen. **Individual dose:** Pour 1 cup of boiling water over 2g of shredded moss and infuse. Drink several times a day. **Risks:** Iceland moss is not known to have any serious side effects.
Onion (*Allium cepa*)	Taken orally, onion **may be of some use** as a treatment attempt for a lack of appetite. **Daily dose:** 2oz of fresh or 1oz of dried onion. **Individual dose:** Express the juice from a fresh onion and take 1 dessertspoon three times daily. Use ready-formulated preparations as instructed by the manufacturer/prescriber. **Risks:** Gastrointestinal intolerance is rare but possible.
Orange peel (*Citrus sinensis*)	Taken orally, orange peel **may be of some use** as a treatment attempt for a lack of appetite. **Daily dose:** 10–15g peel. **Individual dose:** Pour 1 cup of hot water over 5g and infuse. Take half an hour before meals. **Risks:** Orange peel is not known to have any serious side effects.
Pollen from various flowering plants	Taken orally, pollen **may be of some use** as an attempted treatment for a lack of appetite. Pollen is an appetite stimulant. **Daily dose:** 30–40g; micronized pollen (see instructions on the label), take 3–4g. Use ready-formulated preparations as instructed by the manufacturer/prescriber. **Risks:** Pollen must not be taken by persons who are allergic to it, as the reactions may be intense (including asthma attacks).

Active ingredient/preparation	*Rating*

Sour orange peel
(*Citrus aurantium* ssp. *aurantium*)

Taken orally, the peel of sour (Seville) oranges **may be of some use** as a treatment attempt for a lack of appetite and digestive disorders.
Daily dose: 4–6g peel, 2–3g tincture. To prepare a tea drink, pour boiling water over 2g of peel; 30–40 drops of tincture on sugar.
Risks: Photosensitization (persons with a light complexion should avoid direct sunlight after taking sour orange peel, or they may suffer allergic skin reactions).

Soybean phospholipids
(*Glycine max*)

Taken orally, these **may be of some use** as an attempt to improve the subjective condition of persons lacking an appetite.
Daily dose: Use ready-formulated preparations as instructed by the manufacturer/prescriber.
Risks: Gastric problems, soft stools, and diarrhea are occasionally encountered.

White horehound
(*Marrubium vulgare*)

Taken orally, white horehound **may be of some use** as a treatment attempt for a lack of appetite, digestive disorders, and a feeling of fullness. The constituent marrubic acid is a cholagogue.
Daily dose: 4.5g herb.
Individual dose: Pour 1 cup of boiling water over 1.5g of herb and infuse.
Risks: White horehound is not known to have any serious side effects.

Wormwood
(*Artemisia absinthium*)

Taken orally, wormwood **may be of some use** as a treatment attempt for a lack of appetite and digestive disorders. Contains bitter principles and volatile oil.
Daily dose: 3–5g herb.
Individual dose: Pour 1 cup of hot water over 1.5–2g of dried herb and infuse. Use ready-formulated preparations as instructed by the manufacturer/prescriber.
Risks: Do not use oil of wormwood. The isolated essential oil can damage the nervous system and impair intellectual faculties. Many countries therefore forbid alcoholic solutions and the pure oil.

Active ingredient/preparation	Rating
Yarrow shoot and flowers (*Achillea millefolium*)	Taken orally, yarrow **may be of some use** as a treatment attempt for a lack of appetite, digestive disorders, and spasms. Yarrow is a cholagogue and antispasmodic. **Daily dose:** 4.5g aerial parts, 3g yarrow flowers. To prepare a tea drink, pour hot water over 1.5g of aerial parts or 1g of flowers. Use ready-formulated preparations as instructed by the manufacturer/ prescriber. **Risks:** Not to be taken by persons who are allergic to compositae.

Liver disease

Causes and symptoms

The liver is the largest gland in the human body. It has a number of digestive and metabolic functions and also plays a key role in the circulatory and hormonal systems. It is instrumental in the detoxification of drugs and many other toxic and waste products that are either produced within the body or assimilated from the environment. There is a particularly wide range of diseases that involve the liver.

Orthodox treatment

- Fatty degeneration of the liver, through alcohol abuse or excessive use of drugs, can normally be reversed by cutting out alcohol and the drugs in question.
- Cases of hepatitis A usually recover without specific treatment. In hepatitis of types B and C, and also of types D and E, modern methods of treatment, e.g. using interferons (anti-viral proteins produced within the body), are still at the clinical testing stage. In most cases, the acute phase of hepatitis subsides within four to eight weeks without any special treatment and the majority of cases will recover completely within three to six months. Active immunization can be useful in preventing hepatitis A and B.

- There is presently no treatment that is 100 percent effective for cirrhosis, a condition of progressive scarring of the liver, so a liver transplant is sometimes the only recourse.
- Surgery and chemotherapy are occasionally effective against primary liver cancer.

Complementary therapies

Various naturopathic remedies are claimed to be effective for treating liver diseases. There is no formal evidence, however, that these work against hepatitis B, C, and E, nor against cirrhosis, serious autoimmune diseases, and cancer of the liver.

Nutritional therapies, and sometimes botanicals, can be successful against certain conditions affecting the liver. Overall, however, complementary therapies are not important except in a supporting role, e.g. for alleviating discomfort or for lessening the withdrawal symptoms of alcoholism.

Treatment plan and limited trial

Before administering a complementary treatment, every therapist should propose a treatment plan (*see* page xxiii) that sets out a clear time frame and defines the goal that the treatment is designed to achieve. Treatment should then be tried for a limited term to test the patient's response.

Caution

Always consult a physician to obtain a thorough examination before embarking on any alternative or complementary treatment for symptoms that may be associated with a liver disease. If you do not, you risk forgoing a vital orthodox treatment, or of exposing others unnecessarily to an infection form of hepatitis.

Complementary treatments for liver disease

Treatment	Rating	Point of delivery/risks
Acupressure This treatment (*see* page 769), otherwise known as pressure-point massage, is claimed to lessen pain and nausea during alcohol withdrawal (*see* page 66), to release tension, and to improve general well-being. Acupressure is also claimed to impart vital energy (*see* Life force, page 928).	**Inappropriate** as the sole treatment for liver disease. **May be of some use** as a short-term, supportive treatment attempt aimed at easing symptoms during alcohol withdrawal. The easing of symptoms and long recidivation-free periods claimed in field studies probably apply to only a proportion of patients (*see* Placebo, page xxi).	**Suitable for DIY** Qualified guidance is recommended. Therapists should be properly qualified and should propose a treatment plan. **Risks:** Unlikely provided treatment is carried out competently.
Acupuncture Acupuncture in its various forms (*see* page 772) aims to encourage the flow of energy (*see* page 927), to lessen pain during alcohol withdrawal, or to strengthen the liver directly and hasten its regeneration. The acupuncture points chosen can vary from one practitioner to another.	**Inappropriate** as the sole treatment for liver disease. **May be of some use** as a short-term, supportive treatment attempt, e.g. for relief of pain during alcohol withdrawal, and as a means of strengthening the liver and hastening its regeneration. Case reports and field studies claim efficacy; however, success is probably seen in only a proportion of patients (*see* Placebo, page xxi).	**Requires a qualified practitioner** Acupuncturists should be properly qualified and should propose a treatment plan. No credence should be given to anyone promising immediate or total success. **Risks:** Probably rare provided treatment is carried out competently.

Treatment	Rating	Point of delivery/risks
Anthroposophical medicine In acute inflammatory liver disease, doctors who practice AM (*see* page 781) prescribe a diet and potentized tin; in degenerative conditions, the composition Hepatodoron is given.	**May be of some use** as a short-term, supportive treatment attempt. Case reports claim efficacy for these two types of preparation; however, success is probably seen in only a proportion of patients (*see* Placebo, page xxi).	**Requires a qualified practitioner** Practitioners should be properly qualified and should propose a treatment plan. **Risks:** Allergies and intolerance are possible.
Aromatherapy Essential oils (*see* page 786) are used to soothe and relax, or to invigorate, thereby improving general well-being. The essences may be taken orally, used externally as massage oils or bathing emulsions, or inhaled as vapors.	**Inappropriate** as the sole treatment for liver disease. **May be of some use** as a short-term, supportive treatment attempt aimed at invigorating or soothing the patient. Some case reports claim efficacy; however, success is probably seen in only a small proportion of patients (*see* Placebo, page xxi).	**Suitable for DIY** Qualified guidance is recommended. The effects of individual essential oils differ widely. **Risks:** Allergies or intolerance are possible. Some oils are carcinogenic in test systems and possibly in humans.
Bioresonance therapy Bioresonance therapists use electrical devices in an attempt to discover the causes of illness and claim to be able to weaken or turn around pathogenic energies and disease related vibrations (*see* page 794).	**Inappropriate** as the sole treatment for liver disease. Possibly acceptable as a short-term, supportive treatment attempt in persistent cases when simpler, more established methods have been unsuccessful. Some case reports claim efficacy; however, success is probably seen, if at all, in only a small proportion of patients (*see* Placebo, page xxi).	**Requires a qualified practitioner** Practitioners should be properly qualified and should propose a treatment plan. No credence should be given to anyone promising immediate or total success. **Risks:** Fairly unlikely.

Treatment	Rating	Point of delivery/risks
Cell therapy Injecting or ingesting products extracted from the tissues and organs of animals is said to have a rejuvenating and revitalizing effect and to enhance the healing of human tissues and organs (*see* page 796).	**Not advised** Based on present knowledge, there is inadequate evidence of the efficacy and mode of action of these costly and relatively risky procedures.	**Risks:** Injecting foreign proteins into the body can provoke (possibly fatal) allergic reactions. Also, pathogens such as those that cause bovine spongiform encephalopathy (BSE) or other serious infections may be introduced.
Electroacupuncture according to Voll By taking readings of the electrical conductivity of the skin (*see* page 802), therapists claim to be able to derive an insight into diseased areas of the body, pathogenic foci (*see* page 928), and stress factors (*see* Toxins, page 929). The factors presumed to be instrumental in the causation of liver disease can then be addressed.	**Inappropriate** as the sole treatment for liver disease. Possibly acceptable as a short-term, supportive treatment attempt when simpler, more established methods have been unsuccessful. Some case reports claim efficacy; however, success is probably seen, if at all, in only a small proportion of patients (*see* Placebo, page xxi).	**Requires a qualified practitioner** Practitioners should be properly qualified and should propose a treatment plan. No credence should be given to anyone promising immediate or total success. **Risks:** A second opinion must always be obtained from a qualified physician before any attempt is made to "eliminate foci" (e.g. by surgery).
Electroneural therapy according to Croon According to the theory, readings taken at various reactive sites on the skin highlight diseased areas within the body. Based on these readings, targeted electrostimulative measures can be undertaken to address factors presumed to be instrumental in the causation of liver disease (*see* page 806).	**Inappropriate** as the sole treatment for liver disease. Possibly acceptable as a short-term, supportive treatment attempt when simpler, more established methods have been unsuccessful. Some case reports claim efficacy; however, success is probably seen, if at all, in only a small proportion of patients (*see* Placebo, page xxi).	**Requires a qualified practitioner** Practitioners should be properly qualified and should propose a treatment plan. No credence should be given to anyone promising immediate or total success. **Risks:** Proponents themselves warn that treatment should not be given in acute inflammatory conditions.

Treatment	*Rating*	*Point of delivery/risks*
Eliminative methods, bloody Bloody cupping (*see* page 815) is said to improve general well-being and to boost the body's own regulatory systems.	**Not advised** The efficacy and mode of action of this invasive and sometimes risky procedure are unproven.	**Risks:** Bloody cupping can cause infection and scarring. Furthermore, it should not be carried out on persons with bleeding disorders.
Eliminative methods, unbloody Unbloody cupping (*see* page 817) is supposed to energize (*see* page 927) the patient and to improve the body's own regulatory systems.	**Inappropriate** as the sole treatment for liver disease. **May be of some use** as a short-term, supportive treatment attempt aimed at alleviating pain during alcohol withdrawal, for instance. Some case reports claim efficacy; however, success is probably seen in only a proportion of patients (*see* Placebo, page xxi).	**Suitable for DIY** Unbloody cupping is best carried out under the guidance of a qualified practitioner. **Risks:** Unlikely provided treatment is carried out competently.
Flower remedies Flower remedies (*see* page 828) are said to restore emotional balance and assist the body's psychic ability to heal itself.	**Inappropriate** as the sole treatment for liver disease. **May be of some use** as a short-term, supportive treatment attempt aimed at soothing and relaxing. Some case reports claim efficacy; however, success is probably seen in only a proportion of patients (*see* Placebo, page xxi).	**Suitable for DIY** Qualified guidance is recommended. Practitioners should be properly qualified and should propose a treatment plan. **Risks:** Possible intolerance.

Treatment	Rating	Point of delivery/risks
Homeopathy Highly diluted (potentized) solutions (*see* page 831) are believed to be able to redress vital energy imbalances. Organo- and functiotropic (*see* page 833) homeopathy is claimed to be effective for dealing directly with liver disease.	**Inappropriate** as the sole treatment for liver disease. **May be of some use** as a supportive treatment attempt and for helping the patient come to terms emotionally with his/her condition. Some case reports claim efficacy; however, success is probably seen in only a proportion of patients (*see* Placebo, page xxi).	**Requires a qualified practitioner** Homeopaths should be properly qualified and should propose a treatment plan. Ready-formulated preparations are suitable for do-it-yourself. **Risks:** Allergies and intolerance are possible.
Hypnosis and self-hypnosis In the relaxed and generally altered state of awareness that is induced in hypnosis or self-hypnosis (*see* page 837), physical conditions can be addressed and pain alleviated. Hypnosis is often used in combination with other psycho- and behavioral therapies in order to help the patient change his/her lifestyle.	**Inappropriate** as the sole treatment for liver disease. **May be of some use** as a short-term, supportive treatment attempt for relaxing the patient and easing symptoms during alcohol withdrawal, and for helping the patient to achieve a change in his/her lifestyle. Case reports claim efficacy; however, success is probably seen in only a proportion of patients (*see* Placebo, page xxi).	**Requires a qualified practitioner** Hypnotherapists should be properly qualified and should propose a treatment plan. No credence should be given to anyone promising immediate or total success. **Risks:** Unlikely provided treatment is carried out competently.
Magnetic field therapy The use of magnetic field generators, magnetic strips, bracelets, and other objects (*see* page 841) allegedly encourages cell metabolism and so hastens recovery.	**Inappropriate** Based on present knowledge, there is inadequate evidence of the efficacy and mode of action of magnetic field therapy in liver disease.	Operation of magnetic field equipment **requires a qualified practitioner**. **Risks:** Magnetic field equipment can cause implanted cardiac pacemakers to malfunction.

Treatment	Rating	Point of delivery/risks
Massage Classical massage (*see* page 847) can ease muscular and emotional tension, and thereby hasten recovery.	**Inappropriate** as the sole treatment for liver disease. **Useful** as a short-term, supportive treatment attempt aimed at relaxing the patient. Case reports claim efficacy; however, success is probably seen in only a proportion of patients (*see* Placebo, page xxi).	**Suitable for DIY** Qualified guidance is recommended. Masseurs/masseuses should propose a treatment plan. **Risks:** Some people are sensitive to manual stimuli; others find it hard to tolerate close physical contact.
Nutritional therapies The vitamins and secondary plant nutrients that an organic diet (*see* page 4) provides are believed to exercise a multitude of positive effects. Patients suffering from alcoholism are often undersupplied with vitamins (*see* page 900).	**Useful** as a longer-term, individually directed measure and as a way of combating vitamin deficiency.	**Suitable for DIY** Qualified guidance is recommended. In advanced stages the optimum diet should be discussed with a doctor. **Risks:** Avoid imbalanced or intolerable diets. They can cause deficiencies with serious consequences. Children are particularly at risk.
Physical therapies Ascending-temperature sitz baths, body wraps, hot packs (*see* pages 871–8), etc., are said to improve the hepatic circulation.	**Inappropriate** as the sole treatment for liver disease. **May be of some use** as a short-term treatment attempt aimed at improving general well-being. Case reports and field studies claim efficacy; however, success is probably seen in only a proportion of patients (*see* Placebo, page xxi).	**Suitable for DIY** Qualified guidance is recommended. An individual plan of treatment should be defined in association with the treating physician. **Risks:** Skin damage may be caused to persons with diminished temperature sensation when extreme temperatures are applied.

Treatment	_Rating_	_Point of delivery/risks_
Probiotics The introduction of certain bacteria into the gut is claimed to bring the intestinal flora back into balance, to have an immune system modulating effect, and to hasten the breakdown of poisons and fusel alcohols in the colon (_see_ page 878).	**Inappropriate** as the sole treatment for liver disease. **May be of some use** as a short-term, supportive treatment attempt aimed at reducing the production of fusel alcohols in the colon. Experiments have shown that probiotics might indeed achieve this aim. Case reports claim efficacy; however, success is probably seen in only a proportion of patients (_see_ Placebo, page xxi).	**Requires a qualified practitioner** Practitioners should be properly qualified and should propose a treatment plan. Non-prescription formulations are suitable for do-it-yourself. **Risks:** Fairly unlikely provided treatment is carried out competently.
Reflex therapies Connective tissue massage and colonic massage (_see_ page 883) are claimed to improve the hepatic circulation.	**Inappropriate** as the sole treatment for liver disease. **May be of some use** as a short-term, supportive treatment attempt aimed at improving the hepatic circulation or at alleviating pain. Case reports claim efficacy; however, success is probably seen in only a proportion of patients (_see_ Placebo, page xxi).	**Requires a qualified practitioner** Practitioners should be properly qualified and should propose a treatment plan. **Risks:** Some people are sensitive to manual stimulation or close physical contact.

Treatment	Rating	Point of delivery/risks
Relaxation techniques Autogenic training (*see* page 888), muscle relaxation according to Jacobson (*see* page 893), and various biofeedback techniques (*see* page 891) are said to relieve muscle tension and inner unrest and, in combination with psychotherapy, might be instrumental in easing alcohol withdrawal.	**Inappropriate** as the sole treatment for liver disease. **May be of some use** as a short-term, supportive treatment attempt aimed at relaxing the patient and facilitating alcohol withdrawal. Case reports claim efficacy; however, success is probably seen in only a proportion of patients (*see* Placebo, page xxi).	**Suitable for DIY** Once a sound understanding of the technique has been acquired from a trainer in group sessions or through individual tuition, patients can perform exercises themselves. Therapists should propose a treatment plan **Risks:** Fairly unlikely.
TENS The use of low frequency electrical currents on the surface of the skin (*see* page 886) is said to energize (*see* page 927) the patient, release energy blockages (*see* page 927), ease pain, and improve the circulation.	**Inappropriate** as the sole treatment for liver disease. **May be of some use** as a short-term, supportive treatment attempt aimed at improving the circulation and easing pain. Case reports and field studies claim efficacy; however, success is probably seen in only a proportion of patients (*see* Placebo, page xxi).	**Requires a qualified practitioner** Practitioners should be properly qualified and should propose a treatment plan. **Risks:** Some people react sensitively to electrical stimuli or rubber electrodes.
Vitamins and trace elements The antioxidative properties of beta-carotene, vitamins C and E, and selenium are claimed to modulate the immune system (*see* page 10) and exercise a multitude of beneficial effects. Vitamin tablets are said to counter vitamin deficiency caused by damage to the liver (*see* page 900).	**Inappropriate** as the sole treatment for liver disease. **May be of some use** in vitamin deficiency caused by liver disease. Based on present knowledge, no definitive recommendations regarding dosages of vitamins with antioxidative properties can be given.	**Suitable for DIY** Qualified guidance is recommended though not essential. **Risks:** Intolerance and overdosage are possible. Recent studies imply that beta-carotene might increase the risk of cancer.

Herbal remedy for liver disease

Active ingredient/preparation	Rating
Milk thistle seeds (*Silybum marianum*)	Taken internally, milk thistle **may be of some use** as a treatment attempt for toxic liver damage, e.g. in Amanita (agaric) poisoning. **Of little use** as a supportive treatment for liver regeneration in chronic inflammatory liver disease, e.g. liver cirrhosis. It does not provide any protection against substances that adversely affect the liver, such as alcohol. Only abstinence protects against progressive liver disease. **Daily dose:** 12–15g seeds (for preparing infusions). **Individual dose:** Pour 5oz of hot water over 3–5g, strain, and drink with meals. Use ready-formulated preparations as instructed by the manufacturer/prescriber. **Risks:** There are various accounts of milk thistle having a laxative effect. There is also evidence that it may cause severe allergic (even anaphylactic) reactions.

Vomiting

Causes and symptoms

Vomiting may be caused by many infectious and non-infectious diseases. However, psychological factors, environmental influences, and toxins may be instrumental in its causation. Vomiting also occurs frequently during pregnancy.

Orthodox treatment

Doctors often try to reduce or prevent vomiting through the use of drugs, as treating the cause is not always an effective means of stopping it. Fluids and salts must be replaced. Psychotherapy or counselling may prove useful in certain patients who suffer chronically from bouts of vomiting.

Complementary therapies

There is evidence to suggest that certain complementary treatments may indeed be effective against nausea and vomiting.

Treatment plan and limited trial

Before administering a complementary treatment, every therapist should propose a treatment plan (*see* page xxiii) that sets out a clear time frame and defines the goal that the treatment is designed to achieve. Treatment should then be tried for a limited term to test the patient's response.

Caution

Always consult a physician if vomiting is recurrent or persistent, as it may suggest the presence of a serious physical ailment.

Complementary treatments for vomiting

Treatment	Rating	Point of delivery/risks
Acupressure This treatment (*see* page 769), otherwise known as pressure-point massage, is claimed to prevent or ease nausea and vomiting. The pressure points chosen may differ from one practitioner to another. Special bracelets and poultices are sometimes used.	**Useful** for prevention and as a treatment attempt. Observational studies and case reports ascribe a degree of efficacy in the treatment of nausea and vomiting (*see* Placebo, page xxi).	**Suitable for DIY** Qualified guidance is recommended. Therapists should be properly qualified. **Risks:** Unlikely provided treatment is carried out competently.

Treatment	Rating	Point of delivery/risks
Acupuncture Acupuncture in its various forms (*see* page 772) aims to prevent or alleviate nausea and vomiting. The acupuncture points chosen can vary from one practitioner to another.	**Useful** for prevention and as a treatment attempt. Observational studies and case reports ascribe a degree of efficacy in the treatment of nausea and vomiting (*see* Placebo, page xxi).	**Requires a qualified practitioner** Acupuncturists should be properly qualified and should propose a treatment plan. **Risks:** Probably rare provided treatment is carried out competently.
Aromatherapy Essential oils (*see* page 786) are used to soothe and relax, or to invigorate, thereby reducing nausea.	**Of little use** Acceptable as a supportive treatment attempt aimed at soothing and relaxing. Some case reports claim efficacy; however, success is probably seen in only a small proportion of patients (*see* Placebo, page xxi).	**Suitable for DIY** Qualified guidance is recommended. The effects of individual essential oils differ widely. **Risks:** Allergies or intolerance are possible. Some oils are carcinogenic in test systems and possibly in humans.
Flower remedies Flower remedies (*see* page 828) are said to restore emotional balance and assist the body's psychic ability to heal itself.	**Of little use** Acceptable as a short-term, supportive treatment attempt aimed at soothing and relaxing. Some case reports claim efficacy; however, success is probably seen in only a small proportion of patients (*see* Placebo, page xxi).	**Suitable for DIY** Qualified guidance is recommended. Practitioners should be properly qualified and should propose a treatment plan. **Risks:** Possible intolerance.

Treatment	Rating	Point of delivery/risks
Homeopathy The highly diluted (potentized) solutions (*see* page 831) used in organo- and functiotropic (*see* page 833) homeopathy are claimed to be effective for dealing with nausea and vomiting.	**Of little use** Acceptable as a supportive treatment attempt. Some case reports claim efficacy; however, success is probably seen in only a proportion of patients (*see* Placebo, page xxi).	**Requires a qualified practitioner** Homeopaths should be properly qualified and should propose a treatment plan. Ready-formulated preparations are suitable for do-it-yourself. **Risks:** Allergies and intolerance are possible.
Hypnosis and self-hypnosis In the relaxed and generally altered state of awareness that is induced in hypnosis or self-hypnosis (*see* page 837), physical and emotional conditions can be addressed to counter retching.	**Of little use** Acceptable in persistent cases as a preventive measure when simpler, more established methods have been unsuccessful. Some case reports claim efficacy; however, success is probably seen in only a proportion of patients treated (*see* Placebo, page xxi).	**Requires a qualified practitioner** Hypnotherapists should be properly qualified and should propose a treatment plan. **Risks:** Unlikely provided treatment is carried out competently.
Massage Ice massage is claimed to act via reflex channels (see page 881) to ease or eliminate nausea and vomiting.	**Maybe of some use** as a treatment attempt for vomiting. Some case reports claim efficacy; however, success is probably seen in only a proportion of patients (*see* Placebo, page xxi).	**Requires a qualified practitioner** Masseurs/masseuses should be properly qualified and should propose a treatment plan. **Risks:** Some people are sensitive to manual stimuli; others find it hard to tolerate close physical contact.

Treatment	Rating	Point of delivery/risks
Reflex therapies Various therapies such as acupressure (*see* page 769), connective tissue massage (*see* page 883), and ice massage (*see* page 878), are claimed to act via reflex channels (*see* page 881) to ease or eliminate nausea and vomiting.	**May be of some use** as a treatment attempt for vomiting. Some case reports claim efficacy; however, success is probably seen in only a proportion of patients (*see* Placebo, page xxi).	**Requires a qualified practitioner** Practitioners should be properly qualified and should propose a treatment plan. **Risks:** Some people cannot tolerate cold, pressure applied during massage, or close physical contact.
Relaxation techniques Autogenic training (*see* page 888), muscle relaxation according to Jacobson (*see* page 893), and various biofeedback techniques (*see* page 891) are said to relieve muscle tension and inner unrest, and might be instrumental in countering retching.	**May be of some use** in persistent cases as a supportive treatment attempt aimed at relaxing the patient. Case reports claim efficacy; however, success is probably seen in only a proportion of patients (*see* Placebo, page xxi).	**Suitable for DIY** Once a sound understanding of the technique has been acquired from a trainer in group sessions or through individual tuition, patients can perform exercises themselves. Therapists should propose a treatment plan. **Risks:** Fairly unlikely.
TENS The use of low frequency electrical currents (*see* page 886) on the surface of the skin is said to lessen or eliminate nausea and vomiting.	**May be of some use** as a treatment attempt for vomiting. A small number of controlled clinical studies, observational studies, and case reports ascribe a degree of efficacy to this treatment for nausea and vomiting. Case reports claim efficacy; however, success is probably seen in only a proportion of patients (*see* Placebo, page xxi).	**Requires a qualified practitioner** Practitioners should be properly qualified and should propose a treatment plan. **Risks:** Some people react sensitively to electrical stimuli or rubber electrodes.

Herbal remedy for vomiting

Active ingredient/preparation	Rating
Ginger root (*Zingiber officinale*)	Taken orally, ginger root **may be of some use** as a treatment attempt for digestive disorders and travel sickness. **Daily dose:** 1–3g root. To be chewed occasionally throughout the day. Can also be prepared as in infusion or decoction (0.25–1g to 1 cup of hot water three times daily). Use ready-formulated preparations as instructed by the manufacturer/prescriber. **Risks:** Patients with gall stones should ask their doctor before taking ginger root. Not to be used for morning sickness.

Wind (meteorism and flatulence)

Causes and symptoms

Meteorism is a buildup of air or gas in the gut. Flatulence is a distension of the stomach and/or bowel through the buildup of gas, producing a bloated feeling and an embarrassing release of wind. The conditions have many causes including nervousness and other psychological factors; they may be symptomatic of a physical disease or the consequence of food intolerance. They also may have no significance at all and may simply be related to the food consumed most recently.

Orthodox treatment

Acute attacks of wind can be treated with medical preparations to bind the gas.

Complementary therapies

The principal approach of most complementary therapies is to reduce the symptoms. Meteorism and flatulence are often seen as having a constitutional causation (*see* Constitution, page 927), so treatments are offered accordingly.

Treatment plan and limited trial

Before administering a complementary treatment, every therapist should propose a treatment plan (*see* page xxiii) that sets out a clear time frame and defines the goal that the treatment is designed to achieve. Treatment should then be tried for a limited term to test the patient's response.

Caution

Patients with persistent or chronic symptoms should visit their doctor for a thorough investigation, followed by a specific treatment.

Complementary treatments for wind (meteorism and flatulence)

Treatment	Rating	Point of delivery/risks
Acupressure This treatment (*see* page 769), otherwise known as pressure-point massage, is claimed to release tension and ease wind when pressure is applied to the appropriate points.	**May be of some use** as a short-term treatment attempt. Some case reports claim efficacy; however, success is probably seen in only a proportion of patients (*see* Placebo, page xxi).	**Suitable for DIY** Qualified guidance is recommended. Therapists should be properly qualified. **Risks:** Unlikely provided treatment is carried out competently.
Acupuncture Acupuncture in its various forms (*see* page 772) aims to encourage the flow of energy (*see* page 927) or to act directly to ease wind.	**May be of some use** as a short-term treatment attempt. Some case reports claim efficacy; however, success is probably seen in only a proportion of patients (*see* Placebo, page xxi).	**Requires a qualified practitioner** Practitioners should be properly qualified and should propose a treatment plan. **Risks:** Probably rare provided treatment is carried out competently.

Treatment	Rating	Point of delivery/risks
Anthroposophical medicine For treating wind, AM (*see* page 781) uses special diets and compositions.	**May be of some use** as a short-term treatment attempt. Case reports claim efficacy; however, success is probably seen in only a proportion of patients (*see* Placebo, page xxi).	**Requires a qualified practitioner** Practitioners should be properly qualified and should propose a treatment plan. **Risks:** Allergies and intolerance are possible.
Bioresonance therapy Bioresonance therapists use electrical devices in an attempt to discover the causes of illness and claim to be able to weaken or turn around pathogenic energies and disease related vibrations (*see* page 794).	**Of little use** Possibly acceptable as a short-term treatment attempt in persistent cases when simpler, more established methods have been unsuccessful. Some case reports claim efficacy; however, success is probably seen, if at all, in only a small proportion of patients (*see* Placebo, page xxi).	**Requires a qualified practitioner** Practitioners should be properly qualified and should propose a treatment plan. No credence should be given to anyone promising immediate or total success. **Risks:** Fairly unlikely.
Cell therapy Injecting or ingesting products extracted from the tissues of newborn animals or animal fetuses is said to have a rejuvenating and revitalizing effect and to enhance the healing of human tissues and organs (*see* page 796).	**Not advised** Based on present knowledge, there is inadequate evidence of the efficacy and mode of action of these costly and relatively risky procedures.	**Risks:** Injecting foreign proteins into the body can provoke (possibly fatal) allergic reactions. Also, pathogens such as those that cause bovine spongiform encephalopathy (BSE) or other serious infections may be introduced.

Treatment	Rating	Point of delivery/risks
Electroacupuncture according to Voll By taking readings of the electrical conductivity of the skin (*see* page 802), therapists claim to be able to derive an insight into diseased areas of the body, pathogenic foci (*see* page 928), and stress factors (*see* Toxins, page 929). The factors presumed to be instrumental in the causation of wind can then be addressed.	**Of little use** Possibly acceptable as a short-term, supportive treatment attempt when simpler, more established methods have been unsuccessful. Some case reports claim efficacy; however, success is probably seen, if at all, in only a small proportion of patients (*see* Placebo, page xxi).	**Requires a qualified practitioner** Practitioners should be properly qualified and should propose a treatment plan. No credence should be given to anyone promising immediate or total success. **Risks:** A second opinion must always be obtained from a qualified physician before any attempt is made to "eliminate foci" (e.g. by surgery).
Electroneural therapy according to Croon According to the theory, readings taken at various reactive sites on the skin highlight diseased areas within the body. Based on these readings, targeted electrostimulative measures can be undertaken to address factors presumed to be instrumental in the causation of wind (*see* page 806).	**Of little use** Possibly acceptable as a short-term, supportive treatment attempt in persistent cases when simpler, more established methods have been unsuccessful. Some case reports claim efficacy; however, success is probably seen, if at all, in only a small proportion of patients (*see* Placebo, page xxi).	**Requires a qualified practitioner** Practitioners should be properly qualified and should propose a treatment plan. No credence should be given to anyone promising immediate or total success. **Risks:** Proponents themselves warn that treatment should not be given in acute inflammatory conditions.
Eliminative methods, unbloody Unbloody cupping (*see* page 817) is supposed to relax patients with wind and to improve the body's regulatory systems. Enemas are used to hasten evacuation of the bowel.	**Of little use** Acceptable as a short-term treatment attempt. Some case reports and field studies claim efficacy; however, success is probably seen, if at all, in only a proportion of patients (*see* Placebo, page xxi).	**Suitable for DIY** Unbloody cupping is best carried out under the guidance of a qualified practitioner. **Risks:** Unlikely provided treatment is carried out competently.

Treatment	Rating	Point of delivery/risks
Enzyme therapy The enzymes used (*see* page 824) are claimed, *inter alia*, to exert an influence on digestion.	**Of little use** Some case reports claim efficacy for this little researched therapy; however, success is probably seen in only a small proportion of patients (*see* Placebo, page xxi).	**Requires a qualified practitioner** Practitioners should propose a treatment plan. Non-prescription preparations are suitable for do-it-yourself. **Risks:** Allergies or intolerance are possible.
Flower remedies Flower remedies (*see* page 828) are said to restore emotional balance and assist the body's psychic ability to heal itself.	**Of little use** Acceptable as a short-term treatment attempt aimed at soothing and relaxing. Some case reports claim efficacy; however, success is probably seen in only a proportion of patients (*see* Placebo, page xxi).	**Suitable for DIY** Qualified guidance is recommended. Practitioners should propose a treatment plan. **Risks:** Possible intolerance.
Homeopathy Highly diluted (potentized) solutions (*see* page 831) are believed to be able to redress vital energy imbalances and strengthen the body's defences. Organo- and functiotropic (*see* page 833) homeopathy is claimed to be effective for dealing with symptoms.	**May be of some use** as a supportive treatment attempt in persistent cases. Some case reports and field studies claim efficacy; however, success is probably seen in only a proportion of patients (*see* Placebo, page xxi).	**Requires a qualified practitioner** Homeopaths should be properly qualified and should propose a treatment plan. Ready-formulated preparations are suitable for do-it-yourself. **Risks:** Allergies and intolerance are possible.

Treatment	Rating	Point of delivery/risks
Hypnosis and self-hypnosis In the relaxed and generally altered state of awareness that is induced in hypnosis or self-hypnosis (*see* page 837), physical and mental conditions can be addressed. Hypnosis is often used in combination with other psycho- and behavioral therapies.	**Of little use** Acceptable as a short-term, supportive treatment attempt aimed at soothing and relaxing and bringing about a change of behavior when symptoms persist. Case reports claim efficacy; however, success is probably seen in only a proportion of patients treated (*see* Placebo, page xxi).	**Requires a qualified practitioner** Hypnotherapists should be properly qualified and should propose a treatment plan. No credence should be given to anyone promising immediate or total success. **Risks:** Unlikely provided treatment is carried out competently.
Manual therapies Chiropractors and osteopaths (*see* page 844) use a series of manipulations to realign allegedly displaced vertebrae. This is said to ease dysfunctions, release energy blockages (*see* page 927), and address factors that may be at the root of the problem.	**Of little use** Possibly acceptable as a short-term treatment attempt when wind is due to a change of posture. Some case reports claim efficacy for these potentially risky procedures; however, success is probably seen, if at all, in only a small proportion of patients (*see* Placebo, page xxi).	**Requires a qualified practitioner** Practitioners should be properly qualified and should propose a treatment plan. **Risks:** Manipulation of the head and cervical vertebrae can cause serious injury. Osteoporosis is one of several risk factors.
Massage Classical massage (*see* page 847) is said to relax and invigorate, and to make tissues more reactive.	**May be of some use** as a short-term treatment attempt. Some case reports claim efficacy; however, success is probably seen in only a proportion of patients (*see* Placebo, page xxi).	**Requires a qualified practitioner** Masseurs/masseuses should be properly qualified and should propose a treatment plan. **Risks:** Some people are sensitive to manual stimuli; others find it hard to tolerate close physical contact.

Treatment	Rating	Point of delivery/risks
Nutritional therapies An organic diet (*see* page 4) is beneficial owing to its high content of secondary plant constituents. Foods that cause wind, such as cabbage or legumes, should be avoided (*see* pages 858–67).	**Useful** as an individually directed supportive measure. Elimination and rotation diets may be of some assistance in identifying the cause of food allergies.	**Suitable for DIY** Qualified guidance is recommended. See your doctor before starting an elimination or rotation diet. **Risks:** Avoid imbalanced or intolerable diets. They can cause deficiencies with serious consequences. Children are particularly at risk.
Physical therapies Exercise therapy (*see* page 868), hot water bottles, hot wraps and packs, alternating temperature foot baths (*see* pages 871–8) and medicinal mineral waters are said to relax or invigorate the patient, easing symptoms.	**Useful** as a short-term treatment attempt. Some case reports and field studies claim efficacy; however, success is probably seen in only a proportion of patients (*see* Placebo, page xxi).	**Suitable for DIY** Qualified guidance is recommended. The effects of these treatments differ widely from person to person. Their use should be guided by the success achieved. **Risks:** Skin damage may be caused to persons with diminished temperature sensation when extreme temperatures are applied.
Probiotics The introduction of certain bacteria into the gut is claimed to bring the intestinal flora back into balance and to have a beneficial effect on the digestive system (*see* page 878).	**May be of some use** as a short-term treatment attempt for persistent cases. Some case reports claim efficacy; however, success is probably seen in only a proportion of patients (*see* Placebo, page xxi).	**Requires a qualified practitioner** Practitioners should be properly qualified and should propose a treatment plan. Non-prescription formulations are suitable for do-it-yourself. **Risks:** Fairly unlikely provided treatment is carried out competently.

Treatment	Rating	Point of delivery/risks
Reflex therapies Reflex zone massage, colonic massage, reflexology (*see* page 883), and TENS (*see* page 886) are claimed to act via reflex channels (*see* page 881) to relax the patient and alleviate symptoms.	**Useful** as a short-term treatment attempt. Some observational studies, case studies, and individual case reports claim efficacy; however, success is probably seen in only a proportion of patients (*see* Placebo, page xxi).	**Suitable for DIY** Qualified guidance is essential. The effects of the various procedures can vary significantly from one person to another. **Risks:** Some people are sensitive to electrical stimuli and rubber electrodes; others find it hard to tolerate manual stimulation or close physical contact.
Relaxation techniques Autogenic training (*see* page 888), muscle relaxation according to Jacobson (*see* page 893), and various biofeedback techniques (*see* page 891) are said to relieve tension and inner unrest, and might be instrumental in reducing the tendency for the person to swallow air.	**Useful** as a short-term treatment attempt aimed at relaxing the patient and reducing the swallowing of air. Case reports claim efficacy; however, success is probably seen in only a proportion of patients (*see* Placebo, page xxi).	**Suitable for DIY** Once a sound understanding of the technique has been acquired from a trainer, patients can perform exercises themselves. Therapists should propose a treatment plan. **Risks:** Fairly unlikely.

Herbal remedies for wind (meteorism and flatulence)

Active ingredient/preparation	Rating
Caraway oil (*Carum carvi*)	Taken orally, caraway oil is **useful** as a treatment attempt for flatulence and a feeling of fullness, as well as for mild gastrointestinal spasm. Caraway oil is an antispasmodic and antimicrobial. **Individual dose:** 3–6 drops of oil on sugar, taken at mealtimes. **Risks:** Gastrointestinal problems may be caused by continuous high dosages and following prolonged use. Following skin contact, caraway oil may cause skin or respiratory allergies.

Active ingredient/preparation	*Rating*
Caraway seeds (*Carum carvi*)	Taken orally, caraway seeds **may be of some use** as a treatment attempt for flatulence and a feeling of fullness. Their action is antispasmodic and antimicrobial. **Daily dose:** 1.5–6g seeds. **Individual dose:** Pour 1 cup of hot water over 1.5g of crushed seeds and infuse. **Risks:** Gastrointestinal problems may occur at high dosages and following prolonged use.
Cinchona bark (*Cinchona succirubra* and *pubescens*)	Taken orally, cinchona bark **may be of some use** as a treatment attempt for flatulence and a feeling of fullness. It encourages the secretion of digestive juices and saliva. **Daily dose:** 1–3g bark. **Individual dose:** Pour boiling water over 1g of bark, infuse for ten minutes, strain, and drink half an hour before meals. Alternatively, 30–40 drops of tincture on sugar. **Risks:** Increased bleeding and hypersensitive reactions are possible. Cinchona bark should not be used during pregnancy, nor by individuals suffering from an allergy. Cinchona bark intensifies the action of anticoagulants. It should not be taken for long periods of time, as it may give rise to symptoms of cinchonism (characterized by tinnitus, headaches, visual disturbances, and nausea). In the UK it may only be sold to practitioners.
Cinnamon bark (*Cinnamomum verum*)	Taken orally, cinnamon bark **may be of some use** as a treatment attempt for digestive disorders and a feeling of fullness. **Daily dose:** 2–4g dried inner bark. **Individual dose:** Pour 1 cup of hot water over 1g of dried inner bark and infuse. Alternatively, 2–8 days of volatile oil on sugar. **Risks:** Allergic skin and mucosal reactions are relatively common. Not to be used during pregnancy or by persons who are allergic to cinnamon or balsam of Tolú.

Active ingredient/preparation	Rating
Dandelion (*Taraxacum officinale*)	Taken orally, dandelion **may be of some use** as a treatment attempt for flatulence and a feeling of fullness. **Dosage:** Three times daily pour 1 cup of hot water over 2–3g of herb and infuse. **Risks:** Contact allergies can occur (rarely). Not to be taken by persons with occlusion of the bile duct, gall bladder empyema, or intestinal occlusion. If you have gall stones, ask your doctor before taking dandelion.
Fennel oil (*Foeniculum vulgare*)	Taken orally, fennel oil **may be of some use** as a treatment attempt for flatulence, a feeling of fullness, and spasms. Fennel oil is a digestive stimulant and, at higher concentrations, an antispasmodic. **Daily dose:** 0.1–0.6ml volatile oil. 4–24 drops on sugar. Fennel honey: 0.5 ml oil per 2lbs honey solution, 1 tablespoon taken several times daily. **Risks:** Fennel oil may cause skin and allergic respiratory reactions. Do not use for prolonged periods (more than a couple of weeks) without consulting your doctor. **Caution:** Fennel honey and syrup have a relatively high sugar content; this increases the risk of dental caries, especially in children. Do not use fennel oil for infants and young children, nor during pregnancy.
Fennel seeds (*Foeniculum vulgare*)	Taken orally, fennel seeds **may be of some use** as a treatment attempt for flatulence, a feeling of fullness, and spasms. Fennel is a digestive stimulant and, in high concentrations, an antispasmodic. **Daily dose:** 5–7g seeds. **Individual dose:** Pour hot water over 1–2 teaspoons of slightly crushed seeds and infuse. Use ready-formulated preparations as instructed by the manufacturer/prescriber. **Risks:** Use of the oil may cause skin and respiratory allergies. During pregnancy use only as an infusion, not as the volatile oil. Do not use for prolonged periods (more than a couple of weeks) without consulting your doctor.

Active ingredient/preparation	*Rating*
Gentian root (*Gentiana lutea*)	Taken orally, gentian **may be of some use** as a treatment attempt for a lack of appetite, a feeling of fullness, and flatulence. It encourages the secretion of saliva and gastric juices. **Daily dose:** 2–4g herb or 1–3g tincture. **Individual dose:** As a decoction, 1g of root to 1 cup of boiling water, leave to steep for five to ten minutes and drink half an hour before meals. Alternatively, 1–3g of tincture. Use ready-formulated preparations as instructed by the manufacturer/prescriber. **Risks:** May cause headaches. Not to be taken by persons with a gastric or duodenal ulcer. In experiments with bacteria, gentian root was found to have gene-mutating properties. However, these results may not be relevant to the treatment situation.
Lemon balm leaves (*Melissa officinalis*)	Taken orally, lemon balm **may be of some use** as a treatment attempt for functional gastric disorders such as flatulence. It calms the nervous system and relieves digestive tensions. **Daily dose:** 8–10g. **Individual dose:** Pour 1 cup of hot water over 1.5–4.5g of herb and infuse. **Risks:** The volatile oil contained in lemon balm may cause allergic reactions.
White horehound (*Marrubium vulgare*)	Taken orally, white horehound **may be of some use** as a treatment attempt for digestive disorders and a feeling of fullness. The constituent marrubic acid is a cholagogue. **Daily dose:** 4.5g herb. **Individual dose:** Pour 1 cup of boiling water over 1.5g of herb and infuse. **Risks:** White horehound is not known to have any serious side effects.

Worms

Causes and symptoms

Worms are parasites found in animals and humans. There are three main types: threadworms, roundworms, and tapeworms. They enter the body via infected food or through poor personal hygiene, and may evoke various symptoms, including inflammation and sores.

Orthodox treatment

Anthelmintics are generally used to treat worm infestations.

Complementary therapies

The main complementary approach is either to tackle the infestation directly or to stimulate the immune system. There is not sufficient evidence that these procedures work.

Treatment plan and limited trial

Before administering a complementary treatment, every therapist should propose a treatment plan (*see* page xxiii) that sets out a clear time frame and defines the goal that the treatment is designed to achieve. Treatment should then be tried for a limited term to test the patient's response.

Caution

Complementary medicine can offer no substitute for modern anthelmintics.

Complementary treatments for worms

Treatment	Rating	Point of delivery/risks
Homeopathy Some homeopaths claim that highly diluted (potentized) solutions (*see* page 831) can be used to help the body to overcome worm infestations.	**Of little use** as the sole measure. The efficacy of homeopathic remedies and the way in which they might work in dealing with worm infestations have not been convincingly demonstrated.	**Requires a qualified practitioner** Homeopaths should be properly qualified and should propose a treatment plan. **Risks:** Allergies and intolerance are possible.
Probiotics The introduction of certain bacteria into the gut is claimed to bring the intestinal flora back into balance and to boost the body's defence systems (*see* page 878).	**Of little use** Possibly acceptable as a short-term treatment attempt when more established methods have been unsuccessful. Some case reports claim efficacy; however, success is probably seen in only a proportion of patients (*see* Placebo, page xxi).	**Requires a qualified practitioner** Practitioners should be properly qualified and should propose a treatment plan. Non-prescription formulations are suitable for do-it-yourself. **Risks:** Fairly unlikely provided treatment is carried out competently.

Herbal remedies for worms

Active ingredient/preparation	Rating
Larkspur flowers (*Delphinium consolida*)	**Not advised** as a vermifuge. Evidence of efficacy is lacking. **Risks:** Larkspur roots, seeds, and leaves (probably not the flowers) contain alkaloids which slow down the heartbeat, lower blood pressure, and even lead to cardiac arrest at higher doses.

Active ingredient/preparation	Rating
Male fern leaves and root (*Dryopteris filix-mas*)	**Not advised** as a treatment for helminthic disease. **Risks:** Male fern is poisonous and can lead to cardiac arrhythmia, visual disturbances (even blindness), vertigo, vomiting, cramps, etc. It must therefore never be used internally; also, its external use cannot be advised owing to a lack of efficacy. **Caution:** Male fern must only be used, if at all, under medical supervision. Use has been superseded by less toxic (conventional) agents.
Melon tree leaves (*Carica papaya*)	**Not advised** for the treatment of parasitic diseases and as a vermifuge. Evidence of efficacy is lacking.

Metabolic disorders

Diabetes

Causes and symptoms

Diabetes mellitus is characterized by high levels of glucose in the blood (hyperglycemia). It is caused by a deficiency of insulin, a hormone that is produced in the pancreas, either because this organ is no longer able to produce insulin or because the insulin that is produced is not effective. Apart from diabetic coma—an acute and life-threatening risk—diabetes is associated with a number of longer-term complications, including atherosclerosis (which can affect, *inter alia*, the coronary arteries and brain—*see* page 420), scarring of the retina (leading to blindness), kidney problems (including chronic kidney failure), loss of limbs, and neuropathies (*see* page 140).

Diabetes tends to be linked to genetic factors but may also be caused by viruses and tumors. Lifestyle may play a prominent role in its etiology.

There are two types of diabetes: insulin-dependent diabetes mellitus (IDDM or Type I diabetes), which affects some 10–15 percent of diabetics, and non-insulin-dependent diabetes mellitus (NIDDM or Type II diabetes), which chiefly affects older people. Sufferers may have a wide assortment of symptoms. High blood glucose levels are associated with frequent urination and thirst, and with marked weight loss despite normal or even increased food intake.

Orthodox treatment

The principal objective in treating diabetes is to achieve and maintain effective control over the concentration of glucose in the blood by keeping to a healthy way of eating, by adopting a modified lifestyle and, where necessary, by daily injections of insulin or through oral drugs.

Complementary therapies

Many complementary therapists see diabetes mellitus as the result of toxins (*see* page 929), foci (*see* page 928), or an energy imbalance (*see* page 927). The treatments suggested will be geared accordingly.

Claims of efficacy made for various complementary treatments for diabetes mellitus are usually not well substantiated. The only effective treatments are offered by mainstream medicine. Other than by conventional means, there is no way of preventing diabetes and its longer term complications.

Treatment plan and limited trial

Before administering a complementary treatment, every therapist should propose a treatment plan (*see* page xxiii) that sets out a clear time frame and defines the goal that the treatment is designed to achieve. Treatment should then be tried for a limited term to test the patient's response.

Cautions

Persons receiving only complementary medical treatment for diabetes mellitus risk receiving a lower level of care than is required, and are more prone to longer-term complications, which may possibly lead to blindness, loss of limbs, and other serious complications.

An orthodox physician must be consulted if there is any suspicion whatsoever of diabetes mellitus. Only mainstream therapy can prevent a life-threatening coma and longer term diabetic complications. Complementary therapies are suitable merely as adjuncts to orthodox treatment.

Complementary treatments for diabetes

Treatment	Rating	Point of delivery/risks
Acupuncture Acupuncture in its various forms (*see* page 772) aims to encourage the flow of energy (*see* page 927), to ease pain directly, or to influence the hormone system.	**Inappropriate** as a treatment for diabetes. **May be of some use** as a short-term treatment attempt, e.g. for easing pain (*see* Neuropathy, page 140). Case reports claim efficacy; however, success is probably seen in only a proportion of patients (*see* Placebo, page xxi).	**Requires a qualified practitioner** Practitioners should be properly qualified and should propose a treatment plan. **Risks:** Probably rare provided treatment is carried out competently.
Anthroposophical medicine Doctors who practice AM (*see* page 781) try to prevent diabetic complications such as arteriosclerosis (*see* page 420) and infections.	**Inappropriate** as a treatment for diabetes. Acceptable as a supportive or preventive measure. Some case reports claim efficacy; however, success is probably seen in only a proportion of patients (*see* Placebo, page xxi).	**Requires a qualified practitioner** Practitioners should be properly qualified and should propose a treatment plan. **Risks:** Allergies and intolerance are possible.
Aromatherapy Essential oils (*see* page 786) are used to soothe and relax, or to invigorate, thereby improving the body's own regulatory systems. The essences may be taken orally, used externally as massage oils or bathing emulsions, or inhaled as vapors.	**Inappropriate** as a treatment for diabetes. Possibly acceptable as a short-term, supportive treatment attempt aimed at soothing and relaxing. Some case reports claim efficacy; however, success is probably seen in only a small proportion of patients (*see* Placebo, page xxi).	**Suitable for DIY** Qualified guidance is recommended. The effects of individual essential oils differ widely. **Risks:** Allergies or intolerance are possible. Some oils are carcinogenic in test systems and possibly in humans.

Treatment	Rating	Point of delivery/risks
Bioresonance therapy Bioresonance therapists use electrical devices in an attempt to discover the causes of illness and claim to be able to weaken or turn around pathogenic energies and disease related vibrations (*see* page 794).	**Inappropriate** as a treatment for diabetes. Possibly acceptable as a short-term, supportive treatment attempt. Some case reports claim efficacy; however, success is probably seen, if at all, in only a small proportion of patients (*see* Placebo, page xxi).	**Requires a qualified practitioner** Practitioners should be properly qualified and should propose a treatment plan. No credence should be given to anyone promising immediate or total success. **Risks:** Fairly unlikely.
Cell therapy Injecting or ingesting products extracted from the tissues of newborn animals or animal fetuses is said to have a rejuvenating and revitalizing effect and to enhance the healing of human tissues and organs (*see* page 796).	**Not advised** Based on present knowledge, there is inadequate evidence of the efficacy and mode of action of these costly and relatively risky procedures.	**Risks:** Injecting foreign proteins into the body can provoke (possibly fatal) allergic reactions. Also, pathogens such as those that cause bovine spongiform encephalopathy (BSE) or other serious infections may be introduced.
Electroacupuncture according to Voll By taking readings of the electrical conductivity of the skin (*see* page 802), therapists claim to be able to derive an insight into diseased areas of the body, pathogenic foci (*see* page 928), and stress factors (*see* Toxins, page 929). The factors presumed to be instrumental in the causation of diabetes can then be addressed.	**Inappropriate** as a treatment for diabetes. Possibly acceptable as a short-term, supportive treatment attempt. Some case reports claim efficacy; however, success is probably seen, if at all, in only a small proportion of patients (*see* Placebo, page xxi).	**Requires a qualified practitioner** Practitioners should be properly qualified and should propose a treatment plan. No credence should be given to anyone promising immediate or total success. **Risks:** A second opinion must always be obtained from a qualified physician before any attempt is made to "eliminate foci" (e.g. by surgery).

Treatment	Rating	Point of delivery/risks
Electroneural therapy according to Croon According to the theory, readings taken at various reactive sites on the skin highlight diseased areas within the body. Based on these readings, targeted electrostimulative measures can be undertaken to address factors presumed to be instrumental in the causation of diabetes (*see* page 806).	**Inappropriate** as a treatment for diabetes. Possibly acceptable as a short-term, supportive treatment attempt. Some case reports claim efficacy; however, success is probably seen, if at all, in only a small proportion of patients (*see* Placebo, page xxi).	**Requires a qualified practitioner** Practitioners should be properly qualified and should propose a treatment plan. No credence should be given to anyone promising immediate or total success. **Risks:** Proponents themselves warn that treatment should not be given in acute inflammatory conditions.
Eliminative methods, bloody Bloody cupping (*see* page 815) is said to improve the body's own regulatory systems and to boost general well-being.	**Not advised** The efficacy and mode of action of this invasive procedure are unproven.	**Risks:** Bloody cupping can cause infection and scarring. Furthermore, it should not be carried out in persons with bleeding disorders.
Flower remedies Flower remedies (*see* page 828) are said to restore emotional balance and assist the body's psychic ability to heal itself.	**Inappropriate** as a treatment for diabetes. Possibly acceptable as a short-term, supportive treatment attempt aimed at soothing and relaxing. Some case reports claim efficacy; however, success is probably seen in only a small proportion of patients (*see* Placebo, page xxi).	**Suitable for DIY** Qualified guidance is recommended. Practitioners should propose a treatment plan. **Risks:** Possible intolerance.

Treatment	*Rating*	*Point of delivery/risks*
Homeopathy Highly diluted (potentized) solutions (*see* page 831) are believed able to redress vital energy imbalances. Organo- and functiotropic (*see* page 833) homeopathy is claimed to act directly to counter diabetes.	**Inappropriate** as a treatment for diabetes. Possibly acceptable as a supportive treatment attempt aimed at easing symptoms. Some case reports claim efficacy; however, success is probably seen in only a proportion of patients (*see* Placebo, page xxi).	**Requires a qualified practitioner** Homeopaths should be properly qualified and should propose a treatment plan. Ready-formulated preparations are suitable for do-it-yourself. **Risks:** Allergies and intolerance are possible.
Massage Classical massage (*see* page 847) reportedly eases muscular and emotional tension.	**Inappropriate** as a treatment for diabetes. **May be of some use** as a supportive measure aimed at soothing and relaxing. Case reports claim efficacy; however, success is probably seen in only a proportion of patients (*see* Placebo, page xxi).	**Requires a qualified practitioner** Masseurs/masseuses should be properly qualified. **Risks:** Some people are sensitive to manual stimuli; others find it hard to tolerate close physical contact.
Nutritional therapies An organic diet (*see* page 4) provides the body with essential and secondary plant nutrients that are believed to exercise a multitude of positive effects (*see* pages 858–67).	**Inappropriate** as the sole measure in the treatment of insulin-dependent diabetics. **Useful** as one of the supportive measures necessary in diabetes mellitus.	**Suitable for DIY** Diets should be discussed individually with the treating physician. **Risks:** Avoid imbalanced or intolerable diets. They can cause deficiencies with serious consequences. Children are particularly at risk. Curative fasting should not be attempted without medical supervision.

Treatment	Rating	Point of delivery/risks
Physical therapies Skin care with total washings, warm brushing, Kneipp treatments (*see* page 871), and exercise therapy (*see* page 868) are claimed to encourage metabolic processes, to invigorate the patient, and to improve his/her general well-being.	**Inappropriate** as a treatment for diabetes. **Useful** as a short-term, supportive treatment attempt aimed at invigorating the patient and improving his/her general well-being. Some case reports and field studies claim efficacy; however, success is probably seen in only a proportion of patients (*see* Placebo, page xxi).	**Suitable for DIY** Qualified guidance is recommended though not essential. **Risks:** Skin damage may be caused to persons with diminished temperature sensation when extreme temperatures are applied.
Reflex therapies Reflex zone massage (*see* page 883), reflexology (*see* page 883), and TENS (*see* page 886) are claimed to be relaxing, and to act via reflex channels (*see* page 881) to ease pain.	**Inappropriate** as a treatment for diabetes. **May be of some use** as a short-term, supportive treatment attempt aimed at alleviating pain (*see* Neuropathy, page 140). Case reports and clinical studies (TENS) claim efficacy; however, success is probably seen in only a small proportion of patients (*see* Placebo, page xxi).	**Suitable for DIY** Qualified guidance is essential. Therapists should propose a treatment plan. **Risks:** Some people are sensitive to electrical stimuli and rubber electrodes; others find it hard to tolerate manual stimulation or close physical contact.
Relaxation techniques Autogenic training (*see* page 888), muscle relaxation according to Jacobson (*see* page 893), and various biofeedback techniques (*see* page 891) are said to relieve muscle tension and inner unrest, and might be instrumental in helping diabetics come to terms better with their condition.	**Inappropriate** as a treatment for diabetes. **May be of some use** as a supportive measure aimed at soothing and relaxing, and at helping the patient come to terms better with his/her condition. Some case reports claim efficacy; however, success is probably seen in only a proportion of patients (*see* Placebo, page xxi).	**Suitable for DIY** Once a sound understanding of the technique has been acquired from a trainer in group sessions or through individual tuition, patients can perform exercises themselves. Therapists should be properly qualified. **Risks:** Fairly unlikely.

Treatment	Rating	Point of delivery/risks
Vitamins and trace elements The antioxidative properties of beta-carotene, vitamins C and E, and selenium are, it is supposed, instrumental in countering the formation of free radicals (*see* page 902) and in boosting the body's antioxidative defence systems (*see* page 900).	**Inappropriate** as a treatment for diabetes. **May be of some use** as a short-term, supportive treatment attempt. No definitive recommendations can be made based on present knowledge.	**Suitable for DIY** Medical supervision is recommended though not essential. **Risks:** Intolerance and overdosage are possible. Recent studies imply that beta-carotene might increase the risk of cancer.

Herbal remedies for diabetes

Active ingredient/preparation	Rating
Bean pod tea (*Phaseolus vulgaris*)	**Of little use.** There is some doubt as to its therapeutic value in diabetes. Its action is mildly diuretic. **Daily dose:** 5–15g tea. **Individual dose:** As a tea drink, 5g tea to 1 cup of boiling water. **Risks:** Bean pod tea is not known to have any serious side effects.
Guar meal (from *Cyamopsis tetragonolobus*)	**May be of some use** as a supportive treatment attempt for smoothing blood glucose peaks after meals. Cereal muesli is also useful. This type of product slows the absorption of carbohydrates. **Dosage:** As instructed by the manufacturer/prescriber. **Risks:** Gastrointestinal problems (flatulence, a feeling of fullness, diarrhea) are possible. Guar meal may also agglomerate dangerously in the gullet and intestine. It is thus essential to swallow plenty of liquid with it. Guar meal should not be used in patients with esophageal disease or intestinal obstruction.

Active ingredient/preparation	Rating
Seedless bean pods (*Phaseolus vulgaris*)	**Of little use** in diabetes. Mildly diuretic action. **Daily dose:** 5–15g dried pods. **Individual dose:** As a tea drink, 2–3g dried pods to 1 cup of boiling water. **Risks:** Bean pods are not known to have any serious side effects.

High cholesterol

Causes and symptoms

A high level of cholesterol in the blood has long been considered a risk factor for cardiovascular disease. Additional attention has to be paid to such factors as age, sex, lifestyle, eating habits, the person's previous medical history and family history of cardiac and vascular disease. As a consequence of this approach to risk assessment, doubt has been cast on the validity of the accepted cholesterol limits for deciding whether medical intervention is necessary—except when the values are very high. Fat-related disorders sometimes become manifest as excessively high levels of blood fats, i.e. cholesterol and triglycerides. Some are attributable to genetic factors, others to hormone disturbance or some other predisposing diseases. Lifestyle factors such as diet, lack of exercise, and chronic stress may also have a contributory role.

Most fats in the blood occur in the form of lipoproteins, more specifically as chylomicrons, very low density lipoproteins (VLDL), low density lipoproteins (LDL) and high density lipoproteins (HDL). Fat-related disorders are classified into five major types all according to typical lipoprotein patterns. A person's risk of developing arteriosclerosis, for instance, may be unchanged, slightly raised, or significantly raised depending on the particular type of disorder. The risk of developing other diseases such as pancreatitis, or of fat becoming deposited in various tissues will not necessarily run parallel to the arteriosclerosis risk.

Currently the upper limit for total cholesterol is variable according to individual circumstances, age, and sex. Doctors must advise patients individually whether their cholesterol level needs to be investigated further and, possibly, reduced.

Orthodox treatment

The generally accepted advice for dealing with fat-related disorders is to maintain a healthy pattern of eating. This is a fairly flexible concept, however, and will inevitably be interpreted to reflect national and cultural predilections. The normal recommendation is to take in less than 30 percent of one's daily calories as fats, approximately 60 percent as carbohydrates, and the remainder as proteins. This intake pattern should enable cholesterol levels to be reduced by some 5–10 percent.

Cholesterol levels can also be reduced through regular sustained exercise. Lipid-lowering drugs are widely prescribed in cases where this measure is found to be inadequate. Except in clear-cut cases of cholesterol levels way above the normal limits and of patients with a genetic predisposition to fat-related disease, experts still disagree as to when this type of medication should be given.

Complementary therapies

Complementary therapies incorporate many of the principles accepted in orthodox medicine. Apart from exercise and a reduction in the daily intake of calories, much emphasis is placed on dietary elements such as antioxidants and secondary plant constituents not normally featured in calculations of calorie content. Some herbal remedies also have cholesterol lowering properties. Of the numerous other proposed remedies, many are simply supportive in nature.

Treatment plan and limited trial

Before administering a complementary treatment, every therapist should propose a treatment plan (*see* page xxiii) that sets out a clear time frame and defines the goal that the treatment is designed to achieve. Treatment should then be tried for a limited term to test the patient's response.

Cautions

A cholesterol level that is way above the normal limit may be symptomatic of a serious ailment. A qualified medical diagnosis must therefore be obtained in such cases.

Complementary treatments for high cholesterol levels

Treatment	Rating	Point of delivery/risks
Acupuncture Acupuncture in its various forms (*see* page 772) aims to encourage the flow of energy (*see* page 927) or to act directly to reduce feelings of hunger.	**Of little use** Acceptable as a short-term, supportive treatment attempt aimed at reducing feelings of hunger and at facilitating weight reduction. Case reports and field studies claim efficacy; however, success is probably seen in only a proportion of patients (*see* Placebo, page xxi).	**Requires a qualified practitioner** Practitioners should be properly qualified and should propose a treatment plan. **Risks:** Probably rare provided treatment is carried out competently.
Anthroposophical medicine In patients with fat-related disorders, doctors who practice AM (*see* page 781) carry out liver therapy and prescribe herbal drugs, e.g. artichoke because of its cholesterol reducing properties.	**May be of some use** as a short-term, supportive treatment attempt aimed at lowering cholesterol and triglyceride levels when more established methods have been unsuccessful. Case reports claim efficacy; however, success is probably seen in only a proportion of patients (*see* Placebo, page xxi).	**Requires a qualified practitioner** Practitioners should be properly qualified and should propose a treatment plan. **Risks:** Allergies and intolerance are possible.

Treatment	Rating	Point of delivery/risks
Homeopathy Highly diluted (potentized) solutions (*see* page 831) are believed to be able to redress vital energy imbalances. Organo- and functiotropic (*see* page 833) homeopathy is claimed to act directly to influence metabolic functions.	**Of little use** Acceptable as a short-term, supportive treatment attempt aimed at lowering cholesterol and triglyceride levels when more established methods have been unsuccessful. Case reports claim efficacy; however, success is probably seen in only a proportion of patients (*see* Placebo, page xxi).	**Requires a qualified practitioner** Homeopaths should be properly qualified and should propose a treatment plan. Ready-formulated preparations are suitable for do-it-yourself. **Risks:** Allergies and intolerance are possible.
Hypnosis and self-hypnosis In the relaxed and generally altered state of awareness that is induced in hypnosis or self-hypnosis (*see* page 837), inner unrest can, it is claimed, be relieved and stress reduced, so that a beneficial effect is exercised on cholesterol and triglyceride levels.	**May be of some use** as a supportive measure aimed at stress reduction, which possibly has a beneficial effect on triglyceride and cholesterol levels. Some case reports claim efficacy; however, success is probably seen in only a proportion of patients (*see* Placebo, page xxi).	**Requires a qualified practitioner** Hypnotherapists should be properly qualified and should propose a treatment plan. No credence should be given to anyone promising immediate or total success. **Risks:** Unlikely provided treatment is carried out competently.
Nutritional therapies An organic diet (*see* page 4) provides the body with essential and secondary plant nutrients that are believed to be capable, *inter alia*, of lowering cholesterol levels and reducing body weight.	**Useful** as an individually directed measure. Controlled studies, observational studies, and case reports ascribe a degree of efficacy to organic diets in the lowering of cholesterol and triglyceride levels.	**Suitable for DIY** Qualified guidance is recommended though not essential. **Risks:** Avoid imbalanced or intolerable diets. They can cause deficiencies with serious consequences. Children are particularly at risk.

Treatment	Rating	Point of delivery/risks
Physical therapies Exercise therapy (*see* page 868) in the form of regular, sustained exercise is said to lower cholesterol and triglyceride levels.	Sustained exercise and sports are **useful** as a means of lowering cholesterol and triglyceride levels. Observational and controlled studies ascribe a degree of efficacy to this form of treatment in some of the patients examined.	**Suitable for DIY** Qualified guidance is recommended though not essential. **Risks:** Risk of sporting injuries.
Relaxation techniques Autogenic training (*see* page 888), muscle relaxation according to Jacobson (*see* page 893), and various biofeedback techniques (*see* page 891) are said to relieve muscle tension and inner unrest, thereby exercising a beneficial effect on cholesterol and triglyceride levels.	**May be of some use** as a supportive measure aimed at stress reduction, this having a beneficial effect on cholesterol and triglyceride levels. Some case reports claim efficacy; however, success is probably seen in only a proportion of patients (*see* Placebo, page xxi).	**Suitable for DIY** Once a sound understanding of the technique has been acquired from a trainer, patients can perform exercises themselves. Therapists should be properly qualified. **Risks:** Fairly unlikely.
Vitamins and trace elements The antioxidative properties of beta-carotene, vitamins C and E, and selenium are believed to exercise a multitude of beneficial effects and to be capable, *inter alia*, of lowering cholesterol values (*see* page 900).	**Useful** when taken as part of an organic diet (*see* page 4). **May be of some use** as a supportive measure. Studies ascribe a degree of success to this form of treatment in the lowering of cholesterol and triglyceride values in some of the patients examined. Dosage recommendations differ widely and are probably set to rise.	**Suitable for DIY** Qualified guidance is recommended though not essential. **Risks:** Intolerance and overdosage are possible. Recent studies imply that beta-carotene might increase the risk of cancer.

Herbal remedies for high cholesterol

Active ingredient/preparation	Rating
Garlic corms (*Allium sativum*)	**Useful** as a supportive treatment (with diet) for high cholesterol. **Dosage:** As instructed by the manufacturer/prescriber, otherwise 600–1200mg dry extract or 4g fresh corms (2–4 small cloves). **Risks:** Gastric and allergic problems are possible but rare.
Garlic oil maceration products	**Of little use**, as the chemical compositions of the preparations differ widely and no general daily dosage recommendations can be given. Manufacturers' recommendations range from 18mg to 1.2g. **Risks:** Gastric and allergic problems are possible but rare.
Globe artichoke leaf extract (*Cynara scolymus*)	**May be of some use** as a supportive treatment attempt for disorders of fat metabolism. **Daily dose:** 1–4g of drug. **Individual dose:** As a tea drink, 1–2g of drug to 1 cup of hot water. Use ready-formulated preparations as instructed by the manufacturer/prescriber. **Risks:** Contact eczema (skin irritation after contact with the leaves) is possible. Not to be used by persons with biliary tract occlusion or gall stones.
Soy lecithin (*Glycine max*)	**Of little use**. This is a rarely used and (at most) supportive treatment for mild disorders of fat metabolism, in association with (or after) dietary measures to prevent hardening of the arteries. Soy lecithin reportedly changes the LDL/HDL ratio and so possibly has positive effects on blood lipids. **Dosage:** As instructed by the manufacturer/prescriber. **Risks:** Soy lecithin is not known to have any serious side effects.

Thyroid disorders (goiter, hyperthyroidism, and hypothyroidism)

Causes and symptoms

The three main thyroid disorders are hyperthyroidism (overactive thyroid), hypothyroidism (underactive thyroid), and goiter. Hyperthyroidism and hypothyroidism may be accompanied by general or localized swelling. Symptoms vary widely depending on the nature of the disorder and the size of the thyroid. Hyperthyroidism, for instance, is associated with increased anxiety, a fast heartbeat, tremors, profuse sweating, weight loss, an increased appetite, muscle weakness, tiredness, heat intolerance, bulging eyes, and clammy skin. In hypothyroidism patients complain of a lack of energy, weight gain, and fatigue; they may also have a hoarse voice and slow speech, exhibit a change in facial features, and have hair that is thin and dishevelled. Life-threatening crises can arise in both these types of thyroid disorder. Thyroid tumors, on the other hand, may remain relatively symptom-free for long periods.

Orthodox treatment

Orthodox treatment will be chosen to suit the particular clinical picture and will involve thyroid hormone treatments, inhibitors to stop hormone production, anti-inflammatory drugs, and beta-blockers. Surgery and radiation may be required in certain circumstances.

Complementary therapies

There is no substitute for proper conventional treatment. Complementary treatments are no more than palliative, at least for severe thyroid disorders.

Treatment plan and limited trial

Before administering a complementary treatment, every therapist should propose a treatment plan (*see* page xxiii) that sets out a clear time frame and defines the goal that the treatment is designed to achieve. Treatment should then be tried for a limited term to test the patient's response.

Cautions

Severe thyroid disorders need specialist medical attention, so the role of any complementary procedures will be purely supportive. Unless a proper medical diagnosis is obtained, the sufferer will perhaps receive inadequate or inappropriate treatment for what is essentially a life-threatening disorder.

Complementary treatments for thyroid disorders

Treatment	Rating	Point of delivery/risks
Acupuncture Acupuncture in its various forms (*see* page 772) aims to encourage the flow of energy (*see* page 927) or to exercise a direct effect on the thyroid and on metabolic processes.	**Of little use** Possibly acceptable as a short-term treatment attempt. Some case reports claim efficacy; however, success is probably seen in only a small proportion of patients (*see* Placebo, page xxi).	**Requires a qualified practitioner** Practitioners should be properly qualified and should propose a treatment plan. **Risks:** Probably rare provided treatment is carried out competently.
Anthroposophical medicine AM (*see* page 781) suggests the use of Thyreodoron ointment for treating goiter. If the thyroid is over- or underactive, various compositions will be described depending on the constitution (*see* page 927) of the patient.	**Of little use** Acceptable as a short-term treatment attempt in the initial stages of thyroid disease. Case studies claim efficacy; however, success is probably seen in only a proportion of patients (*see* Placebo, page xxi).	**Requires a qualified practitioner** Practitioners should be properly qualified and should propose a treatment plan. **Risks:** Allergies and intolerance are possible.

Treatment	Rating	Point of delivery/risks
Bioresonance therapy Bioresonance therapists use electrical devices in an attempt to discover the causes of illness and claim to be able to weaken or turn around pathogenic energies and disease related vibrations (*see* page 974).	**Of little use** Possibly acceptable as a short-term, supportive treatment attempt when simpler, more established methods have been unsuccessful. Some case reports claim efficacy; however, success is probably seen, if at all, in only a small proportion of patients (*see* Placebo, page xxi).	**Requires a qualified practitioner** Practitioners should be properly qualified and should propose a treatment plan. No credence should be given to anyone promising immediate or total success. **Risks:** Fairly unlikely.
Cell therapy Injecting or ingesting products extracted from the tissues of newborn animals or animal fetuses is said to have a rejuvenating and revitalizing effect and to enhance the healing of human tissues and organs (*see* page 796).	**Not advised** Based on present knowledge, there is inadequate evidence of the efficacy and mode of action of these costly and relatively risky procedures.	**Risks:** Injecting foreign proteins into the body can provoke (possibly fatal) allergic reactions. Also, pathogens such as those that cause bovine spongiform encephalopathy (BSE) or other serious infections may be introduced.
Electroacupuncture according to Voll By taking readings of the electrical conductivity of the skin, therapists claim to be able to address factors presumed to be instrumental in the causation of symptoms (*see* page 802).	**Not advised** The efficacy and mode of action of this relatively complex procedure have not been satisfactorily demonstrated.	**Risks:** A second opinion must always be obtained from a qualified physician before any attempt is made to "eliminate foci" (e.g. by surgery).

Treatment	Rating	Point of delivery/risks
Electroneural therapy according to Croon According to the theory, readings taken at various reactive sites on the skin can be used as a basis for targeted electrostimulative measures carried out to address the factors presumed to be instrumental in the causation of symptoms (see page 806).	**Not advised** The efficacy and mode of action of this relatively complex procedure have not been satisfactorily demonstrated.	**Risks:** Proponents themselves warn that treatment should not be given in acute inflammatory conditions.
Eliminative methods, unbloody Unbloody cupping (*see* page 817) is supposed to energize (*see* page 927) the patient, to improve the body's regulatory systems, and to alleviate symptoms.	**Of little use** Acceptable as a short-term, supportive treatment attempt aimed at alleviating symptoms. Case reports claim efficacy; however, success is probably seen in only a proportion of patients (*see* Placebo, page xxi).	**Suitable for DIY** Qualified guidance is essential. Practitioners should propose a treatment plan. **Risks:** Unlikely provided treatment is carried out competently.
Flower remedies Flower remedies (*see* page 828) are said to restore emotional balance and assist the body's psychic ability to heal itself.	**Of little use** Acceptable as a short-term, supportive treatment attempt aimed at soothing and relaxing. Some case reports claim efficacy; however, success is probably seen in only a proportion of patients (*see* Placebo, page xxi).	**Suitable for DIY** Qualified guidance is recommended. Practitioners should propose a treatment plan. **Risks:** Possible intolerance.

Treatment	Rating	Point of delivery/risks
Homeopathy Highly diluted (potentized) solutions (*see* page 831) are believed to be able to redress vital energy imbalances. Organo- and functiotropic (*see* page 833) homeopathy is claimed to act directly to counter thyroid disease.	**May be of some use** as a supportive treatment attempt aimed at alleviating symptoms. Some case reports claim efficacy; however, success is probably seen, if at all, in only a small proportion of patients (*see* Placebo, page xxi).	**Requires a qualified practitioner** Homeopaths should be properly qualified and should propose a treatment plan. Ready-formulated preparations are suitable for do-it-yourself. **Risks:** Allergies and intolerance are possible.
Nutritional therapies An organic diet (*see* page 4) provides the body with essential and secondary plant nutrients that are believed to exercise a multitude of positive effects.	**Useful** as an individually directed supportive measure. Iodine should be given if a deficiency has been diagnosed.	**Suitable for DIY** Qualified guidance is recommended though not essential. **Risks:** Avoid imbalanced or intolerable diets. They can cause deficiencies with serious consequences. Children are particularly at risk.

Treatment	Rating	Point of delivery/risks
Physical therapies In the case of an overactive thyroid, local cold treatments such as compresses around the neck, torso, and lower legs, walking in water, and upper body washes are claimed to suppress activity. If the thyroid is underactive, alternating temperature washes, walking in water, ascending temperature foot, arm, full immersion, or brush baths (*see* pages 871–8) are said to improve the circulation. Exercise therapy (*see* page 868) is beneficial in both cases. In goiter, alternating temperature total washes and cold upper body washes, walking in water, and healing earth packs at night are said to bring relief.	**Useful** as a supportive treatment attempt. Some case reports claim efficacy; however, success is probably seen in only a proportion of patients (see Placebo, page xxi).	**Suitable for DIY** Qualified guidance is recommended. Practitioners should be properly qualified and should propose a treatment plan. There may be wide differences in the effects of the various procedures. Each treatment should therefore be reviewed and, if necessary, discontinued or replaced by another one. **Risks:** Skin damage may be caused to persons with diminished temperature sensation when extreme temperatures are applied.
Relaxation techniques Autogenic training (*see* page 888) is said to relieve the muscular tension and unrest typically encountered in thyroid disease.	**Useful** as a supportive treatment attempt aimed at alleviating unrest. Field studies claim efficacy; however, success is probably seen in only a small proportion of patients (*see* Placebo, page xxi).	**Suitable for DIY** Once a sound understanding of the technique has been acquired from a trainer, patients can perform exercises themselves. Therapists should be properly qualified. **Risks:** Fairly unlikely.

Treatment	Rating	Point of delivery/risks
Vitamins and trace elements The antioxidative properties of beta-carotene, vitamins C and E, and selenium are said to be responsible for a number of beneficial effects (*see* page 900).	**Of little use** No definitive recommendations can be given based on present knowledge. Recommended dosages vary considerably and are probably set to rise.	**Suitable for DIY** Qualified guidance is recommended though not essential. **Risks:** Intolerance and overdosage are possible. Recent studies imply that beta-carotene might increase the risk of cancer.

Herbal remedies for thyroid disorders

Active ingredient/preparation	Rating
Bugleweed (*Lycopus europaeus*)	**May be of some use** as a supportive treatment attempt for a slightly overactive thyroid attended with nervous symptoms. **Daily dose:** 1–2g of herb. **Individual dose:** For a tea drink, 0.5g. Use ready-formulated preparations as instructed by the manufacturer/prescriber. Bodyweight and age must be taken into account for working out the dosage. It should therefore only be taken on doctor's orders. **Risks:** Thyroid enlargement may occasionally occur. Do not use with any other thyroid preparation. Do not stop taking teas or drugs containing *Lycopus* abruptly; instead, reduce the dose gradually, otherwise the clinical picture may worsen. Not to be taken by persons with an underactive thyroid or with thyroid enlargement not involving functional disturbance.
Motherwort (*Leonurus cardiaca*)	**May be of some use** as a supportive treatment attempt for thyroid disorders attended by nervous heart complaints. **Daily dose:** 4.5g herb. **Individual dose:** Pour 1 cup of hot water over 1.5g of herb, steep for five minutes, strain, and drink. Drink 1 cup twice daily. Use ready-formulated preparations as instructed by the manufacturer/prescriber. **Risks:** Motherwort is not known to have any serious side effects.

Sexual organs and secondary sexual characteristics

Breast disorders (mastopathy and mastodynia)

Causes and symptoms

Mastodynia is a painful tenseness of the breasts that occurs at puberty when the breasts start to develop and prior to menstrual periods as a result of hormonal changes. The breasts can become extremely sensitive. Pain and tenseness may also be caused by swellings and lumps (mastopathy) in the breasts during the monthly cycle. In most cases lumpiness is due to the formation or small, liquid filled cysts (a condition known as cystic mastopathy or fibrocystic disease); the cysts are most noticeable just before menstrual bleeding commences and will mostly disappear by the third day of the menstrual cycle. These complaints tend not to occur after menopause (*see* page 672).

Orthodox treatment

Mastodynia and mastopathy are mostly treated with hormone containing gels. In some women the contraceptive pill can also be used to bring effective relief from symptoms.

Complementary therapies

Complementary medicine offers a number of remedies. These are claimed to bring relief by relaxing the patient, by exploiting energy links (*see* page 928), or by removing the root cause of complaints through direct action against foci (*see* page 928), toxins (*see* page 929), or energy imbalances (*see* page 927). Some herbal treatments may affect the hormonal balance and so offer effective relief from symptoms.

Treatment plan and limited trial

Before administering a complementary treatment, every therapist should propose a treatment plan (*see* page xxiii) that sets out a clear time frame and defines the goal that the treatment is designed to achieve. Treatment should then be tried for a limited term to test the patient's response.

Cautions

A doctor must be consulted if a lump is discovered in the breast. Complementary medicine has no effective treatment for breast cancer; its procedures are suitable at most as adjuncts to orthodox treatment. Unless a proper medical diagnosis is obtained, the sufferer will perhaps receive inadequate or inappropriate treatment for what may be an extremely serious medical condition.

Complementary treatments for breast disorders

Treatment	Rating	Point of delivery/risks
Acupressure This treatment (*see* page 769), otherwise known as pressure-point massage, is claimed to ease sore breasts and improve general well-being. Acupressure is also used to impart vital energy (*see* Life force, page 928).	**May be of some use** as a short-term treatment attempt aimed at alleviating soreness. Some case reports claim efficacy; however, success is probably seen in only a proportion of patients (*see* Placebo, page xxi).	**Suitable for DIY** Qualified guidance is recommended. Therapists should be properly qualified. **Risks:** Unlikely provided treatment is carried out competently.

Treatment	Rating	Point of delivery/risks
Acupuncture Acupuncture in its various forms (*see* page 772) aims to encourage the flow of energy (*see* page 927) or to ease sore breasts directly. The acupuncture points chosen can vary from one practitioner to another.	**May be of some use** as a short-term treatment attempt for swollen or sore breasts. Case reports claim efficacy; however, success is probably seen in only a proportion of patients (*see* Placebo, page xxi).	**Requires a qualified practitioner** Acupuncturists should be properly qualified and should propose a treatment plan. **Risks:** Probably rare provided treatment is carried out competently.
Bioresonance therapy Bioresonance therapists use electrical devices in an attempt to discover the causes of illness and claim to be able to weaken or turn around pathogenic energies and disease related vibrations (*see* page 794).	**Of little use** Possibly acceptable as a short-term treatment attempt for persistent problems when simpler, more established methods have been unsuccessful. Some case reports claim efficacy; however, success is probably seen, if at all, in only a small proportion of patients (*see* Placebo, page xxi).	**Requires a qualified practitioner** Practitioners should be properly qualified and should propose a treatment plan. No credence should be given to anyone promising immediate or total success. **Risks:** Fairly unlikely.
Cell therapy Injecting or ingesting products extracted from the tissues of newborn animals or animal fetuses is said to have a rejuvenating and revitalizing effect and to enhance the healing of human tissues and organs (*see* page 796).	**Not advised** Based on present knowledge, there is inadequate evidence of the efficacy and mode of action of these costly and relatively risky procedures.	**Risks:** Injecting foreign proteins into the body can provoke (possibly fatal) allergic reactions. Also, pathogens such as those that cause bovine spongiform encephalopathy (BSE) or other serious infections may be introduced.

Treatment	Rating	Point of delivery/risks
Electroacupuncture according to Voll By taking readings of the electrical conductivity of the skin (*see* page 802), therapists claim to be able to derive an insight into diseased areas of the body, pathogenic foci (*see* page 928), and stress factors (*see* Toxins, page 929). The factors presumed to be instrumental in the causation of breast disorders can then be addressed.	**Of little use** Possibly acceptable as a short-term treatment attempt when simpler, more established methods have been unsuccessful. Some case reports claim efficacy; however, success is probably seen, if at all, in only a small proportion of patients (*see* Placebo, page xxi).	**Requires a qualified practitioner** Practitioners should be properly qualified and should propose a treatment plan. No credence should be given to anyone promising immediate or total success. **Risks:** A second opinion must always be obtained from a qualified physician before any attempt is made to "eliminate foci" (e.g. by surgery).
Electroneural therapy according to Croon According to the theory, readings taken at various reactive sites on the skin highlight diseased areas within the body. Based on these readings, targeted electrostimulative measures can be undertaken to address factors presumed to be instrumental in the causation of breast disorders (*see* page 806).	**Of little use** Possibly acceptable as a short-term treatment attempt when simpler, more established methods have been unsuccessful. Some case reports claim efficacy; however, success is probably seen, if at all, in only a small proportion of patients (*see* Placebo, page xxi).	**Requires a qualified practitioner** Practitioners should be properly qualified and should propose a treatment plan. No credence should be given to anyone promising immediate or total success. **Risks:** Proponents themselves warn that treatment should not be given in acute inflammatory conditions.

Treatment	Rating	Point of delivery/risks
Eliminative methods, unbloody Unbloody cupping (*see* page 817) is supposed to ease sore breasts and improve the body's own regulatory systems.	**Of little use** Acceptable as a short-term, supportive treatment attempt. Some case reports claim efficacy; however, success is probably seen in only a proportion of patients (*see* Placebo, page xxi).	**Suitable for DIY** Unbloody cupping is best carried out under the guidance of a qualified practitioner. **Risks:** Unlikely provided treatment is carried out competently.
Enzyme therapy The enzymes used (*see* page 824) are said to dispel and destroy "immune complexes" that course in the blood and that are responsible, for instance, for sustaining inflammatory processes and various other disorders.	**Of little use** Some case reports claim efficacy for this little researched therapy; however, success is probably seen in only a small proportion of patients (*see* Placebo, page xxi).	**Requires a qualified practitioner** Practitioners should propose a treatment plan. Non-prescription preparations are suitable for do-it-yourself. **Risks:** Allergies or intolerance are possible.
Flower remedies Some flower therapists see breast disorders as an expression of emotional disharmony. Flower remedies (*see* page 828) are said to restore emotional balance and assist the body's psychic ability to heal itself.	**Of little use** Acceptable as a short-term, supportive treatment attempt aimed at soothing and relaxing. Some case reports claim efficacy; however, success is probably seen in only a proportion of patients (*see* Placebo, page xxi).	**Suitable for DIY** Qualified guidance is recommended. Practitioners should propose a treatment plan. **Risks:** Possible intolerance.

Treatment	Rating	Point of delivery/risks
Homeopathy Highly diluted (potentized) solutions (*see* page 831) are believed to be able to redress vital energy imbalances. Organo- and functiotropic (*see* page 833) homeopathy is claimed to act directly to alleviate breast disorders.	**May be of some use** as a supportive treatment attempt when more established methods have been unsuccessful. Some case reports claim efficacy; however, success is probably seen in only a proportion of patients (*see* Placebo, page xxi).	**Requires a qualified practitioner** Homeopaths should be properly qualified and should propose a treatment plan. Ready-formulated preparations are suitable for do-it-yourself. **Risks:** Allergies and intolerance are possible.
Manual therapies Chiropractors and osteopaths (*see* page 844) use a series of manipulations to realign allegedly displaced vertebrae. This is said to reduce soreness, ease tension, release energy blockages (*see* page 927), and alleviate other symptoms.	**Of little use** Possibly acceptable as a short-term treatment attempt in persistent cases when less risky, more established methods have been unsuccessful. Some case reports claim efficacy; however, success is probably seen, if at all, in only a small proportion of patients (*see* Placebo, page xxi).	**Requires a qualified practitioner** Practitioners should be properly qualified and should propose a treatment plan. **Risks:** Manipulation of the head and cervical vertebrae can cause serious injury. Osteoporosis is one of several risk factors.
Nutritional therapies An organic diet (*see* page 4) provides the body with essential and secondary plant nutrients that are believed to exercise a multitude of positive effects.	**May be of some use** as a general supportive measure.	**Suitable for DIY** Qualified guidance is recommended though not essential. **Risks:** Avoid imbalanced or intolerable diets. They can cause deficiencies with serious consequences. Children are particularly at risk.

Treatment	Rating	Point of delivery/risks
Physical therapies Ascending temperature arm baths (*see* page 874), wraps (*see* page 877), and exercise therapy (*see* page 868) are said to invigorate the patient, improve the circulation, and ease symptoms.	**May be of some use** as a short-term treatment attempt. Case reports claim efficacy; however, success is probably seen in only a proportion of patients (*see* Placebo, page xxi).	**Suitable for DIY** Qualified guidance is recommended though not essential. **Risks:** Skin damage may be caused to persons with diminished temperature sensation when extreme temperatures are applied.
Reflex therapies Reflex zone massage (*see* page 883), reflexology (*see* page 883), and TENS (*see* page 886) are claimed to act via reflex channels (*see* page 881) to ease breast soreness and alleviate pain and other symptoms.	**May be of some use** as a short-term treatment attempt aimed at alleviating symptoms. Case reports claim efficacy; however, success is probably seen in only a proportion of patients (*see* Placebo, page xxi).	**Suitable for DIY** Qualified guidance is essential. **Risks:** Some people are sensitive to electrical stimuli and rubber electrodes; others find it hard to tolerate manual stimulation or close physical contact.
Relaxation techniques Autogenic training (*see* page 888), muscle relaxation according to Jacobson (*see* page 893), and various biofeedback techniques (*see* page 891) are said to relieve tension and inner unrest, and might be instrumental in helping patients to become more aware of their physical and emotional states.	**May be of some use** as a supportive treatment attempt aimed at soothing and relaxing. Some case reports claim efficacy; however, success is probably seen in only a proportion of patients (*see* Placebo, page xxi).	**Suitable for DIY** Once a sound understanding of the technique has been acquired from a trainer in group sessions or through individual tuition, patients can perform exercises themselves. Therapists should be properly qualified. **Risks:** Fairly unlikely.

Treatment	Rating	Point of delivery/risks
Vitamins and trace elements Some manufacturers claim that vitamins A and E are helpful in easing breast symptoms (*see* page 900).	**May be of some use** No definitive recommendations can be given based on present knowledge.	**Suitable for DIY** Qualified guidance is recommended though not essential. **Risks:** Intolerance and overdosage are possible.

Herbal remedies for breast disorders

Active ingredient/preparation	Rating
Agnus castus fruit (*Vitex agnus-castus*)	Taken orally, agnus castus **can be useful** as a treatment attempt for mastodynia and other breast problems, premenstrual syndrome (PMS), and also as an attempt to increase milk production. **Dosage:** As instructed by the manufacturer/prescriber. **Risks:** Irregular bleeding, increased menstrual blood loss, and perpetual bleeding from the uterus with associated anemia are possible but rare. Skin itchiness may also occasionally occur. If the breasts feel tender, consult your doctor to discover the cause. Not to be used during pregnancy and breastfeeding.
Bugleweed (*Lycopus europaeus*)	Taken orally, bugleweed is **of little use** as a treatment attempt for mastodynia. **Daily dose:** 1–2g of herb. **Individual dose:** For a tea drink, 0.5g to 1 cup of hot water. Use ready-formulated preparations as instructed by the manufacturer/prescriber. Do not stop taking bugleweed abruptly; instead, reduce the dose gradually. **Risks:** Thyroid enlargement may occasionally occur. Do not use with any other thyroid preparation. Not to be taken by persons with an overactive thyroid or with thyroid enlargement not involving functional disturbance.

Fertility problems

Causes and symptoms

The reason for a couple's infertility may lie with the man or with the woman. If attempts at conceiving are unsuccessful, it will be necessary for both partners to seek expert medical advice.

There are many reasons why a couple may be unable to conceive. Their problem may be emotional or psychosocial in origin or may be due to a hormonal disturbance or other physical ailment, or to certain environmental factors, intoxicants, or immune phenomena. Infertility, if it persists, may damage the couple's relationship. Apart from the sexuality and partnership aspect, infertility can impact other areas, affecting, for example, work performance and job satisfaction, as well as the quality of life and even health.

Orthodox treatment

The key to any orthodox treatment that is attempted will be a thorough physical examination of both partners. Attention will also be paid to possible psychological factors. Depending on the condition that is diagnosed, an antimicrobial, anti-inflammatory, or hormone treatment may be advised. Certain problems can be eliminated by surgery. Experts' opinions differ regarding the suitability and efficacy of some of the measures that are advocated. Psychotherapy and counselling may have a useful role.

Complementary therapies

Some complementary therapists attempt to act directly on the reproductive organs or functions, through energy links (*see* page 928), for instance. Others see infertility as being caused by toxins (*see* page 929), immune disorders, foci (*see* page 928), or an energy imbalance (*see* page 927), and propose treatments accordingly.

Treatment plan and limited trial

Before administering a complementary treatment, every therapist should propose a treatment plan (*see* page xxiii) that sets out a clear time frame and defines the goal that the treatment is designed to achieve. Treatment should then be tried for a limited term to test the patient's response.

Cautions

No complementary procedure is suitable for use on its own against infertility. Complementary therapies can have a role as adjuncts to orthodox medical treatment. Unless a couple receive proper medical examinations to discover whether there is a physical cause for their infertility, they may be offered inappropriate treatment.

Complementary treatments for fertility problems

Treatment	Rating	Point of delivery/risks
Acupressure This treatment (*see* page 769), otherwise known as pressure-point massage, is claimed to encourage various functions in the genital region and to release tension. Acupressure is also used as a restorative measure that is intended to impart vital energy (*see* Life force, page 928) to the body.	**Inappropriate** as the sole treatment for infertility. Acceptable as a short-term, supportive treatment attempt aimed at soothing and relaxing the patient and improving the circulation. Case reports claim efficacy; however, success is probably seen in only a proportion of patients (*see* Placebo, page xxi).	**Suitable for DIY** Qualified guidance is recommended. Therapists should be properly qualified. **Risks:** Unlikely provided treatment is carried out competently.

Treatment	Rating	Point of delivery/risks
Acupuncture Acupuncture in its various forms (*see* page 772) aims to encourage the flow of energy (*see* page 927) or to act directly by exercising a beneficial effect on the hormone system. The acupuncture points chosen can vary from one practitioner to another.	**Inappropriate** as the sole treatment for infertility. **May be of some use** as a short-term treatment attempt in cases where infertility is of hormonal or emotional origin. Some case reports and field studies claim efficacy; however, success is probably seen in only a proportion of patients (*see* Placebo, page xxi).	**Requires a qualified practitioner** Acupuncturists should be properly qualified and should propose a treatment plan. **Risks:** Probably rare provided treatment is carried out competently.
Anthroposophical medicine Constitutional (*see* page 927) or dialog therapy is supposed to have a beneficial effect on the woman's ability to conceive (*see* page 781).	**Inappropriate** as the sole treatment for infertility. **May be of some use** as a short-term treatment attempt. Some case reports claim efficacy; however, success is probably seen in only a proportion of patients (*see* Placebo, page xxi).	**Requires a qualified practitioner** Practitioners should be properly qualified and should propose a treatment plan. **Risks:** Allergies and intolerance are possible.
Aromatherapy Essential oils (*see* page 786) are used to soothe and relax, or to invigorate the patient. The essences may be taken orally, used externally as massage oils or bathing emulsions, or inhaled as vapors.	**Inappropriate** as the sole treatment for infertility. **May be of some use** as a supportive measure aimed at soothing and relaxing, or invigorating the patient. Some case reports claim efficacy; however, success is probably seen in only a small proportion of patients (*see* Placebo, page xxi).	**Suitable for DIY** Qualified guidance is recommended. The effects of individual essential oils differ widely. **Risks:** Allergies or intolerance are possible. Some oils are carcinogenic in test systems and possibly in humans.

Treatment	Rating	Point of delivery/risks

Bioresonance therapy
Bioresonance therapists use electrical devices in an attempt to discover the causes of illness and claim to be able to weaken or turn around pathogenic energies and disease related vibrations (*see* page 794).

Inappropriate as the sole treatment for infertility.
Possibly acceptable as a short-term, supportive treatment attempt when simpler, more established methods have been unsuccessful. Some case reports claim efficacy; however, success is probably seen, if at all, in only a small proportion of patients (*see* Placebo, page xxi).

Requires a qualified practitioner
Practitioners should be properly qualified and should propose a treatment plan. No credence should be given to anyone promising immediate or total success.
Risks: Fairly unlikely.

Cell therapy
Injecting or ingesting products extracted from the tissues of newborn animals or animal fetuses is said to have a rejuvenating and revitalizing effect and to enhance the healing of human tissues and organs (*see* page 796).

Not advised
Based on present knowledge, there is inadequate evidence of the efficacy and mode of action of these costly and relatively risky procedures.

Risks: Injecting foreign proteins into the body can provoke (possibly fatal) allergic reactions. Also, pathogens such as those that cause bovine spongiform encephalopathy (BSE) or other serious infections may be introduced.

Electroacupuncture according to Voll
By taking readings of the electrical conductivity of the skin (*see* page 802), therapists claim to be able to derive an insight into diseased areas of the body, pathogenic foci (*see* page 928), and stress factors (*see* Toxins, page 929). The factors presumed to be instrumental in the causation of fertility problems can then be addressed.

Inappropriate as the sole treatment for infertility.
Possibly acceptable as a short-term, supportive treatment attempt when simpler, more established methods have been unsuccessful. Some case reports claim efficacy; however, success is probably seen, if at all, in only a small proportion of patients (*see* Placebo, page xxi).

Requires a qualified practitioner
Practitioners should be properly qualified and should propose a treatment plan. No credence should be given to anyone promising immediate or total success.
Risks: A second opinion must always be obtained from a qualified physician before any attempt is made to "eliminate foci" (e.g. by surgery).

Treatment	Rating	Point of delivery/risks
Electroneural therapy according to Croon According to the theory, readings taken at various reactive sites on the skin highlight diseased areas within the body. Based on these readings, targeted electrostimulative measures can be undertaken to address factors presumed to be instrumental in the causation of fertility problems (*see* page 806).	**Inappropriate** as the sole treatment for infertility. Possibly acceptable as a short-term, supportive treatment attempt when simpler, more established methods have been unsuccessful. Some case reports claim efficacy; however, success is probably seen, if at all, in only a small proportion of patients (*see* Placebo, page xxi).	**Requires a qualified practitioner** Practitioners should be properly qualified and should propose a treatment plan. No credence should be given to anyone promising immediate or total success. **Risks:** Proponents themselves warn that treatment should not be given in acute inflammatory conditions.
Eliminative methods, bloody Bloody cupping (*see* page 815) is said to improve the body's own regulatory systems and to invigorate patients with fertility problems.	**Not advised** The efficacy of this invasive method is unproven.	**Risks:** Bloody cupping can cause infection and scarring. Furthermore, it should not be carried out in persons with bleeding disorders.
Eliminative methods, unbloody Unbloody cupping (*see* page 817) is said to improve the body's own regulatory systems and to invigorate patients with fertility problems.	**Inappropriate** as the sole treatment for infertility. Possibly acceptable as a short-term, supportive treatment attempt in persistent cases. Some case reports claim efficacy; however, success is probably seen in only a proportion of patients (*see* Placebo, page xxi).	**Suitable for DIY** Unbloody cupping is best carried out under the guidance of a qualified practitioner. **Risks:** Unlikely provided treatment is carried out competently.

Treatment	Rating	Point of delivery/risks
Flower remedies Some flower therapists see infertility as an expression of emotional disharmony. Flower remedies (*see* page 828) are said to restore emotional balance and assist the body's psychic ability to heal itself.	**Inappropriate** as the sole treatment for infertility. **May be of some use** as a short-term, supportive treatment attempt aimed at soothing and relaxing. Some case reports claim efficacy; however, success is probably seen in only a proportion of patients (*see* Placebo, page xxi).	**Suitable for DIY** Qualified guidance is recommended. Practitioners should propose a treatment plan. **Risks:** Possible intolerance.
Homeopathy Highly diluted (potentized) solutions (*see* page 831) are believed to be able to redress vital energy imbalances. Organo- and functiotropic (*see* page 833) homeopathy is claimed to be effective for dealing directly with fertility problems.	**Inappropriate** as the sole treatment for infertility. **May be of some use** as a supportive treatment attempt aimed at helping the patient come to terms emotionally with his/her problem. Field studies, case reports, and case studies claim efficacy for homeopathic treatments; however, success is probably seen in only a proportion of patients (*see* Placebo, page xxi).	**Requires a qualified practitioner** Homeopaths should be properly qualified and should propose a treatment plan. Ready-formulated preparations are suitable for do-it-yourself. **Risks:** Allergies and intolerance are possible.
Massage Classical massage (*see* page 847) and lymphatic drainage (*see* page 850) can, it is said, soothe or invigorate the patient, as well as ease muscular and emotional tension. Inappropriate as the sole treatment for infertility.	**Inappropriate** as the sole treatment for infertility. **May be of some use** as a supportive treatment attempt aimed at soothing and relaxing. Case reports claim efficacy in the treatment of infertility; however, success is probably seen in only a proportion of patients (*see* Placebo, page xxi).	**Requires a qualified practitioner** Masseurs/masseuses should be properly qualified and should propose a treatment plan. **Risks:** Some people are sensitive to manual stimuli; others find it hard to tolerate close physical contact.

Treatment	Rating	Point of delivery/risks
Nutritional therapies An organic diet (*see* page 4) provides the body with essential and secondary plant nutrients that are believed to exercise a multitude of positive effects.	**Inappropriate** as the sole treatment for infertility. **Useful** as a general supportive measure.	**Suitable for DIY** Qualified guidance is recommended though not essential. **Risks:** Avoid imbalanced or intolerable diets. They can cause deficiencies with serious consequences. Children are particularly at risk.
Physical therapies Ascending temperature sitz baths, mud baths, partial washings, or brushings (*see* pages 871–8) are said to relax the patient and improve the circulation.	**Inappropriate** as the sole treatment for infertility. **Useful** as a supportive measure aimed at soothing and relaxing. Case reports claim efficacy in the treatment of infertility; however, success is probably seen in only a proportion of patients (*see* Placebo, page xxi).	**Suitable for DIY** Qualified guidance is recommended though not essential. **Risks:** Skin damage may be caused to persons with diminished temperature sensation when extreme temperatures are applied.
Reflex therapies Reflex zone massage (*see* page 883), reflexology (*see* page 883), and TENS (*see* page 886) are claimed to act via reflex channels (*see* page 881) to relax the patient, to improve the circulation, and to have a beneficial effect on various body functions.	**Inappropriate** as the sole treatment for infertility. **Useful** as a short-term, supportive treatment attempt aimed at soothing and relaxing the patient and at improving the circulation. Case reports claim efficacy in the treatment of infertility; however, success is probably seen in only a proportion of patients (*see* Placebo, page xxi).	**Suitable for DIY** Qualified guidance is essential. **Risks:** Some people are sensitive to electrical stimuli and rubber electrodes; others find it hard to tolerate manual stimulation or close physical contact.

Treatment	Rating	Point of delivery/risks
Relaxation techniques Autogenic training (*see* page 888), muscle relaxation according to Jacobson (*see* page 893), and various biofeedback techniques (*see* page 891) are said to relieve muscle tension and inner unrest, and might be instrumental in helping the patient to become more aware of his/her emotional states.	**Inappropriate** as the sole treatment for infertility. **May be of some use** as a supportive treatment attempt aimed at soothing and relaxing the patient and easing muscular tension. Some case reports claim efficacy; however, success is probably seen in only a proportion of patients (*see* Placebo, page xxi).	**Suitable for DIY** Once a sound understanding of the technique has been acquired from a trainer in group sessions or through individual tuition, patients can perform exercises themselves. Therapists should be properly qualified. **Risks:** Fairly unlikely.
Vitamins and trace elements Through its antioxidative properties, vitamin E is believed to achieve a number of beneficial effects in the body and, according to some manufacturers, to be capable of assisting in the treatment of infertility (*see* page 900).	**Inappropriate** as the sole treatment for infertility. **Useful** when vitamin deficiency has been diagnosed.	**Suitable for DIY** Qualified guidance is recommended though not essential. **Risks:** Intolerance and overdosage are possible.

Herbal remedies for female fertility problems

Active ingredient/preparation	Rating
Agnus castus fruit (*Vitex agnus-castus*)	Taken orally for its estrogenic action, agnus castus is **of little use** as a treatment attempt for female fertility problems. **Dosage:** As instructed by the manufacturer/prescriber. **Risks:** Irregular bleeding, increased menstrual blood loss, and perpetual bleeding from the uterus with associated anemia are possible. Skin itchiness may also occasionally occur. If the breasts feel tender, consult your doctor to discover the cause. Not to be used during pregnancy and breastfeeding.

Active ingredient/preparation	*Rating*
Black cohosh root (*Cimicifuga racemosa*)	Taken orally for its estrogenic action, black cohosh is **of little use** as a treatment attempt for female fertility problems. However, as an estrogenic it is useful in painful pre- and post-menstrual conditions as well as in unrest and nervous excitability during menopause. **Dosage:** As instructed by the manufacturer/ prescriber. **Risks:** Gastrointestinal problems are possible. On account of its estrogenic action, black cohosh must not be used by women with certain types of tumor (those said to be estrogen-binding). Black cohosh is potentially dangerous in high doses. It must not be used during pregnancy.

Infections of the sexual organs, discharge

Causes and symptoms

Infections of the sexual organs are caused by a wide range of bacteria, viruses, and fungi. The pathogen is often sexually transmitted, thriving well in the moist environment of the vagina, especially when resistance to disease is lowered; also, coli bacteria are easily transferred inadvertently from the anus to the vagina on toilet paper. Symptoms of infected sexual organs will include redness, swelling, burning, itchiness, or discharge, possibly accompanied by inflammation of the bladder (cystitis), and of the penis or prostate in men and the labia or vagina in women.

Orthodox treatment

Generally an oral or topical preparation will be needed to clear the infection. A condom or femidom affords the best protection against sexually transmitted diseases.

Complementary therapies

Complementary medicine offers methods that usually have only a subordinate role in the treatment of genital infections, e.g. as a means of providing relief from discomfort. Depending on the therapist's particular approach, attempts will be made to relax the patient, to address symptoms via energy links (*see* page 928), to modulate the immune system (*see* page 10), or to eliminate foci (*see* page 928), toxins (*see* page 929), or energy imbalances (*see* page 927).

Treatment plan and limited trial

Before administering a complementary treatment, every therapist should propose a treatment plan (*see* page xxiii) that sets out a clear time frame and defines the goal that the treatment is designed to achieve. Treatment should then be tried for a limited term to test the patient's response.

Cautions

In infections of the genitalia, there is no complementary therapy that can match the success of orthodox antibiotic therapy. Genital infections that do not receive appropriate treatment may go on to cause serious complications.

Complementary treatments for infections of the sexual organs

Treatment	Rating	Point of delivery/risks
Acupressure This treatment (*see* page 769), otherwise known as pressure-point massage, is used to alleviate symptoms of infections of the sexual organs.	**Of little use** Acceptable as a short-term treatment attempt aimed at easing symptoms of minor infections. Some case reports claim efficacy; however, success is probably seen in only a proportion of patients (*see* Placebo, page xxi).	**Suitable for DIY** Qualified guidance is recommended. Therapists should be properly qualified. **Risks:** Unlikely provided treatment is carried out competently.
Acupuncture Acupuncture in its various forms (*see* page 772) aims to encourage the flow of energy (*see* page 927) or to act directly to ease symptoms of infections of the sexual organs.	**Of little use** Acceptable as a short-term, supportive treatment attempt aimed at easing symptoms of minor infections. Field studies claim efficacy; however, success is probably seen in only a small proportion of patients (*see* Placebo, page xxi).	**Requires a qualified practitioner** Acupuncturists should be properly qualified and should propose a treatment plan. **Risks:** Probably rare provided treatment is carried out competently.
Aromatherapy Essential oils (*see* page 786) are used to soothe and relax, or to invigorate, thereby possibly contributing to an easing of symptoms. The essences may be taken orally, used externally as massage oils or bathing emulsions, or inhaled as vapors.	**Of little use** Acceptable as a short-term, supportive treatment attempt aimed at soothing and relaxing. Some case reports claim efficacy; however, success is probably seen in only a proportion of patients (*see* Placebo, page xxi).	**Suitable for DIY** Qualified guidance is recommended. The effects of individual essential oils differ widely. **Risks:** Allergies or intolerance are possible. Some oils are carcinogenic in test systems and possibly in humans.

Treatment	Rating	Point of delivery/risks
Bioresonance therapy Bioresonance therapists use electrical devices in an attempt to discover the causes of illness and claim to be able to weaken or turn around pathogenic energies and disease related vibrations (*see* page 794).	**Of little use** Possibly acceptable as a short-term, supportive treatment attempt for chronic symptoms when more established methods have been unsuccessful. Some case reports claim efficacy; however, success is probably seen, if at all, in only a small proportion of patients (*see* Placebo, page xxi).	**Requires a qualified practitioner** Practitioners should be properly qualified and should propose a treatment plan. No credence should be given to anyone promising immediate or total success. **Risks:** Fairly unlikely.
Cell therapy Injecting or ingesting products extracted from the tissues of newborn animals or animal fetuses is said to have a rejuvenating and revitalizing effect and to enhance the healing of human tissues and organs (*see* page 796).	**Not advised** Based on present knowledge, there is inadequate evidence of the efficacy and mode of action of these costly and relatively risky procedures.	**Risks:** Injecting foreign proteins into the body can provoke (possibly fatal) allergic reactions. Also, pathogens such as those that cause bovine spongiform encephalopathy (BSE) or other serious infections may be introduced.
Electroacupuncture according to Voll By taking readings of the electrical conductivity of the skin (*see* page 802), therapists claim to be able to derive an insight into diseased areas of the body, pathogenic foci (*see* page 928), and stress factors (*see* Toxins, page 929). The factors presumed to be instrumental in the causation of infections can then be eliminated.	**Of little use** Possibly acceptable as a short-term, supportive treatment attempt when simpler, more established methods have been unsuccessful. Some case reports claim efficacy; however, success is probably seen, if at all, in only a small proportion of patients (*see* Placebo, page xxi).	**Requires a qualified practitioner** Practitioners should be properly qualified and should propose a treatment plan. No credence should be given to anyone promising immediate or total success. **Risks:** A second opinion must always be obtained from a qualified physician before any attempt is made to "eliminate foci" (e.g. by surgery).

Treatment	*Rating*	*Point of delivery/risks*
Electroneural therapy according to Croon According to the theory, readings taken at various reactive sites on the skin highlight diseased areas within the body. Based on these readings, targeted electrostimulative measures can be undertaken to eliminate factors presumed to be instrumental in the causation of infections (*see* page 806).	**Of little use** Possibly acceptable as a short-term, supportive treatment attempt when simpler, more established methods have been unsuccessful. Some case reports claim efficacy; however, success is probably seen, if at all, in only a small proportion of patients (*see* Placebo, page xxi).	**Requires a qualified practitioner** Practitioners should be properly qualified and should propose a treatment plan. No credence should be given to anyone promising immediate or total success. **Risks:** Proponents themselves warn that treatment should not be given in acute inflammatory conditions.
Eliminative methods, unbloody Unbloody cupping (*see* page 817) is supposed to ease pain and improve the body's own regulatory systems.	**Of little use** Acceptable as a short-term, supportive treatment attempt aimed at alleviating pain. Some case reports claim efficacy; however, success is probably seen in only a small proportion of patients (*see* Placebo, page xxi).	**Suitable for DIY** Unbloody cupping is best carried out under the guidance of a qualified practitioner. **Risks:** Unlikely provided treatment is carried out competently.
Flower remedies Taking flower remedies (*see* page 828) in infections of the sexual organs is said to restore emotional balance and assist the body's psychic ability to heal itself.	**Of little use** Acceptable as a short-term, supportive treatment attempt aimed at soothing and relaxing. Some case reports claim efficacy; however, success is probably seen in only a proportion of patients (*see* Placebo, page xxi).	**Suitable for DIY** Qualified guidance is recommended. Practitioners should propose a treatment plan. **Risks:** Possible intolerance.

Treatment	Rating	Point of delivery/risks
Homeopathy Highly diluted (potentized) solutions (*see* page 831) are believed to be able to redress vital energy imbalances and strengthen the body's defences. Organo- and functiotropic (*see* page 833) homeopathy is claimed to be effective for dealing directly with infections of the sexual organs.	**May be of some use** as a supportive treatment attempt. Some case reports claim efficacy; however, success is probably seen in only a proportion of patients (*see* Placebo, page xxi).	**Requires a qualified practitioner** Homeopaths should be properly qualified and should propose a treatment plan. Ready-formulated preparations are suitable for do-it-yourself. **Risks:** Allergies and intolerance are possible.
Manual therapies Chiropractors and osteopaths (*see* page 844) use a series of manipulations to realign vertebrae allegedly displaced as a result of the infection. This is said to reduce pain, release energy blockages (*see* page 927), and to have a beneficial effect on the infection.	**Of little use** Possibly acceptable as a short-term, supportive treatment attempt for persistent symptoms when less risky, more established methods have been unsuccessful. Some case reports claim efficacy; however, success is probably seen, if at all, in only a small proportion of patients (*see* Placebo, page xxi).	**Requires a qualified practitioner** Practitioners should be properly qualified and should propose a treatment plan. **Risks:** Manipulation of the head and cervical vertebrae can cause serious injury. Osteoporosis is one of several risk factors.
Nutritional therapies An organic diet (*see* page 4) provides the body with essential and secondary plant nutrients that are believed to be capable, *inter alia*, of boosting the immune system.	**Useful** as a supportive general measure.	**Suitable for DIY** Qualified guidance is recommended though not essential. **Risks:** Avoid imbalanced or intolerable diets. They can cause deficiencies with serious consequences. Children are particularly at risk.

Treatment	Rating	Point of delivery/risks
Physical therapies Warm or hot sitz and full immersion baths, and mud baths, are claimed to reduce swelling, inhibit inflammation, and ease pain (*see* pages 871–8).	**May be of some use** as a short-term, supportive treatment attempt. Some case reports and field studies claim efficacy; however, success is probably seen in only a proportion of patients (*see* Placebo, page xxi).	**Suitable for DIY** Qualified guidance is recommended though not essential. **Risks:** Skin damage may be caused to persons with diminished temperature sensation when extreme temperatures are applied.
Probiotics The introduction of certain bacteria into the gut is claimed to bring the intestinal flora back into balance and to have a beneficial effect on the immune system (*see* page 878).	**Of little use** Acceptable as a short-term treatment attempt in persistent cases or as a means of preventing fungal infections. Case reports claim efficacy; however, success is probably seen in only a proportion of patients (*see* Placebo, page xxi).	**Requires a qualified practitioner** Practitioners should be properly qualified and should propose a treatment plan. Non-prescription formulations are suitable for do-it-yourself. **Risks:** Fairly unlikely provided treatment is carried out competently.
Reflex therapies Connective tissue massage, reflexology (*see* page 883), and TENS (*see* page 886) are claimed to act via reflex channels (*see* page 881) to improve the circulation and ease symptoms.	**Of little use** Possibly acceptable as a short-term, supportive treatment attempt. Some case reports claim efficacy; however, success is probably seen in only a proportion of patients (*see* Placebo, page xxi).	**Requires a qualified practitioner** Practitioners should be properly qualified and should propose a treatment plan. **Risks:** Some people are sensitive to electrical stimuli and rubber electrodes; others find it hard to tolerate manual stimulation or close physical contact.

Treatment	Rating	Point of delivery/risks
Relaxation techniques Autogenic training (*see* page 888), muscle relaxation according to Jacobson (*see* page 893), and various biofeedback techniques (*see* page 891) are said to relieve muscle tension and inner unrest, and might help the patient to become more aware of his/her physical and emotional states.	**May be of some use** as a short-term treatment attempt in persistent cases when the procedure chosen is perceived as being pleasant and effective. Case reports claim efficacy; however, success is probably seen in only a proportion of patients (*see* Placebo, page xxi).	**Suitable for DIY** Once a sound understanding of the technique has been acquired from a trainer in group sessions or through individual tuition, patients can perform exercises themselves. Therapists should be properly qualified. **Risks:** Fairly unlikely.

Herbal remedies for infections of the sexual organs

Treatment with herbal remedies is no substitute for appropriate antibiotic treatment. However, in some infections supportive use of herbal baths or ointments may be useful.

Active ingredient/preparation	Rating
German camomile flowers (*Chamomilla recutita*)	**Only useful** as an externally applied supportive treatment attempt for infection and mild inflammatory conditions of the anal/genital region, for superficial inflammation, and lesions to the skin and mucosa, including the mouth. **Daily dose:** 10–15g flowerheads. **Individual dose:** As a tea drink, mix 3g of flowerheads with 1 cup of hot water and add to the bathwater (sitz bath). Also for wraps, poultices, or rinses. Use ready-formulated preparations as instructed by the manufacturer/prescriber. **Risks:** Allergic skin reactions may occur in isolated cases.

Active ingredient/preparation	Rating
Witch hazel leaves and bark (*Hamamelis virginiana*)	**Only useful** as an attempted external treatment for superficial skin inflammation and lesions. Its action is astringent and anti-inflammatory. **Dosage:** 0.1–1g of herb to a cup of hot water as an infusion, one to three times daily. **Individual dose:** To prepare a decoction for adding to bathwater or for embrocation, cover 5g of leaves and bark with 1 cup of water, bring to a boil, simmer, and strain. Use ready-formulated preparations as instructed by the manufacturer/prescriber. **Risks:** Skin irritation may occur in isolated cases.

Menopause

Causes and symptoms

Menopause occurs as a result of a gradual winding down in the production of hormones by the ovaries. Periods are more irregular, of shorter duration, and with less blood loss. The changes in hormone secretion can produce subjective and physical symptoms, such as hot flushes and night sweats, vaginal dryness, dry wrinkled skin, feelings akin to panic attacks, dizziness, lack of energy, palpitations, irritability, decreased sexual interest, and depression. Gradual bone demineralization occurs in most women during and after menopause (*see* Osteoporosis, page 195).

What impact the "change" has and how long it takes to run its course will depend on the genetic, cultural, emotional, and biographical context in which it occurs.

Orthodox treatment

Various preparations will help to reduce symptoms, including lubricants to overcome vaginal dryness and vitamins and minerals for lackluster hair and hair loss. Much publicity has been given to hormone replacement therapy (HRT). Estrogen can be used to improve skin tone, stop hot flushes, improve blood flow to the mucous membranes and help ward off osteoporosis. A doctor should be consulted to see whether there is any benefit to be derived from HRT.

Complementary therapies

Some therapists consider problems experienced during menopause to be due to toxins (*see* page 929), immune disorders, foci (*see* page 928), or energy imbalances (*see* page 927), and gear their treatments accordingly.

Treatment plan and limited trial

Before administering a complementary treatment, every therapist should propose a treatment plan (*see* page xxiii) that sets out a clear time frame and defines the goal that the treatment is designed to achieve. Treatment should then be tried for a limited term to test the patient's response.

Caution

Complementary medicine can offer no effective alternative to hormone replacement therapy as a means of preventing osteoporosis.

Complementary treatments for problems during menopause

Treatment	Rating	Point of delivery/risks
Acupressure This treatment (*see* page 769), otherwise known as pressure-point massage, is claimed to ease complaints during menopause. Acupressure is also used as a restorative treatment intended to impart vital energy (*see* Life force, page 928).	**May be of some use** as a short-term treatment attempt aimed at easing symptoms. Some case reports and field studies claim efficacy; however, success is probably seen in only a proportion of patients (*see* Placebo, page xxi).	**Suitable for DIY** Qualified guidance is recommended. Therapists should be properly qualified. **Risks:** Unlikely provided treatment is carried out competently.
Acupuncture Acupuncture in its various forms (*see* page 772) aims to encourage the flow of energy (*see* page 927) or to act directly to ease symptoms. The acupuncture points chosen can vary from one practitioner to another.	**May be of some use** as a short-term treatment attempt aimed at alleviating symptoms. Some case reports and field studies claim efficacy; however, success is probably seen in only a proportion of patients (*see* Placebo, page xxi).	**Requires a qualified practitioner** Practitioners should be properly qualified and should propose a treatment plan. **Risks:** Probably rare provided treatment is carried out competently.
Anthroposophical medicine Through anthroposophical psychotherapy and potentized preparations, doctors who practice AM (*see* page 781) aim to help women through menopause without the need for hormone replacement.	**May be of some use** as a supportive measure. Some case reports claim efficacy for the drugs used; however, success is probably seen in only a small proportion of patients (*see* Placebo, page xxi).	**Requires a qualified practitioner** Practitioners should be properly qualified and should propose a treatment plan. **Risks:** Allergies and intolerance are possible.

Treatment	Rating	Point of delivery/risks
Aromatherapy Essential oils (*see* page 786) are used to soothe and relax, or to invigorate, thereby contributing to an easing of symptoms. The essences may be taken orally, used externally as massage oils or bathing emulsions, or inhaled as vapors.	**May be of some use** as a short-term, supportive treatment attempt aimed a soothing and relaxing. Case reports claim efficacy; however, success is probably seen in only a proportion of patients (*see* Placebo, page xxi).	**Suitable for DIY** Qualified guidance is recommended. The effects of individual essential oils differ widely. **Risks:** Allergies or intolerance are possible. Some oils are carcinogenic in test systems and possibly in humans.
Bioresonance therapy Bioresonance therapists use electrical devices in an attempt to discover the causes of illness and claim to be able to weaken or turn around pathogenic energies and disease related vibrations (*see* page 794).	**Of little use** Possibly acceptable as a short-term treatment attempt in persistent cases when simpler, more established methods have been unsuccessful. Some case reports claim efficacy; however, success is probably seen, if at all, in only a small proportion of patients (*see* Placebo, page xxi).	**Requires a qualified practitioner** Practitioners should be properly qualified and should propose a treatment plan. No credence should be given to anyone promising immediate or total success. **Risks:** Fairly unlikely.
Cell therapy Injecting or ingesting products extracted from the tissues of newborn animals or animal fetuses is said to have a rejuvenating and revitalizing effect and to enhance the healing of human tissues and organs (*see* page 796).	**Not advised** Based on present knowledge, there is inadequate evidence of the efficacy and mode of action of these costly and relatively risky procedures.	**Risks:** Injecting foreign proteins into the body can provoke (possibly fatal) allergic reactions. Also, pathogens such as those that cause bovine spongiform encephalopathy (BSE) or other serious infections may be introduced.

Treatment	Rating	Point of delivery/risks
Electroacupuncture according to Voll By taking readings of the electrical conductivity of the skin (*see* page 802), therapists claim to be able to derive an insight into diseased areas of the body, pathogenic foci (*see* page 928), and stress factors (*see* Toxins, page 929). The factors presumed to be instrumental in the causation of climacteric problems can then be addressed.	**Of little use** Possibly acceptable as a short-term, supportive treatment attempt when simpler, more established methods have been unsuccessful. Some case reports claim efficacy; however, success is probably seen, if at all, in only a small proportion of patients (*see* Placebo, page xxi).	**Requires a qualified practitioner** Practitioners should be properly qualified and should propose a treatment plan. No credence should be given to anyone promising immediate or total success. **Risks:** A second opinion must always be obtained from a qualified physician before any attempt is made to "eliminate foci" (e.g. by surgery).
Electroneural therapy according to Croon According to the theory, readings taken at various reactive sites on the skin highlight diseased areas within the body. Based on these readings, targeted electrostimulative measures can be undertaken to address factors presumed to be instrumental in the causation of climacteric problems (*see* page 806).	**Of little use** Possibly acceptable as a short-term, supportive treatment attempt when simpler, more established methods have been unsuccessful. Some case reports claim efficacy; however, success is probably seen, if at all, in only a small proportion of patients (*see* Placebo, page xxi).	**Requires a qualified practitioner** Practitioners should be properly qualified and should propose a treatment plan. No credence should be given to anyone promising immediate or total success. **Risks:** Proponents themselves warn that treatment should not be given in acute inflammatory conditions.

Treatment	Rating	Point of delivery/risks
Eliminative methods, bloody Bloody cupping (*see* page 815) is said to improve the body's own regulatory systems during menopause and to ease symptoms.	**Of little use** Acceptable as a supportive measure when more established, less invasive methods have been unsuccessful. Some case reports and field studies claim efficacy; however, success is probably seen in only a proportion of patients (*see* Placebo, page xxi).	**Requires a qualified practitioner** Practitioners should be properly qualified and should propose a treatment plan. No credence should be given to anyone promising immediate or total success. **Risks:** Bloody cupping can cause infection and scarring. Furthermore, it should not be carried out in persons with bleeding disorders.
Eliminative methods, unbloody Unbloody cupping (*see* page 817) is said to improve the body's own regulatory systems during menopause, to energize (*see* page 927) the patient, and to ease symptoms.	**May be of some use** as a short-term treatment attempt aimed at alleviating pain. Some case reports claim efficacy; however, success is probably seen in only a proportion of patients (*see* Placebo, page xxi).	**Suitable for DIY** Unbloody cupping is best carried out under the guidance of a qualified practitioner. **Risks:** Unlikely provided treatment is carried out competently.
Flower remedies Flower remedies (*see* page 828) are said to restore emotional balance and, during menopause, to improve general well-being.	**May be of some use** as a short-term treatment attempt aimed at soothing and relaxing. Some case reports claim efficacy; however, success is probably seen in only a proportion of patients (*see* Placebo, page xxi).	**Suitable for DIY** Qualified guidance is recommended. Practitioners should propose a treatment plan. **Risks:** Possible intolerance.

Treatment	*Rating*	*Point of delivery/risks*
Homeopathy Highly diluted (potentized) solutions (*see* page 831) are believed to be able to redress vital energy imbalances. Organo- and functiotropic (*see* page 833) homeopathy is claimed to be effective for dealing with individual symptoms.	**May be of some use** as a treatment attempt for persistent complaints when more established methods have been unsuccessful. Case reports and field studies claim efficacy; however, success is probably seen in only a proportion of patients (*see* Placebo, page xxi).	**Requires a qualified practitioner** Homeopaths should be properly qualified and should propose a treatment plan. Ready-formulated preparations are suitable for do-it-yourself. **Risks:** Allergies and intolerance are possible.
Hypnosis and self-hypnosis In the relaxed and generally altered state of awareness that is induced in hypnosis or self-hypnosis (*see* page 837), physical conditions can be addressed and pain eased. Some professionally organized courses in self-hypnosis are now available. Hypnosis is often used in combination with other psycho- and behavioral therapies to effect a change of lifestyle or to help the patient come to terms better with her condition.	**Of little use** Acceptable as a short-term, supportive treatment attempt aimed at relaxing the patient and effecting a change of lifestyle when simpler, more established methods have been unsuccessful. Some case reports claim efficacy; however, success is probably seen in only a proportion of patients (*see* Placebo, page xxi).	**Requires a qualified practitioner** Hypnotherapists should be properly qualified and should propose a treatment plan. No credence should be given to anyone promising immediate or total success. **Risks:** Unlikely provided treatment is carried out competently.

Treatment	*Rating*	*Point of delivery/risks*
Manual therapies Chiropractors and osteopaths (*see* page 844) use a series of manipulations to re-align allegedly displaced vertebrae. This is said to ease pain, release energy blockages (*see* page 927), and eliminate factors presumed to be instrumental in the causation of symptoms.	**Of little use** Possibly acceptable as a short-term treatment attempt in persistent cases when less risky, more established methods have been unsuccessful. Some case reports claim efficacy; however, success is probably seen, if at all, in only a small proportion of patients (*see* Placebo, page xxi).	**Requires a qualified practitioner** Practitioners should be properly qualified and should propose a treatment plan. **Risks:** Manipulation of the head and cervical vertebrae can cause serious injury. Osteoporosis frequently occurs during menopause and is a significant risk factor.
Massage Classical massage (*see* page 847) and lymphatic drainage (*see* page 850) can soothe the patient, as well as ease muscular and emotional tension.	**May be of some use** as a supportive treatment attempt aimed at relaxing the patient. Some case reports and field studies claim efficacy; however, success is probably seen in only a proportion of patients (*see* Placebo, page xxi).	**Requires a qualified practitioner** Masseurs/masseuses should be properly qualified and should propose a treatment plan. **Risks:** Only gentle massaging techniques should be used on parts of the body affected by osteoporosis.
Nutritional therapies An organic diet (*see* page 4) provides the body with essential and secondary plant nutrients that are believed to exercise a multitude of positive effects and to be capable, *inter alia*, of boosting the immune system.	**Useful** as a supportive measure. Reducing the intake of sugar may help to prevent diet-related tiredness and lack of concentration.	**Suitable for DIY** Qualified guidance is recommended though not essential. **Risks:** Avoid imbalanced or intolerable diets. They can cause deficiencies with serious consequences. Children are particularly at risk.

Treatment	Rating	Point of delivery/risks
Physical therapies Various hydrotherapeutic techniques, brushings, mud baths (*see* pages 871–8) and exercise therapy (*see* page 868) are said to relax the patient and provide extra vitality.	**Useful** as a supportive measure aimed at relaxing the patient and providing extra vitality. Exercise in particular is an effective form of treatment. Case reports claim efficacy; however, success is probably seen in only a proportion of patients (*see* Placebo, page xxi).	**Suitable for DIY** Qualified guidance is recommended though not essential. Therapists should propose a treatment plan. **Risks:** Skin damage may be caused to persons with diminished temperature sensation when extreme temperatures are applied.
Reflex therapies Reflex zone massage (*see* page 883), reflexology (*see* page 883), and TENS (*see* page 886) are claimed to act via reflex channels (*see* page 881) to energize (*see* page 927) the patient and so improve blood flow in the genital region.	**May be of some use** as a short-term, supportive treatment attempt for circulation problems or pain. Case reports and field studies claim efficacy; however, success is probably seen in only a proportion of patients (*see* Placebo, page xxi).	**Suitable for DIY** Qualified guidance is essential. **Risks:** Some people are sensitive to electrical stimuli and rubber electrodes; others find it hard to tolerate manual stimulation or close physical contact.
Relaxation techniques Autogenic training (*see* page 888), muscle relaxation according to Jacobson (*see* page 893), and various biofeedback techniques (*see* page 891) are said to relieve muscle tension and inner unrest, and might be instrumental in helping patients become more aware of their physical and emotional states.	**Useful** as a supportive measure aimed at soothing and relaxing, and at helping patients come to terms better with their symptoms and other problems. Some case reports claim efficacy; however, success is probably seen in only a proportion of patients (*see* Placebo, page xxi).	**Suitable for DIY** Once a sound understanding of the technique has been acquired from a trainer in group sessions or through individual tuition, patients can perform exercises themselves. Therapists should be properly qualified. **Risks:** Fairly unlikely.

Treatment	Rating	Point of delivery/risks
Vitamins and trace elements Vitamins C, E, niacin, multivitamins, etc., are able, manufacturers claim, to ease symptoms and arrest the ageing process (*see* page 900).	**Of little use** except in cases where a vitamin deficiency has been diagnosed. Otherwise, no definitive recommendations can be made based on present knowledge.	**Suitable for DIY** Qualified guidance is recommended though not essential. **Risks:** Intolerance and overdosage are possible.

Herbal remedies for problems during menopause

Active ingredient/preparation	Rating
Agnus castus fruit (*Vitex agnus-castus*)	**May be of some use** as a treatment attempt for problems during menopause. **Dosage:** As instructed by the manufacturer/prescriber. **Risks:** Irregular bleeding, increased menstrual blood loss, and perpetual bleeding from the uterus with associated anemia are possible. Skin itchiness may also occasionally occur. If the breasts feel tender, consult your doctor to discover the cause.
Black cohosh root (*Cimicifuga racemosa*)	On account of its estrogenic action, black cohosh **may be of some use** as a treatment attempt for certain neurovegetative complaints (unrest, nervous agitation, hot flushes) during menopause. **Dosage:** As instructed by the manufacturer/prescriber. **Risks:** Gastrointestinal problems are possible. On account of its estrogenic action (LH suppression, binding to estrogen receptors), black cohosh must not be used by women with certain forms of breast cancer (estrogen-binding tumors). Black cohosh is potentially dangerous in high doses.

Premenstrual syndrome (PMS)

Causes and symptoms

PMS ranges widely in nature from abdominal pains before and during menstruation, to tenderness and swelling of the breasts (*see* Breast disorders, page 648), depression (*see* page 100), low self-esteem, moodiness and irritability (*see* Anxiety and worry, page 84), lack of concentration, insomnia (*see* page 109), and headaches (*see* page 23). The causes are not entirely understood. It is thought that it may be due, *inter alia*, to a disturbed secretion of hormones in the interval between menstruation and ovulation, as well as to psychological and psychosocial influences, environmental factors, vitamin deficiency, and disorders of fat metabolism.

Problems during menstruation can likewise have a variety of causes, including general ailments, stress and worry, crash dieting (*see* Obesity, page 6) and other attempts to lose weight, various medications, environmental poisons, and addictive substances.

Orthodox treatment

Relaxation techniques (*see* page 888), various relaxing physiotherapeutic procedures (*see* page 867) and regular exercise can help to reduce symptoms. Menstrual irregularity usually responds to hormonal treatment. Psychotherapy and counselling may be useful.

Complementary therapies

Herbal medications and/or physical therapies are used widely. Some complementary therapists try to act directly on the organs and organ functions that are associated with menstruation, e.g. by exploiting energy links (*see* page 928). PMS and menstrual irregularity are frequently interpreted, depending on the therapist's leaning, as being due to toxins (*see* page 929), immune imbalance, foci (*see* page 928), or a poor balance of energies (*see* page 927). Treatments are suggested accordingly.

Treatment plan and limited trial

Before administering a complementary treatment, every therapist should propose a treatment plan (*see* page xxiii) that sets out a clear time frame and defines the goal that the treatment is designed to achieve. Treatment should then be tried for a limited term to test the patient's response.

Caution

As period and cyclic problems may have a serious physical cause, it is vital that you visit your doctor if you have any unexpected or unexplained symptoms.

Complementary treatments for premenstrual syndrome

Treatment	Rating	Point of delivery/risks
Acupressure This treatment (*see* page 769), otherwise known as pressure-point massage, is claimed to alleviate pain, cramps, and PMS. Acupressure is also used as a restorative measure intended to impart vital energy (*see* Life force page 928) to the body.	**May be of some use** as a short-term treatment attempt aimed at easing pain, cramps, and PMS. Case reports claim efficacy; however, success is probably seen in only a proportion of patients (*see* Placebo, page xxi).	**Suitable for DIY** Qualified guidance is recommended. Therapists should be properly qualified. **Risks:** Unlikely provided treatment is carried out competently.
Acupuncture Acupuncture in its various forms (*see* page 772) aims to relax the patient, rectify hormone balance, and alleviate PMS, and other menstrual problems. The acupuncture points chosen can vary from one practitioner to another.	**May be of some use** as a short-term treatment attempt for PMS and menstrual problems. Case reports, field studies, and clinical studies (PMS) ascribe a degree of efficacy to this treatment in some patients.	**Requires a qualified practitioner** Acupuncturists should be properly qualified and should propose a treatment plan. **Risks:** Probably rare provided treatment is carried out competently.

Treatment	*Rating*	*Point of delivery/risks*
Anthroposophical medicine Potentized magnesium or Tabacum preparations are said to ease acute symptoms. The long-term remedy Menodoron is supposed to prevent cramps and nausea and to help regulate the monthly cycle (*see* page 781).	**Of little use** Acceptable as a short-term treatment attempt for PMS and menstrual disorders. Some studies claim efficacy; however, success is probably seen in only a small proportion of patients (*see* Placebo, page xxi).	**Requires a qualified practitioner** Practitioners should be properly qualified and should propose a treatment plan. **Risks:** Allergies and intolerance are possible.
Aromatherapy Essential oils (*see* page 786) are used to soothe and relax, or to invigorate, thereby possibly leading to an easing of PMS and menstrual complaints. The essences may be taken orally, used externally as massage oils or bathing emulsions, or inhaled as vapors.	**Of little use** Acceptable as a short-term, supportive treatment attempt aimed at soothing and relaxing. Some case reports claim efficacy in the treatment of menstrual problems; however, success is probably seen in only a proportion of patients (*see* Placebo, page xxi).	**Suitable for DIY** Qualified guidance is recommended. The effects of individual essential oils differ widely. **Risks:** Allergies or intolerance are possible. Some oils are carcinogenic in test systems and possibly in humans.
Bioresonance therapy Bioresonance therapists use electrical devices in an attempt to discover the causes of illness and claim to be able to weaken or turn around pathogenic energies and disease related vibrations (*see* page 794).	**Of little use** Possibly acceptable as a short-term treatment attempt in persistent cases when more established methods have been unsuccessful. Some case reports claim efficacy; however, success is probably seen, if at all, in only a small proportion of patients (*see* Placebo, page xxi).	**Requires a qualified practitioner** Practitioners should be properly qualified and should propose a treatment plan. No credence should be given to anyone promising immediate or total success. **Risks:** Fairly unlikely.

Treatment	Rating	Point of delivery/risks

Cell therapy
Injecting or ingesting products extracted from the tissues of newborn animals or animal fetuses is said to have a rejuvenating and revitalizing effect and to enhance the healing of human tissues and organs (*see* page 796).

Not advised
Based on present knowledge, there is inadequate evidence of the efficacy and mode of action of these costly and relatively risky procedures.

Risks: Injecting foreign proteins into the body can provoke (possibly fatal) allergic reactions. Also, pathogens such as those that cause bovine spongiform encephalopathy (BSE) or other serious infections may be introduced.

Electroacupuncture according to Voll
By taking readings of the electrical conductivity of the skin (*see* page 802), therapists claim to be able to derive an insight into diseased areas of the body, pathogenic foci (*see* page 928), and stress factors (*see* Toxins, page 929). The factors presumed to be instrumental in the causation of symptoms can then be addressed.

Of little use
Possibly acceptable as a short-term treatment attempt for persistent conditions when simpler, more established methods have been unsuccessful. Some case reports claim efficacy; however, success is probably seen, if at all, in only a small proportion of patients (*see* Placebo, page xxi).

Requires a qualified practitioner
Practitioners should be properly qualified and should propose a treatment plan. No credence should be given to anyone promising immediate or total success.
Risks: A second opinion must always be obtained from a qualified physician before any attempt is made to "eliminate foci" (e.g. by surgery).

Electroneural therapy according to Croon
According to the theory, readings taken at various reactive sites on the skin highlight diseased areas within the body. Based on these readings, targeted electrostimulative measures can be undertaken to address factors presumed to be instrumental in the causation of symptoms (*see* page 806).

Of little use
Possibly acceptable as a short-term treatment attempt in persistent cases when simpler, more established methods have been unsuccessful. Some case reports claim efficacy; however, success is probably seen, if at all, in only a small proportion of patients (*see* Placebo, page xxi).

Requires a qualified practitioner
Practitioners should be properly qualified and should propose a treatment plan. No credence should be given to anyone promising immediate or total success.
Risks: Proponents themselves warn that treatment should not be given in acute inflammatory conditions.

Treatment	Rating	Point of delivery/risks
Eliminative methods, bloody Bloody cupping (*see* page 815) is said to have an additional eliminative effect and to improve the body's own regulatory systems.	**Not advised** The efficacy of this relatively invasive method for dealing with menstrual problems is unproven.	**Requires a qualified practitioner** Practitioners should be properly qualified and should propose a treatment plan. **Risks:** Bloody cupping can cause infection and scarring. Furthermore, it should not be carried out in persons with bleeding disorders.
Eliminative methods, unbloody Unbloody cupping (*see* page 817) is supposed to alleviate menstrual pain, to improve the body's own regulatory systems, and to energize (*see* page 927) the patient.	**Of little use** Acceptable as a short-term, supportive treatment attempt aimed at alleviating pain. Case reports claim efficacy; however, success is probably seen in only a proportion of patients (*see* Placebo, page xxi).	**Suitable for DIY** Unbloody cupping is best carried out under the guidance of a qualified practitioner. **Risks:** Unlikely provided treatment is carried out competently.
Flower remedies For some flower therapists, menstrual problems are an expression of emotional disharmony. Flower remedies (*see* page 828) are said to restore emotional balance and assist the body's psychic ability to heal itself.	**Of little use** Acceptable as a short-term treatment attempt aimed at soothing and relaxing. Some case reports claim efficacy; however, success is probably seen in only a proportion of patients (*see* Placebo, page xxi).	**Suitable for DIY** Qualified guidance is recommended. Practitioners should propose a treatment plan. **Risks:** Possible intolerance.

Treatment	Rating	Point of delivery/risks
Homeopathy Highly diluted (potentized) solutions (*see* page 831) are believed to be able to redress vital energy imbalances. Organo- and functiotropic (*see* page 833) homeopathy is claimed to be effective for dealing directly with menstrual problems.	**May be of some use** as a treatment attempt for PMS and other menstrual problems. Some case reports and field studies claim efficacy; however, success is probably seen, if at all, in only a proportion of patients (*see* Placebo, page xxi).	**Requires a qualified practitioner** Homeopaths should be properly qualified and should propose a treatment plan. Ready-formulated preparations are suitable for do-it-yourself. **Risks:** Allergies and intolerance are possible.
Manual therapies Chiropractors and osteopaths (*see* page 844) use a series of manipulations to realign allegedly displaced vertebrae. This is said to reduce pain, release energy blockages (*see* page 927), and address factors that may be at the root of symptoms.	**Of little use** Acceptable as a short-term treatment attempt in persistent cases when less risky, more established methods have been unsuccessful. Some case reports claim efficacy; however, success is probably seen, if at all, in only a small proportion of patients (*see* Placebo, page xxi).	**Requires a qualified practitioner** Practitioners should be properly qualified and should propose a treatment plan. **Risks:** Manipulation of the head and cervical vertebrae can cause serious injury. Osteoporosis is one of several risk factors.
Massage Classical massage (*see* page 847) and lymphatic drainage (*see* page 850) can invigorate the patient, as well as ease muscular and emotional tension.	**Of little use** Acceptable as a short-term, supportive treatment attempt aimed at relaxing the patient. Case reports claim efficacy in the treatment of menstrual problems; however, success is probably seen in only a proportion of patients (*see* Placebo, page xxi).	**Requires a qualified practitioner** Masseurs/masseuses should be properly qualified and should propose a treatment plan. **Risks:** Some people are sensitive to manual stimuli; others find it hard to tolerate close physical contact.

Treatment	Rating	Point of delivery/risks
Nutritional therapies An organic diet (*see* page 4) provides the body with essential and secondary plant nutrients that are believed to exercise a multitude of positive effects.	**Useful** as a supportive and preventive measure.	**Suitable for DIY** Qualified guidance is recommended though not essential. **Risks:** Avoid imbalanced or intolerable diets. They can cause deficiencies with serious consequences. Children are particularly at risk.
Physical therapies Ascending temperature foot baths, sitz baths, semi-immersion baths and full immersion baths (*see* pages 871–8), possibly incorporating herbal additives or mud treatments, loosening-up exercises, or general physical exercise are said to relax the patient, ease cramps, and improve the circulation.	**May be of some use** as a treatment attempt for various conditions. Case reports and field studies claim efficacy; however, success is probably seen in only a proportion of patients (*see* Placebo, page xxi).	**Suitable for DIY** Qualified guidance is recommended though not essential. **Risks:** Skin damage may be caused to persons with diminished temperature sensation when extreme temperatures are applied.
Reflex therapies Heat treatments, reflex zone massage (*see* page 883), reflexology (*see* page 883), and TENS (*see* page 886) are claimed to act via reflex channels (*see* page 881) to ease pain, relax the patient, and exercise a beneficial effect on various physical functions.	**May be of some use** as a short-term treatment attempt aimed at alleviating pain and cramps. Some case reports and field studies claim efficacy; however, success is probably seen in only a proportion of patients (*see* Placebo, page xxi).	**Suitable for DIY** Qualified guidance is essential. **Risks:** Some people are sensitive to electrical stimuli and rubber electrodes; others find it hard to tolerate manual stimulation or close physical contact.

Treatment	Rating	Point of delivery/risks
Relaxation techniques Autogenic training (*see* page 888), muscle relaxation according to Jacobson (*see* page 893), and various biofeedback techniques (*see* page 891) are said to relieve muscle tension and inner unrest, and might be instrumental in helping patients become more aware of their physical and emotional states.	**Useful** as a supportive treatment attempt aimed at soothing and relaxing. Case reports and field studies claim efficacy; however, success is probably seen in only a proportion of patients (*see* Placebo, page xxi).	**Suitable for DIY** Once a sound understanding of the technique has been acquired from a trainer in group sessions or through individual tuition, patients can perform exercises themselves. Therapists should be properly qualified. **Risks:** Fairly unlikely.
Vitamins and trace elements Vitamins E and B6 are claimed to reduce pain and other menstrual problems (*see* page 900).	**Of little use** Acceptable as a short-term treatment attempt. Case reports, field studies, and initial clinical studies claim efficacy for this treatment; however, success is probably seen in only a proportion of patients (*see* Placebo, page xxi).	**Suitable for DIY** Qualified guidance is recommended though not essential. **Risks:** Intolerance and overdosage are possible. Vitamin B6 in high doses can cause serious side effects.

Herbal remedies for premenstrual syndrome

Active ingredient/preparation	Rating
Agnus castus fruit (*Vitex agnus-castus*)	**May be of some use** as a treatment attempt for menstrual problems or premenstrual syndrome. Suitable for self-medication. **Dosage:** As instructed by the manufacturer/ prescriber. **Risks:** Irregular bleeding, increased menstrual blood loss, and perpetual bleeding from the uterus with associated anemia are possible. Skin itchiness may also occasionally occur. If the breasts feel tender, consult your doctor to discover the cause. Not to be used during pregnancy and breastfeeding.

Active ingredient/preparation	*Rating*
Black cohosh root (*Cimicifuga racemosa*)	Taken orally for its estrogenic action, black cohosh **may be of some use** for alleviating pain before and during menstruation. Suitable for self-medication. **Dosage:** As instructed by the manufacturer/ prescriber. **Risks:** Gastrointestinal problems are possible. On account of its estrogenic action, black cohosh must not be used by women with certain forms of breast cancer (estrogen-binding tumors). Black cohosh is potentially dangerous in high doses. It must not be used during pregnancy.
Evening primrose oil (*Oenothera biennis*)	**May be of some use** as a supportive treatment attempt for menstrual disorders. As yet there have not been any long-term controlled studies that would permit a definitive assessment to be made of the therapeutic benefits of evening primrose oil. Nevertheless, many women find this remedy helpful. **Risks:** Patients taking potentially epileptogenic agents, e.g. certain neuroleptic agents (phenothiazines), should not receive simultaneous treatment with evening primrose oil. Nausea, digestive problems, headaches, abdominal pain, and skin hypersensitivity may occasionally be experienced.
Lavender flowers (*Lavandula angustifolia*)	When added to bathwater, lavender flowers **may be of some use** supportively for addressing menstrual and associated problems. Has a calming effect. **Dosage:** 4oz flowers to 2 quarts of hot water, made up to a full immersion bath. **Risks:** Lavender flowers are not known to have any serious side effects.

Active ingredient/preparation	Rating
Lemon balm leaves (*Melissa officinalis*)	**May be of some use** as a supportive treatment attempt for menstrual disorders. Suitable for self-medication. **Daily dose:** 8–10g dried herb. **Individual dose:** As an infusion, 1.5–2.5g of dried herb to 1 cup of hot water. Can also be used as an addition to bathwater (for its calming, relaxing effect) 2–4oz dried herb to 2 quarts of hot water, strained, then made up to a full immersion bath. **Risks:** The essential oil can cause allergic reactions.
Shepherd's purse (*Capsella bursa-pastoris*)	Taken orally, shepherd's purse **may be of some use** as a treatment attempt for menstrual problems such as menorrhagia and metrorrhagia. **Daily dose:** 3–12g dried herb. **Individual dose:** As a tea drink, 2–3g of dried herb to 1 cup of hot water. **Risks:** Shepherd's purse is not known to have any serious side effects.
Silverweed (*Potentilla anserina*)	**May be of some use** as a treatment attempt for menstrual problems, also used with lavender, yarrow, and lemon balm for premenstrual bathing. Silverweed has an astringent action on the uterus. **Daily dose:** 4–6g dried herb. **Individual dose:** Pour 1 cup of hot water over 2g or dried herb, infuse for ten minutes, strain, and drink several times a day. **Risks:** Stomach irritation is possible.
Yarrow flowers and leaves (*Achillea millefolium*)	**May be of some use** as a treatment attempt for cramplike complaints. **Daily dose:** 4.5g dried herb. **Individual dose:** As an infusion, 1.5g of dried leaves or 1g of dried flowers to 1 cup of hot water. Can also be added to bathwater (for its calming, relaxing effect): 2–4oz of dried herb to 2 quarts of hot water, infuse for five to ten minutes, strain, and make up to a full immersion bath. **Risks:** Contact allergies (allergic skin reactions) are possible. Not to be used by persons known to be allergic to compositae.

Sexual problems

Causes and symptoms

Female sexual problems may include a lack of interest in sex, painful intercourse, and difficulty in reaching orgasm. Typical male problems are a lack of libido, erection difficulties, and problems with orgasm. Sexual problems are rarely due to physical causes alone; indeed, emotional stress, psychosocial problems, cultural and moral factors, any medication being taken, alcohol, and environmental influences can all contribute to sexual problems.

Apart from the causes outlined above there may be other factors, such as a circulation problem or diabetes mellitus (*see* page 627), which make it difficult, for instance, to achieve an erection.

Orthodox treatment

Treatments for sexual problems are varied and often inadequately researched. They are often flavor of the month, as typified by the therapies advocated to persons with erection difficulties; sometimes surgery is advised, sometimes a course of medication—then again a prosthetic appliance or other mechanical aid may be recommended, while a short time later the emphasis may be on psychotherapy or counselling.

In order for a therapy to have any chance of success it is important for partners actually to admit that there is a sexual problem (itself often a taboo) and to come to terms with it honestly and realistically. Sometimes, e.g. in diabetes mellitus (*see* page 627), it will be necessary to address the underlying cause.

Complementary therapies

Often the success of a complementary therapy is documented in just a single case report. Nevertheless, some therapies may help when they are part of an overall program of treatment.

Treatment plan and limited trial

Before administering a complementary treatment, every therapist should propose a treatment plan (*see* page xxiii) that sets out a clear time frame and defines the goal that the treatment is designed to achieve. Treatment should then be tried for a limited term to test the patient's response.

Cautions

As sexual problems may be the result of a severe disease or personality disorder, a doctor should always be consulted to enable a medical assessment to be made of the symptoms.

Complementary treatments for sexual problems

Treatment	Rating	Point of delivery/risks
Acupuncture Acupuncture in its various forms (*see* page 772) aims to encourage the flow of energy (*see* page 927) or to act directly on the sexual organs. The acupuncture points chosen can vary from one practitioner to another.	**May be of some use** as a short-term treatment attempt. Case reports claim efficacy; however, success is probably seen in only a small proportion of patients (*see* Placebo, page xxi).	**Requires a qualified practitioner** Acupuncturists should be properly qualified and should propose a treatment plan. **Risks:** Probably rare provided treatment is carried out competently.
Anthroposophical medicine Treatments for sexual problems used by doctors who practice AM (*see* page 781) include biographical work, anthroposophical psychotherapy, and constitutional drug therapies.	**May be of some use** as a longer-term treatment attempt. Case reports claim efficacy; however, success is probably seen in only a proportion of patients (*see* Placebo, page xxi).	**Requires a qualified practitioner** Practitioners should be properly qualified and should propose a treatment plan. **Risks:** Allergies and intolerance are possible.

Treatment	Rating	Point of delivery/risks
Aromatherapy Essential oils (*see* page 786) are used to soothe and relax, or to invigorate. The essences may be taken orally, used externally as massage oils or bathing emulsions, or inhaled as vapors.	**Of little use** Acceptable as a short-term, supportive treatment attempt aimed at invigorating, or soothing and relaxing the patient. Some case reports claim efficacy; however, success is probably seen in only a proportion of patients (*see* Placebo, page xxi).	**Suitable for DIY** Qualified guidance is recommended. The effects of individual essential oils differ widely. **Risks:** Allergies or intolerance are possible. Some oils are carcinogenic in test systems and possibly in humans.
Bioresonance therapy Bioresonance therapists use electrical devices in an attempt to discover the causes of illness and claim to be able to weaken or turn around pathogenic energies and disease related vibrations (*see* page 794).	**Of little use** Possibly acceptable as a short-term, supportive treatment attempt when simpler, more established methods have been unsuccessful. Some case reports claim efficacy; however, success is probably seen, if at all, in only a small proportion of patients (*see* Placebo, page xxi).	**Requires a qualified practitioner** Practitioners should be properly qualified and should propose a treatment plan. No credence should be given to anyone promising immediate or total success. **Risks:** Fairly unlikely.
Cantharidin Pulverized, dried Spanish fly is reported to increase sexual arousal and potency.	**Not advised** Evidence of the mode of action and therapeutic usefulness of this toxic substance is lacking.	**Risks:** Cantharidin can damage the kidneys, cause cramps and, especially when used systemically, can prove fatal.
Cell therapy Injecting or ingesting products extracted from the tissues of newborn animals or animal fetuses is said to have a rejuvenating and revitalizing effect and to enhance the healing of human tissues and organs (*see* page 796).	**Not advised** Based on present knowledge, there is inadequate evidence of the efficacy and mode of action of these costly and relatively risky procedures.	**Risks:** Injecting foreign proteins into the body can provoke (possibly fatal) allergic reactions. Also, pathogens such as those that cause bovine spongiform encephalopathy (BSE) or other serious infections may be introduced.

Treatment	Rating	Point of delivery/risks
Electroacupuncture according to Voll By taking readings of the electrical conductivity of the skin (*see* page 802), therapists claim to be able to derive an insight into diseased areas of the body, pathogenic foci (*see* page 928), and stress factors (*see* Toxins, page 929). The factors presumed to be instrumental in the causation of sexual problems can then be addressed.	**Of little use** Possibly acceptable as a short-term, supportive treatment attempt in persistent cases when simpler, more established methods have been unsuccessful. Some case reports claim efficacy; however, success is probably seen, if at all, in only a small proportion of patients (*see* Placebo, page xxi).	**Requires a qualified practitioner** Practitioners should be properly qualified and should propose a treatment plan. No credence should be given to anyone promising immediate or total success. **Risks:** A second opinion must always be obtained from a qualified physician before any attempt is made to "eliminate foci" (e.g. by surgery).
Electroneural therapy according to Croon According to the theory, readings taken at various reactive sites on the skin highlight diseased areas within the body. Based on these readings, targeted electrostimulative measures can be undertaken to address factors presumed to be instrumental in the causation of sexual problems (*see* page 806).	**Of little use** Possibly acceptable as a short-term, supportive treatment attempt when simpler, more established methods have been unsuccessful. Some case reports claim efficacy; however, success is probably seen, if at all, in only a small proportion of patients (*see* Placebo, page xxi).	**Requires a qualified practitioner** Practitioners should be properly qualified and should propose a treatment plan. No credence should be given to anyone promising immediate or total success. **Risks:** Proponents themselves warn that treatment should not be given in acute inflammatory conditions.

Treatment	Rating	Point of delivery/risks
Eliminative methods, bloody Bloody cupping (*see* page 815) in the genital region is said to improve the body's own regulatory systems and counter sexual problems.	**Of little use** Possibly acceptable in persistent cases as a short-term treatment attempt when more established, less invasive methods have been unsuccessful. Some case reports and field studies claim efficacy; however, success is probably seen in only a proportion of patients (*see* Placebo, page xxi).	**Requires a qualified practitioner** Practitioners should be properly qualified and should propose a treatment plan. **Risks:** Bloody cupping can cause infection and scarring. Furthermore, it should not be carried out in persons with bleeding disorders.
Eliminative methods, unbloody Cantharide poultices (*see* page 812) are said to eliminate "bad humors" and "poisons". Unbloody cupping (*see* page 817) in the genital region is said to improve the body's own regulatory systems and to energize (*see* page 927) the patient, thus possibly countering sexual problems.	Cantharide poultices are **not advised**. Unbloody cupping is **of little use** but is acceptable as a short-term, supportive treatment attempt in persistent cases. Some case reports claim efficacy; however, success is probably seen in only a small proportion of patients (*see* Placebo, page xxi).	Unbloody cupping is **suitable for DIY**. Qualified guidance is recommended. Treatment with cantharide poultices **requires a qualified practitioner**. **Risks:** Unlikely with unbloody cupping provided treatment is carried out competently. Cantharide poultices can cause second-degree burns.
Flower remedies Some flower therapists see sexual problems as an expression of emotional disharmony. Flower remedies (*see* page 828) are said to restore emotional balance and assist the body's psychic ability to heal itself.	**May be of some use** as a short-term, supportive treatment attempt aimed at soothing and relaxing. Some case reports claim efficacy; however, success is probably seen in only a small proportion of patients (*see* Placebo, page xxi).	**Suitable for DIY** Qualified guidance is recommended. Practitioners should propose a treatment plan. **Risks:** Possible intolerance.

Treatment	Rating	Point of delivery/risks
Homeopathy Highly diluted (potentized) solutions (*see* page 831) are believed to be able to redress vital energy imbalances and strengthen the body's defences. Organo- and functiotropic (*see* page 833) homeopathy is claimed to be effective for dealing directly with sexual problems.	**May be of some use** as a supportive treatment attempt. Case reports claim efficacy; however, success is probably seen in only a proportion of patients (*see* Placebo, page xxi).	**Requires a qualified practitioner** Homeopaths should be properly qualified and should propose a treatment plan. Ready-formulated preparations are suitable for do-it-yourself. **Risks:** Allergies and intolerance are possible.
Hypnosis and self-hypnosis In the relaxed and generally altered state of awareness that is induced in hypnosis or self-hypnosis (*see* page 837), physical and mental conditions can be addressed. Hypnosis is often used in combination with other psycho- and behavioral therapies.	**May be of some use** in persistent cases as a supportive treatment attempt aimed at soothing and relaxing the patient and at rendering him/her more accessible emotionally when simpler, more established methods have been unsuccessful. Some case reports claim efficacy; however, success is probably seen in only a proportion of patients (*see* Placebo, page xxi).	**Requires a qualified practitioner** Hypnotherapists should be properly qualified and should propose a treatment plan. No credence should be given to anyone promising immediate or total success. **Risks:** Unlikely provided treatment is carried out competently.
Manual therapies Chiropractors and osteopaths (*see* page 844) use a series of manipulations to realign allegedly displaced vertebrae, e.g. in the pelvic region, and to release muscular tension, thereby perhaps eliminating the sexual problems.	**Of little use** Acceptable as a short-term treatment attempt when less risky, more established methods have been unsuccessful. Some case reports claim efficacy; however, success is probably seen, if at all, in only a small proportion of patients (*see* Placebo, page xxi).	**Requires a qualified practitioner** Practitioners should be properly qualified and should propose a treatment plan. **Risks:** Spinal manipulations can cause serious injury. Osteoporosis is one of several risk factors.

Treatment	Rating	Point of delivery/risks
Massage Classical massage (*see* page 847) is claimed to invigorate the patient as well as ease muscular and emotional tension.	**May be of some use** as a supportive measure. Case reports claim efficacy in the treatment of sexual problems; however, success is probably seen in only a proportion of patients (*see* Placebo, page xxi).	**Suitable for DIY** Qualified guidance is recommended. **Risks:** Some people are sensitive to manual stimuli; others find it hard to tolerate close physical contact.
Nutritional therapies An organic diet (*see* page 4) provides the body with essential and secondary plant nutrients that are believed to exercise a multitude of positive effects.	**Useful** as an individually directed supportive measure.	**Suitable for DIY** Qualified guidance is recommended though not essential. **Risks:** Avoid imbalanced or intolerable diets. They can cause deficiencies with serious consequences. Children are particularly at risk.
Physical therapies Partial washings, sitz baths (*see* page 874), brushings, etc, are supposed to invigorate the patient and improve the circulation and the body's own regulatory systems.	**May be of some use** as a supportive treatment attempt aimed at relaxing the patient, improving the circulation and helping him/her feel more positive about his/her body. Case reports claim efficacy; however, success is probably seen in only a proportion of patients (*see* Placebo, page xxi).	**Suitable for DIY** Qualified guidance is recommended though not essential. **Risks:** Skin damage may be caused to persons with diminished temperature sensation when extreme temperatures are applied.

Treatment	Rating	Point of delivery/risks
Reflex therapies Reflex zone massage (*see* page 883), reflexology (*see* page 883), and TENS (*see* page 886) are claimed to act via reflex channels (*see* page 881) to encourage the circulation and increase sexual desire.	**May be of some use** as a short-term treatment attempt aimed at soothing and relaxing the patient, improving the circulation, and helping him/her feel more positive about his/her body. Some case reports claim efficacy; however, success is probably seen in only a proportion of patients (*see* Placebo, page xxi).	**Suitable for DIY** Qualified guidance is essential. **Risks:** Some people are sensitive to electrical stimuli and rubber electrodes; others find it hard to tolerate manual stimulation or close physical contact.
Relaxation techniques Autogenic training (*see* page 888), muscle relaxation according to Jacobson (*see* page 893), and various biofeedback techniques (*see* page 891) are said to relieve tension and to be instrumental in helping patients become better aware of their physical and emotional states.	**May be of some use** as a supportive treatment attempt aimed at soothing and relaxing. Case reports claim efficacy; however, success is probably seen in only a proportion of patients (*see* Placebo, page xxi).	**Suitable for DIY** Once a sound understanding of the technique has been acquired from a trainer, patients can perform exercises themselves. Therapists should be properly qualified. **Risks:** Fairly unlikely.

Herbal remedies for sexual problems

Active ingredient/preparation	Rating
Spanish fly, sometimes in combination with other agents for increasing male sex drive	**Not advised.** Such remedies have not been shown to overcome erection difficulties or increase libido. **Risks:** Tincture of Spanish fly (cantharidin) can produce severe gastrointestinal complaints, central nervous system disorders, and cardiovascular problems (including circulatory collapse). It severely irritates the skin, causing inflammation and blistering, particularly on sensitive mucosa (e.g. in the genital region).

Active ingredient/preparation	Rating
Yohimbé bark (*Corynanthe yohimbe*)	**Useful** for treating certain forms of erectile dysfunction. **Risks:** States of agitation, tremor, sleeplessness, hypertension, and tachycardia are possible. Not to be used by persons with kidney or liver damage. It interacts adversely with many psychotropic drugs.

Cancer

Causes and symptoms

Cancer is a general term used to denote the unrestrained growth of cells in various tissues and organs. Just as cancer differs widely in its causes and forms, so also do the patient's prospects of recovery and the therapies that are available. Cancer is one of the modern lifestyle diseases. In some European countries as many as one person in four will suffer from some form of cancer at some time in his life. There is no single cause of cancer; indeed, many factors are implicated in its causation, including genetic predisposition, lifestyle, general demeanor, and environmental factors.

Many cancers start with few, if any, symptoms. As many as half of all cancers will be associated with pain even at a very early stage. When a cancer has become advanced and incurable, about a third of patients will suffer from severe, chronic pain. The individual clinical picture depends largely on the way in which the primary cancer and its metastases interfere with the normal structures and functioning of the body.

Orthodox treatment

A very precise diagnosis will be required in order to provide a realistic prognosis and help decide on the best treatment. Depending on the form of cancer and its severity, the commonly used orthodox treatments will include surgery, radiation or immune therapy, and/or chemotherapy. These treatments can be effective against some forms of cancer and less so against others.

Complementary therapies

A number of complementary therapies are used for cancer, though they have not been the subject of rigorous investigation and there is no compelling evidence that they are effective. The principal objective of treatment is to provide support in alleviating the various symptoms and to help the body and mind fight the disease. Some complementary treatments are aimed at preventing cancer, although, again, the claims made are not backed up with hard evidence.

Treatment plan and limited trial

Before administering a complementary treatment, every therapist should propose a treatment plan (*see* page xxiii) that sets out a clear time frame and defines the goal that the treatment is designed to achieve. Treatment should then be tried for a limited term to test the patient's response.

Caution

In potentially curable forms of cancer, complementary treatments should be used in support, not in lieu, of conventional treatments. When the objective is to ease pain, for instance, weigh up carefully the relief that can be provided by an appropriate dose of morphine against a complementary approach with the same aim.

Complementary treatments for cancer

Treatment	Rating	Point of delivery/risks
Acupressure This treatment (*see* page 769), otherwise known as pressure-point massage, is used in cancer patients to alleviate pain, release tension, improve general well-being, and lessen nausea resulting from chemo- or radiotherapy.	**Inappropriate** as a treatment for cancer. **Useful** as a short-term, supportive treatment attempt aimed at easing pain and reducing nausea. Case reports and field studies claim efficacy in the reduction of pain and nausea; however, success is probably seen in only a proportion of patients (*see* Placebo, page xxi).	**Suitable for DIY** Qualified guidance is recommended. Therapists should be properly qualified. **Risks:** Acupressure must not be carried out on damaged skin or on parts of the body where metastases have formed.
Acupuncture Acupuncture in its various forms (*see* page 772) is used to alleviate pain, nausea, and vomiting resulting from chemo- or radiotherapy, to reduce muscular tension, to energize (*see* page 927) the patient, and to release energy blockages (*see* page 927). The acupuncture points chosen can vary from one practitioner to another.	**Inappropriate** as a treatment for cancer. **Useful** as a short-term, supportive treatment attempt aimed at reducing nausea, vomiting, and muscle pain. Controlled clinical studies ascribe a degree of efficacy in the treatment of mild forms of nausea. Some field studies and case reports claim efficacy in the treatment of pain in the muscles and joints; however, success is probably seen in only a proportion of patients (*see* Placebo, page xxi).	**Requires a qualified practitioner** Acupuncturists should be properly qualified and should propose a treatment plan. **Risks:** Probably rare provided treatment is carried out competently.

Treatment	Rating	Point of delivery/risks
Anthroposophical medicine AM (*see* page 781) makes significant use of psychotherapeutic approaches, of mistletoe preparations, and of various other compositions. The aim is to stop the tumor from growing and to modulate the immune system (*see* page 10). Injections of dilute mistletoe extract are sometimes given by conventional doctors.	**Inappropriate** as the sole treatment for cancer. Mistletoe injections **may be of some use** as a supportive treatment attempt aimed at improving quality of life and general well-being. Field and case studies claim efficacy; however, success is probably seen in only a proportion of patients (*see* Placebo, page xxi). Whether mistletoe preparations are able to inhibit tumor growth directly is debatable.	**Requires a qualified practitioner** Practitioners should be properly qualified and should propose a treatment plan. **Risks:** Allergies and intolerance are possible.
Aromatherapy Essential oils (*see* page 786) are used to soothe and relax. The essences may be taken orally, used externally as massage oils or bathing emulsions, or inhaled as vapors.	**Inappropriate** as a treatment for cancer. **May be of some use** as a short-term, supportive treatment attempt aimed at soothing and relaxing the patient and improving his/her general well-being. Case reports claim efficacy; however, success is probably seen in only a proportion of patients (*see* Placebo, page xxi).	**Suitable for DIY** Qualified guidance is recommended. The effects of individual essential oils differ widely. **Risks:** Allergies or intolerance are possible. Some oils are carcinogenic in test systems and possibly in humans.

Treatment	Rating	Point of delivery/risks
Bioresonance therapy Bioresonance therapists use electrical devices in an attempt to discover the causes of illness and claim to be able to weaken or turn around pathogenic energies and disease related vibrations (*see* page 794).	**Inappropriate** as a treatment for cancer. Possibly acceptable as a short-term, supportive treatment attempt aimed at alleviating individual symptoms when more established methods have been unsuccessful. Some case reports claim efficacy; however, success is probably seen, if at all, in only a small proportion of patients (*see* Placebo, page xxi). No credence should be given to claims that bioresonance therapy can provide a successful cure for cancer.	**Requires a qualified practitioner** Practitioners should be properly qualified and should propose a treatment plan. **Risks:** Fairly unlikely.

Treatment	*Rating*	*Point of delivery/risks*

Cell therapy
Injecting or ingesting products extracted from the tissues or organs of animals is said to modulate the immune system (*see* page 796) and to enhance the healing of human tissues and organs. The thymus preparations sometimes used to treat cancer are also claimed to counter poor physical performance, depression, and fatigue, and to improve general well-being (*see* page 798).

Inappropriate as a treatment for cancer. Possibly acceptable as a short-term, supportive treatment attempt aimed at easing individual symptoms and at modulating the immune system when less risky, more established methods have been unsuccessful. Fresh cell therapy is **not advised**. Case studies claim efficacy for thymus preparations for easing symptoms and improving general well-being; however, success is probably seen in only a small proportion of patients (*see* Placebo, page xxi). Study findings pertaining to the immune system modulating action of thymus therapy are contradictory. No credence should be given to rumors of alleged cures.

Requires a qualified practitioner
Practitioners should be properly qualified and should propose a treatment plan. No credence should be given to anyone promising immediate or total success.
Risks: Injecting foreign proteins into the body can provoke (possibly fatal) allergic reactions. Also, pathogens such as those that cause bovine spongiform encephalopathy (BSE) or other serious infections may be introduced.

Treatment	Rating	Point of delivery/risks
Electroacupuncture according to Voll By taking readings of the electrical conductivity of the skin (*see* page 802), therapists claim to be able to derive an insight into diseased areas of the body, pathogenic foci (*see* page 928), and stress factors (*see* Toxins, page 929). The factors presumed to be instrumental in the causation of cancer can then be addressed.	**Inappropriate** as a treatment for cancer. Possibly acceptable as a short-term, supportive treatment attempt aimed at alleviating individual symptoms when more established methods have been unsuccessful. Some case reports claim efficacy; however, success is probably seen, if at all, in only a small proportion of patients (*see* Placebo, page xxi). No credence should be given to claims that EAV can provide a successful cure for cancer.	**Requires a qualified practitioner** Practitioners should be properly qualified and should propose a treatment plan. No credence should be given to anyone promising immediate or total success. **Risks:** A second opinion must always be obtained from a qualified physician before any attempt is made to "eliminate foci" (e.g. by surgery).
Electroneural therapy according to Croon According to the theory, readings taken at various reactive sites on the skin highlight diseased areas within the body. Based on these readings, targeted electrostimulative measures can be undertaken to address factors presumed to be instrumental in the causation of cancer (*see* page 806).	**Inappropriate** as a treatment for cancer. **Of little use** Possibly acceptable as a short-term, supportive treatment attempt aimed at alleviating individual symptoms when more established methods have been unsuccessful. Some case reports claim efficacy; however, success is probably seen, if at all, in only a small proportion of patients (*see* Placebo, page xxi). No credence should be given to claims that ENT can provide a successful cure for cancer.	**Requires a qualified practitioner** Practitioners should be properly qualified and should propose a treatment plan. No credence should be given to anyone promising immediate or total success. **Risks:** Proponents themselves warn that treatment should not be given in acute inflammatory conditions.

Treatment	Rating	Point of delivery/risks
Eliminative methods, unbloody Unbloody cupping (*see* page 817) is often used to address cancer pains. This is said to improve the body's own regulatory systems, to energize (*see* page 927) the patient and, as a reflex therapy, to be effective in the relief of pain.	**Inappropriate** as a treatment for cancer. **May be of some use** as a short-term, supportive treatment attempt aimed at alleviating pain. Some case reports claim efficacy; however, success is probably seen in only a proportion of patients (*see* Placebo, page xxi).	**Suitable for DIY** Unbloody cupping is best carried out under the guidance of a qualified practitioner. **Risks:** Unlikely provided treatment is carried out competently.
Enzyme therapy Enzymes (*see* page 824) extracted from plant and animal tissues reportedly inhibit inflammation and modulate the immune system.	**Inappropriate** as a treatment for cancer. No credence should be given to claims that enzyme therapy can provide a successful cure for cancer.	**Requires a qualified practitioner** Practitioners should propose a treatment plan. Non-prescription preparations are suitable for do-it-yourself. **Risks:** Allergies or intolerance are possible.
Flower remedies Flower remedies (*see* page 828) are said to restore emotional balance and assist the body's psychic ability to heal itself. Some flower therapists claim to have treated cancer successfully.	**Inappropriate** as a treatment for cancer. **May be of some use** as a short-term, supportive treatment attempt aimed at reducing anxiety and despondency. Some case reports claim efficacy; however, success is probably seen in only a proportion of patients (*see* Placebo, page xxi). No credence should be given to claims that flower remedies can provide a successful cure for cancer.	**Suitable for DIY** Qualified guidance is recommended. **Risks:** Possible intolerance.

Treatment	Rating	Point of delivery/risks
Homeopathy In classical homeopathy, highly diluted (potentized) solutions (*see* page 831) are believed to be able to redress vital energy imbalances. Organo- and functiotropic (*see* page 833) homeopathy is also claimed to be effective as a means of dealing with symptoms, e.g. nausea resulting from chemo- or radiotherapy.	**Inappropriate** as a treatment for cancer. **May be of some use** as a supportive treatment attempt, e.g. for nausea resulting from chemo- or radiotherapy. Case reports claim efficacy; however, success is probably seen in only a proportion of patients (*see* Placebo, page xxi). No credence should be given to claims that homeopathic remedies can provide a successful cure for cancer.	**Requires a qualified practitioner** Homeopaths should be properly qualified and should propose a treatment plan. Ready-formulated preparations are suitable for do-it-yourself. **Risks:** Allergies and intolerance are possible.
Hypnosis and self-hypnosis In the relaxed and generally altered state of awareness that is induced in hypnosis or self-hypnosis (*see* page 837), anxiety can be lessened, hope can be reinforced, and the patient can be helped to come to terms with his/her condition.	**Inappropriate** as a treatment for cancer. **May be of some use** as a short-term, supportive treatment attempt aimed at alleviating pain and reinforcing hope. Case reports claim efficacy; however, success is probably seen in only a proportion of patients (*see* Placebo, page xxi).	**Requires a qualified practitioner** Hypnotherapists should be properly qualified and should propose a treatment plan. **Risks:** Unlikely provided treatment is carried out competently.
Magnetic field therapy The use of magnetic field generators, magnetic strips, bracelets, and other objects (*see* page 841) allegedly encourages cell metabolism and so relieves pain.	**Inappropriate** Based on present knowledge, there is inadequate evidence of the efficacy and mode of action of magnetic field therapy in the treatment of cancer.	Operation of magnetic field equipment **requires a qualified practitioner**. **Risks:** Magnetic field equipment can cause implanted cardiac pacemakers to malfunction.

Treatment	*Rating*	*Point of delivery/risks*
Manual therapies Chiropractors and osteopaths (*see* page 844) use a series of manipulations to realign allegedly displaced vertebrae and head joints, including the jaw. This is said to reduce pain. These procedures are sometimes used holistically (*see* page 928) to release blocked energy (*see* page 927).	**Inappropriate** as a treatment for cancer. **Useful** as a short-term, supportive treatment attempt aimed at alleviating pain in the muscles and joints. Some case reports claim efficacy; however, success is probably seen, if at all, in only a small proportion of patients (*see* Placebo, page xxi). For all other symptoms, the efficacy of these treatments is unproven.	**Requires a qualified practitioner** Practitioners should be properly qualified and should propose a treatment plan. **Risks:** Manipulation of the head and cervical vertebrae can cause serious injury. These treatments must not be carried out on parts of the body affected by osteoporosis or cancer.
Massage Classical massage (*see* page 847) can invigorate the patient, as well as ease muscular and emotional tension and alleviate muscle pains.	**Inappropriate** as a treatment for cancer. **Useful** as a short-term, supportive treatment attempt aimed at soothing the patient and easing muscle pains. Case reports and field studies claim efficacy; however, success is probably seen in only a proportion of patients (*see* Placebo, page xxi).	**Requires a qualified practitioner** Masseurs/masseuses should be properly qualified. **Risks:** Some people are sensitive to manual stimuli; others find it hard to tolerate close physical contact. This treatment must not be carried out on parts of the body affected by osteoporosis or cancer.

Treatment	*Rating*	*Point of delivery/risks*
Nutritional therapies An organic diet (*see* page 4) provides the body with essential and secondary plant nutrients that, in association with certain vitamin preparations, may have a role in fending off some of the mechanisms that lead to cancer. Fasting briefly is said to have an anti-inflammatory effect, to improve the body's own regulatory systems, and to influence tumor growth (*see* page 864).	**Inappropriate** as a treatment for cancer. **Useful** as a supportive treatment attempt when the individual tolerates the diet chosen. Whether dietary measures can be used successfully to prevent gastric, colonic, or breast cancer is unclear. No credence should be given to claims that nutritional therapies can provide a successful cure for cancer.	**Suitable for DIY** Qualified guidance is recommended though not essential. No credence should be given to anyone promising immediate or total success. **Risks:** Avoid imbalanced or intolerable diets. They can cause deficiencies with serious consequences. Children are particularly at risk.
Physical therapies Heat and cold treatments, bathing, and exercise therapy (*see* pages 867–78) are claimed to relax, strengthen, or invigorate the patient, or ease pain. An individual plan of treatment should be defined in association with the treating physician.	**Inappropriate** as a treatment for cancer. **Useful** as a supportive treatment attempt aimed at alleviating pain, or when the procedure is perceived as being pleasant and stimulating. Case reports and field studies claim efficacy; however, success is probably seen in only a proportion of patients (*see* Placebo, page xxi).	**Suitable for DIY** Qualified guidance is recommended. Practitioners should be properly qualified and should propose a treatment plan. **Risks:** Skin damage may be caused to persons with diminished temperature sensation when extreme temperatures are applied.
Probiotics The introduction of certain bacteria into the gut is claimed to bring the intestinal flora back into balance and to have a beneficial effect on the immune system (*see* page 878).	**Inappropriate** as a treatment for cancer. **Useful** as a supportive treatment attempt after chemotherapy as a means of correcting any imbalance in the intestinal flora. No credence should be given to claims that probiotics can provide a successful cure for cancer.	**Requires a qualified practitioner** Practitioners should be properly qualified and should propose a treatment plan. Non-prescription formulations are suitable for do-it-yourself. **Risks:** Fairly unlikely provided treatment is carried out competently.

Treatment	Rating	Point of delivery/risks
Reflex therapies Reflex zone massage (*see* page 883), reflexology (*see* page 883), and TENS (*see* page 886) are claimed to act via reflex channels (*see* page 881) to soothe the patient, alleviate pain, and lessen nausea and vomiting.	**Inappropriate** as a treatment for cancer. **Useful** as a short-term, supportive treatment attempt aimed at alleviating pain, soothing the patient, and improving general well-being. Case reports and field studies claim efficacy; however, success is probably seen in only a proportion of patients (*see* Placebo, page xxi).	**Suitable for DIY** Qualified guidance is essential. Practitioners should be properly qualified and should propose a treatment plan. **Risks:** Some people are sensitive to electrical stimuli and rubber electrodes; others find it hard to tolerate manual stimulation or close physical contact.
Relaxation techniques Autogenic training (*see* page 888), muscle relaxation according to Jacobson (*see* page 893), and various biofeedback techniques (*see* page 891) are said to relieve muscle tension and inner unrest, and might be instrumental in dealing with feelings of despondency.	**Inappropriate** as a treatment for cancer. **Useful** as a short-term, supportive treatment attempt aimed at easing muscle tension, anxiety, and feelings of despondency.	**Suitable for DIY** Once a sound understanding of the technique has been acquired from a trainer, patients can perform exercises themselves. Therapists should be properly qualified. **Risks:** Fairly unlikely.

Treatment	Rating	Point of delivery/risks
Vitamins and trace elements The painkilling properties of vitamin B6 are thought to contribute to pain relief. The antioxidative properties of beta-carotene and vitamins C and E are, it is supposed, instrumental in countering the formation of free radicals (*see* page 900), in boosting the body's own antioxidative defences, and in fending off mechanisms that might lead to certain forms of cancer.	**Inappropriate** as a treatment for cancer. **Useful** in vitamin deficiency. High doses of vitamins (vitamins B6, C, E, and beta-carotene) **may be of some use** as a preventive measure. Findings are at present contradictory and do not enable any definitive recommendations to be made. Field studies ascribe a degree of efficacy to vitamin B6 in the treatment of pain.	**Suitable for DIY** Qualified guidance is recommended though not essential. Recommended doses vary widely but are probably set to rise. **Risks:** Intolerance and overdosage are possible. Vitamin B6 in high doses can cause serious side effects. Recent studies imply that beta-carotene might increase the risk of cancer.

Herbal remedies for cancer

Active ingredient/preparation	Rating
Echinacea coneflowers (*Echinacea purpurea*)	**May be of some use** as an immune system stimulant. **Dosage:** As instructed by the manufacturer/prescriber. **Risks:** Do not use in progressive systemic diseases such as tuberculosis, leukosis, collagenosis, multiple sclerosis, or if allergic.
Echinacea pallida **root**	**May be of some use** as a supportive treatment attempt at immune stimulation therapy for flus. Preparations of *Echinacea augustifolia* (root and coneflowers) and *Echinacea purpurea* (root) are **of little use**. **Dosage:** As instructed by the manufacturer/prescriber. **Risks:** Do not use in progressive systemic diseases such as tuberculosis, multiple sclerosis, leukosis, collagenosis, and others. Do not use for more than eight weeks.

Active ingredient/preparation	Rating

Mistletoe injections
(*Viscum album* for injection)

May be of some use as a supportive and palliative treatment and for immune stimulation therapy.
Dosage: As instructed by the manufacturer/prescriber.
Standardized mistletoe preparations enable an accurately controlled dose to be administered and are thus the preparations of choice.
Risks: Shivering attacks, a raised temperature, headaches, chest and heart problems, circulatory disorders, allergic reactions. Liver-damaging properties have also been reported. Always consult your doctor before using mistletoe. Do not use in highly febrile, inflammatory disease.
Caution: The berries must not be used.

Thuja
(*Thuja occidentalis*)

May be of some use as it encourages the body's defence system. It may be used, for instance, as a supportive treatment for malignant tumors. Parts used: dried young twigs.
Dosage: As instructed by the manufacturer/prescriber.
Risks: Cramps, visual disturbance, cardiac arrhythmia, and symptoms of kidney and liver damage are possible. Contains thujone, which is toxic, so do not exceed manufacturers' recommended doses (see package labels and inserts).

AIDS

Causes and symptoms

Acquired Immune Deficiency Syndrome (AIDS) is an immune disorder that is strongly linked with the human immunodeficiency virus (HIV). HIV is spread through infected blood or by an exchange of body fluids during unprotected sexual intercourse, as well as through infected syringes, needles, and blood products. The virus and the body's response to it gradually weaken the immune system, so the normal means of protection against infection is lost. HIV infection progresses in stages, starting with the sufferer being a symptom-free carrier, and developing (possibly) at a later stage into full-blown AIDS. Once AIDS has developed, sufferers are susceptible to a wide assortment of opportunistic infections, including many fungal infections and pneumonia. These infections are caused by agents to which a person without AIDS would not normally be susceptible. People with AIDS also fall victim to a number of tumors, neurological disorders, and various other complaints and sequelae.

While orthodox treatments are usually effective against the opportunistic infections, all attempts at actually treating HIV infection itself are in their infancy. At present there is no cure for AIDS.

Orthodox treatment

Treatment of HIV infection focuses on the use of antibiotic, anti-viral and anti-fungal agents. At the time of writing, there is no general consensus regarding the optimum time at which treatment should commence and the period for which it should be continued.

Various antibiotic and chemotherapies are used to prevent and treat opportunistic infections.

Complementary therapies

Despite many claims to the contrary, there is as yet no evidence that complementary therapies are beneficial in dealing with the HIV virus. Some treatments are useful only for relieving symptoms such as anxiety, pain, or nausea. In many patients the decision to try a complementary treatment heightens the will for it to succeed. Apart from that, many patients see complementary therapies as a way of improving their quality of life.

Treatment plan and limited trial

Before administering a complementary treatment, every therapist should propose a treatment plan (*see* page xxiii) that sets out a clear time frame and defines the goal that the treatment is designed to achieve. Treatment should then be tried for a limited term to test the patient's response.

Caution

Give no credence to anyone claiming to be able to cure AIDS.

Complementary treatments for AIDS

Treatment	Rating	Point of delivery/risks
Acupressure This treatment (*see* page 769), otherwise known as pressure-point massage, is used by AIDS patients to alleviate pain, release tension, improve general well-being, and reduce nausea due to chemo- or radiotherapy.	**Inappropriate** as a treatment for AIDS. **Useful** as a short-term treatment attempt aimed at reducing pain and nausea. Case reports claim efficacy; however, success is probably seen in only a proportion of patients (*see* Placebo, page xxi).	**Suitable for DIY** Qualified guidance is recommended. Therapists should be properly qualified. **Risks:** Acupressure must not be carried out on damaged skin or on parts of the body affected by tumors.
Acupuncture Acupuncture in its various forms (*see* page 772) is used in AIDS patients to alleviate pain, to reduce nausea and vomiting, and to ease muscular tension. In early stages of the disease, acupuncture is claimed to energize (*see* page 927) the patient, release blocked energy (*see* page 927), and increase the body's own ability to withstand disease.	**Inappropriate** as a treatment for AIDS. **Useful** as a short-term treatment attempt aimed at reducing nausea, vomiting, and muscular pain. Studies ascribe a degree of efficacy to this treatment in patients with mild forms of nausea. Case reports and field studies claim efficacy in the treatment of pain; however, success is probably seen in only a proportion of patients (*see* Placebo, page xxi).	**Requires a qualified practitioner** Acupuncturists should be properly qualified and should propose a treatment plan. **Risks:** Acupressure must not be carried out on damaged skin or on parts of the body affected by tumors. Disposable needles are a must owing to the risk of infection.
Anthroposophical medicine Mistletoe preparations play a prominent role in current therapeutic approaches. Other important treatments include art therapy, biographical work, and anthroposophically based spiritual care (*see* page 781).	**Inappropriate** as a treatment for AIDS. **May be of some use** as a supportive treatment attempt. The empirical basis for recommendations is lacking. There is no doubt, however, that the attention given to the patient's spiritual needs is beneficial.	**Requires a qualified practitioner** Practitioners should be properly qualified and should propose a treatment plan. **Risks:** Allergies and intolerance are possible.

Treatment	Rating	Point of delivery/risks
Aromatherapy Essential oils (*see* page 786) are used to soothe and relax, or to invigorate, thereby improving the quality of life of HIV-positive and AIDS patients.	**Inappropriate** as a treatment for AIDS. **May be of some use** as a treatment attempt aimed at soothing and relaxing the patient and improving his/her general well-being. Claims of efficacy probably apply to only a proportion of patients (*see* Placebo, page xxi).	**Suitable for DIY** Qualified guidance is recommended. The effects of individual essential oils differ widely. **Risks:** Allergies or intolerance are possible. Some oils are carcinogenic in test systems and possibly in humans.
Bioresonance therapy Bioresonance therapists use electrical devices in an attempt to discover the causes of illness and claim to be able to weaken or turn around pathogenic energies and disease related vibrations (*see* page 794).	**Inappropriate** as a treatment for AIDS. Possibly acceptable as a short-term treatment attempt aimed at improving general well-being when simpler, more established methods have been unsuccessful. Some case reports claim efficacy; however, success is probably seen, if at all, in only a small proportion of patients (*see* Placebo, page xxi).	**Requires a qualified practitioner** Practitioners should be properly qualified and should propose a treatment plan. No credence should be given to anyone promising immediate or total success. **Risks:** Fairly unlikely.
Cell therapy Injecting or ingesting products extracted from the tissues of newborn animals or animal fetuses is said to have a rejuvenating and revitalizing effect and to enhance the healing of human tissues and organs (*see* page 796).	**Not advised** Based on present knowledge, there is inadequate evidence of the efficacy and mode of action of these costly and relatively risky procedures.	**Risks:** Injecting foreign proteins into the body can provoke (possibly fatal) allergic reactions. Also, pathogens such as those that cause bovine spongiform encephalopathy (BSE) or other serious infections may be introduced.

Treatment	Rating	Point of delivery/risks
Electroacupuncture according to Voll By taking readings of the electrical conductivity of the skin (*see* page 802), therapists claim to be able to derive an insight into diseased areas of the body, pathogenic foci (*see* page 928), and stress factors (*see* Toxins, page 929). The factors presumed to be instrumental in the causation of AIDS can then be addressed.	**Inappropriate** as a treatment for AIDS. Possibly acceptable as a short-term treatment attempt aimed at improving general well-being when simpler, more established methods have been unsuccessful. Some case reports claim efficacy; however, success is probably seen, if at all, in only a small proportion of patients (*see* Placebo, page xxi).	**Requires a qualified practitioner** Practitioners should be properly qualified and should propose a treatment plan. No credence should be given to anyone promising immediate or total success. **Risks:** A second opinion must always be obtained from a qualified physician before any attempt is made to "eliminate foci" (e.g. by surgery).
Electroneural therapy according to Croon According to the theory, readings taken at various reactive sites on the skin highlight diseased areas within the body. Based on these readings, targeted electrostimulative measures can be undertaken to address factors presumed to be instrumental in the causation of AIDS (*see* page 806).	**Inappropriate** as a treatment for AIDS. Possibly acceptable as a short-term treatment attempt aimed at improving general well-being when simpler, more established methods have been unsuccessful. Some case reports claim efficacy; however, success is probably seen, if at all, in only a small proportion of patients (*see* Placebo, page xxi).	**Requires a qualified practitioner** Practitioners should be properly qualified and should propose a treatment plan. No credence should be given to anyone promising immediate or total success. **Risks:** Proponents themselves warn that treatment should not be given in acute inflammatory conditions.
Eliminative methods, unbloody Unbloody cupping (*see* page 817) is sometimes used to ease pain. This treatment is said to energize (*see* page 927) the patient and improve the body's own regulatory systems.	**Inappropriate** as a treatment for AIDS. **May be of some use** as a short-term treatment attempt aimed at alleviating pain. Some case reports claim efficacy; however, success is probably seen in only a proportion of patients (*see* Placebo, page xxi).	**Suitable for DIY** Unbloody cupping is best carried out under the guidance of a qualified practitioner. **Risks:** Unlikely provided treatment is carried out competently.

Treatment	Rating	Point of delivery/risks
Enzyme therapy The enzymes used (*see* page 841) are said to dispel and destroy "immune complexes" that course in the blood and that are responsible, for instance, for sustaining inflammatory processes.	**Of little use** as a treatment for AIDS. Some case reports claim efficacy for this little researched therapy; however, success is probably seen in only a small proportion of patients (*see* Placebo, page xxi).	**Requires a qualified practitioner** Practitioners should propose a treatment plan. Non-prescription preparations are suitable for do-it-yourself. **Risks:** Allergies or intolerance are possible.
Flower remedies Flower remedies (*see* page 828) are said to restore emotional balance and assist the body's psychic ability to heal itself.	**Inappropriate** as a treatment for AIDS. May be of some use as a short-term treatment attempt aimed at soothing and relaxing. Some case reports claim efficacy; however, success is probably seen in only a proportion of patients (*see* Placebo, page xxi).	**Suitable for DIY** Qualified guidance is recommended. Practitioners should propose a treatment plan. **Risks:** Possible intolerance.
Homeopathy Highly diluted (potentized) solutions (*see* page 831) are believed to be able to redress vital energy imbalances and strengthen the body's defences. Organo- and functiotropic (*see* page 833) homeopathy is claimed to be effective for dealing with symptoms.	**Inappropriate** as a treatment for AIDS. Reports of HIV disappearing after homeopathic treatment are pure hearsay. **May be of some use** as a short-term treatment attempt directed against the symptoms and aimed at helping the body to deal better with the infection. Several case reports claim efficacy in the treatment of symptoms; however, success is probably seen in only a proportion of patients (*see* Placebo, page xxi).	**Requires a qualified practitioner** Homeopaths should be properly qualified and should propose a treatment plan. No credence should be given to anyone promising immediate or total success. **Risks:** Allergies and intolerance are possible.

Treatment	Rating	Point of delivery/risks
Hypnosis and self-hypnosis In the relaxed and generally altered state of awareness that is induced in hypnosis or self-hypnosis (*see* page 837), worries can be dispelled and the patient can be helped to come to terms better with his/her condition. Hypnosis is often used in combination with other psycho- and behavioral therapies.	**Inappropriate** as a treatment for AIDS. **May be of some use** as a short-term, supportive treatment attempt aimed at dispelling worries and at helping the patient come to terms better with his/her condition. Some case reports claim efficacy; however, success is probably seen in only a proportion of patients (*see* Placebo, page xxi).	**Requires a qualified practitioner** Hypnotherapists should be properly qualified and should propose a treatment plan. **Risks:** Unlikely provided treatment is carried out competently.
Magnetic field therapy The use of magnetic field generators, magnetic strips, bracelets, and other objects (*see* page 841) allegedly encourages cell metabolism and so relieves pain.	**Of little use** Based on present knowledge, there is inadequate evidence of the efficacy and mode of action of magnetic field therapy in AIDS.	Operation of magnetic field equipment **requires a qualified practitioner**. **Risks:** Magnetic field equipment can cause implanted cardiac pacemakers to malfunction.
Manual therapies Chiropractors and osteopaths (*see* page 844) use a series of manipulations to realign allegedly displaced vertebrae. This is said to reduce pain and release energy blockages (*see* page 927).	**Inappropriate** as a treatment for AIDS. **May be of some use** as a short-term treatment attempt aimed at alleviating pain in the muscles and joints. Some case reports claim efficacy; however, success is probably seen, if at all, in only a small proportion of patients (*see* Placebo, page xxi).	**Requires a qualified practitioner** Practitioners should be properly qualified and should propose a treatment plan. **Risks:** Manipulation of the head and cervical vertebrae can cause serious injury. These procedures must not be carried out on parts of the body that are damaged or affected by osteoporosis.

Treatment	Rating	Point of delivery/risks
Massage Classical massage (*see* page 847) can invigorate the patient, as well as ease muscular and emotional tension and alleviate muscle pains.	**Inappropriate** as a treatment for AIDS. **May be of some use** as a short-term treatment attempt aimed at relaxing the patient and alleviating muscle pains. Several case reports claim efficacy; however, success is probably seen in only a small proportion of patients (*see* Placebo, page xxi).	**Suitable for DIY** Qualified guidance is recommended. Masseurs/masseuses should propose a treatment plan. **Risks:** Some people are sensitive to manual stimuli; others find it hard to tolerate close physical contact. Parts of the body that are damaged must not be massaged.
Nutritional therapies An organic diet (*see* page 4) provides the body with essential and secondary plant nutrients that are believed to exercise a multitude of positive effects and to be capable, *inter alia*, of boosting the immune system (*see* page 10).	**Inappropriate** as a treatment for AIDS. **Useful** as an individually directed supportive measure. Claims of improvements having been achieved through macrobiotics (*see* page 861) are unsubstantiated.	**Suitable for DIY** Qualified guidance is recommended though not essential. **Risks:** Avoid imbalanced or intolerable diets. They can cause deficiencies with serious consequences. Children are particularly at risk.
Physical therapies Heat and cold treatments, baths (*see* pages 871–8), and exercise therapy (*see* page 868) can be used to relax, strengthen, or invigorate the patient, to ease pain, and to help the patient come to terms better with his/her condition.	**Inappropriate** as a treatment for AIDS. **Useful** as a short-term treatment attempt aimed at alleviating pain. Several case reports claim efficacy; however, success is probably seen in only a proportion of patients (*see* Placebo, page xxi).	**Suitable for DIY** Qualified guidance is recommended. Therapists should be properly qualified. **Risks:** Skin damage may be caused to persons with diminished temperature sensation when extreme temperatures are applied.

Treatment	Rating	Point of delivery/risks
Probiotics The introduction of certain bacteria into the gut is claimed to bring the intestinal flora back into balance and to have a beneficial effect on the immune system (*see* page 878).	**Inappropriate** as a treatment for AIDS. Acceptable as a short-term treatment attempt following chemo-therapy, as a means of rebalancing the intestinal flora or of treating diarrhea. Case reports and field studies claim efficacy; however, success is probably seen in only a proportion of patients (*see* Placebo, page xxi).	**Requires a qualified practitioner** Practitioners should be properly qualified and should propose a treatment plan. Non-prescription formulations are suitable for do-it-yourself. **Risks:** Fairly unlikely provided treatment is carried out competently.
Reflex therapies Reflex zone massage (*see* page 883), reflexology (*see* page 883), and TENS (*see* page 886) are claimed to act via reflex channels (*see* page 881) to ease pain, relax the patient, influence a number of physical functions, and reduce nausea and vomiting.	**Inappropriate** as a treatment for AIDS. **Useful** as a short-term treatment attempt aimed at alleviating pain, nausea, and vomiting. Several case reports claim efficacy; however, success is probably seen in only a proportion of patients (*see* Placebo, page xxi).	**Suitable for DIY** Qualified guidance is essential. **Risks:** Some people are sensitive to electrical stimuli and rubber electrodes; others find it hard to tolerate cold, manual stimulation, or close physical contact.
Relaxation techniques Autogenic training (*see* page 888), muscle relaxation according to Jacobson (*see* page 893), and various biofeedback techniques (*see* page 891) are said to relieve muscle tension and inner unrest, and might be instrumental in combating despondency.	**Inappropriate** as a treatment for AIDS. **Useful** as a supportive treatment attempt aimed at soothing and relaxing when the procedure chosen is perceived to be pleasant and effective. Some case reports and field studies claim efficacy; however, success is probably seen in only a proportion of patients (*see* Placebo, page xxi).	**Suitable for DIY** Once a sound understanding of the technique has been acquired from a trainer, patients can perform exercises themselves. Therapists should be properly qualified. **Risks:** Fairly unlikely.

Treatment	Rating	Point of delivery/risks
Vitamins and trace elements The painkilling properties of vitamin B6 are thought to contribute to pain relief. Beta-carotene and vitamins C and E are, it is supposed, instrumental in countering the formation of free radicals and in modulating the immune system (*see* page 10). They may also have a preventive role (*see* page 900).	**Inappropriate** as a treatment for AIDS. **Useful** in dietary vitamin deficiency. There is no evidence that high doses of vitamins delay the onset of AIDS or prolong life.	**Suitable for DIY** Qualified guidance is recommended though not essential. **Risks:** Intolerance and overdosage are possible. Vitamin B6 in high doses can cause serious side effects. Recent findings imply that beta-carotene might increase the risk of cancer.

Herbal remedies for AIDS

Active ingredient/preparation	Rating
Echinacea coneflowers (*Echinacea purpurea*)	**May be of some use** as a supportive measure for stimulating the immune system. **Dosage:** As instructed by the manufacturer/prescriber. **Risks:** Do not use in progressive systemic diseases such as tuberculosis, leukosis, collagenosis, multiple sclerosis, or if allergic.
***Echinacea pallida* root**	**May be of some use** as a supportive treatment attempt at immune stimulation therapy in grippal infections. Preparations of *Echinacea angustifolia* (root and coneflowers) and *Echinacea purpurea* (root) are **of little use**. **Dosage:** As instructed by the manufacturer/prescriber. **Risks:** Do not use in progressive systemic diseases. Do not use for more than eight weeks.

Active ingredient/preparation	Rating

Mistletoe injections
(*Viscum album* for injection)

May be of some use as a supportive and palliative treatment and for immune stimulation therapy. Mistletoe reportedly has a T-lymphocyte stimulating action.
Dosage: As instructed by the manufacturer/prescriber. Standardized mistletoe preparations enable an accurately controlled dose to be administered and are thus the preparations of choice.
Risks: Shivering attacks, a raised temperature, headaches, chest and heart problems, circulatory disorders, allergic reactions. Not suitable for self-medication; always consult your doctor before using mistletoe. Do not use in acute inflammatory disease.
Caution: The berries must not be used.

St. John's wort
(*Hypericum perforatum*)

May be of some use as a supportive treatment attempt. There have been individual reports of subjective improvements in patients, in some cases associated with weight gain. However, even high-dose therapy (e.g. 3 x 40 drops daily, 2 x 2 ampules per week) has failed to prolong life expectancy demonstrably. Subjective reports of a mood-improving effect are attributable to the known antidepressive action of St. John's wort.
Dosage: As instructed by the manufacturer/prescriber.
Risks: Photosensitization (persons with a light complexion should keep out of bright sunlight after taking St. John's wort, or they may suffer allergic skin irritation).

Thuja drops
(*Thuja occidentalis*)

May be of some use as thuja encourages the body's defence system. It may be used, for instance, as a supportive treatment. Parts used: dried young twigs.
Dosage: As instructed by the manufacturer/prescriber.
Risks: Cramps, visual disturbance, cardiac arrhythmia, and symptoms of kidney and liver damage are possible. Contains thujone, which is toxic, so do not exceed manufacturers' recommended doses (see package labels and inserts).

Ailments of the elderly

Elderly people are a lucrative target group. Some complementary practitioners have come to realize this and, in addition to their usual therapies, are keen to offer "rejuvenating" and "revitalizing" treatments and products. They also have a tendency to play on the fears of elderly people, whether about growing old, becoming ill or dying, or becoming despondent. Only by becoming familiar with the limitations of complementary medicine can one lessen the chance of being taken in, at great expense, by fraudulent claims about rejuvenation or "cure all" remedies.

At the other extreme, advanced age should on no account be a reason for failing to obtain potentially beneficial treatment; nor for withholding such a treatment from the patient. Often, a complementary approach will be tried in support of an overall treatment plan: to help motivate or relax, to help alleviate symptoms, or to ease pain.

Treatment plan and limited trial

Before administering a complementary treatment, every therapist should propose a treatment plan (*see* page xxiii) that sets out a clear time frame and defines the goal that the treatment is designed to achieve. Treatment should then be tried for a limited term to test the patient's response.

Cautions

Complementary therapies should only be administered by practitioners skilled in the treatment of the elderly. A thorough medical checkup should be carried out before an elderly person undergoes any complementary therapy, so as not to preclude what might be a more appropriate orthodox treatment.

Old skin, being thinner, is very delicate. Also, blood vessels may have become sclerotic. Special care is thus needed during massage and the practice of certain physical techniques. Some techniques should be avoided altogether; for example, osteoporosis, which affects virtually every elderly woman and most elderly men, represents a relative contraindication to spinal manipulation.

Complementary treatments for the elderly

Treatment	Rating	Point of delivery/risks
Acupressure This treatment (*see* page 769), otherwise known as pressure-point massage, is claimed to alleviate tension, pain, and other symptoms when pressure is applied to the appropriate points. Acupressure is also used for its general restorative effect. The pressure points chosen may differ from one practitioner to another.	**May be of some use**, when administered by an experienced person, as a short-term treatment attempt for various conditions, especially pain, and for soothing and relaxing the patient. Case reports claim efficacy; however, success is probably seen in only a proportion of patients (*see* Placebo, page xxi).	**Suitable for DIY** Qualified guidance is recommended. Friends or relatives can subsequently administer acupressure. **Risks:** Unlikely provided treatment is carried out competently. Osteoporosis is one of several risk factors. The skin of elderly persons is sometimes very easily damaged. Only gentle acupressure should be applied.

Treatment	Rating	Point of delivery/risks
Acupuncture Acupuncture in its various forms (*see* page 772) is used in elderly persons to ease pain and other symptoms. The acupuncture points chosen can vary from one practitioner to another.	**May be of some use**, when administered by an experienced person, as a short-term treatment attempt for various conditions, especially pain, and for soothing and relaxing the patient. Claims of efficacy probably only apply to a proportion of patients (*see* Placebo, page xxi).	**Requires a qualified practitioner** Acupuncturists should be properly qualified and should propose a treatment plan. **Risks:** Probably rare provided treatment is carried out competently. The skin of elderly persons is sometimes very easily damaged. The tissue is much thinner and more susceptible to mechanical damage, and blood vessels may be affected by arteriosclerosis. Deep needling techniques increase the risk of injury and complications.
Anthroposophical medicine Doctors who practice AM (*see* page 781) recognize that elderly persons are more difficult to "regulate" and often respond less well to individual therapies than children or young adults. Commonly used therapeutic approaches include dialog, various forms of massage, and "compositions." The special doctor–patient rapport is a significant factor in the treatment of serious illness.	**May be of some use** as a treatment attempt for chronic conditions, psychosomatic ailments, and pain. Case reports claim efficacy; however, success is probably seen in only a proportion of patients (*see* Placebo, page xxi).	**Requires a qualified practitioner** Practitioners should be properly qualified and should propose a treatment plan. **Risks:** Probably rare provided treatment is carried out competently. Allergies and intolerance are possible with some compositions.

Treatment	Rating	Point of delivery/risks
Aromatherapy Essential oils (*see* page 786) are used to soothe and relax, or to invigorate, thereby improving the patient's general well-being and contributing to an easing of symptoms. The essences may be taken orally, used externally as massage oils or bathing emulsions, or inhaled as vapors.	**May be of some use** as a treatment attempt aimed at soothing and relaxing. Some case reports claim efficacy; however, success is probably seen in only a proportion of patients (*see* Placebo, page xxi). There is at present no evidence that aromatherapy can be targeted directly at specific ailments.	**Suitable for DIY** Qualified guidance is recommended. The effects of individual essential oils differ widely. **Risks:** Allergies or intolerance are possible. Some oils are carcinogenic in test systems and possibly in humans.
Bioresonance therapy Bioresonance therapists use electrical devices in an attempt to discover the causes of illness and claim to be able to weaken or turn around pathogenic energies and disease related vibrations (*see* page 794). This procedure is frequently used for treating allergies.	**Of little use** Possibly acceptable as a short-term treatment attempt, especially for psychosomatic ailments, when simpler, more established methods have been unsuccessful. Some case reports claim efficacy; however, success is probably seen, if at all, in only a small proportion of patients (*see* Placebo, page xxi).	**Requires a qualified practitioner** Practitioners should be properly qualified and should propose a treatment plan. **Risks:** Fairly unlikely.
Cell therapy Injecting or ingesting products extracted from the tissues of newborn animals or animal fetuses is said to have a rejuvenating and revitalizing effect and to enhance the healing of human tissues and organs (*see* page 796).	**Not advised** Based on present knowledge, there is inadequate evidence of the efficacy and mode of action of these costly and relatively risky procedures. The claimed rejuvenating effect of cell therapy is unsubstantiated.	**Risks:** Injecting foreign proteins into the body can provoke (possibly fatal) allergic reactions. Also, pathogens such as those that cause bovine spongiform encephalopathy (BSE) or other serious infections may be introduced.

Treatment	Rating	Point of delivery/risks
Chelation therapy The chelating agent EDTA (*see* page 800) is able, it is claimed, to bind calcareous deposits and heavy metals in the blood vessels. These are subsequently eliminated from the body.	**Not advised** Studies were unable to substantiate the claimed therapeutic efficacy of this risky procedure. The complementary therapy has nothing to do with the conventional method of dealing with heavy metal intoxications.	**Risks:** EDTA can cause a deficit of calcium and essential heavy metals and, in extreme cases, can lead to cardiac arrhythmia, respiratory failure, cramps, and death.
Electroacupuncture according to Voll By taking readings of the electrical conductivity of the skin (*see* page 802), therapists claim to be able to derive an insight into diseased areas of the body, pathogenic foci (*see* page 928), and stress factors (*see* Toxins, page 929). The factors presumed to underlie individual symptoms can then be addressed.	**Of little use** Possibly acceptable as a short-term, supportive treatment attempt for persistent complaints when simpler, more established methods have been unsuccessful. Some case reports claim efficacy; however, success is probably seen, if at all, in only a small proportion of patients (*see* Placebo, page xxi).	**Requires a qualified practitioner** Practitioners should be properly qualified and should propose a treatment plan. No credence should be given to anyone promising immediate or total success. **Risks:** A second opinion must always be obtained from a qualified physician before any attempt is made to "eliminate foci" (e.g. by surgery).
Electroneural therapy according to Croon According to the theory, readings taken at various reactive sites on the skin highlight diseased areas within the body. Based on these readings, targeted electrostimulative measures can be undertaken to address factors presumed to underlie individual symptoms (*see* page 806).	**Of little use** Possibly acceptable as a short-term, supportive treatment attempt for persistent complaints when simpler, more established methods have been unsuccessful. Some case reports claim efficacy; however, success is probably seen, if at all, in only a small proportion of patients (*see* Placebo, page xxi).	**Requires a qualified practitioner** Practitioners should be properly qualified and should propose a treatment plan. No credence should be given to anyone promising immediate or total success. **Risks:** Proponents themselves warn that treatment should not be given in acute inflammatory conditions.

Treatment	Rating	Point of delivery/risks
Eliminative methods, bloody Bloody cupping (*see* page 815) and cantharide poultices (*see* page 812) are said to alleviate pain, modulate the immune system (*see* page 10), and improve the body's own regulatory systems.	Cantharide poultices are **not advised**. Bloody cupping is **of little use**. It is possibly acceptable for treating persistent symptoms such as pain when more established, less invasive methods have been unsuccessful.	**Requires a qualified practitioner** Practitioners should be properly qualified, should have experience in treatment of the elderly, and should propose a treatment plan. **Risks:** These procedures are painful. The skin of elderly persons is sometimes very easily damaged. The tissue is much thinner and more susceptible to mechanical damage, and blood vessels may be affected by arteriosclerosis. Bloody cupping can cause infection and scarring. Furthermore, it should not be carried out in persons with bleeding disorders. Cantharide poultices can cause second-degree burns. Problems with wound healing are more common in the elderly than in other age groups.

Treatment	Rating	Point of delivery/risks
Eliminative methods, unbloody Sweating (*see* page 877) and enemas (*see* page 819) are claimed to improve the body's own regulatory systems or to modulate the immune system (*see* page 10). Unbloody cupping (*see* page 817) is claimed to provide relief from pain.	Sweating **may be of some use** in dealing with the common cold; and unbloody cupping **may be of some use** in providing relief from pain. All other eliminative methods are **of little use**; there is no evidence that the benefits outweigh the risks involved.	**Suitable for DIY** Unbloody cupping requires a qualified practitioner initially, but can subsequently by carried out by friends or relatives. **Risks:** Sweating may overwork the circulation. Unbloody cupping is painful and, in the elderly, can cause skin and vascular damage. Enemas may lead to constipation, disturb the electrolyte balance and, when improperly administered, damage the colonic mucosa.
Enzyme therapy The enzymes used (*see* page 824) are said to dispel and destroy "immune complexes" that course in the blood and that are responsible, for instance, for causing autoimmune diseases and for sustaining the inflammatory processes.	**Of little use** Some case reports claim efficacy for this little researched therapy; however, success is probably seen in only a small proportion of patients (*see* Placebo, page xxi).	**Requires a qualified practitioner** Practitioners should propose a treatment plan. **Risks:** Allergies or intolerance are possible. In elderly patients the risk of hemorrhage is higher, as blood clotting and the vascular system undergo changes with age.

Treatment	Rating	Point of delivery/risks
Flower remedies Flower remedies (*see* page 828) are said to restore emotional balance and assist the body's psychic ability to heal itself.	**May be of some use** as a short-term treatment attempt aimed at soothing and relaxing and at helping the patient to deal better with personal problems and emotional states. Case reports claim efficacy; however, success is probably seen in only a proportion of patients (*see* Placebo, page xxi).	**Suitable for DIY** Qualified guidance is essential. Practitioners should propose a treatment plan. **Risks:** Possible intolerance.
Homeopathy Highly diluted (potentized) solutions (*see* page 831) are believed to be able to redress vital energy imbalances. Organo- and functiotropic (*see* page 833) homeopathy is claimed to be effective for dealing directly with symptoms.	**May be of some use** as a treatment attempt for chronic conditions and for rectifying impaired well-being. Some case reports claim efficacy; however, success is probably seen in only a proportion of patients (*see* Placebo, page xxi).	**Requires a qualified practitioner** Homeopaths should be properly qualified and should propose a treatment plan. Ready-formulated preparations are suitable for do-it-yourself. **Risks:** Allergies and intolerance are possible.
Hypnosis and self-hypnosis In the relaxed and generally altered state of awareness that is induced in hypnosis (*see* page 837), physical and mental conditions can be addressed and relief from pain possibly provided.	**May be of some use** as a short-term treatment attempt for pain or persistent psychosomatic ailments when simpler, more established methods have been unsuccessful. Some case reports claim efficacy; however, success is probably seen in only a proportion of patients (*see* Placebo, page xxi).	**Requires a qualified practitioner** Hypnotherapists should be properly qualified and should propose a treatment plan. **Risks:** Unlikely provided treatment is carried out competently.

Treatment	Rating	Point of delivery/risks

Magnetic field therapy
The use of magnetic field generators, magnetic strips, bracelets, and other objects (*see* page 841) allegedly encourages cell metabolism and so eases a multitude of symptoms.

Inappropriate
Based on present knowledge, there is inadequate evidence of the efficacy and mode of action of magnetic field therapy in the elderly. Claims of efficacy in the treatment of osteoporosis have not been properly substantiated.

Operation of magnetic field equipment **requires a qualified practitioner**.
Risks: Magnetic field equipment can cause implanted cardiac pacemakers to malfunction. Before any treatment is carried out, the possible risks should be discussed with a cardiologist.

Manual therapies
Chiropractors and osteopaths (*see* page 844) use a series of manipulations to realign allegedly displaced vertebrae. This is said to reduce pain, release energy blockages (*see* page 927), and address factors that may be at the root of various diseases and symptoms.

Of little use
Possibly acceptable as a short-term treatment attempt aimed at easing persistent pain or tension. Some case reports claim efficacy for these potentially risky procedures; however, success is probably seen, if at all, in only a small proportion of patients (*see* Placebo, page xxi).

Requires a qualified practitioner
Practitioners should be properly qualified, should have considerable experience in treatment of the elderly, and should propose a treatment plan.
Risks: Manipulation of the head and cervical vertebrae can cause serious injury. Osteoporosis is one of several risk factors. The spine and joints of elderly persons may have undergone degenerative change and may be particularly vulnerable.

Treatment	Rating	Point of delivery/risks
Massage Classical massage (*see* page 847) and lymphatic drainage (*see* page 850) can invigorate the patient, as well as ease muscular and emotional tension. Ice massage (*see* page 878) is claimed to ease pain and other symptoms, to relieve muscle tension, and to soothe and relax.	**May be of some use** as a short-term treatment attempt aimed at easing persistent tension. Some case reports claim efficacy; however, success is probably seen in only a proportion of patients (*see* Placebo, page xxi).	**Suitable for DIY** Qualified guidance is essential. Friends or relatives can subsequently administer massages. **Risks:** The skin of elderly persons is sometimes very easily damaged. The tissue is much thinner and more susceptible to mechanical damage. Osteoporosis is one of several risk factors. Some people are also sensitive to cold.
Nutritional therapies An organic diet (*see* page 4) provides the body with essential and secondary plant nutrients that are believed to exercise a multitude of positive effects and to be capable, *inter alia*, of boosting the immune system.	**Useful** as an individually directed supportive measure provided that the diet is balanced and appealing. Since vitamin requirements in the elderly are often higher, or because dietary intake of vitamins is insufficient, vitamin supplementation may be beneficial. There are presently insufficient data to enable definitive dosage recommendations to be made.	**Suitable for DIY** Qualified guidance is recommended though not essential. **Risks:** Avoid imbalanced or intolerable diets. They can cause deficiencies with serious consequences.

Treatment	Rating	Point of delivery/risks
Physical therapies Procedures such as brushing, whole body washing, various hydrotherapeutic treatments , Kneipp treatments (*see* pages 871–8), etc, are claimed to invigorate, relax, improve the circulation, and ease pain and other symptoms. Saunas (*see* page 876) are claimed to improve the body's own regulatory systems or to modulate the immune system (*see* page 10).	**Useful** as a means of relaxing or invigorating the patient and improving his/her circulation; also as a treatment attempt aimed at alleviating pain. The effects achieved with the various treatments differ widely from patient to patient. Some case reports claim efficacy; however, success is probably seen in only a proportion of patients (*see* Placebo, page xxi). Regular saunas **may be of some use** for strengthening the immune system.	**Suitable for DIY** Qualified guidance is recommended. **Risks:** Skin damage may be caused to persons with diminished temperature sensation when extreme temperatures are applied. Electrostimulative techniques can cause implanted cardiac pacemakers to malfunction and adversely affect artificial joints. Saunas may overwork the circulation.
Probiotics The introduction of certain bacteria into the gut is claimed to bring the intestinal flora back into balance and to have a beneficial effect on various diseases and symptoms (*see* page 878).	**Of little use** Acceptable as a short-term treatment attempt for medication induced constipation. Case reports claim efficacy; however, success is probably seen in only a proportion of patients (*see* Placebo, page xxi).	**Requires a qualified practitioner** Practitioners should be properly qualified and should propose a treatment plan. Non-prescription formulations are suitable for do-it-yourself. **Risks:** Fairly unlikely provided treatment is carried out competently.

Treatment	*Rating*	*Point of delivery/risks*
Reflex therapies Reflex zone massage (*see* page 883) and cold sprays are claimed to act via reflex channels (*see* page 881) to ease pain and other symptoms, to relieve muscle tension, and to soothe and relax.	**Useful** as a short-term treatment attempt aimed at alleviating muscle tension, pain, and other symptoms, or as a pleasant, relaxing experience. These procedures are all of roughly equal merit, though the actual benefits derived from them may differ considerably from one person to another. Case reports claim efficacy; however, success is probably seen in only a proportion of patients (*see* Placebo, page xxi).	**Suitable for DIY** Qualified guidance is essential. Practitioners should be properly qualified and should propose a treatment plan. **Risks:** Some people are sensitive to cold; others find it hard to tolerate manual stimulation or close physical contact. The skin of elderly persons is sometimes very easily damaged. The tissue is much thinner and more susceptible to mechanical damage. Osteoporosis is one of several risk factors.
Relaxation techniques Autogenic training (*see* page 888), muscle relaxation according to Jacobson (*see* page 893), and various biofeedback techniques (*see* page 891) are said to relieve muscle tension and inner unrest, and might be instrumental in helping the patient to become more aware of his/her physical and emotional states.	**Useful** for relaxing the patient and for helping him/her become more aware of his/her physical and emotional states. Some case reports claim efficacy; however, success is probably seen in only a proportion of patients (*see* Placebo, page xxi).	**Suitable for DIY** Once a sound understanding of the technique has been acquired from a trainer in group sessions or through individual tuition, patients can perform exercises themselves. Therapists should be properly qualified. **Risks:** Fairly unlikely.

Treatment	Rating	Point of delivery/risks
TENS The use of low frequency electrical currents (*see* page 886) on the surface of the skin is said to act to release blocked energy (*see* page 927) and, as a reflex therapy, to ease pain.	**May be of some use** as a short-term treatment attempt aimed at alleviating pain. Controlled clinical studies and case reports confirm the efficacy of TENS in the treatment of pain (*see* Placebo, page xxi).	**Requires a qualified practitioner** Practitioners should be properly qualified and should propose a treatment plan. **Risks:** TENS may cause implanted cardiac pacemakers to malfunction. Potential risks should be discussed with a cardiologist before treatment is started.
Vitamins and trace elements The antioxidative properties of beta-carotene, vitamins C and E, and selenium are, it is supposed, instrumental in countering the formation of free radicals (*see* page 902), in boosting the body's antioxidative defence systems, and in achieving a multitude of other beneficial effects (*see* page 900).	**Useful** in the form of an organic diet (*see* page 4) that has a high content of fruit and vegetables, and in the form of vitamin supplements when vitamin deficiency has been diagnosed. Vitamins and trace elements with anti-oxidative properties **may be of some use** as a preventive measure. There are at present insufficient data to allow concrete dosage recommendations to be made.	**Suitable for DIY** Qualified guidance is recommended though not essential. Elderly persons may benefit from taking higher vitamin doses than those previously recommended. **Risks:** Intolerance and overdosage are possible. Recent studies imply that beta-carotene might increase the risk of cancer.

Herbal remedies for the elderly

Active ingredient/preparation	Rating

Garlic corms
(*Allium sativum*)

Only useful as a supportive measure for raised blood fat values and as a preventive measure against age-related vascular changes. Garlic is an antibacterial and anti-fungal; it also lowers blood fats. It thins the blood and thus possibly also improves its flow properties.
Mean daily dose: 600–1200mg dry powder or 4g fresh corms (2–4 small cloves). Use ready-formulated preparations as instructed by the manufacturer/prescriber.
Risks: Gastric and allergic problems and asthma are possible but rare.

Garlic oil maceration products

Of little use, as the chemical compositions of the preparations differ widely and no general daily dosage recommendations can be given.
Dosage: As instructed by the manufacturer/prescriber.
Risks: Gastric problems and asthma are possible. There have been reports of paralytic symptoms following excessively high doses.

Ginkgo extract
(*Ginkgo biloba*)

Useful as a treatment attempt for circulatory problems, in conjunction with physical measures designed to improve walking distance. Also useful in poor cerebral perfusion with signs of weak cerebral function and vertigo. Memory and learning ability may improve.
Dosage: As instructed by the manufacturer/prescriber.
Risks: Mild gastrointestinal problems, headaches, and allergic skin reactions are possible. Not to be taken by persons who are hypersensitive to ginkgo. Injectable ginkgo preparations have been withdrawn owing to hypersensitivity reactions.

Active ingredient/preparation	*Rating*
Ginseng, Asiatic (*Panax ginseng*)	Asiatic ginseng **may be of some use** as a tonic for exhaustion, debility, and poor performance in the elderly. In various tests it was seen to improve the ability of rodents to withstand stress, though the importance of these findings for humans is unclear. There is no effective difference between red and white ginseng. The red color of red ginseng comes from its being preserved with steam. **Dosage:** As instructed by the manufacturer/prescriber. **Risks:** High dosages can lead to agitation and sleeplessness. Ginseng products should not be taken by persons with high blood pressure or arteriosclerosis (both common in the elderly), as they may increase blood pressure even further. Prolonged use can produce "ginseng abuse syndrome": morning diarrhea, sleeplessness, and depression. Asiatic ginseng should be avoided by individuals who are highly energetic, nervous, hysteric, manic, or schizophrenic; it should not be taken with stimulants including coffee and antipsychotic drugs.
Ginseng, Siberian (*Eleutherococcus senticosus*)	**May be of some use** as a tonic for exhaustion, debility, and poor performance in the elderly; also as an immune system stimulant. **Dosage:** As instructed by the manufacturer/prescriber (generally for up to three months). **Risks:** Hypertension, headaches, vertigo, and mastalgia are possible. Long-term use may result in loose morning stools, sleeplessness, and depression. Not to be taken by persons with high blood pressure. Siberian ginseng should be avoided by individuals who are highly energetic, nervous, hysteric, manic, or schizophrenic; it should not be taken with stimulants including coffee and antipsychotic drugs.

Active ingredient/preparation	*Rating*

Hawthorn leaves and blossom
(*Crataegus monogyna* and *laevigata*)

Useful as a treatment attempt for age-related mild heart failure when there is not yet a need for other medications.
Daily dose: 1g herb.
Individual dose: Pour hot water over 0.3g of herb. Infuse for 15 minutes and strain. Drink 1 cup several times daily. Use ready-formulated preparations as instructed by the manufacturer/prescriber.
Risks: Consult a doctor if heart failure and water retention in the legs have not cleared up after six weeks. A doctor must be consulted if there are severe symptoms (pain near the heart, in the arms, upper abdomen, or neck). Hawthorn may in some cases cause nausea, headaches, and vertigo. Remedies containing hawthorn may possibly potentiate the action and thus the toxicity of digitalis. Hawthorn must not be used, therefore, together with cardiac tonics that contain digitalis. It is not suitable for self-medication.

Rosemary wine
(*Rosmarinus officinalis*)

May be of some use as a measure to improve the circulation; also for addressing problems with the joints. This is a traditional remedy against senility.
Dosage: As instructed by the manufacturer/prescriber.
Risks: Gastric problems and allergic reactions on account of the volatile oil.

Soy lecithin
(*Glycine max*)

Of little use. This is a rarely used and (at most) supportive treatment for mild age-related disorders of fat metabolism, combined with (or after) dietary measures to prevent hardening of the arteries. Soy lecithin is reported to affect cholesterol favorably and possibly has blood fat-lowering properties.
Dosage: As instructed by the manufacturer/prescriber.
Risks: Soy lecithin is not known to have any serious side effects.

Children's ailments

Complementary therapies for children's ailments are becoming a thriving aspect of pediatric practice. In particular, natural remedies, complementary treatments, etc. are offered for chronic skin conditions, allergies, and susceptibility to infection, as well as for other common problems such as abdominal pain and headaches.

However, there is little evidence to support claims that complementary procedures actually provide significant benefit. There have been few, if any, controlled studies into the various treatments available. Often, claims that a treatment is efficacious are based on nothing more than the odd outcome report. The data that are available have in many cases been derived from studies in adults.

Based on current findings, complementary procedures cannot substitute for orthodox pediatric medicine in the treatment of most childhood diseases.

Treatment plan and limited trial

Before administering a complementary treatment, every therapist should propose a treatment plan (*see* page xxiii) that sets out a clear time frame and defines the goal that the treatment is designed to achieve. Treatment should then be tried for a limited term to test the patient's response.

Caution

Complementary therapies should only be administered by practitioners skilled in the treatment of children. If the practitioner is not skilled in pediatric medicine, any decision to seek a complementary treatment should only be made after consultation with an orthodox doctor or pediatrician in order to find the cause of the child's symptoms.

Serious physical ailments should be excluded as the cause of symptoms before therapy commences. Some complementary practitioners advise against immunizations; discuss this issue with your doctor.

Complementary treatments for children's ailments

Treatment	Rating	Point of delivery/risks
Acupressure This treatment (*see* page 769), otherwise known as pressure-point massage, is claimed to ease tension and alleviate pain and other symptoms in children when pressure is applied to the appropriate points. The pressure points chosen may differ from one practitioner to another.	**May be of some use** as a short-term treatment attempt, e.g. aimed at alleviating pain, colic, and various psychosomatic ailments. Some case reports claim efficacy; however, success is probably seen in only a proportion of children (*see* Placebo, page xxi).	**Suitable for DIY** by adults. Qualified guidance is essential. Therapists should have considerable experience in the treatment of children and should propose a treatment plan. **Risks:** Unlikely provided treatment is carried out competently. Serious organic causes of illness must be ruled out before treatment is started.

Treatment	*Rating*	*Point of delivery/risks*
Acupuncture In children, acupuncture in its various forms (*see* page 772) is used to ease symptoms. The acupuncture points chosen can vary from one practitioner to another. Special acupuncture needles are used in infants and young children.	**May be of some use** as a short-term treatment attempt, e.g. for asthma, allergies, headaches and migraines, pain in the muscles, bones, and joints, sleeplessness, and various psychosomatic ailments. Some case reports claim efficacy; however, success is probably seen in only a proportion of children (*see* Placebo, page xxi).	**Requires a qualified practitioner** Acupuncturists should be properly qualified, should have considerable experience in the treatment of children, and should propose a treatment plan. **Risks:** Probably rare provided treatment is carried out competently. Serious organic causes of illness must be ruled out before treatment is started.
Anthroposophical medicine Doctors who practice AM (*see* page 781) consider that, in children, regulation is especially easy to achieve, which is why many diseases and symptoms are said to respond well to this treatment. When diseases are of longer duration, parents are frequently actively involved in the treatment. Tender loving care is one of the cornerstones of AM in children.	**May be of some use** as a short-term treatment attempt for chronic conditions such as skin disease or rheumatism. Some case reports claim efficacy; however, success is probably seen in only a proportion of children (*see* Placebo, page xxi).	**Requires a qualified practitioner** Practitioners should be properly qualified, should have considerable experience in the treatment of children, and should propose a treatment plan. **Risks:** Allergies and intolerance are possible. Possible causes of the child's condition must be sought by a doctor or pediatrician.

Children's ailments   745

Treatment	*Rating*	*Point of delivery/risks*
Aromatherapy Essential oils (*see* page 786) are used to soothe and relax, or to invigorate the child, so improving his/her well-being and contributing to an easing of symptoms. The essences may be taken orally, used externally as massage oils or bathing emulsions, or inhaled as vapors. When breast-feeding mothers receive aromatherapy, the effect is said to be transmitted to their offspring.	**May be of some use** as a short-term treatment attempt aimed at soothing and relaxing. Some case reports claim efficacy; however, success is probably seen in only a proportion of children (*see* Placebo, page xxi). There is no evidence to substantiate claims that aromatherapy can be directed against specific ailments or symptoms.	**Suitable for DIY** with adult assistance. Qualified guidance is recommended. The effects of individual essential oils differ widely. **Risks:** Allergies or intolerance are possible. Some oils are carcinogenic in test systems and possibly in humans. Serious organic causes of illness must be ruled out before treatment is started.
Bioresonance therapy Bioresonance therapists use electrical devices in an attempt to discover the causes of illness and claim to be able to weaken or turn around pathogenic energies and disease related vibrations (*see* page 794). This treatment is frequently used for treating allergies.	**Of little use** Possibly acceptable as a short-term treatment attempt, especially for psychosomatic ailments when simpler, more established methods have been unsuccessful. Some case reports claim efficacy; however, success is probably seen, if at all, in only a small proportion of children (*see* Placebo, page xxi). Despite the popularity of this procedure for the treatment of allergies, its efficacy is unproven.	**Requires a qualified practitioner** Practitioners should be properly qualified and should propose a treatment plan. No credence should be given to anyone promising immediate or total success. **Risks:** Fairly unlikely. Serious organic causes of illness must be ruled out before treatment is started.

Treatment	Rating	Point of delivery/risks
Cell therapy Injecting or ingesting products extracted from the tissues of newborn animals or animal fetuses is said to have a rejuvenating and revitalizing effect and to enhance the healing of human tissues and organs (*see* page 796).	**Not advised** Based on present knowledge, there is inadequate evidence of the efficacy and mode of action of these costly and relatively risky procedures.	**Risks:** Injecting foreign proteins into the body can provoke (possibly fatal) allergic reactions. Also, pathogens such as those that cause bovine spongiform encephalopathy (BSE) or other serious infections may be introduced.
Chelation therapy The chelating agent EDTA (*see* page 800) is able, it is claimed, to bind calcareous deposits and heavy metals in the blood vessels. These are subsequently eliminated from the body.	**Not advised** Studies were unable to substantiate the claimed therapeutic efficacy of this risky procedure. The complementary therapy has nothing to do with the conventional method of dealing with heavy metal intoxications.	**Risks:** EDTA can cause a deficit of calcium and essential heavy metals and, in extreme cases, can lead to cardiac arrhythmia, respiratory failure, cramps, and death.
Electroacupuncture according to Voll By taking readings of the electrical conductivity of the skin (*see* page 802), therapists claim to be able to derive an insight into diseased areas of the body, pathogenic foci (*see* page 928), and stress factors (*see* Toxins, page 929). The factors presumed to underlie individual symptoms can then be addressed.	**Of little use** Possibly acceptable as a short-term, supportive treatment attempt for persistent complaints when simpler, more established methods have been unsuccessful. Some case reports claim efficacy; however, success is probably seen, if at all, in only a small proportion of children (*see* Placebo, page xxi).	**Requires a qualified practitioner** Practitioners should be properly qualified, should have considerable experience in the treatment of children, and should propose a treatment plan. **Risks:** A second opinion must always be obtained from a qualified physician before any attempt is made to "eliminate foci" (e.g. by surgery). Serious organic causes of illness must be ruled out before treatment is started.

Treatment	*Rating*	*Point of delivery/risks*
Electroneural therapy according to Croon According to the theory, readings taken at various reactive sites on the skin highlight diseased areas within the body. Based on these readings, targeted electrostimulative measures can be undertaken to address factors presumed to underlie individual symptoms (*see* page 806).	**Of little use** Possibly acceptable as a short-term, supportive treatment attempt for persistent complaints when simpler, more established methods have been unsuccessful. Some case reports claim efficacy; however, success is probably seen, if at all, in only a small proportion of children (*see* Placebo, page xxi).	**Requires a qualified practitioner** Practitioners should be properly qualified, should have considerable experience in the treatment of children, and should propose a treatment plan. **Risks:** Proponents themselves warn that treatment should not be given in acute inflammatory conditions. Serious organic causes of illness must be ruled out before treatment is started.
Eliminative methods, bloody Bloody cupping (*see* page 815) is said to alleviate pain, modulate the immune system, and improve the body's own regulatory systems.	**Not advised** There is no evidence that this invasive and, in children, particularly risky procedure has any effect.	**Risks:** Bloody cupping is painful and can cause infection and scarring. Furthermore, it should not be carried out in children with bleeding disorders.
Eliminative methods, unbloody Sweating (*see* page 877) and colonic irrigation (*see* page 819) are said to improve the body's own regulatory systems or to modulate the immune system (*see* page 10). Unbloody cupping (*see* page 817) is claimed to ease pain.	**Of little use** There is no evidence that the benefits outweigh the possible risks.	**Suitable for DIY** with adult assistance. Unbloody cupping requires the guidance of a qualified practitioner. **Risks:** Unlikely provided treatment is carried out competently. Unbloody cupping is painful and can damage the skin. Enemas can cause constipation and an electrolyte imbalance.

Treatment	_Rating_	_Point of delivery/risks_
Enzyme therapy The enzymes used (_see_ page 824) are said to dispel and destroy "immune complexes" that course in the blood and that are responsible, for instance, for causing autoimmune diseases and for sustaining inflammatory processes.	**Of little use** Some case reports claim efficacy for this little researched therapy; however, success is probably seen in only a small proportion of children (_see_ Placebo, page xxi).	**Requires a qualified practitioner** Practitioners should propose a treatment plan. Non-prescription preparations are suitable for do-it-yourself. **Risks:** Allergies or intolerance are possible. Serious organic causes of illness must be ruled out before treatment is started.
Flower remedies Flower remedies (_see_ page 828) are said to restore emotional balance and assist the body's psychic ability to heal itself.	**May be of some use** as a short-term treatment attempt aimed at soothing and relaxing. Case reports claim efficacy; however, success is probably seen in only a proportion of children (_see_ Placebo, page xxi).	**Suitable for DIY** with adult assistance. Qualified guidance is essential. **Risks:** Possible intolerance and allergies. Serious organic causes of illness must be ruled out before treatment is started.
Homeopathy Highly diluted (potentized) solutions (_see_ page 831) are believed to be able to redress vital energy imbalances. Organo- and functiotropic (_see_ page 883) homeopathy is claimed to be effective for dealing with symptoms.	**May be of some use** as a short-term treatment attempt for chronic conditions as a means of improving general well-being. Some case reports claim efficacy; however, success is probably seen in only a proportion of children (_see_ Placebo, page xxi).	**Requires a qualified practitioner** Homeopaths should be properly qualified, should have considerable experience in the treatment of children, and should propose a treatment plan. Ready-formulated preparations are suitable for do-it-yourself. **Risks:** Allergies and intolerance are possible. Serious organic causes of illness must be ruled out before treatment is started.

Treatment	Rating	Point of delivery/risks
Hypnosis and self-hypnosis In the relaxed and generally altered state of awareness that is induced in hypnosis (*see* page 837), physical and mental conditions can be addressed and pain possibly alleviated. Since young children cannot usually be hypnotized, this treatment is generally only used for children 12 years old and over.	**Of little use** Possibly acceptable as a short-term treatment attempt for persistent psychosomatic ailments or for behavioral, learning or eating disorders. Some case reports claim efficacy; however, success is probably seen in only a proportion of children (*see* Placebo, page xxi).	**Requires a qualified practitioner** Hypnotherapists should be properly qualified, should have considerable experience in the treatment of children, and should propose a treatment plan. **Risks:** Unlikely provided treatment is carried out competently. Serious organic causes of illness must be ruled out before treatment is started.
Magnetic field therapy The use of magnetic field generators, magnetic strips, bracelets, and other objects (*see* page 841) allegedly encourages cell metabolism and so eases a multitude of symptoms.	**Inappropriate** Based on present knowledge, there is inadequate evidence of the efficacy and mode of action of magnetic field therapy in children's ailments.	Operation of magnetic field equipment **requires a qualified practitioner**, who should have considerable experience in the treatment of children and should propose a treatment plan. **Risks:** Serious organic causes of illness must be ruled out before treatment is started.

Treatment	Rating	Point of delivery/risks
Manual therapies Chiropractors and osteopaths (*see* page 844) use a series of manipulations to realign allegedly displaced vertebrae. This is said to reduce pain, release energy blockages (*see* page 927), and eliminate factors that may be instrumental in the causation of a number of diseases and symptoms.	**Of little use** Possibly acceptable as a short-term treatment attempt, e.g. for acute wryneck or for chronic muscular tension, in children of school age. Some case reports claim efficacy for these potentially risky procedures; however, success is probably seen, if at all, in only a small proportion of children (*see* Placebo, page xxi).	**Requires a qualified practitioner** Practitioners should be properly qualified, should have considerable experience in the treatment of children, and should propose a treatment plan. **Risks:** Manipulation of the head and cervical vertebrae can cause serious injury. Serious organic causes of illness must be ruled out before treatment is started.
Massage Classical massage (*see* page 847) and lymphatic drainage (*see* page 850) can invigorate the patient, as well as ease muscular and emotional tension.	**May be of some use** as a short-term treatment attempt for chronic muscular tension. Some case reports claim efficacy; however, success is probably seen in only a proportion of children (*see* Placebo, page xxi).	**Suitable for DIY** by adult. Qualified guidance is essential. **Risks:** Some people are sensitive to manual stimuli. Serious organic causes of illness must be ruled out before treatment is started.

Treatment	Rating	Point of delivery/risks
Nutritional therapies An organic diet (*see* page 4) provides the body with essential and secondary plant nutrients that are believed to exercise a multitude of positive effects and to be capable, *inter alia*, of boosting the immune system (*see* page 10).	**Useful** as an individually directed supportive measure. Case reports suggest that an organic diet might exhibit a degree of efficacy in the treatment of skin conditions. Elimination diets may be of some assistance in identifying the causes of food induced allergies.	**Suitable for DIY** with adult assistance. Qualified guidance is essential. See your doctor before starting an elimination diet. **Risks:** Avoid imbalanced or intolerable diets. They can cause deficiencies with serious consequences. Children are particularly at risk. Infants and young children should not be put on special diets unless a doctor or pediatrician has been consulted. Serious organic causes of illness must be ruled out before treatment is started.
Physical therapies Warm and cold wraps, baths, or Kneipp treatments are said to hasten recovery from the common cold and to tone up the system (*see* pages 871–8). Saunas are said to improve the body's own regulatory systems or to modulate the immune system (*see* page 876).	**Useful** for toning up the system and as a treatment attempt for acute or chronic colds. Regular saunas, in moderation, are **useful** for boosting the immune system in children four years old and above. Case reports claim efficacy; however, success is probably seen in only a proportion of children (*see* Placebo, page xxi).	**Suitable for DIY** by an adult. Qualified guidance is recommended. These procedures should only be attempted in children four to five years old and over. **Risks:** Children should not perceive the temperatures chosen as unpleasant. Serious organic causes of illness must be ruled out before treatment is started.

Treatment	Rating	Point of delivery/risks
Probiotics The introduction of certain bacteria into the gut is claimed to bring the intestinal flora back into balance and to have a beneficial effect against various diseases and symptoms (*see* page 878).	**May be of some use** as a short-term treatment attempt for chronic skin conditions, rheumatoid arthritis, allergies, or digestive problems. Some case reports claim efficacy; however, success is probably seen in only a proportion of children (*see* Placebo, page xxi).	**Requires a qualified practitioner** Practitioners should be properly qualified, should have considerable experience in the treatment of children, and should propose a treatment plan. **Risks:** Fairly unlikely provided treatment is carried out competently. Serious organic causes of illness must be ruled out before treatment is started.
Reflex therapies Various forms of reflex zone massage (see page 883) can invigorate the patient, as well as ease muscular and emotional tension.	**Maybe of some use** as a short-term treatment attempt for chronic muscular tension. Some case reports claim efficacy; however, success is probably seen in only a proportion of children (*see* Placebo, page xxi).	**Requires a qualified practitioner** Practitioners should be properly qualified and should propose a treatment plan. **Risks:** Some people are sensitive to manual stimuli. Serious organic causes of illness must be ruled out before treatment is started.
Relaxation techniques Autogenic training (*see* page 888), muscle relaxation according to Jacobson (*see* page 893), and various biofeedback techniques (*see* page 891) are said to relieve muscle tension and inner unrest, and might be instrumental in helping the child to become more aware of his/her physical and emotional states.	**Useful** as a means of relaxing children about ten years old and above. Some case reports claim efficacy; however, success is probably seen in only a proportion of children (*see* Placebo, page xxi).	**Suitable for DIY** Once a sound understanding of the technique has been acquired from a trainer in group sessions or through individual tuition, children can perform exercises themselves. Therapists should be properly qualified. **Risks:** Fairly unlikely. Serious organic causes of illness must be ruled out by a doctor or pediatrician.

Treatment	Rating	Point of delivery/risks
TENS The use of low frequency electrical currents (*see* page 886) on the surface of the skin is said to release energy blockages (*see* page 927) and, as a reflex therapy, to reduce pain.	**May be of some use** as a short-term treatment attempt aimed at alleviating pain. Some case reports claim efficacy; however, success is probably seen in only a proportion of children (*see* Placebo, page xxi).	**Requires a qualified practitioner** Practitioners should be properly qualified, should have considerable experience in the treatment of children, and should propose a treatment plan. **Risks:** Some children react sensitively to electrical stimuli or rubber electrodes. Serious organic causes of illness must be ruled out before treatment is started.
Vitamins and trace elements The antioxidative properties of beta-carotene, vitamins C and E, and selenium are, it is supposed, instrumental in countering the formation of free radicals (*see* page 902), in boosting the body's own antioxidative defences, and in exercising a multitude of other beneficial effects (*see* page 900).	**Useful** in the form of an organic diet (*see* page 4) with a high content of fruit and vegetables. **Of little use** when given in the form of vitamin supplements. No definitive recommendations can be given based on present knowledge.	**Suitable for DIY** with adult assistance. Qualified guidance is recommended though not essential. **Risks:** Intolerance and overdosage are possible. Recent findings imply that beta-carotene might increase the risk of cancer.

Herbal remedies for children's ailments

Reliable data on children's dosages are available for only a very small number of the herbal remedies listed here. However, even at the quoted dosages, adverse effects are unlikely as long as the child shows no signs of hypersensitivity and the herb is used for a limited period only (approximately three to four weeks unless advised otherwise).

Active ingredient/preparation	Rating
Bilberries (*Vaccinium myrtillus*)	Taken orally, bilberries **may be of some use** a treatment attempt for unspecific acute diarrhea. Has an astringent action. **Daily dose:** 20–60g berries. **Individual dose:** To prepare a tea drink, pour 1 pint of water over 5–10g of berries, bring to a boil and simmer for 30 minutes, strain, and drink 1 cup slowly; alternatively, chew 1 dessertspoon of bilberries several times a day. Do not use for more than three to four days. Be sure to consult your doctor if the diarrhea persists. **Risks:** Bilberries are not known to have any serious side effects.
Carbo coffea (*Coffea arabica*)	Taken orally, this remedy **may be of some use** as a treatment attempt for unspecific acute diarrhea. It has an astringent action on the gut and supposedly binds organisms that cause diarrhea. **Daily dose:** 9g. **Individual dose:** Stir 3g in cold water or juice and drink. Use ready-formulated preparations as instructed by the manufacturer/prescriber. **Risks:** Carbo coffeae is not known to have any serious side effects.
Cowslip root (*Primula veris*)	Taken orally, cowslip **may be of some use** as a treatment attempt for respiratory catarrh. It has a mucolytic and expectorant action. **Daily dose:** 0.5–1.5g root. **Individual dose:** To prepare a decoction, bring 0.5g of root to a boil with 1 cup of cold water, allow it to stand for five minutes, and strain. Use ready-formulated preparations as instructed by the manufacturer/prescriber. **Risks:** Cowslip may cause stomach and bowel problems, and allergic reactions in sensitive individuals.

Active ingredient/preparation	Rating
Echinacea coneflowers (*Echinacea purpurea*)	**May be of some use** as an immune stimulant and as a supportive measure for treating recurrent infections of the lungs, respiratory tract, and bladder. **Dosage:** As instructed by the manufacturer/prescriber. **Risks:** Do not use in progressive systemic diseases such as tuberculosis, leukosis, collagenosis, multiple sclerosis, or if allergic.
Echinacea pallida **root**	**May be of some use** as a supportive attempt at immune stimulation therapy to fend off colds and flus. Preparations of *Echinacea angustifolia* (root and coneflowers) and *Echinacea purpurea* (root) are **of little use**. **Dosage:** As instructed by the manufacturer/prescriber. **Risks:** Do not use in progressive systemic diseases. Do not use for more than eight weeks.
Echinacin ointment (from *Echinacea pallida*)	**May be of some use** as an external treatment attempt for slow to heal surface wounds, possibly also as a treatment attempt for skin allergies. Echinacin ointment is a vulnerary and possibly an immune stimulant. **Dosage:** As instructed by the manufacturer/prescriber. **Risks:** Allergic reactions are possible.
Fennel honey (*Foeniculum vulgare*)	**May be of some use** as a mucolytic. Contains approximately 0.5g fennel oil per 2 lbs honey. **Daily dose:** 10–20g, eg in hot milk or tea. Use ready-formulated preparations as instructed by the manufacturer/prescriber. **Risks:** Fennel honey is not known to have any serious side effects, though gastric or intestinal complaints may occasionally occur.

Active ingredient/preparation	Rating

Flea seeds (dark psyllium)
(*Plantago psyllium* and *indica*)

Taken orally, flea seeds **may be of some use** as a treatment attempt for constipation and irritable bowel. They help regulate the bowel muscles. Take with plenty of fluid.
Daily dose: 10–30g.
Individual dose: 3–5g to be taken with 1 glass of cold water or juice. Use ready-formulated preparations as instructed by the manufacturer/prescriber.
Risks: Flea seeds can cause allergic reactions. Not to be taken by persons with narrowing of the esophagus or of the gastrointestinal tract.

German camomile flowers
(*Chamomilla recutita*)

Useful as a treatment attempt for inflammation and for treating wounds. Use for drinking, add it to bathwater and use it in wraps. German camomile is an anti-inflammatory, antispasmodic, and antibacterial.
Daily dose: 10–12g dried flowers.
Individual dose: 3g to 5fl ozs hot water. Drink several times a day. Alternatively, apply as a wrap or compress, or add to bathwater.
Risks: Allergic reactions are possible in rare cases.

Horse chestnut extract
(*Aesculus hippocastanum*)

May be of some use as an external treatment attempt for soft tissue swellings and swollen, contused ankles.
Dosage: As instructed by the manufacturer/prescriber.
Risks: Horse chestnut extract can cause itchiness and/or gastrointestinal irritation.

Horsetail
(*Equisetum arvense*)

May be of some use as an external treatment attempt for superficial wounds that are slow to heal. The extract is useful as an addition to bathwater and also for eczema and neurodermatitis.
Dosage: For a partial immersion bath, dilute 2–4oz to approximately $^1/_2$–1 gallon of hot water, then add to the bathwater. Use ready-formulated preparations as instructed by the manufacturer/prescriber.
Risks: Used externally, horsetail is not known to have any serious side effects.

Active ingredient/preparation	Rating

Iceland moss
(*Cetraria islandica, Lichen islandicus*)

Taken orally, Iceland moss **may be of some use** as a treatment attempt for an irritable dry cough. Has a soothing and mildly antibacterial action.
Daily dose: 4–6g herb.
Individual dose: Pour 5fl oz of boiling water over 2g of shredded moss and infuse. Use ready-formulated preparations as instructed by the manufacturer/prescriber.
Risks: Frequent use of Iceland moss pastilles can cause gastric and intestinal problems.

Ivy leaves, ivy leaf extract
(*Hedera helix*)

Taken orally, ivy leaves and extract **may be of some use** as a treatment attempt for respiratory catarrh, for symptomatic treatment of chronic inflammation of the bronchial system and as a supportive measure in the treatment of whooping cough. Antispasmodic and expectorant action.
Daily dose: 0.3g herb.
Individual dose: Pour 1 cup of hot water over 0.1g of herb and infuse. Use ready-formulated preparations as instructed by the manufacturer/prescriber.
Risks: Gastric and intestinal problems are possible.

Kava root
(*Piper methysticum*)

Taken orally, kava **may be of some use** as a treatment attempt for nervous anxiety, tension, and restlessness, also possibly for nocturnal bedwetting. It must be borne in mind, however, that bedwetting is often a sign of emotional or mental stress, so the use of drugs and herbal remedies may not constitute the right approach.
Dosage: As instructed by the manufacturer/prescriber.
Risks: Not to be taken for longer than three months except on a doctor's advice. Even in recommended dosages, kava affects vision and the ability to react. Prolonged use may result in a yellowing of the skin, allergic skin reactions, difficulty in focusing the eyes and pupil dilation.

Active ingredient/preparation	Rating

Lemon balm leaves
(*Melissa officinalis*)

Taken orally, lemon balm **may be of some use** as an external treatment attempt for cold sores (*Herpes simplex*). So far there have not been sufficient scientific studies that show lemon balm to be effective.
Dosage: As instructed by the manufacturer/prescriber.
Risks: Lemon balm is not known to have any serious side effects.

Linseed
(*Linum usitatissimum*)

Taken orally, linseed **may be of some use** as a treatment attempt for constipation and diverticulitis. It has a demulcent action.
Daily dose: 15–20g of seeds.
Individual dose: Take 5g of seeds with plenty of liquid. Use ready-formulated preparations as instructed by the manufacturer/prescriber.
Risks: May cause other drugs taken simultaneously to be absorbed more slowly. Not to be taken by persons with any form of intestinal obstruction or occlusion.

Licorice root
(*Glycyrrhiza glabra*)

May be of some use as a treatment attempt for upper respiratory catarrh. Has an expectorant and antitussive action.
Daily dose: 5–15g root.
Individual dose: For a decoction, cover 3–5g of root with 1 cup of cold water, bring to a boil, simmer gently for 15 minutes, and strain. Syrup: take ½ to 1 teaspoon with water before meals.
Risks: Prolonged use and high dosages may lead to edema, potassium deficiency, and high blood pressure. Do not take for longer than four to six weeks without consulting a doctor.

Mallow leaves and flowers
(*Malva sylvestris* and *neglecta*)

Taken orally, mallow **may be of some use** for an irritable dry cough. It has a soothing effect.
Daily dose: 5g herb (leaves and flowers).
Individual dose: To prepare a tea drink, pour 5fl oz of cold water over 1–2g of dried herb, bring to a boil, simmer gently for ten minutes, strain, and drink. Sweeten with honey and add lemon juice, for instance.
Risks: Mallow is not known to have any serious side effects.

Active ingredient/preparation	*Rating*

Marigold flowers
(*Calendula officinalis*)

May be of some use as a treatment attempt for superficial wounds that are slow to heal (apply externally or drink). Marigold is a vulnerary and anti-inflammatory. Marigold leaves receive a negative assessment due to their lack of efficacy.
Daily dose: 2–5g herb.
Individual dose: To prepare an infusion (for drinking or as a poultice), pour hot water over 1–2g of florets, allow to infuse for ten minutes and strain. Use ready-formulated preparations as instructed by the manufacturer/prescriber.
Risks: Marigold can cause allergic skin reactions.

Marsh mallow root and leaves
(*Althaea officinalis*)

Taken orally, marsh mallow **may be of some use** as a treatment attempt for a dry cough. Has a soothing action.
Daily dose: 5g dried leaf or 6g dried root.
Individual dose: 1 cup of cold water to 1–2g of dried leaf or root. Allow to stand for 2 hours, then heat and drink. Use ready-formulated preparations as instructed by the manufacturer/prescriber.
Risks: Marsh mallow may slow down the absorption and action of other drugs taken simultaneously.

Meadowsweet flowers and leaves
(*Filipendula ulmaria*)

Taken orally, meadowsweet **may be of some use** as a supportive treatment attempt for pain, fever, and the common cold.
Daily dose: 2.5–3.5g meadowsweet flowers or 4–5g leaves.
Individual dose: 1.5g of flowers or leaves to 5fl oz of boiling water. Use ready-formulated preparations as instructed by the manufacturer/prescriber.
Risks: Meadowsweet should not be taken by children known to be sensitive to salicylates (e.g. if they are allergic to aspirin), and should be used with caution by children with asthma.

Active ingredient/preparation	*Rating*
Mint oil (from *Mentha arvense*)	As a volatile oil, mint oil **may be of some use** for the external treatment of contusion pain. Can also be used to massage away headaches. Has a cooling and relaxing effect. **Dosage:** As instructed by the manufacturer/prescriber. **Risks:** May cause severe skin irritation. Do not apply to the nose and face of infants and young children.
Mullein (*Verbascum densiflorum*)	**May be of some use** as a treatment attempt for catarrh of the airways attended by coughing. Has a soothing, expectorant action. **Daily dose:** 3–4g herb. **Individual dose:** Pour 5fl oz of boiling water over 1g of herb and infuse. Sweeten with honey, for instance, and add lemon juice. **Risks:** Possible gastric intolerance.
Oil of cloves (from *Caryophylli atheroleum*)	As a rinse (1–2 drops in a glass of warm water), oil of cloves **may be of some use** as a treatment attempt for inflammation of the mucosa of the mouth and throat; also for acute painkilling from a toothache. It has a local analgesic and antispasmodic action, as well as inhibiting bacterial growth. To apply, soak cottonwool or a cotton swab in undiluted volatile oil and apply to the painful tooth as required. It may sting when applied. **Risks:** Can have an irritant or numbing effect on the surrounding gum.

Active ingredient/preparation	*Rating*
Pale psyllium (*Plantago ovata* and *ispaghula*)	Taken orally, pale psyllium **may be of some use** as a treatment attempt for constipation and conditions requiring a looser stool; and as a supportive measure in diarrhea and irritable bowel syndrome. **Dosage:** As instructed by the manufacturer/prescriber. **Risks:** Can lead to hypersensitivities and may slow down absorption of various drugs (take half to one hour apart). Not to be used in persons with intestinal occlusion, poor diabetic control, or pathological narrowing of the gastrointestinal tract. In insulin-dependent diabetics, consider reducing the insulin dose (ask your doctor). Consult a doctor if diarrhea persists (for more than three to four days).
Pansy (*Viola tricolor*)	Pansy (or heartsease) **may be of some use** as a treatment attempt. For external or internal use in mild scaly skin infections and cradlecap. **Daily dose:** 4–5g dried herb. **Individual dose:** Pour 5fl oz of hot water over 1.5g of dried herb and infuse; do this three times a day. Also for poultices, rinses, or baths. **Risks:** Allergic reactions are possible.
Peppermint oil (from *Mentha piperita*)	**May be of some use** as a cooling external treatment for contusion pains or as a remedy for massaging away a headache. It has a cooling effect. **Daily dose:** 3–4 drops in water (for inhalation) or a few drops for massaging. Use ready-formulated preparations as instructed by the manufacturer/prescriber. **Risks:** Gastric problems and allergic skin reactions are possible. Do not apply to the nose and face of infants and young children.
Pumpkin seeds (*Cucurbita pepo*)	Taken orally, pumpkin seeds **may be of some use** as a treatment attempt for an irritable bladder. Children taking pumpkin seeds must be kept under regular medical review. **Dosage:** As instructed by the manufacturer/prescriber. **Risks:** Gastric and intestinal problems are possible.

Active ingredient/preparation	Rating

St. John's wort
(*Hypericum perforatum*)

Taken orally, St. John's wort **may be of some use** as an attempt to treat bedwetting, though its claimed beneficial effect has not been fully substantiated. St. John's wort is otherwise used for nervous system problems, such as muscle pain, depression, and anxiety.
Daily dose: 2–4g dried herb. **Individual dose:** Infuse 1–1.5g of dried herb with 1 cup of boiling hot water. Use ready-formulated preparations as instructed by the manufacturer/prescriber.
Risks: Photosensitization (persons with a light complexion should avoid bright sunlight after taking St. John's wort, or they may suffer allergic skin irritation).

St. John's wort oil
(*Hypericum perforatum*)

May be of some use as an external treatment attempt for first-degree burns. The oil has an anti-inflammatory action. Apply diluted to inflamed or injured skin.
Risks: Photosensitization following prolonged use (persons with a light complexion should avoid bright sunlight after taking St. John's wort, or they may suffer allergic skin irritation).

Sundew
(*Drosera rotundifolia*)

Taken orally, sundew **may be of some use** as a treatment attempt for whooping cough and dry cough. It relaxes the airways and relieves irritation.
Daily dose: 3g herb.
Individual dose: Pour 5fl oz of hot water over 1–1.5g of flowerheads and infuse. Use ready-formulated preparations as instructed by the manufacturer/prescriber.
Risks: Gastric intolerance is possible.

Active ingredient/preparation	*Rating*

Thuja
(*Thuja occidentalis*)

May be of some use, as it encourages the body's defence system. It may be used, for instance, as a supportive treatment for malignant tumors. Parts used: dried young twigs.
Dosage: As instructed by the manufacturer/prescriber.
Risks: Cramps, visual disturbance, cardiac arrhythmia, and symptoms of kidney and liver damage are possible. Contains thujone, which is toxic, so do not exceed manufacturers' recommended doses (see package labels and inserts).

Thyme, common
(*Thymus vulgaris*)

May be of some use as a treatment attempt for symptoms of bronchitis, whooping cough, and catarrh of the upper airways. Has an antispasmodic, expectorant, and antibacterial action.
Daily dose: 10g herb.
Individual dose: Pour 1 cup of hot water over 2.5g of dried herb and infuse. Use ready-formulated preparations as instructed by the manufacturer/prescriber.
Risks: Gastric intolerance is possible.

Uva-ursi leaves
(*Arctostaphylos uva-ursi*)

May be of some use as a treatment attempt for inflammation of the efferent urinary tract; also as a treatment attempt for an irritable bladder. Uva-ursi has an antibacterial and antimicrobial action.
Daily dose: 10g of dried leaves.
Individual dose: Pour 5fl oz of hot water over 3g of dried leaves, infuse for five minutes, and strain. Drink 1 cup several times a day between meals. Use ready-formulated preparations as instructed by the manufacturer/prescriber.
Risks: Nausea, vomiting, skin irritation, and shortness of breath are possible. Not to be taken by children under 12 years. Not to be taken with agents that acidify the urine. Use for a maximum of one week and not more than five times a year.

Active ingredient/preparation	Rating

Uzara root
(*Xysmalobium undulatum*)

Taken orally, uzara root **may be of some use** as a treatment attempt for acute diarrhea. **Risks:** Not to be taken with digitalis glycosides (which are used for treating a weak heart). Not to be taken for longer than three to four days without consulting your doctor. Be sure to see your doctor if the diarrhea persists.

Valerian root
(*Valeriana officinalis*)

Taken orally, valerian is **useful** as an attempt to promote natural sleep and relieve worry. **Daily dose:** For a tea drink, infuse 2–3g of fresh or dried root with boiling water. Tincture: 15–20 drops one to three times daily. Full bath: 4oz fresh or dried root to 2 quarts of hot water, then strain and add to the bathwater. Use ready-formulated preparations as instructed by the manufacturer/prescriber.
Risks: Headaches, restlessness, and cardiac effects are possible. Only *Valeriana officinalis* should be taken. Ready-formulated preparations frequently contain 3–5 percent so-called valepotriates, which reportedly cause cell damage, especially in the liver.

Willow bark, willow bark extract
(*Salix fragilis*)

Taken internally, willow bark and willow bark extract **may be of some use** as a treatment attempt for fevers and headaches. Willow bark is a febrifuge, analgesic, and anti-inflammatory agent. **Daily dose:** 6–12g bark. **Individual dose:** 2g of bark to 5fl oz of boiling water. Use ready-formulated preparations as instructed by the manufacturer/prescriber.
Risks: Skin reactions and allergies (asthma attacks) are possible. Do not use in febrile infections or chickenpox.

Yarrow flowers and leaves
(*Achillea millefolium*)

Only useful for adding to bathwater in the supportive treatment of inflammation in the genital region or for wounds that are slow to heal. For baths use in the form of an extract or as leaves and flowers. **Dosage:** 2oz dried herb or 1oz yarrow leaves to 9fl oz of hot water, made up to a full-immersion bath.
Risks: Contact dermatitis and allergic skin reactions are possible.

Active ingredient/preparation	*Rating*

Yeast dried
(*Saccharomyces cerevisiae*)

Taken orally, dried yeast **may be of some use** as a treatment attempt for acute diarrhea and for preventing "travel tummy" and diarrhea often associated with tube feeding. **Dosage:** For children over two years and adults five days before departure, 250–500mg daily (prophylaxis), 250–500mg daily (therapy). For diarrhea from tube feeding: 500mg per quart nutrient solution. Use ready-formulated preparations as instructed by the manufacturer/prescriber. **Risks:** Has a hypertensive action when taken with MAO inhibitors (type of antidepressant drug). Not to be taken by persons known to be hypersensitive to yeast. It can cause flatulence. Occasionally there will be hypersensitivity with itchiness and Quincke's edema.

PART 2

The therapies used in complementary medicine

Acupressure and shiatsu

Rating
Useful as short-term attempt to treat headaches, neck and back pains, tension, nausea, vomiting, and psychosomatic illness.
May be of some use for inducing relaxation and providing relief from colds and diarrhea.
Not advised as the sole treatment for persistent complaints unless a conventional physician has diagnosed the patient's condition and made a proper risk–benefit assessment.

Method

Acupressure and its Japanese variant shiatsu are point-massaging techniques that are designed to soothe, invigorate, or provide pain relief.

Rationale and historical perspective

Acupressure is now popular in the West as a do-it-yourself treatment for fatigue and as a means of relaxation and disease prevention. Like shiatsu, acupressure applies pressure not only to selected points along so-called meridians (*see* page 772) but also to sites of pain and to associated trigger points (*see* page 929). Applying pressure to and massaging these points is thought to rebalance energy forces that have been thrown out of kilter by stress, weakness, or an unhealthy lifestyle. This, it is claimed, reinforces the body's self-healing powers and relieves symptoms of illness. While acupressure is generally applied only with the fingertips and nails, shiatsu practitioners often use the hands, elbows and feet to apply pressure—techniques that can be painful.

How it works

Acupressure and shiatsu share the same theoretical background as acupuncture (*see* page 772).

Indications

Many of the proponents of acupressure and shiatsu maintain that these treatments are effective against virtually any type of complaint. In the West, the complaints for which they are most frequently administered are nausea, vomiting, travel sickness, sleeplessness, and pain—especially in the head, neck, and back. The treatments are also used palliatively to provide relief in other conditions such as cancer.

Reputable practitioners use acupressure and shiatsu primarily to treat reversible conditions, i.e. those where there is a mild disturbance rather than a full functional breakdown.

Proof it works

So far proof that acupressure and shiatsu work has only been adduced for a small number of indications. The results of the first controlled clinical studies to be undertaken are now beginning to appear. Claims that acupressure is efficacious in nausea, vomiting and travel sickness are supported by good evidence from controlled clinical trials. For insomnia and pain it probably only works for a proportion of patients treated.

Risks, cautions, and contraindications

When carried out by an expert, acupressure and shiatsu carry few risks. The treatments should not be attempted, however, when the skin is inflamed or diseased, nor in patients with cardiovascular disorders, tumors or osteoporosis. During pregnancy, care must be taken not to stimulate points that are associated with the uterus. Regular use of acupressure or shiatsu to treat persistent complaints carries with it the risk that symptoms which should be interpreted as a warning of a serious disease will be eradicated and that, as a consequence, the opportunity to undertake more appropriate measures against that disease will be lost.

Duration of treatment

Depending on the symptoms, anything from a one-off treatment to lifelong therapy (e.g. self-treatment of migraines) may be required.

Finding the right therapist

Therapists offering acupressure and shiatsu should be professionally qualified. Although in most cases this will give a certain assurance as to the standard of treatment that the patient can expect, it will not necessarily follow that the treatment given will be the most appropriate for dealing with the patient's condition.

A reputable therapist will generally not offer treatment for a persistent complaint until the patient has consulted a doctor for a conventional diagnosis. With the patient he/she will define a treatment goal and propose a short-term treatment plan (*see* page xxiii) to be used to check the efficacy of the particular acupressure or shiatsu treatment. No credence should be given to therapists promising an immediate or complete cure (*see* Practitioner checklist, page xxv). Once acupressure techniques have been learned, they are also suitable for self-treatment or for massaging a partner. Professional guidance is advised, though not absolutely necessary.

A number of professional foundations exist for acupressure and shiatsu. Courses in acupressure are often available from organizations that promote acupressure or traditional Chinese medicine (*see* page 895), as well as at various adult education centers.

Point-massaging techniques are often carried out by masseurs, who should at least have a formal qualification in massaging.

Acupuncture

> **Rating**
>
> **Useful** as short-term attempt to treat pain, tension, and vomiting; also for limiting the amounts of painkillers used.
>
> **May be of some use** as a supportive treatment during rehabilitation following a stroke, during withdrawal therapy (heroin, alcohol, nicotine), in asthma, tinnitus (ringing in the ears), angina pectoris pain, and premenstrual syndrome (PMS). Acceptable as a means of addressing energy blockage (*see* page 927).
>
> **Not advised** as the sole treatment for persistent complaints unless a conventional physician has diagnosed the patient's condition and made a proper risk–benefit assessment.

Method

Inserting needles into acupuncture points along special channels (meridians) throughout the body is said to free blocked energy (*see* Energy blockage, page 927) and provide relief from a wide range of symptoms. Some patients find acupuncture a painful procedure.

Rationale and historical perspective

In the Western world acupuncture is probably the most popular and well-known of the oriental medical procedures, having been in and out of vogue ever since the 17th century. In traditional Chinese medicine (TCM) (*see* page 895), where it has its origins, it has always had its place. In complementary medicine it is currently Europe's "number-one hit."

Acupuncture techniques have been handed down through the millennia in a metaphorical language often perceived as alien to the Western way of thinking. Chinese acupuncturists classify pathological symptoms based on a system of eight diagnostic criteria arranged in four interacting pairs: yin and yang, internal and external, fullness and emptiness, hot and cold.

The type of stimulus needed to effect treatment is determined individually for each patient. If there is an "excess" (fullness, hotness, blockage), a strong stimulus is required; this is created by inserting the acupuncture needles slowly and withdrawing them quickly (to draw out the excess), a technique which is supposed to have a soothing, "cooling" effect. In the case of a "deficit" (emptiness, coldness, fragility), a gently invigorating, "warming" stimulus is required; this is achieved by inserting the needles quickly and withdrawing them slowly (to impart fullness).

According to traditional beliefs, the vital energy chi circulates through all living things in channels or meridians each of which is connected to a principal organ or body structure to form an invisible circulatory system. Disease and illness are believed to be caused when the circulation of chi becomes blocked and stagnant, throwing the body out of balance and making it disharmonious. Disharmony can be corrected by a change of lifestyle and through stimulation of acupoints to encourage the body's self-healing powers.

In acupuncture, the twelve principal meridians (the kidney, bladder, liver, gallbladder, heart, small intestine, spleen, stomach, lung, colon, circulation, and triple burner meridians), each of which is linked to a vital organ, are arranged as yin and yang dualities; there are also a series of secondary meridians. The principal meridians are linked to form an endless chain through which chi flows in a 24-hour cycle. These meridian linkages are said to generate five "elements", "functional cycles" or "phrases of change" in the body, which again are associated with various organs. Chinese doctors formerly used golden or silver needles to regulate the flow of chi along these energy pathways, as precious metals were thought to possess special powers. Western acupuncturists generally use flexible steel needles .01–.02 inch thick and ¹⁄₂–8 inches long. Some acupuncturists stimulate the acupoints additionally with heat, beads, small rods, or clips, or intensify the effect with electrical impulses. Many schools have their own distinctive needling and twirling techniques, the differences being seen not only in terms of the equipment they use but also in the number of meridian points they employ and the positions of these on the body. An acupuncture point, when stimulated, can elicit a general, local, or specific response.

Some schools consider the principal organs of the human body to be linked to specific points on the head, mouth, nose, hand, and foot, so treatment can be effected through pressing or needling at these points.

Acupuncture has now achieved considerable international diversity and its Western proponents have added tremendous variety to the ancient technique. There are now two conflicting cultures. While TCM-oriented therapists insist on maintaining the authenticity of the centuries-old concepts of disease, diagnosis, and therapy, those who advocate the Western style of acupuncture aim to see it used to complement the principles of modern mainstream medicine. Many positions lie between these two extremes.

TCM-style acupuncture

TCM defines illness not as the end-product of a chain of circumstances and events but as a discrete process that can be influenced by encouraging the body to heal itself, e.g. by rebalancing the flow of chi energy. Chinese diagnosis is always a prelude to differentiated, individually attuned therapies; the chosen acupoints, as also the needling and stimulation techniques used, can change from one treatment session to the next. In present-day China acupuncturists practice their art, as indeed their ancestors before them did, not as a monotherapy but in association with other therapeutic techniques, preventive as well as curative—possibly including some mainstream conventional ones.

Western acupuncture

Western acupuncture blends Chinese methods with empirical techniques that have been developed for Western patients. In other words, it is a pragmatic combination of various acupuncture concepts and techniques plus notions of disease and diagnosis that are accepted in modern mainstream medicine. For example, Western acupuncture recognizes various acupoint constellations for typically Western diagnoses. In order to counter the criticism that acupuncture is merely a form of suggestion, its proponents are in the process of applying modern scientific principles in an attempt not only to show empirically that their treatment works but also to gain an insight into *how* it works.

Some variants of acupuncture

Moxibustion

Moxibustion is a form of treatment in which a combination of heat and aromatic substances applied to specific sites or broader areas along the meridians is said to penetrate deep into the body and produce an invigorating and "warming" effect. The acupuncture points are stimulated by burning moxa, a cotton-like preparation of the dried leaves of Chinese wormwood, at the exposed tip of the acupuncture needle. Patients can self-administer the moxibustion technique provided that an acupuncturist has first marked the appropriate application points on the skin with a marker.

A variety of methods can be used:

- Moxa cigars are sticks of moxa rolled up in thin paper. The practitioner brings the glowing tip of a cigar to within $^1/_4$ inch of the acupuncture point and, once the patient has clearly sensed the heat from the cigar, moves the tip away again slightly from the skin. This procedure is repeated until the application points visibly redden.
- During treatment with moxa cones, a slice of fresh ginger is placed on the skin to act as a heat insulator. Fresh ginger is said to create an additional warming effect by releasing its own stimulants. The moxa cone is placed on the ginger and lit. As soon as the patient feels the heat, the moxa cone is moved on to the next point.

Moxibustion is used primarily to treat chronic forms of

bronchitis, bronchial asthma, diarrhea, depression, and debilitation following chronic illness.

Ear acupuncture

Ear acupuncture is based on the idea that the organs of the human body are linked to specific regions on the earlobe and can be treated by various needling or pressure techniques. Stimuli are provided by acupuncture needles, small beads, or glass rods. Certain types of needles can be implanted and left *in situ* for several days. They resemble small drawing pins, are attached to the chosen acupoints with small strips of bandage and are activated by pressing or twirling.

The various forms of ear acupuncture are used mainly to treat pain and soreness caused by fractures or other injuries, rheumatism, neuralgia, phantom pain, and circulatory problems. Ear acupuncture is also claimed to be beneficial in the treatment of psychological problems and addictions.

Modern forms of acupuncture

Electroacupuncture is a variation in which an electrical device is used to deliver a very small current through the needle to assist point stimulation. This method is now widely used to treat chronic pain. Transcutaneous electric nerve stimulation (TENS) (*see* page 886) is another technique in which very small currents are delivered to the patient. Certain elements of electroacupuncture according to Voll (*see* page 802) are also based in part on this principle.

Injection acupuncture uses a variety of materials, ranging from local anesthetics to the patient's own urine, that are injected into acupuncture points to alleviate pain or modulate the immune system.

Since the 1960s, needles have given way in some cases to lasers, particularly for children and needle-shy adults.

How acupuncture works

There are a number of possible explanations, some hypothetical, some empirical.

- Groups studying pain have shown that needling activates a system of pain control partly via the neural pathways and partly by inducing the body to release its own natural painkillers—endorphins. These processes mostly occur in the central nervous system and influence many of the body's functions and emotional states.
- Inserting needles at the relevant sites has been shown to reduce tension measurably in muscles associated with those sites.
- Acupuncture is able to produce a soothing and relaxing effect on the psyche and the autonomic nervous system. Some practitioners use the technique for patients with emotional blockages to initiate or support psychotherapy.
- Acupuncture is claimed to improve the circulation via the autonomic nervous system.

Research so far conducted has failed to show how the acupoints differ in terms of their metabolism and tissue structures from other, comparable, sites.

Indications

Some therapists maintain that acupuncture can be used to treat virtually any complaint. Responsible therapists use acupuncture primarily to treat reversible conditions, i.e. those where there is a mild disturbance rather than a full functional breakdown.

The World Health Organization in Geneva has drawn up a catalog of more than 40 conditions which, it suggests, can be treated with acupuncture techniques. The catalog includes infectious diseases such as acute conjunctivitis and bronchitis, and conditions such as retinitis, glaucoma, and intestinal occlusion. It should be appreciated, however, that the WHO document was conceived not as a list of acknowledged indications but rather as an attempt to suggest a widely available, low-cost treatment for use in certain countries faced with problems of poverty and a general lack of medical facilities.

In the West, acupuncture is mostly used to treat pain, mild psychosomatic and functional disorders and so-called energy blockages (*see* page 927). It is also being used by an increasing number of doctors to treat asthma, non-specific neck and back pains, rheumatism, and urinary tract problems.

Proof it works

There have so far been several hundred controlled clinical studies (*see* page xix) and other research projects into acupuncture; their quality has differed widely. To these can be added a considerable number of outcome studies and case reports (*see* page xx), as well as results of countless Russian and Chinese studies which have up until recently remained inaccessible to Western researchers.

Some of these trials suggest that acupuncture is effective for headaches, back pain, and aching joints. There is also evidence to suggest that it can perhaps be of some benefit in the treatment of addictions and various psychosomatic disorders. However, the results are often contradictory. It generally remains to be explained, for instance, how various practical aspects (e.g. the selection of acupuncture points, the duration of therapy, the interval between treatment sessions) can affect the treatment outcome. Research into the different ways in which the different acupuncture techniques work has been inconclusive. In many cases questions as to the degree of efficacy that was allegedly achieved in various indications are largely unresolved.

Some experts say that, even though there does seem to be sufficient anecdotal support for the efficacy of acupuncture in quite a range of indications, there is still just as little scientific proof *that* it works as there is explanation of *how* it works. They argue that the sometimes spectacular results achieved with acupuncture may be due to an impressive placebo effect (*see* page xxi).

Risks, cautions, and contraindications

Lasting ill effects are probably rare, providing that a competent needling technique is used, the therapist has an appropriate knowledge of anatomy, and strict hygiene rules are followed. Nevertheless, complications do sometimes occur during or after acupuncture.

- Patients who are emotionally fragile or of a weak disposition are prone to fainting during the insertion of the needles. This complication affects about 5 percent of all patients during their initial acupuncture session(s). Patients should therefore lie down to have the needles inserted.
- Deep needling techniques can cause injury to organs such as the heart, lungs, bladder, spinal cord, nerves, eyes, and blood vessels. Also, acupuncture needles can break, requiring surgery to remove the fragments.
- Although acupuncturists usually deny this, there *is* an infection risk, e.g. with a hepatitis virus, if needles have not been properly sterilized. Patients should insist on the proper use of disposable needles.
- Acupuncture should not be attempted in cases of severe polyneuropathy or with parapalegic patients, nor following certain forms of neurosurgery and with persons with massive tissue changes caused by radiotherapy.
- Acupuncture is inappropriate for patients with bleeding disorders.
- In pregnancy the stimulation of acupoints associated with hormone regulation might cause complications.
- Semi-permanent ear needles can cause local infections owing to limited perfusion of the earlobe cartilage with blood.
- Moxibustion can burn the skin and must not be used on the face and head, nor near mucous membranes. Acupuncturists themselves advise against using moxibustion in febrile conditions, acute infection, high blood pressure, bleeding and menstruation; also, for patients who are highly agitated or suffering from insomnia.

Duration of treatment

Five to ten treatment sessions are suggested for acute disorders, 15 to 20 for chronic ones. The frequency of sessions will be set individually and depend on the therapist and the disorder being treated: sometimes several times a week to start with, usually reducing to weekly sessions. When symptoms are chronic or recurrent, therapists suggest that the treatment is repeated every three to six months.

Finding the right therapist

An acupuncturist should be qualified and accredited with a professional body. In most cases accreditation will give some assurance as to the quality of training received and the standard of treatment that the patient can expect, but will not necessarily ensure that the therapy given is appropriate to the patient's condition. A reputable therapist will generally not offer treatment until the patient has consulted a physician for a conventional diagnosis. With the patient he/she will define a treatment goal and propose a treatment plan (*see* page xxiii) to be used to monitor the patient's progress. No credence should be given to therapists promising a quick or complete cure (*see* Practitioner checklist, page xxv).

Responsible acupuncturists will insert needles with the patient lying down (at least during the initial sessions), as the treatment may cause susceptible persons to faint. To prevent infections, the acupuncturist should use disposable needles.

Anthroposophical medicine (AM)

Rating

Certain therapeutic "packages" **may be of some use** as a short-term attempt to treat chronic ailments (particularly those of the digestive system), rheumatism, allergies, skin diseases, and psychiatric disorders; also, AM **may be of some use** as a supportive treatment for cancer.

Not advised as the sole treatment for persistent complaints unless a conventional physician has diagnosed the patient's condition and made a proper risk–benefit assessment.

Method

Anthroposophical therapies involve the use of various mineral, vegetable and animal derived drugs, mostly in homeopathic dilutions (*see* Homeopathy, page 831) as well as special diets, "curative eurhythmy," art therapy and psychotherapeutic approaches.

Rationale and historical perspective

In the early 1920s, Rudolf Steiner (1861–1925), the founder of anthroposophy and the Waldorf School movement, propounded a new approach to human medicine in association with Dutch physician Ita Wegman. They drew on the philosophical doctrine of anthroposophy which, as well as incorporating certain scientific elements, has esoteric and religious components, including the idea of reincarnation. With their novel therapeutic concept Steiner and Wegman were aiming to complement orthodox medicine, not fight against it.

Steiner's notions of disease and healing represent a discrete system of thought with its own terminology which, for anyone not conversant with anthroposophy, can be difficult to comprehend. Steiner considered human existence to consist of four constituent elements: the physical body (the tangible, flesh and blood entity), the etheric body (the force that drives us), the astral body (feelings), and the ego (human spirit).

- In Steiner's plan the physical body is governed by the laws of physics and chemistry and is seen as representing the mineral kingdom in man.
- The etheric body or vital body is a superordinate level of material forces; it gives the physical body its powers of nutrition, growth, regeneration, and reproduction, and represents the vegetable kingdom in man.
- The third body, the astral body or soul body, exists as the vector of consciousness. It represents the animal kingdom.
- The ego or human spirit generates the force that binds the human form together, the force that makes us conscious of our own being and individuality.

In the philosophy of Steiner and Wegman, the human form consists of three main bodily regions:

- the upper pole, with it focus around the skull, the sense organs and central nervous system; the "nerve–sense system," located in this upper pole, is the instrument of perception, thought, and consciousness
- the lower pole, which includes the abdomen and extremities and is the region of movement, of metabolism, and of exchanges, as exemplified by the digestive, excretory, and reproductive apparatus and by the muscles; the "motor–digestive system," located here, is the instrument of the will
- a middle or unifying region that contains the heart and lungs; this is the region that reintroduces harmony and balance between the upper and lower poles and is the center of feeling or affect.

This tripartite system is repeated throughout the physical being. Any upset in its balance causes illness.

Illness, in the anthroposophical interpretation, is not simply the failure of an organ to function as it should. Rather, illness occurs when a natural process encroaches into the wrong pole or region and equilibration cannot be achieved through the rhythmic healing powers of the middle, harmonizing region. A disease tendency in the "nerve–sense system" is seen as a hardening, sclerosis, or crystallization. Conditions such as spasms of the digestive tract and stone formation are construed as typical examples of the way in which a hardening tendency in the "nerve–sense system" has descended too far into the lower pole.

The "motor–digestive system," through its dynamism and ability to generate heat, is associated with inflammation and pus formation. From an anthroposophical standpoint, conditions such as migraines or middle-ear infection (otitis media) are examples of how the digestive processes can overshoot and ascend to the upper pole to cause diseases there.

Therapy in the anthroposophical medical sense means bringing a body lacking in balance back into equilibrium. The starting point for therapy, which is always constitution-oriented, is an in-depth dialog between the physician and his/her patient to discover the patient's constitutional type. In every initial consultation the physician will examine the patient's physical type, gait, comportment, temperament, and social and cultural situation, and will explore aspects such as sleep patterns, dreams, likes and dislikes with regard to food, reactions to weather, and the like. The dialog will be followed by treatment with, *inter alia*, mineral-, vegetable- and animal-derived medications, frequently in homeopathic dilutions. Anthroposophical remedies can be swallowed, injected, or applied topically. Preparations formulated with a combination of ingredients are referred to as "compositions."

Anthroposophical teachings draw parallels between man and the universe. Human organs can thus be addressed at a very fundamental level to encourage regeneration and healing. If, for example, the etheric body is predominant in a patient, he or she may go on to develop an imbalance which the ego and astral body are unable to redress. Preparations from the kingdom of minerals and metals are said to assist in limiting and reforming the associated vital processes. Other preparations are used in the belief that they can stimulate weak vital processes.

Hepatodoron, a preparation that is used to improve liver functions, is composed of leaves from the wild strawberry and grapevine. The grapevine and other sugar producing plants symbolize and mirror liver functions. The best known anthroposophical remedy is mistletoe—now used by many to treat cancer. While scientific medicine ascribes to the active principle of mistletoe an immune system modulating effect (*see* page 10), anthroposophical practitioners see this plant as a powerful countertype to cancer, as it shuns—both temporally and spatially—the growth laws by which other plants are governed; its berries ripen in winter, the plant itself does not touch the ground, and it does not grow toward the light.

In addition to appropriate remedies and special forms of massage (rhythmic massage), anthroposophical medicine utilizes various healing procedures (including curative eurhythmy, a special form of treatment devised by Steiner), art therapies such as painting, sculpting, music, etc. (which help the patient recover a harmonious life rhythm), and anthroposophically oriented psychotherapy (which incorporates dialog and biographical work). Sometimes, a special diet will be prescribed. Less common nowadays are the (occasionally outlandish) diagnostic tests that were once popular in anthroposophical medicine. In the capillary dynamic blood test, for instance, the patient's blood was diluted and drawn up into filter paper, and a diagnosis was then formulated based on the shapes and color patterns arising.

How it works

The various therapeutic elements of anthroposophical medicine, which are often bundled together in "packages," are supposed to bring man's constituent elements back into harmony and activate the body's natural healing powers.

The mechanisms by which anthroposophical remedies and procedures supposedly work cannot even approximately be described by means of the usual scientific terminology. The way in which such remedies and procedures relate to individual diseases only has meaning within the anthroposophical system of thinking.

Indications

Anthroposophical medicine is chiefly employed to treat chronic diseases of the digestive system, rheumatism, allergies, skin diseases, and psychiatric disorders; and as a supporting treatment for cancer.

Proof it works

The proponents of anthroposophical medicine reject modern clinical investigation approaches outright for ethical reasons. There is no scientific evidence to suggest that anthroposophical medicine has a valid basis, as AM therapies are not rooted in the normal scientific methods of modern orthodox medicine. However, it is assumed that the strong rapport achieved between practitioner and patient may give rise to a powerful placebo effect (*see* page xxi).

Since anthroposophical therapies are frequently administered in the form of "packages" of psychotherapeutic, physical, and medicine-based measures, it is difficult to attribute beneficial effects to any one element of therapy.

Results reportedly showing mistletoe as having certain powers to stimulate the body's defence cells and improve the mental outlook of cancer patients are still being hotly debated.

Risks, cautions, and contraindications

There seem to be few direct risks provided that it can be established that the patient is not suffering from a disease that requires orthodox medical treatment.

In isolated cases the patient may react allergically to individual substances administered. Lead and mercury, taken at low potency for prolonged periods, may cause chronic intoxication.

Duration of treatment

Treatment may last years (or even be lifelong), depending on the patient and his or her medical condition.

Finding the right therapist

Anthroposophically oriented doctors should belong to a recognized foundation. Although in most cases this will give some assurance as to the quality of training that the doctor will have received and the standard of treatment that the patient can expect, it does not necessarily follow that the treatment proposed will be that which is most appropriate to the condition for which the patient is seeking treatment.

A reputable AM practitioner will generally not start treatment without the patient's condition having been diagnosed conventionally. With the patient, the practitioner will define a treatment goal and propose an (initially limited) treatment plan (*see* page xxiii) to be used as a basis for checking that AM therapy is having the desired effect. A reputable practitioner will not promise an instantaneous or total cure (*see* Practitioner checklist, page xxv).

Aromatherapy

Rating

May be of some use as an adjunct to other therapies and for the treatment of psychosomatic illness.

Not advised as the sole treatment for persistent complaints unless a conventional physician has diagnosed the patient's condition and made a proper risk–benefit assessment.

Method

Essential oils are said to increase a person's sense of well-being and to be able to act directly against disease.

Rationale and historical perspective

In aromatherapy, essential oils obtained from the leaves, flowers, fruits, or roots of various plants are inhaled from a vaporizer, swallowed, massaged into the skin, applied as compresses, or used as bath additives. Since the sense of smell is closely associated with areas of the brain that also control emotions, certain aromas are said, for instance, to impart comfort and relaxation.

While the more esoteric of aromatherapists believe that aromas can transmit the "soul" of plants to human patients and so pass on certain vital "information," researchers with a more conventional scientific leaning are looking for links between aromatic oils and the physiology of the human body.

How it works

Little is known about how aromatherapy actually works. There are blatant inconsistencies in the explanations given by the various schools.

Indications

Aromatherapy, its proponents claim, is suitable for treating virtually any type of disease, even diabetes, cancer, and tuberculosis. It is most commonly used to treat stress and its related illnesses.

Proof it works

There is not yet adequate proof that aromatherapy is actually a valid treatment; few controlled clinical studies (*see* page xix) have been published. Claims regarding the efficacy of aromatherapy are for the most part based simply on case reports (*see* page xx).

What has been shown so far is that inhaling nutmeg, thuja, and lemon oil can ease a cough; that pine needle and rosemary oil have stimulating properties when added to bathwater; and that vapors from oils of cassia, cinnamon, camphor, coriander, caraway, crisped mint, pennyroyal, thyme, and sage can be used to freshen up a stuffy room.

That aromatherapy can in some cases be used to treat serious disease is as yet an unproven hypothesis.

Risks, cautions, and contraindications

Aromatherapy can cause allergies and intolerance, nausea, and headaches. Some oils also have the potential of causing cancer in the long run. The overconfidence of some aromatherapists may mean the patient will fail to obtain a proper medical diagnosis and miss the chance of obtaining more appropriate therapy.

Duration of treatment

The duration of treatment will depend on the therapist's own leaning and on the therapeutic goal. Some therapists offer a series of treatments lasting altogether about ten sessions; sometimes they will advise that a series of treatments be repeated.

Finding the right therapist

In most European countries a person does not need any formal training to become an aromatherapist. Reputable aroma-therapists who suspect the patient might be suffering from a serious illness will not offer treatment unless a conventional diagnosis has been obtained from a qualified physician. With the patient they will define a treatment goal and propose a short-term treatment plan (*see* page xxiii) to be used to check the efficacy of the treatment. No credence should be given to therapists promising an immediate or total cure (*see* Practitioner checklist, page xxv). Aromatherapy is suitable as a DIY therapy. Qualified guidance is advised though not absolutely necessary.

Ayurveda

> **Rating**
>
> **May be of some use** as an attempted treatment for psychosomatic ailments or for bringing symptomatic relief in chronic disease.
>
> **Not advised** as the sole treatment for persistent complaints unless a conventional physician has diagnosed the patient's condition and made a proper risk–benefit assessment.

Method

Ayurveda is a system of diagnosis and healing that originated in ancient India and embraces such treatments as nutritional therapy (*see* pages 858–67), eliminative methods (*see* pages 809–24), meditation, and medical herbalism (*see* pages 853–7).

The limited amount of documentation on ayurvedic medicine that is available in the West precludes a definitive assessment of how it works and of its efficacy in individual diseases and illnesses.

Rationale and historical perspective

Ayurveda (from the Sanskrit *ved*—science—and *ayur*—life) forms part of the veda, the scientific, philosophical, and cultural tradition of ancient India, and is the holistic healing system that began there some 4,500 years ago.

Ayurveda was popular in Europe at the time of Hippocrates, the great medical genius of antiquity and founder of the Greek medical tradition (which he based in part on ayurvedic beliefs and philosophies). In modern Europe the prevalent system of ayurveda that is practiced tends to be Maharishi-Ayur-Veda, which became renowned through the Beatles' visit to India and their association with its Guru, Maharishi Marahesh Yogi.

Ayurveda is said to be of divine inspiration; as well as seeking to improve and maintain health, it also searches for the deeper meaning of life. The main elements are a philosophical interpretation of illness, teachings on hygiene and disease prevention, diagnostic and therapeutic systems, and medical herbalism. Ayurveda has its own distinct teachings of internal medicine, gynacology and obstetrics, ENT, ophthalmology, psychiatry, surgery, sexual medicine, and toxicology. Disease is said to enter the body from outside, so attention to the hygiene of body orifices is a key feature of the ayurvedic medical tradition. More than two-thirds of India's population receives treatment from ayurvedic practitioners.

At the heart of ayurvedic healing is the *tridosha* principle, which recognizes three *doshas* or forces (*vata*, *pitta*, and *kapha*). The human being is seen as a microcosm of the universe, whose energies are derived from five natural elements—earth, water, fire, air, and space. The same three *doshas* combine in various proportions to decide a person's spiritual state and constitution. It is the constitution, in turn, that defines the person's strengths and weaknesses, susceptibility to illness, mind–body interrelationship, and reaction to diet, medicines, climatic influences and sensory impressions.

To ensure that the body remains healthy, the *doshas* must be normal and in balance. According to traditional beliefs, a healthy person is one whose attitude to life and relationship with the environment are harmonious and stable. A healthy body also experiences certain daily, monthly, and seasonal rhythms. When the proper balance is upset, the body sends out signals which, if ignored, develop into symptoms of illness.

If one *dosha* becomes dominant or, conversely, weakened, the effect is a build-up of *ama* (toxins and waste products). Ayurvedic therapy is directed towards ridding the body of *ama*, restoring balance and wholeness. Ayurvedic practitioners will start by discovering the nature of the disease and the patient's constitution through a combination of looking, listening, smelling, interrogation, and palpation.

- Pulse-taking, for which the physician uses a three-finger technique, is said to give an insight into the state and constellation of the *doshas*.
- A *prakriti* analysis is claimed to cast light on special factors affecting the patient. *Prakriti* is determined based on astrological constellations and the circumstances of conception and pregnancy, which remain unchanged throughout a person's life. Imbalanced *doshas* are harmonized through a combination of fasting, oil massage, bathing, eliminative methods (*see* pages 809–24) such as vomiting, enemas, and bloodletting, in association with meditation techniques such as yoga, transcendental meditation, and color, aroma, and music therapies. Ayurveda also draws on a store of some 5,000 herbal preparations that are in some cases used in association with minerals and metals. These remedies are intended to benefit the patient and his or her *doshas* not only through the combinations of ingredients they contain but also through their special taste, their physical characteristics, the way they affect the digestive process, and their inner vitality.

Some of the multinational pharmaceutical companies are presently researching Indian herbal remedies in an attempt to isolate and market individual ingredients and ingredient complexes. However, other attempts that there have been at reconciling the ayurvedic philosophy of health and disease with the principles of modern scientific medicine have failed. Aurvedic philosophy has its origins in a remote and ancient culture and does not lend itself readily to modern interpretation.

How it works

Ayurvedic therapy is said to restore equilibrium to imbalanced *doshas* and so remove the basis and driving force of pathological symptoms. These notions are alien to the Western way of thinking, have changed little throughout history, and cannot readily be transposed to a different cultural setting. Many of the principles, however, can be seen as the oriental precurors of modern psychosomatically oriented preventive medicine.

Explanations of the origins of disease by those who practice ayurveda mostly run counter to the teachings of modern scientific medicine. There is a general lack of scientific proof, in the modern mainstream sense, that ayurveda does actually work when used to treat acute conditions. Few of the medicines used by ayurvedic practitioners have been tested to Western medical standards to discover how they work.

Indications

Based on statements made by some of its own proponents, ayurveda can prove beneficial in virtually any disease or illness. It is widely used for psychosomatic and chronic complaints and for general malaise. Many Western practitioners of ayurveda leave the treatment of acute diseases and psychiatric disorders to conventional doctors.

Proof it works

The underlying philosophy of ayurveda is difficult to judge based on accepted modern medical and scientific standards, as it embraces an entirely different culture and philosophy. Pharmacological research into ayurvedic remedies is very much in its infancy. Clinical studies have indicated that some remedies may be of potential benefit in cirrhosis of the liver, inflammation of the joints, and cardivascular diseases.

The Maharishi-Ayur-Veda organization, whose aim is to popularize ayurveda as a holistic treatment method, has presented findings allegedly showing traditional Indian herbal remedies to be beneficial in patients with, *inter alia*, high blood pressure, angina pectoris, cardiac arrhythmia, asthma, digestive disorders, migraines, rheumatism, and paralysis. However, none of the claims has so far been corroborated in controlled clinical studies from independent investigators (*see* page xix).

Risks, cautions, and contraindications

Ayurveda should not be used to treat serious diseases, as its efficacy is so far unproven; anyone relying entirely on ayurvedic diagnosis runs a risk of a serious disease being overlooked and of a treatment that is appropriate in the Western medical sense being given.

Some drug mixtures contain toxic amounts of mercury and other heavy metals. The long-term effects of such preparations have not been documented.

Duration of treatment

Depending on the condition being treated, therapy may last for years or even be lifelong.

Finding the right therapist

An ayurvedic practitioner should be professionally qualified and accredited. Though in most cases this will provide some assurance as to the training the practitioner will have received and the quality of treatment that the patient can expect, it does not automatically follow that the therapy provided will be the one that is most appropriate to the patient's condition.

A reputable therapist will generally not start treatment until, in serious diseases at least, the patient has consulted a doctor for a conventional diagnosis. With the patient he/she will define a treatment goal and propose a short-term treatment plan (*see* page xxiii) to be used to check the treatment for efficacy. No credence should be given to therapists promising a complete or immediate cure (*see* Practitioner checklist, page xxv).

Bioresonance therapy (BRT)

> **Rating**
>
> **May be of some use**. Possibly acceptable as a short-term attempt to treat, in particular, disorders with a psychosomatic component when more established methods have not been successful.
>
> **Not advised** as the sole treatment for persistent complaints unless a conventional physician has diagnosed the patient's condition and made a proper risk–benefit assessment.

Method

Bioresonance therapists use technological support to detect pathological vibrations in the body and then neutralize them or "turn them around" to remove the basis for continued existence of the disease or disorder. Sometimes they aim to cure the disease directly.

Rationale and historical perspective

In the 1970s physician Franz Morell and Erich Rasche, an engineer, developed "moratherapy", subsequently to be renamed "biocommunication" and later "bioresonance therapy" as their equipment grew in complexity.

The rationale underlying this treatment is that disease is caused and sustained by certain pathological vibrations within the body, and that illness and functional disorders are closely associated with the patient's vibration patterns. The instruments used in bioresonance therapy are claimed to tap into these vibrations, modify them and return them to the body in such a way that pathogenic energies are weakened or prevented from arising in the first place.

One treatment variant is the Multicom, an instrument used to treat (allegedly) the sick organism not through the body's own vibrations but through environmental energies that emanate from trace elements, metals, gemstones, drugs, and colors.

How it works

There is no compelling evidence to validate claims made by practitioners that this therapy works, nor indeed about the way in which it works. That BRT can be beneficial is a hypothesis that is at present unproven.

Indications

Bioresonance therapy is claimed to be effective in virtually any type of disorder. Allergies represent the most common indication. However, "allergy" in this context is a term that a frequently confused with unspecific intolerance.

Proof it works

So far there has not been any rigorous testing (*see* page xix) to validate BRT as an effective therapeutic technique. The beneficial effects described in case reports (*see* page xx) possibly only hold true for a proportion of patients treated (*see* Placebo, page xxi).

Risks, cautions, and contraindications

From what is presently known, there seems to be no direct risk attached to treatment with Mora and Multicom devices. However, overconfidence on the part of BRT practitioners may mean that the patient's condition will not be properly diagnosed in the orthodox sense, so he or she will possibly miss the opportunity of receiving more appropriate treatment.

Duration of treatment

Therapy sessions will generally be for about 20 minutes once a week. There will normally be about six treatment sessions in a series.

Finding the right therapist

Particular care is needed when therapists promise a complete or instantaneous care (*see* Practitioner checklist, page xxv). A reputable therapist will usually not start treatment until the patient has consulted a doctor for a conventional diagnosis. With the patient, the therapist will define a treatment goal and propose a short-term treatment plan (*see* page xxiii) to be used as a basis for checking that BRT is having the desired effect.

Bioresonance therapists should be members of a professional organization. Although in most cases this will give a certain assurance as to the quality of training the therapist will have received and the standard of treatment that the patient can expect, it will not necessarily follow that the treatment proposed will be that which is most appropriate to his or her condition.

Cell therapy

Rating
Not advised as a routine treatment or as the sole therapy for a persistent or severe complaint unless the patient has consulted a physician for a diagnosis. In rare situations, a conventional risk–benefit assessment may justify an attempted cell therapy, e.g. for pain, when more established, less costly procedures have been unsuccessful. Fresh cell therapy is not advised in any circumstances.

Method

Various products obtained from animal and—rarely—from human tissues and organs are injected, swallowed, or applied topically and are said to heal a number of chronic complaints, rectify organ dysfunction, modulate the immune system, or act in rejuvenating the body.

Rationale and historical perspective

This form of therapy is supposed to enable the diseased body to repair various functional and structural defects. The rationale at the heart of this treatment is attributed in part to Swiss physician Paul Niehans, who, in the 1930s, injected some of his patients with tissue extracted from newborn animals. Believing that the vitality and youthfulness of the donor animal could be transferred to the recipient, Niehans included rejuvenation in his catalog of indications for what he termed his "fresh cell cure".

Two decades later, a Swedish veterinary surgeon by the name of Sandberg was one of the most successful proponents of thymus therapy. He injected sick persons with an extract of calf thymus in the belief that this important organ, which "prepares" certain white blood cells for their immunological role, is able to communicate its power to the immune system of the recipient. Nowadays, various thymus preparations are used, ranging from complex extracts to highly purified monosubstances.

Preparations are today mostly obtained from cells or cell constituents from animal fetuses, or from newborn or adolescent animals, mostly sheep and calves. A heterologous preparation is one that is obtained from animal tissue, a homologous preparation one that is obtained from human tissue.

Generally, the preparations are extracted from the same organ as that which is diseased in the recipient. There may be wide variability in the proposed therapeutic goals.

- For so-called substitution of deficient cells, intact cells are introduced to replace dead or supposedly deficient cells.
- For regeneration, cell material (mostly comprising cellular constituents, some of which are said to be reduced to the molecular level) is introduced in order to repair damaged cells or stimulate physical functions in the recipient.

- For improving mental outlook or for modulating the immune system, preparations of various organs (but chiefly the thymus) are employed.
- Organ extracts can also be administered in potentized form (*see* page 831).

Fresh, frozen, or lyophilized (freeze-dried) material is normally injected. Other formulations include tablets, pills, or drops that are taken orally (allowed to disperse in the mouth for absorption through the mucous tissues).

How it works

Animal cells are claimed to support the self-healing powers of human tissues, organs, and joints. Cells from juvenile animals are sometimes injected in the belief that the vitality and youthfulness of the donor animal will be communicated to the human recipient. Thymus preparations are thought to modulate the immune system (*see* page 10) and are used in cancer therapy. The alleged rejuvenating effect of fresh cell cures is speculative and unproven clinically.

There is no scientific proof of the claimed ability of this therapeutic procedure to act specifically on diseased organs.

Indications

Manufacturers and users of various cell preparations make the wildest of claims. Some say that certain preparations can favorably influence chronic ailments, exercise an immune modulating effect, work against the ageing process, and even rejuvenate.

Thymus therapy is said to be effective in diseases such as cancer and polyarthritis; it is even claimed to be beneficial in Down's syndrome. Certain other organ extracts, it is claimed, are useful in more than 100 indications, even to the point of protecting against radiation following a nuclear incident.

Proof it works

There have not been many controlled clinical studies (*see* page xix) showing these preparations to be efficacious. For some thymus extracts there have been various minor studies with highly purified thymus factors (monopreparations), though not with complex preparations. These studies supposedly suggest a potentially significant clinical efficacy, but their importance with regard to thymus extracts, used in a large number of preparations, is unclear. The efficacy of organ extracts in joint diseases that is implied in various case reports (*see* page xx) probably only holds true for a proportion of patients receiving treatment (*see* Placebo, page xxi).

Risks, cautions, and contraindications

Cell therapists themselves state that this treatment should not be employed in acute infectious diseases and chronic ailments caused by bacterial foci. The methods are not directed against individual pathogens, being intended rather as a means of regeneration. Cell therapy is not advised in persons who suffer allergic reactions; nor should it be used for four weeks either side of an inoculation.

A present it is impossible to judge definitively whether certain of the therapeutic preparations used might, or might not, transmit pathogens (possibly even the agent that causes BSE if the cell material was obtained from cattle, sheep, and goats carrying the disease). With BSE, the causative agent is not itself detectable in cells obtained from infected animals; it may lie dormant and only become manifest decades later. Any injected foreign protein can provoke severe allergic reactions, even fatal shock. To date there have been numerous reports of fatalities caused by the injection of fresh cells. Many patients show signs of irritation at the injection site.

Duration of treatment

Cell therapeutics are generally injected in a series of treatment sessions the duration and frequency of which will depend on the condition being treated. There should always be an interval of five to eight months between any two treatment series.

Finding the right therapist

Therapists promising an instantaneous or total cure should be viewed with considerable scepticism (*see* Practitioner checklist, page xxv). Even where the therapist has received some level of training, this in no way ensures that the preparations used will be pure, nor that this form of therapy will be appropriate.

A reputable therapist will generally not start treatment until the patient has consulted a qualified physician for a medical assessment. With the patient the therapist should define a treatment goal and propose an initially limited plan of treatment (*see* page xxiii) to be used as a basis for checking that the therapy is having the desired effect.

Chelation therapy

> **Rating**
> **Not advised**. This is a risky and expensive treatment for problems with blood circulation; its efficacy is seriously questioned.

Method

The chelating agent ethylenediamine tetraacetic acid (EDTA), it is claimed, is able to dissolve atheromatous deposits in the body and eliminate heavy metals, so preventing or curing a number of diseases.

Rationale and historical perspective

Since the 1940s, conventional physicians in the USA have performed chelation therapy for lead, copper, manganese, mercury, and zinc poisoning. Since, in the human body, EDTA can form complexes not only with heavy metals but also with calcium, the pioneers of chelation therapy surmised that the substance must also be able to dissolve calcified atheromatous deposits from the walls of blood vessels and so prevent stroke, alleviate angina pectoris, cure smoker's leg, and reduce blood pressure. In the 1980s, the treatment was also introduced in Europe. It involves infusion of EDTA as part of a cocktail of vitamins and trace elements in saline solution. Calcium deposits are allegedly dissolved and flushed from the body through the kidneys.

How it works

There is no evidence to indicate how chelation therapy works, if indeed it does. Various rigorous studies have failed to substantiate its claimed efficacy in circulation disorders.

Indications

Chelation therapy can, it is claimed, be used to treat virtually any disease, including vascular disorders and associated complications, sexual potency problems, diabetes, cancer, and tuberculosis. In mainstream medicine—unlike in complementary medicine—chelation therapy is employed only for heavy metal intoxications.

Proof it works

Evidence that this therapy might be beneficial has so far only been adduced for heavy metal intoxications. At least three controlled clinical studies (*see* page xix) have shown that the benefit claimed in testimonials (*see* page xx) to have been obtained in circulatory disorders is due at most to a placebo effect (*see* page xxi), while accompanying side effects are much more common and pronounced.

Risks, cautions, and contraindications

Chelating agents remove minerals and trace elements from the body. They may affect normal calcium metabolism and cause cessation of breathing, cardiac arrhythmia, or cramps.

The overconfidence shown by some chelation therapists in their ability to diagnose the patient's condition means that he or she might fail to obtain a proper medical diagnosis and miss the opportunity of receiving what might be more appropriate treatment.

Duration of treatment

A course of treatment will generally consist of anything up to 25 sessions.

Finding the right therapist

No credence can be given to practitioners promising a complete or instantaneous care (*see* Practitioner checklist, page xxv).

Electroacupuncture according to Voll (EAV)

Rating

Of little use. Possibly acceptable as a short-term attempt to treat persistent or recurrent complaints when more established treatment methods have been unsuccessful or the patient's condition requires further diagnostic clarification.

Not advised as the sole treatment for persistent complaints unless a conventional physician has diagnosed the patient's condition and made a proper risk–benefit assessment.

Method

Measurement of various electrical properties of the skin, such as its electrical potential, resistance or conductivity at various points, is said to provide an insight into areas of the body that are diseased, and to enable intoxications to be pinpointed and foci (*see* page 928) to be located. Following diagnosis, a pathological condition can be addressed through elimination of the focus, by electroneural stimulation, or through administration of a remedy—usually homeopathic.

Rationale and historical perspective

In the 1950s, German physician Reinhold Voll began working on his diagnostic (*see* page 912) and therapeutic system, EAV (also sometimes known as biometric system diagnosis or regulation therapy)—an amalgam of various complementary medical procedures. Voll initially proceeded from experiments previously carried out by colleagues of his into the electrical properties of acupuncture points. Accepting the teachings of traditional acupuncture (*see* page 772) that, when a person is ill, his or her energy flow is thrown out of balance, he went on to define further points, presuming that, at these points, the flow of energy must be not only measurable but receptive to external influences. Voll commissioned a special device that in his view would help him measure the body's response to neural stimulation and that he could also use to impart energy through such stimuli. By observing changes in skin conductivity caused by delivering minute electrical stimuli, he concluded that he was able to detect early stages of pathogenesis in the body and, through the use of EAV, to support the body's self-healing powers in overcoming disease.

Once, while demonstrating the EAV technique, Voll believed he discovered by accident that medications also in some way modify the skin's resistance, whereupon he also began to investigate whether these could be suitability tested using the same method. He formulated his hypothesis that EAV readings can be used to discover which substances are harmful to the patient, and which beneficial.

During EAV treatment, initial readings covering all of the

body's main subsystems are systematically taken. The patient grasps a negative electrode, shaped like a handle, while the therapist uses a probe (the positive electrode) to investigate the electrical resistance at various points. Assuming the normal state (test person in good health) to be when the needle is deflected roughly halfway along the scale of an ohmmeter, values that are higher than the norm suggest inflammation, an allergic reaction, or intoxication, while those that are lower may indicate that the person is run-down or suffering from a degenerative disease.

The results are recorded on a special card. A second set of readings is then taken at points at which the initial results are said to have revealed pathological changes in the associated organs. If the needle gradually falls back having once attained a value, this is said to indicate a possible focus (*see* page 928).

During this stage of the examination procedure, ampoules (mostly containing homeopathic preparations—*see* page 831) are placed in a metal container or held in the patient's hand to form part of the electrical circuit. Those preparations which, when tested, are seen to return the alleged high or low values to normal are then prescribed for oral use or injection.

Nowadays, most of these procedures are fully computerized.

How it works

According to Voll's theory, the procedure normalizes the body's energy balance (*see* Energy, page 927), thus enabling it to overcome disease. This self-healing potential is supported by certain medications that will have been tested and shown to be beneficial. The procedure is also purportedly able to locate foci said to be responsible for causing and sustaining illness.

There has not been any convincing explanation of the physiological principles that might be at the heart of the claimed beneficial effect of this treatment. Several studies found that the readings of the instrument are not reproducible and depend entirely on artefacts. The existence of foci is also in doubt; the present view is that the focus theory is an inadequately substantiated hypothesis which, some would claim, has already been disproven.

What Voll saw as his normal range of electrical resistance is simply an arbitrary assumption and carries no weight other than in EAV.

Indications

EAV, its users maintain, can detect and combat diseases even before they have become manifest. It is also, they say, a way of detecting exposure to environmental and other toxins and of discovering foci, the removal of which is supposed to prevent or remove the basis of certain diseases and associated conditions. EAV practitioners recommend the treatment for all acute and chronic conditions that have previously eluded diagnosis and successful treatment.

Proof it works

The efficacy of EAV as a therapy has not been satisfactorily researched. There are so far no compelling findings from rigorously controlled studies supporting the method (*see* page xix). The efficacy that is claimed in certain case reports (*see* page xx) as having been achieved cannot presently be assessed and probably holds true for only a proportion of patients treated (*see* page xxi).

Risks, cautions, and contraindications

Provided treatment is carried out competently, there seem to be no direct risks. However, patients must consult a medical practitioner for a second opinion before agreeing to surgical removal of their tonsils, appendix, teeth, ovaries, or prostate, or to any other expensive surgical measures or interventions.

Duration of treatment

A series of treatments will generally consist of between one and 20 sessions.

Finding the right therapist

Patients should be particularly wary of therapists promising an instantaneous or complete cure or who advocate surgery for focal elimination without a second opinion from an orthodox physician.

A reputable EAV therapist will usually not start treatment until the patient has obtained a conventional diagnosis from a qualified doctor. With the patient, he or she will define a treatment goal and propose a short-term treatment plan (*see* page xxiii) to be used as a basis for checking that the treatment is having the desired effect.

If the therapist has some formal qualification, this will in most cases give a certain assurance as to the training he or she will have received and the standard of treatment the patient can expect; however, it will not necessarily follow that the treatment the therapist proposes will be that which is most appropriate to the condition for which the patient is seeking treatment.

Electroneural therapy according to Croon (ENT)

Rating

Of little use. Possibly acceptable as a short-term attempt to treat various painful conditions, circulation disorders, and muscle diseases.

Not advised as the sole treatment for persistent complaints unless a conventional physician has diagnosed the patient's condition and made a proper risk–benefit assessment.

Method

Readings taken at certain reactive sites on the skin are said to help pinpoint diseased parts of the body. Armed with this diagnostic information, therapists are supposedly able to elicit a beneficial effect in a number of conditions by electroneural stimulation.

Rationale and historical perspective

In the 1950s German physician Richard Croon developed an electrical device which he used to take readings at 212 so-called reactive sites located at various points on the skin. These sites, he claimed, differ from other comparable areas of skin in that they exhibit lower electrical resistance and thus higher conductivity than the areas surrounding them. The points in question can be matched to specific organs, as in reflexology.

Croon's electrical device is used to take readings at the reactive sites, which are located chiefly on the head and back and have an approximate diameter of $^3/_4$–$1^1/_4$ inches. Certain key values are plotted on an electroneural somatogram. Then minute, individually dosed currents are delivered to shift the electrical resistance and conductivity of the skin back into the "normal range." The results plotted on the somatogram are claimed to give a diagnostic insight into the person's overall state of health, to be able to locate pathogenic foci (*see* page 928), and to detect possible organ disease (*see* page 914). Nowadays these processes are mostly computerized.

How it works

ENT, its proponents claim, normalizes the electrical situation in the body and enables it to overcome illness and disease. It is also supposed to be able to act directly on diseased organs, in a way akin to reflexology (*see* page 883). So far there has not been a satisfactory explanation of the physiological principles that might be at the heart of the beneficial effect claimed to be achieved with ENT. What Croon saw as his "normal range" of electrical readings is simply an arbitrary assumption.

Even outside the complementary field, however, stimulation therapy is acknowledged to have a beneficial effect, particularly in providing pain relief (*see* TENS, page 886).

Indications

ENT, some of its advocates proclaim, is able to combat any chronically degenerative disease, including asthma, diabetes, multiple sclerosis, and cancer, and is also able to overcome childhood development disorders. Its main indications are headaches, neuralgia, orthopedic problems, and rheumatic disorders.

Proof it works

There has been little research into the efficacy or otherwise of ENT. There have so far not been any compelling results from rigorously controlled studies (*see* page xix). The efficacy that certain field study reports (*see* page xx) claim as having been achieved probably only applies in a proportion of patients treated (*see* Placebo, page xxi).

Risks, cautions, and contraindications

Provided treatment is carried out competently, there seem to be no direct risks. Some of those who use ENT state, however, that it should not be used in cases of acute inflammation, open sores, or highly febrile conditions.

Duration of treatment

A series of treatments will generally consist of 20–40 sessions over a period of two to six weeks. New readings will be taken at all 212 reactive sites after every tenth session.

Finding the right therapist

Patients should be particularly wary of therapists promising an instantaneous or complete cure. A reputable ENT therapist will usually not start treatment until the patient has obtained a conventional diagnosis from a qualified doctor. With the patient, he or she will define a treatment goal and propose a short-term treatment plan (*see* page xxiii) to be used as a basis for checking that the treatment is having the desired effect.

  If the therapist can show that he or she has a formal qualification, this will in most cases give a certain assurance as to the quality of training he or she will have received and the standard of treatment the patient can expect; however, it will not necessarily follow that the treatment the therapist proposes will be that which is most appropriate to the condition for which the patient is seeking treatment.

Eliminative methods

In Europe, before modern science-based medicine began to develop, disease was generally seen as an imbalance of humors (Latin *humores*: fluids of the body), caused by an accumulation of waste products or a change in the patient's humoral make-up. One notable exponent of this theory was Hippocrates of Kos (460–377 BC). At the heart of his concept of healing were the four "cardinal humors": yellow and black bile, blood, and phlegm. An illness, he thought, could be brought to an end by eliminating the "bad humors". Diseased organs would then be purified and healed as more of the poisons were removed from the body via the skin.

Viennese gynacologist Bernhard Aschner repopularized the eliminative approach in the 1920s and, to encourage elimination, proposed procedures such as swallowing toxic substances, inducing vomiting, and inflicting minor injuries. Many of the therapies nowadays used in complementary medicine are based on the notion of poisons or other harmful substances circulating in the body.

Bloodletting

> **Rating**
>
> **Not advised** as a routine treatment. Perhaps acceptable as a short-term, rarely undertaken attempt to treat chronic illness when more established, less invasive therapies have been unsuccessful. At all events a medically qualified practitioner must diagnose the patient's condition and make an orthodox risk–benefit assessment.

Method

Bloodletting, say its proponents, thins the blood, unclogs the circulation, and rids the body of "bad humors."

Rationale and historical perspective

Right up until the 19th century, bloodletting was a commonly practiced technique for treating virtually any disease or condition, since drawing off blood was thought to eliminate the poisons that made a person ill. In modern bloodletting, the therapist inserts a butterfly canula into the patient, then allows about 100–150ml of blood to run off into a beaker. Occasionally, the same amount of saline solution or blood substitute will be infused. Even modern mainstream medicine utilizes procedures that are reminiscent of bloodletting (e.g. hemodilution and apheresis) but operate at a much higher technological level.

How it works

Bloodletting is supposed to bring about a change in the patient's general mental state, to dilute the blood, unclog the circulation, rid the body of alleged pathogenic factors, and improve the supply of oxygen to the body. The changes in the flow properties of blood brought about by bloodletting can be beneficial in a number of circulatory diseases.

The idea of "bad humors" circulating in the body is a concept rooted in an age long since gone.

Indications

For some therapists bloodletting is a panacea that is even recommended as a preventive measure, but it is most frequently reserved for poor circulation, disturbed metabolism, cardio-vascular disorders and lung disease.

Proof it works

There has been little research into whether bloodletting works. There have not been any reliable clinical trial results (*see* page xix). The efficacy claimed in certain case reports (*see* page xx) cannot be substantiated on the basis of modern clinical research findings (*see* Placebo, page xxi).

Risks, cautions, and contraindications

Bloodletting, its proponents warn, should not be attempted in patients with anemia, acute diarrhea, low blood pressure, or general debilitation; nor should it be used in persons with blood clotting disorders.

Duration of treatment

Treatment will last for a length of time that is dependent on the particular approach, the problem being addressed, and the therapeutic goal that has been set.

Finding the right therapist

Therapists who do not insist that the patient should obtain a conventional diagnosis for persistent complaints or who promise a total or immediate cure are not reputable (*see* Practitioner checklist, page xxv). It is advisable to seek treatment only from therapists with a formal qualification. Although in most cases this will give a certain assurance as to the standard of treatment that the patient can expect, it will not necessarily follow that the treatment given will be the most appropriate for dealing with the patient's condition.

With the patient a reputable therapist will define a treatment goal and propose a short-term treatment plan (*see* page xxiii) to be used to check that the therapy is working.

Cantharide poultices

Rating

Not advised as a routine treatment. Perhaps acceptable as a short-term attempt to treat chronic diseases when more established, less invasive therapies have failed. It is essential for the patient to see a medically qualified physician to obtain an orthodox medical diagnosis and a proper risk–benefit assessment.

Method

Cantharide poultices are vesicants, i.e. blistering agents, that are said to rid the body of "bad humors."

Rationale and historical perspective

Vesicants have a history of use in medicine going back thousands of years. The cantharide extracts that are used in this technique are obtained from dried Spanish fly or "blister beetle," which is also known for its alleged aphrodisiac effect. Poultices are applied to the skin, where they induce second-degree burns within an hour or so, producing a water-filled blister. Twenty-four hours later the blister is punctured, the liquid drawn off, and the wound bandaged. Sometimes mustard oil, camphor, or turpentine is used instead of cantharidin. Wounds generally heal without scarring after about ten days.

How it works

Treatment with cantharide poultices is founded on the concept of an eliminative method that will rid the body, purportedly, of "bad humors." It also takes advantage of the reflex principle (*see* Reflex therapies, page 881) through which, it is claimed, the principal organs can be influenced by means of so-called energy links.

The supposedly existence of "bad humors" coursing through the body is a belief from an age gone by.

Indications

Cantharide poultices are claimed to be beneficial in improving a person's mental outlook, stimulating the immune system, relieving pain, breaking down waste products, promoting lymphatic drainage (*see* page 850), and improving the circulation. The treatment is mostly applied for rheumatism, gout, inflammatory diseases, middle-ear infection, and chronic back pain.

Proof it works

Very little research has so far been conducted into the efficacy or otherwise of cantharide poultices. There are no reliable findings from controlled clinical studies (*see* page xix). The efficacy that is sometimes described in case reports and other studies (*see* page xx) as having been achieved against persistent conditions (e.g. painful joints) is very difficult to substantiate and possibly applies to only a proportion of patients receiving treatment (*see* Placebo, page xxi).

Risks, cautions, and contraindications

Cantharide poultices cause transient, but severe, skin lesions. There is probably little significant risk to the patient provided that the cantharidin dosage recommended by the manufacturer (maximum bandage size 2 x 4 inches) is not exceeded. There may be scarring, especially through scratching to relieve itchiness.

Persons with a dark complexion may suffer depigmentation following treatment.

Cantharidin ointment should not be applied to the mucous membranes, nor to broken or diseased skin, open wounds, or inflamed joints. On no account should cantharidin be swallowed, as it may lead to (possibly fatal) kidney damage.

Duration of treatment

The length of time for which poultices are applied will depend on the particular condition being treated.

Finding the right therapist

Patients should be wary of any therapist promising a total or instantaneous cure (*see* Practitioner checklist, page xxv). A responsible therapist will use cantharide poultices very sparingly and judiciously, and not without the patient having consulted a physician for a conventional diagnosis. With the patient he or she will define a goal that the treatment is designed to attain and propose a short-term treatment plan (*see* page xxiii) to be used as a basis for checking that the therapy is having the desired effect.

It is advisable to seek treatment only from a therapist with a medical background. Although in most cases this will give some assurance as to the standard of treatment that the patient can expect, it will not necessarily guarantee that the therapy proposed will be that most appropriate to the condition for which treatment is being sought.

Cupping, bloody

Rating
Of little use as a routine treatment. Possibly acceptable in exceptional cases as a short-term attempt to treat chronic diseases when more established, less invasive therapies have not succeeded in bringing about any improvement.
Not advised as the sole treatment for persistent complaints unless a conventional physician has diagnosed the patient's condition and made a proper risk–benefit assessment.

Method

The skin is superficially incised and small rounded cups, heated beforehand, are placed over the incisions; the vacuum created as the cups cool draws out the patient's blood. Bloody cupping is held to be good for pain relief and improving the patient's mental outlook.

Rationale and historical perspective

Cupping for curative purposes has been a tradition in several cultures, including those of ancient Egypt and Greece.

The amount of blood drawn off under the sterilizable cups can total anything up to 11fl oz. After five to ten minutes the vacuum is released, the cup carefully removed and the wound treated. This procedure is painful.

How it works

Bloody cupping combines elements of the belief in "bad humors," traditional Chinese yin–yang philosophy (*see* page 896), and reflex therapy (*see* page 881).

Indications

For many of its proponents, bloody cupping is a panacea, but its main use is in pain relief.

Proof it works

There has been little research into the efficacy or otherwise of bloody cupping. Nor are there any reliable clinical research findings (*see* page xix). The successes that various case reports and studies (*see* page xx) describe as having been achieved in the relief of pain cannot be scientifically substantiated and probably only hold true for a proportion of patients receiving treatment (*see* Placebo, page xxi).

Risks, cautions, and contraindications

Bloody cupping carries an infection risk if the equipment used to incise the skin is not adequately disinfected beforehand. Patients with bloodclotting disorders must not be treated by bloody cupping.

Duration of treatment

The length of time required for treatment will depend on the condition being treated.

Finding the right therapist

A reputable therapist will insist on the patient obtaining a conventional diagnosis for a persistent condition, and will not promise a total or instantaneous cure (*see* Practitioner checklist, page xxv). It is advisable to seek treatment only from a therapist with a qualified medical background. Although in most cases this will give some assurance as to the quality of training that the therapist will have received and the standard of treatment that the patient can expect, it does not necessarily follow that this treatment will be that most appropriate to the patient's condition.

A responsible therapist will define a treatment goal and propose a short-term treatment plan (*see* page xxiii) to be used as a basis for checking that the therapy is having the desired effect.

Cupping, unbloody

Rating
Possibly of some use as a short-term attempt to provide pain relief.
Not advised as the sole treatment for persistent complaints unless a conventional physician has diagnosed the patient's condition and made a proper risk–benefit assessment.

Method

Small rounded cups are used to stimulate areas of the patient's back. This is said to produce an improvement in mental state as well as correcting energy imbalances and providing relief from pain.

Rationale and historical perspective

The therapist will start by warming the patient's skin with an infrared lamp, then place the cups, heated beforehand, in position; the vacuum created as the cups cool holds the cups firmly in place and causes the capillary blood vessels to dilate, causing small bruises and blisters on the skin.

How it works

Unbloody cupping combines elements of a belief in "bad humors," traditional Chinese yin–yang philosophy (*see* page 896), and reflex therapy (*see* page 881).

Indications

Unbloody cupping is mostly used in pain relief.

Proof it works

There has been little research into the efficacy or otherwise of unbloody cupping. Nor are there any reliable clinical research findings (*see* page xix). The successes that various case reports and studies (*see* page xx) describe as having been achieved in the relief of pain cannot be scientifically substantiated and probably only hold true for a proportion of patients receiving treatment (*see* Placebo, page xxi).

Risks, cautions, and contraindications

The procedure is not thought to carry any risks provided it is applied competently.

Duration of treatment

The length of time required for treatment will depend on the condition being treated.

Finding the right therapist

Therapists should be formally qualified. Although in most cases this will give some assurance as to the standard of treatment that the patient can expect, it does not necessarily follow that this treatment will be that most appropriate to the patient's condition.

A reputable therapist will not treat a persistent or recurrent complaint unless the patient has consulted a physician for a conventional diagnosis. With the patient he or she will define a treatment goal and propose a short-term treatment plan (*see* page xxiii) to be used as a basis for checking that the therapy is having the desired effect. No credence should be given to anyone promising a total or instantaneous cure (*see* Practitioner checklist, page xxv).

Enemas

> **Rating**
> **May be of some use** as a short-term attempt to improve mental outlook in constipation and as a short-term supportive measure for coughs and colds.
> **Not advised** as the sole treatment for persistent complaints. A conventional physician should always have diagnosed the patient's condition and made a proper risk–benefit assessment.

Method

Enemas are claimed to improve mental outlook, detoxify the body, and modulate the immune system (*see* page 10).

Rationale and historical perspective

In days gone by, enemas of water, coffee, tea, milk, or soapsuds were widely used remedies, often being associated with mythical notions of "inner cleansing." Even today, enemas are an important aspect of some complementary practices.

They are nowadays administered using special equipment generally consisting of an irrigator, a catheter, and an evacuation tube to carry away the water and colonic debris. The enema itself should be about 4°F below body temperature. Lubricating the evacuation tube with Vaseline or a suitable cream will help its insertion into the rectum. Enemas can be administered with the patient lying on his or her back or side (knees drawn up), or in a low kneeling, bent-forward position.

The therapist will set up the equipment so that water flows under gentle gravitational pressure into the large intestine, softening any impacted waste. The procedure should be terminated if the patient finds the treatment unpleasant. The water should be retained in the rectum until a strong urge to defecate is felt. The procedure can be repeated if desired.

Colonic hydrotherapy (colonic irrigation)

This is a modern variant of enema treatment that involves flushing the bowel with water in quantities and at temperatures and pressures to suit individual patients' needs. As water is introduced through one tube, water and colonic debris are removed through another, the so-called obturator. Colonic hydrotherapy sessions last about an hour.

How it works

Enemas, it is claimed, help the patient by improving mental outlook, modulating the immune system (*see* page 10), and eliminating toxic substances. The general belief among practitioners is that the intestinal flora not only affect the local immune situation but also can be actively used to modulate the body's entire immune system. This being so, they claim, it must also be possible to use enemas and colonic hydrotherapy successfully in the treatment of diseases and their symptoms outside the gastrointestinal tract.

Indications

Some complementary therapists recommend enemas as a universal remedy for virtually any disease and its associated symptoms. They are often used in an attempt to improve the patient's mental state, to provide support for changed eating habits, and for the treatment of coughs, colds, and constipation.

Proof it works

There has been little research into whether enemas have any beneficial effect. There have not as yet been any reliable clinical studies (*see* page xix). Though certain case reports and some studies (*see* page xx) claim a degree of efficacy, the positive outcome that is described was probably only seen in proportion of patients receiving treatment (*see* Placebo, page xxi).

Risks, cautions, and contraindications

If not properly administered, enemas can damage the intestinal mucosa. Anyone receiving enemas regularly may absorb excessive amounts of water, which can in turn induce problems such as nausea, vomiting, a pulmonary edema, heart failure, or a coma. Colonic hydrotherapy carries a number of significant risks and should only be administered by a highly trained practitioner whose procedures are scrupulously hygienic. There have been a number of fatalities due to colon hydrotherapy equipment not being properly sterilized.

Duration of treatment

The length of treatment can vary according to the patient's condition and needs. Colonic hydrotherapy is usually carried out in a series of ten sessions.

Finding the right therapist

Enemas are suitable for self-treatment.

A reputable colonic hydrotherapist will generally not carry out any treatment until the patient has seen a doctor for a conventional diagnosis. With the patient he or she will define at treatment goal and propose a short-term treatment plan (*see* page xxiii) to be used as a basis for checking that the therapy is having the desired effect. No credence should be given to any therapist promising a total or instantaneous cure (*see* Practitioner checklist, page xxv).

Leeches

> **Rating**
> **Of little use** as a routine treatment. Perhaps acceptable in rare cases as a short-term attempt to treat chronic illness when more established therapies have been unsuccessful or it has not been possible to diagnose the patient's condition.
> **Not advised** as the sole treatment for persistent complaints unless a conventional physician has diagnosed the patient's condition and made a proper risk–benefit assessment.

Method

Leeches are said to clean and detoxify the blood, to relieve congestion, and to exercise a spasmolytic effect.

Rationale and historical perspective

Leeches were used throughout antiquity to treat various ills. Through their indiscriminate use as a catchall remedy and their frequent failure to produce a cure, they gradually fell from favor but have recently made something of a comeback. The medicinal leech *Hirudo medicinalis officinalis* is grown in special breeding centers and is a ringed worm about 5cm long with a sucking disc at both its anterior and its posterior ends. Its anterior mouth has three toothed plates with which it penetrates the skin of its prey, leaving quite visible wounds. The animal's salivary juices contain an anticoagulant substance known as hirudin. Hirudin can nowadays be manufactured genetically. Its chief uses in modern medicine are in the prevention and treatment of thrombosis.

Depending on the condition being treated and the site at which the animals are to be used, a total of between two and twelve leeches will generally be used. They relinquish their tight grip on the skin within about an hour. Because of the risk of infection, they should never be reused.

A leech will consume around ½fl oz of blood; the wound will

produce a further 1–1¹/₂fl oz of blood in the succeeding 24 hours. Since the wounds continue to bleed, it is vital that the patient remains lying after treatment.

How it works

Therapists claim that leeches are able to purify and detoxify the patient's blood, relieve congestion, and exercise a spasmolytic action. These effects are probably due to the fact that hirudin and other principal ingredients have an anti-inflammatory and anticoagulative effect not only at the site of the bite but also systemically. What is more, leeches are said to act directly on various regions of the body through so-called energy links (*see* page 928).

Indications

For some users leeches are a universal remedy. Their most common uses are for vein disorders, acute gout, furuncles in the face, infected insect bites, arthrosis, and certain eye problems.

Proof it works

There has been little research into the overall therapeutic benefit of using leeches. There have been few definitive clinical trials (*see* page xix). Some field surveys and case studies (*see* page xx) maintain that leeches can be used to bring relief from pain. However, the efficacy that is claimed is probably only seen in a proportion of patients (*see* Placebo, page xxi).

Risks, cautions, and contraindications

Leeches must only ever be used once because of their potential for transmitting disease from one person to another. Hemophiliacs must not be treated with leeches. Bleeding may continue unabated in patients with blood-clotting disorders. Leeches should not be introduced to diseased skin, nor used for gangrene. There may be allergic reactions at the points of attachment.

Duration of treatment

The length of treatment will depend on the condition being addressed.

Finding the right therapist

No credence should be given to therapists who promise a total or immediate cure (*see* Practitioner checklist, page xxv). A responsible therapist will not start treatment until the patient has obtained a conventional diagnosis from a practitioner. With the patient the therapist will define a treatment goal and propose a short-term treatment plan (*see* page xxiii) to be used as a basis for checking that the therapy is working.

It is advisable to seek treatment only from therapists who have some formal qualification. Although in most cases this will give a certain assurance as to the training that the therapist has received and the standard of treatment that the patient can expect, it will not necessarily follow that the treatment given will be the most appropriate for dealing with the patient's condition.

Enzyme therapy

Rating

Of little use. Possibly acceptable as an initially limited attempt to treat persistent inflammatory or degenerative conditions when more established and less costly treatments have not produced the desired results.

Not advised as the sole treatment for persistent complaints unless a conventional physician has diagnosed the patient's condition and made a proper risk–benefit assessment.

Method

Plant and animal enzymes are said to act on human blood and tissues and so counter inflammatory and degenerative processes and cancer.

Rationale and historical perspective

The roots of enzyme therapy can be traced back to man's early history. The indigenous inhabitants of Latin American used the pineapple and leaves and fruit of the melon tree, *Carica papaya*, for therapeutic purposes; there are references in the Bible to dates as a useful treatment for sores; and in Europe in the Middle Ages, spurge was a remedy for sores, furuncles, and warts.

It is now known that all of these herbal remedies contain enzymes. Enzymes are protein molecules composed of long amino acid chains that promote and accelerate various chemical reactions in the body that otherwise would not occur or, if they did, would happen only slowly. Enzymes have names ending in "ase".

If the body is unable to produce a certain enzyme, an enzyme supplement may need to be given—for example, when the pancreas is unable to produce the fat-hydrolyzing enzyme esterase, or cannot produce enough of it. Complementary enzyme therapy sets out to achieve more; it claims to be able to treat, or at least arrest, inflammatory and degenerative processes in the body through high-dosed enzyme supplementation, and to be able to speed up wound healing. Modern enzyme therapy evolved as a result of experiments performed by the Scottish physician John Beard who, at the turn of the century, injected cancer patients with extracts of animal pancreas at or near the sites of their malignant growths. Beard allegedly managed to arrest tumor growth and even cause tumors to shrink. In the 1930s, the Viennese researcher Ernst Freund published a paper suggesting that serum obtained from the blood of healthy persons is able to destroy tumor cells but that serum from cancer patients is not. The latter persons, he concluded, must be lacking an "essential substance" that processes this power.

Proceeding from this theory, the Austrian physician Max Wolf discovered in the New York Biological Research Institute that a combination of various proteolytic enzymes (proteases) of animal and plant origin can be used to reinstate the tumor-destroying capability of the blood. In particular, he noticed they had a positive effect in vascular disease, lymphatic edema, and shingles, and on the way in which wounds and inflamed tissues healed.

A group of enzyme preparations is today available that are primarily used for immune-modulation treatment (see page 10) of various types of inflammation, edema, rheumatic disorders, virus infections, and cancer. These enzyme preparations are normally injected or taken in the form of sugar-coated tablets.

How it works

The enzymes and enzyme mixtures employed are said to induce various reactions, some of which have only been studied under laboratory conditions. These preparations are claimed, among other things, to improve blood flow, to reduce clotting, to have an anti-inflammatory effect, and to help reduce swelling and bruising more quickly. They are also, it is said, able to influence the immune system, e.g. by breaking down so-called "immune complexes," substances that are crucial to the functioning of the immune system. The way they work has not been fully elucidated.

Though certain functional aspects of these substances have been studied in the testtube, it remains unclear what their significance might be in healthy and sick persons.

Indications

According to its proponents, enzyme therapy can be employed in almost any condition, including respiratory, vascular, gynacological, dermatological, gastrointestinal, urogenital, cancerous, and age-related conditions. It is also claimed to be a useful way of addressing problems affecting the locomotor system, and of improving post-surgical wound healing.

Proof it works

Medical experts feel there is insufficient evidence to suggest that enzyme therapy actually works. There is a lack of reliable data from rigorous clinical studies (*see* page xix). The extent to which claims made about its efficacy in case reports (*see* page xx) have been borne out cannot be judged at present.

Risks, cautions, and contraindications

Enzyme therapy should not be attempted in persons with blood-clotting disorders or advanced liver or kidney dysfunction. Some patients are allergic to the enzymes used, in which case injection of an enzyme preparation may have life-threatening consequences.

The overconfidence exhibited by some enzyme therapists convinced that they know exactly what is wrong with the patient may mean that he or she will fail to obtain more appropriate treatment.

Duration of treatment

Enzyme preparations are generally taken three times a day before meals. In acute conditions, e.g. following sporting injuries or in chronic painful conditions such as severe rheumatoid arthritis, manufacturers recommend massive-dose therapy with 20–24 tablets three times daily until the symptoms have subsided, which generally takes three to four weeks.

Enemas (*see* page 819) are some therapists' recommended way of delivering higher dosages still. In cancer therapy, preparations are injected directly into the tumor wherever possible. To prevent formation of metastases or recidivation, treatment should be continued, it is advised, for at least three years.

Finding the right therapist

No credence should be given to therapists promising an instantaneous or total cure (*see* Practitioner checklist, page xxv).

A responsible enzyme therapist will generally not start treatment without the patient having obtained a conventional diagnosis. With the patient, he or she will define a treatment goal and propose an initially limited plan of treatment (*see* page xxiii) to be used as a basis for checking that enzyme therapy is producing the desired beneficial effect.

Non-prescription enzyme preparations are suitable for self-treatment.

Flower remedies

> **Rating**
> **Possibly of some use** as an attempted supportive treatment aimed at improving the patient's state of mind and restoring well-being.
> **Not advised** as the sole treatment for persistent complaints unless a conventional physician has diagnosed the patient's condition and made a proper risk–benefit assessment.

Method

Specially preserved infusions of flowers are used in the belief that they can eliminate the causes of disease by improving the harmony of body, mind, and spirit.

Rationale and historical perspective

There are many different types of flower remedies. Of these, the best known are probably those developed by Dr Edward Bach. In 1930 Dr Bach gave up a flourishing medical practice to devote the remaining six years of his life to systematically identifying 38 negative states of mind. Each one of these, he concluded, could be countered with a specific flower remedy. Bach's rather mystical approach to disease (which he saw as the result of conflicts between personality and one's higher self) might best be described as psychosomatically oriented. Physical ailments can be cured by converting character weaknesses into virtues. A combination of the will to get better and the appropriate flower remedy can allegedly overcome any disease. Bach's Rescue Remedy, a blend of cherry plum, clematis, impatiens, rock rose, and star of Bethlehem, is given at times when rapid relief is needed.

In an initial consultation, the flower therapist will decide what remedy is required, either intuitively or through a series of questions that will pinpoint the person's state of mind. The remedies are supplied in small bottles to be taken directly on the tongue or diluted with water and drunk; alternatively they can be massaged into the skin or added to a relaxing bath.

With time, it is claimed, patients can discover how to interpret their own states of mind so precisely that they can formulate the required flower combinations themselves.

How it works

The criteria by which Bach selected his essences of wild flowers and the mechanisms by which his and other flower remedies are said to work have not been properly substantiated. The good results purportedly achieved with flower remedies might possibly be explained in terms of a powerful placebo effect (*see* page xxi).

Indications

For some of the proponents of this therapy, flower remedies act in the capacity of mental purifiers that are able, allegedly, to overcome virtually any physical disease by eliminating negative states of mind. However, responsible therapists will use this form of treatment primarily to improve mental outlook and to assist other therapies.

Proof it works

There have been few, if any, controlled clinical studies to validate whether the therapy does work (*see* page xix). The successes that case reports claim (*see* page xx) cannot be properly substantiated based on present findings; such claims possibly apply to only a proportion of patients receiving treatment (*see* Placebo, page xxi).

Risks, cautions, and contraindications

Flower remedies may (presumably very occasionally) cause intolerance and allergies.

They tend to ignore possible physical causes of disease and may lead to a situation in which the patient fails to obtain a proper diagnosis, and misses the opportunity of receiving more appropriate treatment. Anyone relying solely on Bach Rescue Remedy for the treatment of life-threatening situations such as accidental injury, choking, or myocardial infarction is exposing himself/herself to incalculable risks.

Duration of treatment

Treatment can range between a single series of treatments and lifelong use of flower remedies. Chronic conditions may require several months of treatment.

Finding the right therapist

Therapists promising a total or instantaneous cure should be viewed with great scepticism (*see* Practitioner checklist, page xxv). A reputable flower therapist will generally not start treatment until the patient has obtained a conventional diagnosis. With the patient, the therapist will define a treatment goal and propose an initially limited treatment plan (*see* page xxiii) to be used as a basis for checking that the therapy is having the desired effect.

Anyone who has received qualified instruction can treat himself/herself with flower remedies.

Homeopathy

Method

Highly diluted or potentized drugs are used to encourage the body to better regulate its "disturbed vital force" or to relieve various complaints directly. The substances that are employed in homeopathy are diluted hundreds or thousands of times over, so the effect is in the "message" they carry rather than in the actual constituents of the drug. The dilutant, it is supposed, has a "memory" of the molecules it was once in contact with.

Rationale and historical perspective

In 1790, the German physician Samuel Hahnemann (1755–1843) observed after taking quinine—a popular antimalarial of the day—in small doses for several days, that he actually developed the symptoms of malaria. From here he experimented with vegetable, animal, and mineral substances in healthy volunteers, each time arriving at the same result, namely that the remedies he employed produced exactly the same symptoms as the diseases they were intended to cure. In 1796, Hahnemann published his key homeopathic principle: *"Similia similibus curentur"* or "Like cures like." This law of similars is the cornerstone of homeopathic therapy; it states that an agent that produces the symptoms of an illness can, when taken in minute doses, cure similar symptoms when these are caused by a disease. The word "homeopathy" is derived from the Greek *homios* ("like") and *pathos* ("suffering").

Hahnemann went on to develop the principle of potentization. An animal, mineral, or plant extract is preserved in an alcoholic solution and left to stand for two to four weeks. This solution forms the "mother tincture," which is then diluted to produce the various homeopathic strengths or potencies. Each time the solution is diluted, it is shaken or "succussed". Where the substances are not soluble, the dilutions are added to miniature lactose tablets. It is the process of dilution and succussion that gives the drug its dynamic power.

Successive tenfold dilutions are represented by the letter X, hundredfold dilutions by the letter C, and thousandfold dilutions by the letter M, while Q signifies successive 1:50,000 dilutions. Other dilution factors are sometimes used. Diluting one part mother tincture with nine parts dilutant represents an X1 protenization; diluting the result in turn with nine parts dilutant represents an X2 potentization, and so on. Mathematically, an X6 potency is equivalent to approximately one part mother tincture in a million parts dilutant. The procedure for producing C potencies is similar: one part mother tincture diluted with 99 parts dilutant produces a C1 potency, and so on.

Highly potentized homeopathic preparations are generally given in the form of small sugar pills or "globuli," while lower potencies are given as tablets. Also, preparations may be supplied in ampules or as ointments to be rubbed in.

Classical homeopathy concentrates not on directly combating pathogens causing the disease but on jolting the patient's "vital force" into action. The remedies are thus intended to help the body realize its own self-healing potential. Classical homeopaths select the appropriate remedies after drawing up a sort of personality profile of the patient in an initial session often lasting in excess of an hour. Once details have been gathered regarding the patient's constitution and disease symptoms, the homeopath will choose the appropriate remedy based on the law of similars. Unlike modern mainstream medicine, which largely prescribes drugs to suit a given diagnosis largely irrespective of the patient's profile, classical homeopathy will hardly ever prescribe the same remedy for two patients with the same disease. Conversely, patients who are of largely the same constitutional type will be given the same remedy despite the fact that an orthodox diagnosis has discovered they have different diseases. It is also quite possible that several attempts will be made to treat the patient before the right "similar" has been found.

It can happen, once a person has started taking a homeopathic remedy, that his or her symptoms appear to worsen for a while. This phenomenon, known as "initial aggravation," is taken as being a good sign because, in the logic of homeopathy, it means that the right preparation has been chosen for the patient and his or her particular symptoms.

Several variants of homeopathy have evolved over the years.

Organotropic and functiotropic homeopathy

The off-the-shelf remedies of organotropic and functiotropic homeopathy are not selected according to the patient's constitution or type of vital force disturbance, but tend rather to be symptom oriented. Organotropic means directed toward a specific organ or organ system; functiotropic means directed towards a functional system.

Nosodes

The idea of nosodes was popularized by American Constantin Hering, who in 1830 borrowed this word from the Greek *nosos* ("disease"). A nosode is a product of disease that is used as a remedy. His concept was based on the principles of immunization and homeopathy. Typically, nosodes consist of blood, pus, pathogenic organisms, or cancer cells and are either industrially produced or are tailor-made as "autonosodes" from the patient's own body material. The individual components are sterilized, serially diluted, and given as ampules for drinking or as an injection. Nosodes, it is claimed, encourage the body's own defence system to heal any disease still present and to wash out "poisons."

Homotoxicology

Homotoxicology, which is based on work by the German physician Hans-Heinrich Reckeweg (1905–85) uses classical homeopathic remedies, nosodes, potentized organ extracts, suitably diluted traditional medications, and mixtures of all of these. Homotoxicologists claim that diseases are signs that the body is protecting itself from endogenous and exogenous "poisons." Disease and intoxication processes develop in six progressively worsening stages, but can be arrested and reversed through the use of suitably potentized preparations. Only the final stages of a disease are occasionally incapable of being reversed.

Various modern mainstream drugs allegedly hinder the body in its attempt to rid itself of poisons and cause "counter-poisoning," which is seen as leading to severe illness. Antihomotoxic agents are supposed to mobilize the body's reserves, so enabling it to prevent such poisoning.

Spagyric

Spagyric is partly based on homeopathic principles and proceeds from the notion that human beings, animals, and plants have a "vital energy" that can be released and utilized therapeutically. This energy, which is innate but dormant in plants, is made available as a healing force by fermenting, distilling, and ashing the plant or certain of its component parts, and subsequently reuniting all of these elements. The term is derived from the Greek *span* ("to draw") and *ageirein* ("to bring together"). These types of preparation are believed to release the curative powers inherent in the plant and to enhance their effect. In so-called complex remedies, various plant extracts of allegedly similar therapeutic efficacy are combined; in addition, certain metals, minerals, or animal materials may also be used. The remedies used by spagyric practitioners are said to encourage the body's power of self-healing and to eliminate harmful substances. Spagyric preparations for swallowing or to be applied locally are sometimes prepared by the therapists themselves.

Flower remedies (*see* page 828), electroacupuncture according to Voll (*see* page 802) and numerous preparations used in anthroposophical medicine (*see* page 781) all embody some degree of homeopathic philosophy.

How it works

Low-potency remedies, however much diluted, might be explained in terms of the presence of an active ingredient. However, the way in which highly potentized preparations are thought to act cannot be rationalized in this way. Theoretically, at potencies higher than X24 or C12, there is not a single molecule of mother tincture left in the dilution administered. Nevertheless, homeopathy utilizes even higher potencies than this. Homeopaths believe that their remedies work because "footprints" of the active ingredient are imprinted on each molecule so that, as the mother tincture is diluted many times over, the "energetic memory" of the remedy is passed on to the molecular structure of the dilutant. Unspecified structures in the human body respond to the "message."

Certain experiments have apparently shown some kind of electromagnetic or physiochemical change in water in which a substance has been diluted to the point of disappearance. Biochemical experiments have also shown that homeopathic remedies in certain potency ranges have a different effect from those in others. Others have not been able to replicate such results. The importance of these observations is still unclear, however.

Indications

Potentized homeopathic drugs, many proponents claim, are effective no matter what symptoms are presenting. Homeopathic remedies are most frequently given in chronic diseases, lowered resistance, allergies, and psychosomatic disorders. Reputable homeopaths will attempt to treat only conditions that are essentially curable, i.e. those involving a mild disturbance as opposed to a full functional breakdown; in severe conditions they will offer only supportive treatment.

Proof it works

There is presently insufficient hard evidence to substantiate claims that homeopathy and homeopathic therapies are efficacious for any given condition. Controlled findings that might be considered reliable and of general validity are patchy and incomplete. They are also highly nonuniform as to the results. A wealth of case reports (*see* page xx), field studies, and controlled clinical studies (though these are controversial) suggest that homeopathic remedies are efficacious in a measure that exceeds a pure placebo effect (*see* page xxi). What this means in terms of the general use of homeopathic remedies in the clinical treatment of patients remains unclear.

Risks, cautions, and contraindications

Provided that treatment is carried out competently, there seem to be few direct risks. However, low-potency homeopathic remedies (up to about X8) can—at least theoretically—trigger allergies. Low-potency toxic substances and heavy metals such as arsenic, lead, and mercury can cause chronic intoxication when used continuously in the medium to long term.

The promises made by some homeopaths may mean that a patient will fail to obtain appropriate conventional treatment, or will fail to obtain it early enough.

Duration of treatment

The length of treatment will depend on the disease, the form of treatment administered, the potency of the remedy, and its efficacy in the person receiving treatment. In many cases treatment will continue for many months or even years.

Finding the right therapist

There are doctor homeopaths and non-medically trained homeopaths. Whatever their background, however, they should belong to a registered organization. Although in most cases this will generally give some assurance as to the quality of training the homeopath will have received and the standard of treatment the patient can expect, it does not automatically follow that homeopathy will provide the most appropriate treatment for the condition for which treatment is being sought. Before treatment starts, the homeopath will first ask the patient numerous questions to build up an in-depth picture of his or her constitution and individual disease picture. A reputable homeopath will generally not start treatment without the patient having obtained a conventional diagnosis. With the patient, he or she will define a treatment goal and propose an initially limited treatment plan (*see* page xxiii), to be used as a basis for checking that the treatment is having the desired effect. No credence should be given to any practitioner promising an instantaneous or complete cure (*see* Practitioner checklist, page xxv).

Off-the-shelf organotropic and functiotropic remedies are suitable for self-medication. Professional guidance is recommended, though not absolutely essential.

Hypnosis and self-hypnosis

Rating
Useful as a method of relaxation and of alleviating fear and pain; as an aid during withdrawal from addiction; and as an attempt to treat psychosomatic disorders and alleviate pain (usually supportively).
Not advised as the sole treatment for persistent complaints unless a conventional physician has diagnosed the patient's condition and made a proper risk–benefit assessment.

Method

Hypnosis and self-hypnosis are methods of relaxation that can be helpful for easing muscular tension, inner unrest, and anxiety, and for treating psychosomatic disorders.

Rationale and historical perspective

Hypnosis is a psychotherapeutic technique that has been practiced for thousands of years. In the 19th century it was enormously fashionable and Sigmund Freud studied it before developing his psychoanalytical theories.

Hypnotherapy is based on suggestion; in the state of altered consciousness that is induced, physical conditions can be addressed, pain can be relieved or eliminated, and therapeutic messages about feeling positive and self-confident can be communicated to the patient. Blood pressure, heart rate, circulation, and the vegetative nervous system can all be normalized by hypnosis, and breathing and digestive activity slowed down.

During hypnotherapy, patients are encouraged to lie back comfortably on a couch or reclining chair and to concentrate on the therapist's eyes or an object he or she might be holding. In a calm, monotonous voice, the therapist may suggest that the patient feels heavy and relaxed, and will possibly repeat a series of statements. Once in a deep trance, the patient is ready to take in suggestions affecting his or her mental and physical health. The suggestions will remain in effect for some time and can be reinforced or withdrawn during subsequent sessions. At the end of each session the hypnotherapist will ask the patient to wake up feeling refreshed.

Hypnosis is often combined with other psychotherapeutic techniques. Professional guidance on self-hypnosis may be available.

How it works

Hypnosis is based on the principle of the body and mind forming a single entity. The physical relaxation that is induced by the hypnotherapist through suggestion (by autosuggestion in the case of self-hypnosis) has a restorative and relaxing effect on the mind, enabling various physical functions to be measurably influenced.

Indications

Hypnosis and self-hypnosis can be used to provide relaxation, to relieve stress, anxiety, and pain, and to help with a wide range of problems such as sleeping and eating disorders, addictions to alcohol, tobacco, drugs, etc. It is also often used in support of psychotherapy for psychosomatic ailments. Autogenic training (*see* page 888) can be used supportively to enhance the positive results achieved through hypnotic suggestion.

In children, hypnotherapy may be used to relieve anxiety and restlessness, and overcome associated problems such as bedwetting, stammering, and feelings of inferiority.

Proof it works

Individual case reports, case studies, and outcome studies (*see* page xx) show hypnosis to be an effective means of providing relaxation and reducing pain. In many cases it was shown that a patient receiving hypnotherapy can reduce his or her medication. It is often difficult to assess the specific effect of hypnotherapy, as this is a technique that is sometimes used in conjunction with various other psychotherapeutic measures. Clinical testing of self-hypnosis is still in its infancy. For self-hypnosis to be effective, it is vital that the patient believes that it works.

Risks, cautions, and contraindications

Hypnosis and self-hypnosis should not be used for severe psychosis, depression, and obsessional neurosis; nor in patients with structural changes in the brain caused by a hardening of the blood vessels; nor in patients who are debilitated or have a psychopathic personality.

There are people who do not respond to hypnotherapy and self-hypnosis. Blind people are difficult to hypnotize, while young children and deaf people cannot be hypnotized at all. Anyone afraid of being taken advantage of while in a hypnotic trance can take along someone they trust.

Poorly chosen suggestions can exacerbate existing symptoms.

Courses in hypnosis are sometimes organized by groups akin to sects.

Duration of treatment

How long a course of hypnotherapy will last depends very much on the patient's individual needs. Generally, there will be twice-weekly sessions, reducing after several weeks to once a week or less frequently.

Finding the right therapist

A hypnotherapist should be trained in psychotherapy and belong to a recognized professional organization. Although in most cases this will give some assurance as to the quality of training he or she will have received and the standard of treatment the patient can expect, it does not automatically follow that hypnotherapy will be the most appropriate form of treatment. A reputable hypnotherapist will stick painstakingly to the topics agreed before the start of treatment.

No credence should be given to any therapist promising an instantaneous or complete cure (*see* Practitioner checklist, page xxv).

Magnetic field therapy

> **Rating**
> **Of little use**. Acceptable as an initially limited attempt to treat poorly settling prosthetic implants and bone fractures when more established therapeutic procedures have not produced the desired results.
> **Not advised** as the sole treatment for persistent complaints unless a conventional physician has diagnosed the patient's condition and made a proper risk–benefit assessment.

Method

Magnetic influences are said to speed up cellular metabolism and increase well-being.

Rationale and historical perspective

The use of magnetic metals for treatment purposes can be traced back to the priests of ancient Egypt; in the 4th century BC, Hippocrates, too, described the healing effect of magnetic fields. The belief in mysterious curative force from the cosmos has been enduring and, around the turn of the century, magnetic field therapy was even used in conventional medicine. Magnetic fields, it is claimed, have the power to heal conditions such as migraines or rheumatism, and even to prevent the growth of tumors.

In complementary medicine, various technical aids have been developed to intensify the presumed healing powers of magnetic forces, including special coils for whole body treatment and miniature devices that are implanted near bone fractures to deliver a pulsed electromagnetic field locally. The conviction that magnetic fields alone can have a curative effect has led to the development of various products with a magnetizing effect.

- In some cases, small coils are attached to diseased parts of the body in order for their force fields to act.
- Self-adhesive magnetic strips or foils are also available for application to parts of the body causing pain. They are suitable for self-treatment.
- Magnetic belts, bracelets, etc. can be worn perpetually on the body.

How it works

Manufacturers of magnetic strips, foils, and generators maintain that magnetic field therapy encourages the healing of a number of disorders and even prevents disease from occurring.

Indications

Proponents of magnetic therapy say that it is an effective treatment for more than 30 conditions, including migraines, rheumatic pains, sciatica, circulatory disorders, and inflammation of various etiology, as well as being helpful for healing wounds and bone fractures.

Proof it works

There is no clinical evidence as yet that would corroborate claims by its proponents that magnetic therapy actually works. This treatment method is mostly founded on unproven hypotheses (*see* Placebo, page xxi).

Risks, cautions, and contraindications

Magnetic field devices and strips are not thought to pose any risks as long as the contraindications are heeded. Patients fitted with a heart pacemaker must not undergo magnetic therapy, as it would upset the control system of this delicate instrument.

Duration of treatment

A treatment session lasts about 20 minutes. Normally treatment will be carried out twice or three times a week for a total of ten sessions.

Finding the right therapist

No credence should be given to any therapist promising an instantaneous or total cure (*see* Practitioner checklist, page xxv). Treatment should only be undertaken, if at all, in a specialized clinic under the supervision of a doctor. Although in most cases this will give some assurance as to the quality of training that the therapist will have received and the standard of treatment that the patient can expect, it will not automatically follow that this will be the most appropriate treatment for the patient's condition. Therapists mostly receive their training from equipment manufacturers.

Manual therapies (chiropractic, osteopathy)

> **Rating**
> **May be of some use** as an initially limited attempt to mobilize joints, relax muscles, and alleviate pain, particularly acute low back pain.
> **Not advised** as the sole treatment for persistent complaints unless a conventional physician has diagnosed the patient's condition and made a proper risk–benefit assessment.

Method

Through of series of controlled, usually jerky or levering movements, osteopaths and chiropractors adjust misaligned vertebrae and other bones to ease muscular spasm and dispel pain. Osteopaths tend to use softer techniques, while chiropractors often apply what is called a "high velocity thrust."

Rationale and historical perspective

The practice of manipulating of the spine and skeleton is an ancient one. As statues found in Egypt and Thailand show, it is a form of medicine that has been known for at least 4,000 years. At the end of the 19th century, the American Andrew Taylor Still founded a school of osteopathy to practice this "gentle manipulative technique." At about the same time, the Swiss physician Otto Naegeli published his first book on chirotherapy, and Canadian-born David Daniel Palmer developed chiropractic, a manual therapy involving the adjustment of misaligned vertebrae. It took almost a century of medical debate and rethinking of their therapeutic concept before, in the 1980s, American chiropractors finally received recognition from the American Medical Association.

In the UK, osteopathy achieved respectability with the foundation of the British School of Osteopathy in 1917. With the passing of the Osteopathy Act in 1993, it also received official recognition, being the first non-conventional therapy in the UK to be regulated by law. More than 5 million British citizens a year now visit osteopaths for treatment. Osteopaths and chiropractors usually take a four-year degree course, with some going on to get a master's degree in osteopathy.

How it works

Chiropractors use the hands to adjust malaligned vertebrae and joints back into place through a series of rhythmic or jerky movements to remove the cause of muscular spasm and nerve irritation. The theory is that tension in the muscles restricts the movement of the spinal column and joints and that relieving the strain on the spine through manual realignment can help systems to operate smoothly again. The main difference between osteopathy and chiropractic lies in the method of manipulation used. Chiropractors tend to use brisk movements and manipulations, while osteopaths make more use of soft-tissue techniques, applying leverage and pressure to muscles, bones, and joints to relieve stresses and restore mobility.

Indications

Some proponents of these manual therapies claim that they can be employed to treat virtually any type of disease, though most modern practitioners limit themselves to treating conditions that are thought to be the direct result of malalignment of the bones and joints. Manual therapy is a way of remobilizing the frame and limbs, of easing taut muscles, and of relieving back pain and headaches believed to be caused by misplaced cervical vertebrae.

Proof it works

Several controlled clinical studies (*see* page xix) have shown that relief can be brought to approximately 50–60 percent of patients suffering from back pain and headaches. The results thus appear to be slightly better than those for conventional physical therapies (*see* pages 867–78). But results are contradictory, and recent studies have highlighted the need for better evidence in this area.

Risks, cautions, and contraindications

Treatment carried out on the thoracic and lumbar vertebrae by a trained therapist probably carries little risk, though there have been reported cases of stroke, dislocated or broken vertebrae, prolapsed discs, lesions of the spinal cord, and neuroparalysis. Poor technique in the application of chirotherapeutic manipulations to the head and neck can cause arteries to be seriously injured, stretched, or trapped, the spine to be damaged, or bones fractured. Worldwide, more than 40 fatalities have been reported in the literature.

Chirotherapy should not be used to treat any disorder arising from weakness or disease of the bones or joints themselves (e.g. osteoporosis, rheumatoid arthritis, tumors, or spinal deformity). Manipulations to the neck involving rotational movements are particularly risk-laden in persons over 60 years of age.

Soft-tissue techniques and mobilizations (osteopathy) carry fewer risks than manipulations (chiropractic). Many chiropractors overuse X-rays. As they can cause cancer, it is wise to be cautious about repeated X-rays.

Duration of treatment

One session is sometimes enough. A series of five to ten sessions is usually recommended.

Finding the right therapist

Anyone administering a manual treatment should belong to a professional body. Although in most cases this will give some assurance as to the quality of training that the practitioner will have received and the standard of treatment that the patient can expect, it does not automatically guarantee that a manual treatment will be appropriate to the condition with which the patient is presenting.

A reputable manual therapist will generally not start treatment unless the patient has been diagnosed conventionally and appropriate X-rays have been taken. With the patient, he or she will define a treatment goal and propose an initially limited treatment plan (*see* page xxiii) to be used as a basis for checking that the treatment is having the desired effect. No credence should be given to any therapist promising an instantaneous or total cure (*see* Practitioner checklist, page xxv).

Massage

Classical massage

Rating

Useful as a short-term measure aimed at calming, relaxing, and rehabilitating the patient and providing relief from pain and tension.

Not advised as the sole treatment for persistent complaints unless a conventional physician has diagnosed the patient's condition and made a proper risk–benefit assessment.

Method

Classical massage techniques are said to revitalize the body, encourage self-healing, and impart a feeling of calmness and relaxation.

Rationale and historical perspective

Classical massage is one of the oldest therapies. It is practiced by many cultures, oriental and occidental alike. Massage is a stimulation therapy (*see* page 929) that utilizes stroking (effleurage), kneading (petrissage), rolling, knuckling, pressing, rubbing, percussion (tapotement), shaking, and vibrating movements. A perceptive practitioner will be able to detect even slight tensions and strains and will carefully match the strokes used, and the pressure with which they are applied, to the symptoms and needs of the individual, providing relaxation and refreshment, as well as directly addressing any obvious abnormalities. Massage is also capable of bringing relief from anxiety and tension.

To those who have a disturbed relationship with their body or have had some painful experience massage can bring renewed vigor and a new outlook on life. A good masseur or masseuse will also sometimes be able to release a patient's pent-up emotions; massage thus also has a potentially psychotherapeutic role.

It must be appreciated that massage can on occasion be painful, and the patient may well come away from a treatment session with bruises. However, as long as the practitioner matches the pressure that is applied to the patient's specific constitution, these effects should diminish in the course of treatment.

How it works

Classical massage is dynamic and restorative. The nerve endings that are stimulated in the skin and connective tissue during massage transmit impulses to other parts of the body, so improving blood flow, relaxing muscles, easing knotted tissues, and supporting lymphatic (or waste drainage) systems in the body (*see* Lymphatic drainage, page 850). The primary organs can be acted upon via reflex channels (*see* page 881). Massage also restores a feeling of physical and emotional calmness, and painful "counterstimuli" can be used to dispel pain temporarily.

Indications

Many practitioners see classical massage as a holistic (*see* page 928) system and use it for a wide variety of symptoms and disorders, though its forte is in giving general relaxation, in improving well-being, in treating rheumatic disease, migraines and back pain, in coaxing the tension from muscles, in rehabilitation following injury or surgery to the musculoskeletal system, following paralysis, for heart disease, and for hypertension.

Proof it works

There is little reliable evidence to suggest that classical massage has any disease-specific efficacy. Numerous testimonials, outcome reports, and a few controlled clinical trials (*see* page xx), do, however, underline its general usefulness for bringing relaxation and relief from anxiety, for alleviating pain, and as an aid to rehabilitation.

Risks, cautions, and contraindications

Classical massage should not be used in persons with tumors, febrile infections, arteriosclerosis, a hemorrhagic tendency, or blood circulation problems (such as thrombosis, varicose veins, or phlebitis). Massage is also contraindicated in patients at risk of embolism or those who have recently suffered a heart attack Some patients are oversensitive to manual stimuli or find it hard to accept the close physical contact that is required in classical massage.

Duration of treatment

Classical massage to provide symptomatic treatment will normally be administered in a series of six to twelve sessions taking place twice or three times per week. For relaxation and general restoration, on the other hand, the frequency of treatment sessions will depend on individual requirements.

Finding the right masseur/masseuse

Classical massage should only be performed by a masseur/masseuse who has been fully trained in therapeutic massaging techniques and who is a recognized member of a registered professional body. Although in most cases this will give some assurance as to the quality of training the masseur/masseuse will have received and the standard of treatment the patient can expect, it does not automatically follow that massage will be the most appropriate form of treatment. A reputable masseur/masseuse will generally not treat a persistent or recurrent problem without the patient having obtained a conventional diagnosis. With the client, he or she will define a treatment goal and propose an initially limited treatment plan (*see* page xxiii) to be used as a basis for checking that massage is eliciting the desired beneficial effect. No credence should be given to any practitioner promising an instantaneous or total cure (see Practitioner checklist, page xxv).

Lymphatic drainage

> **Rating**
> **Useful** as a short-term measure aimed at providing relaxation, treating lymphostasis, and as part of a program of aftercare following surgery for cancer.
> **Not advised** as the sole treatment for persistent complaints unless a conventional physician has diagnosed the patient's condition and made a proper risk–benefit assessment.

Method

Lymphatic drainage reportedly improves the elimination of lymph via the lymphatic and venous systems.

Rationale and historical perspective

Lymphatic drainage was first used in the 1930s by a French physician named Vodder. Since then it has undergone some refinement. Lymph transports nutrients from the gut into the bloodstream and has an important role in the immune system.

Lymphatic drainage involves massage administered with gentle, circular movements to encourage the flow of lymph in the right direction for it to be removed from the body.

How it works

Lymphatic drainage increases the transport capacity of the lymph vessels, so speeding up the elimination of the waste products of metabolism. It is also reported to have a calming and pain-relieving function.

Indications

Some proponents of lymphatic drainage see it as a holistic (see page 928) procedure and use it to address an assortment of complaints. It is frequently used for lymphatic swelling (e.g. in the arm) following surgery for cancer, for bruising and accidental bone fractures, for the common cold, post-thrombotic edema, and menstrual disorders. It is also used as an analgesia (e.g. in rheumatism of the joints and soft tissues), as well as for relaxation and improving mental outlook.

Proof it works

Case studies and initial controlled trials suggest that there may be a marked reduction of swelling following breast operations and the like. The efficacy reportedly achieved in hayfever, eczema, neuralgia, and osteoporosis is probably only seen in a proportion of patients receiving treatment (*see* Placebo, page xxi). In numerous testimonials, patients claim to have found relaxation through lymphatic drainage.

Risks, cautions, and contraindications

Lymphatic drainage should not be used in persons with cancer (because of the risk of disseminating malignant cells throughout the body), acute inflammatory disease, or acute thrombosis.

Not all patients are able to accept the close physical contact that is required in lymphatic drainage; some find being touched under their armpits or on their head, neck, groin, or pelvis an unpleasant experience.

Duration of treatment

Treatment is carried out anything from twice a week to daily, as needs dictate; a treatment series normally consists of ten sessions.

Finding the right masseur/masseuse

Lymphatic drainage should be performed by a qualified masseur/masseuse. Although in most cases this will give some assurance as to the quality of training the practitioner will have received and the standard of treatment the patient can expect, it does not automatically follow that lymphatic drainage will be the most appropriate form of treatment. A reputable masseur/masseuse will generally not treat a persistent or recurrent condition without the patient having obtained a conventional diagnosis. With the client, he or she will define a treatment goal and propose an initially limited treatment plan (*see* page xxiii) to be used as a basis for checking that lymphatic drainage is having the desired beneficial effect. No credence should be given to any masseur/masseuse promising an instantaneous or total cure (*see* Practitioner checklist, page xxv).

Medical herbalism (phytotherapy)

Rating

May be of some use for treating some slight to moderately severe forms of cardiovascular disease, sleeplessness, depression, prostate and bladder problems, various skin conditions (e.g. neurodermatitis), menstrual and menopausal complaints, gastrointestinal problems, coughs and colds, bronchitis, sinusitis, certain problems with concentration and memory, sprains, strains and other injuries; also as a means of increasing the body's resistance to disease. Whenever any condition is persistent or recurrent, it is important to consult a doctor for a conventional diagnosis and an individual risk–benefit assessment.

Not advised as the sole treatment for persistent complaints unless a conventional physician has diagnosed the patient's condition and made a proper risk–benefit assessment.

Method

Medical herbalism (phytotherapy) is the use of plants or certain parts thereof for remedial purposes (e.g. as dried herbs or extracts of therapeutic principles). Herbal teas are widely employed. These are prepared as follows:

- Hard parts such as woody stems, bark, and roots are usually prepared as a decoction (cover with water, bring to a boil, simmer for approximately ten minutes, and strain), occasionally as an infusion (pour hot water onto a chopped or sliced herb, allow to steep for about ten minutes, strain, and drink).

- Fruits and seeds are prepared as a decoction: chop or crush the herb, cover with water, bring to a boil, simmer for ten minutes, and strain.
- Leaves, flowers, and other soft arial parts are prepared as infusions: pour hot water onto the dried herb, then steep for about ten minutes before straining and drinking.

Weights and measures: One cup is approximately equivalent to 5fl oz of water, one teaspoon to 5g of dried herb, one heaped teaspoon to 7g of dried herb, one tablespoon to 15g of dried herb.

Teas and tisanes are available in various ready-to-use forms:

- **herbal teas**: chopped, often mixed, herbs
- **tea bags (tisanes)**: very finely chopped and pulverized herbs, usually of acceptable quality
- **tea granules**: teas containing a large amount of carbohydrate (sugar) as excipient, not highly recommended
- **instant teas**: water-soluble, spray-dried tea powders of high quality, a recommended form of tea

Rationale and historical perspective

Herbal medicine is one of the oldest forms of remedial treatment. More than three-quarters of the world's population uses herbal remedies as a significant or exclusive way of treating disease. Western medicine, however, limits itself to some 200–300 known herbs.

Herbs, or at least the parts that are used, contain a wide assortment of constituents, some of which are unique to a given species of plant while others are common across the board. Phytotherapeutic remedies tend to be complex in nature, having more than one constituent. In some instances it is not known which of the many constituents of an herb is actually the one responsible for its remedial effect. In some cases it is presumed that the effect is due to an interplay of several of the herb's constituents. Many phytotherapeutic remedies, however, tend to be standardized to a given content of one or more of their constituents. This is done in an attempt to assure the reproducible quality of the remedy, though there is no guarantee that the standardized constituents are actually the ones exclusively responsible for the herb's curative effect.

A relatively young research arm is currently looking into the question of secondary elements of plants. These include vitamins and other natural constituents such as enzymes and substances that impart taste, smell, or color. It has been shown in animal experiments, for instance, that some secondary elements of plants are able to regulate blood pressure, lower cholesterol levels, and stimulate the immune system, while others have anti-inflammatory, antibacterial or anticancerous properties. Research into the mechanisms by which these secondary elements work and their significance in human medicine is still in its infancy.

How it works

Many herbal preparations are able to intervene in various body functions. They differ from modern synthetic drugs, which generally contain just one or a couple of active ingredients, in that the sheer number of their active principles gives them different, or a wider range of, properties than would be achieved with just a single ingredient. The strength of a herbal remedy is greater than the strength of its individual parts. This is an important principle in medical herbalism—that of "synergism." Medical herbalists believe that the healing properties of a plant lie in its combination of elements and that each element has an active role in the body, quite apart from the active ingredient itself. The elements, working in combination, are also believed to reduce harmful side effects.

Indications

Some herbalists, who should perhaps not be taken too seriously, advise herbal remedies for virtually any type of disease or ailment. There is evidence to suggest that the use of phytotherapeutic remedies may be appropriate in some slight to moderately severe forms of cardiovascular disease, sleeplessness, depression, prostate and bladder problems, various skin conditions (e.g. neurodermatitis), menstrual and menopausal complaints, gastrointestinal problems, coughs and colds, bronchitis, sinusitis, certain problems with concentration and memory, some conditions affecting the brain (e.g. poor perfusion with blood), sprains, strains and other injuries; and also as a means of increasing the body's resistance to disease.

Herbal remedies are also often used as adjuncts to other naturopathic techniques such as nutritional therapy (*see* page 858), exercise (*see* page 868), and hydrotherapy (*see* page 871).

Proof it works

Hitherto, studies on efficacy and risk versus benefit have only been carried out for a relatively small number of remedial plants. For approximately two dozen plant remedies, there is very convincing evidence that they work for defined conditions. In other cases the justification given for using a plant is that it is a traditional remedy, that it seems to have worked before, or that general observations make it seem useful. This empirical approach is difficult to evaluate scientifically and, above all, makes it impossible to draw any comparisons with competing therapies.

Risks, cautions, and contraindications

Not all herbs and phytotherapeutic remedies are safe. Many carry risks or may cause a wide range of unpleasant side effects. Nevertheless, experience has shown that, providing remedies are used sensibly and as instructed, the incidence of side effects and allergies can be kept low, and the possibility of serious side effects occurring is relatively small. Little progress has been made as yet with the systematic recording of the undesirable effects of herbal remedies and phytotherapeutic drugs. There is only scant information regarding the advisability of using herbal remedies during pregnancy and breastfeeding. Plants that must be avoided during pregnancy include, but are not limited to: golden seal, juniper, marjoram, mugwort, pennyroyal, pokeroot, and sage. Any herbal remedy should be discontinued immediately if it is not well tolerated. Even herbal remedies must not be taken to excess, as they may elicit unwanted side effects in the long term. A person with a serious condition or ailment should not take any herbal medicine without expert advice, and must be kept under medical review.

Claims by some herbalists that herbal remedies can cure

virtually any type of disease are fanciful. The consequences of believing such claims may be dire. Allusions to the fact that such remedies have been used for hundreds of years ignore the following facts: that in those days people had a different concept of disease, that it can now no longer be said with certainty exactly what plants were used, and that earlier little heed was given to side effects.

Duration of treatment

The duration of treatment depends on the individual benefits obtained and on the condition for which the patient is seeking treatment.

Finding the right therapist

In the USA, most medical herbalists are members of the professional organizations such as the American Herbalist Guild or the American Herb Association.

A reputable herbalist will generally not treat a chronic condition until the patient has obtained a conventional diagnosis. With the patient, he or she will define a treatment goal and propose an initially limited treatment plan (*see* page xxiii) to be used as a basis for checking that the treatment is having the desired effect. No credence should be given to an herbalist promising an instantaneous or total cure (*see* Practitioner checklist, page xxv).

Certain elements of phytotherapy can be self-administered. Professional guidance is recommended, though not absolutely essential with all treatments.

Nutritional therapies

Hay's diet

> **Rating**
> **May be of some use** as an individual approach to one's own health care and, preventively, as part of an organic philosophy. The "separation" principle that is at the heart of Hay's diet is not sustained, however, by modern concepts of nutrition.
> **Not advised** as the sole treatment for persistent complaints unless a conventional physician has diagnosed the patient's condition and made a proper risk–benefit assessment.

Method

Concentrated carbohydrates should not be consumed with concentrated proteins. Separating foods in this way is supposed not only to keep a person healthy but also to address a number of health problems.

Rationale and historical perspective

Hay's diet was devised by the American physician Howard Hay at the end of the 19th century. Suffering from a kidney condition that was deemed incurable, Hay successfully self-treated it by changing his diet and adhering to certain laws of nutrition which he himself postulated.

Hay believed the following: that protein requires acidic digestive juices, while carbohydrates need alkaline ones; that eating proteins and carbohydrates together at the same meal causes the carbohydrates to remain undigested and to ferment in the gut; and that the fermentation products that arise during pathologically prolonged digestion are a significant cause of illness. He and the many followers who adopted his various nutritional principles believed that concentrated proteins and concentrated carbohydrates should never be eaten at the same meal. Advocates of such separation diets cannot agree as to the length of time which should be allowed to elapse between protein and carbohydrate meals. However, both groups of nutrients may be combined with "neutral" foods. Hay's classifications are as follows:

- Concentrated proteins include the following: meat, fish, and poultry, boiled or otherwise cooked, egg white, soybean meal, milk, up to 55 percent fat cheese, and white wine. Also in this group are cooked spinach and cooked tomatoes, citrus fruits, tropical fruits, and berry, stone, and pomaceous fruits.
- Concentrated carbohydrates include: cereals, flour, durum wheat flour, rice, potatoes, kale, cabbage, salsify, honey, dates, bananas, figs, sugar and maple syrup, peanuts, chestnuts, beer, and apple and pear juice.
- Neutral foods include: oils, fats, butter, sour milk products, more than 55 percent fat cheese, egg yolk, uncooked meat, uncooked fish, olives, most types of vegetables, whortle-berries, raisins, and distilled alcoholic beverages.

Many of his disciples now classify the foods slightly differently.

Hay made an additional distinction between acid-forming (e.g. bread, starch, eggs, cheese) and alkali-forming foods (e.g. vegetables, salads, fresh fruit) which, his separation principle dictates, should be mixed in a 20:80 ratio.

Hay and his adherents hold separation to be a preventive measure that is effective, for instance, against cancer, and a form of treatment for diabetes, nephritis, and dropsy.

How it works

Separation diets are claimed to speed up the digestive process and take some of the load off the gastrointestinal tract. They are also said to prevent the conversion of sugars to acids, poisonous alcohols and gases by fermentation, to stop the putrefaction of proteins, and to inhibit the formation of toxic and cancerogenic degradation products. Hay's concept of digestion is inconsistent with modern principles of nutrition. Simultaneous digestion of proteins and carbohydrates, which Hay claimed could not occur, in actual fact takes place regularly in the gut. Gastric juice is acidic, intestinal fluid on the other hand is alkaline; in both environments there are active enzymes capable of digesting proteins as well as carbohydrates.

Although Hay's separation concept incorporates various unproven hypotheses, this type of diet is actually consistent with the principles of organic nutrition.

Indications

Some therapists advocate Hay's diet as a cure-all for any disease or symptom. Its most widespread use is preventive, however, as an element of organic nutrition (*see* page 4), and as a path to weight reduction and retaining a trim figure.

Proof it works

Controlled clinical studies (*see* page xix) do generally corroborate claims that organic nutrition works in a preventive capacity and is a way of lessening risk factors conducive to many lifestyle diseases.

Risks, cautions, and contraindications

Not all patients can tolerate every style of organic nutrition. Hay's diet should be checked for individual suitability. This form of nutrition should not be attempted with infants and young children, except under the supervision of an experienced pediatrician or nutritionist.

Study findings have not substantiated the claims occasionally made by proponents of Hay's diet that it can cure various serious diseases. Where a condition is recurrent or persistent, the patient should consult his or her doctor for a conventional examination and to receive orthodox treatment where this is called for.

Duration of treatment

Generally, Hay's diet is advocated as a lifelong nutritional commitment.

Finding the right therapist

A reputable nutritionist will generally not start a patient on a Hay's diet until a conventional diagnosis has been obtained. With the patient, he or she will define a treatment goal and propose an initially limited treatment plan (*see* page xxiii) to be used as the basis for checking that the diet is having the desired positive effect. No credence should be given to any therapist promising an instantaneous or complete cure (*see* Practitioner checklist, page xxv).

Macrobiotics

Rating
Possibly of some use for promoting health and as a preventive measure, provided it is not practiced in any of its extreme forms.
Not advised as the sole treatment for persistent complaints unless a conventional physician has diagnosed the patient's condition and made a proper risk–benefit assessment.

Method

This is a form of organic diet based on the belief that every food has yin or yang properties. Macrobiotics is said to promote health and longevity as well as being a prevention and cure for all ills.

Rationale and historical perspective

The term "macrobiotics" has been derived from the Greek *macros* ("long") and *bios* ("life"). Rooted in Zen Buddhism and developed by the Japanese Georges Oshawa (1893–1966), modern macrobiotics is seen as the way to a harmonious lifestyle. For its proponents, macrobiotics is the "biological and physiological implementation of oriental philosophy and medicine."

One of the cornerstones of Oshawa's concept of diet is the principle of yin and yang (*see* Traditional Chinese Medicine, page 895). Foods are classified as yin or yang and the aim is to eat them in a balanced combination. Oshawa considered the optimum balance to be afforded by a 5:1 ratio of yin to yang. According to him, wholegrain cereals already have this balance and are the ideal basis of a macrobiotic diet.

Oshawa defined ten stages on the path to correct eating, on a scale from –3 to +7. The pinnacle is reached with an exclusively cereal diet, when liquids must only be taken in moderate amounts. He advocated in principle the rejection of "denatured" foods such as sugars, sweet drinks, colored products, unfertilized eggs, canned foods, preserves, artificially dressed fruits and vegetables, tea, coffee, and foods from distant sources.

Anyone adhering to this diet, so Oshawa claimed, is as good as immune to disease. Given that the body replaces one-tenth of its blood every day, then, with a proper diet, any disease must be curable within ten days. "Nothing is simpler to cure than cancer," he stated, for instance. "All you need do is adopt stage 7, the most elementary form of diet."

Michio Kushi, Oshawa's disciple, distanced himself from his master's extreme dietary beliefs and steered macrobiotics toward being just a balanced, organic type of diet.

How it works

Kushi's practical advice on nutrition is largely consistent with the modern concept of a healthy diet centered around organic foods. The alleged curative power of a diet based on macrobiotic principles is scientifically unfounded and, in terms of the modern dietary wisdom, can be taken as only hypothetical.

Indications

Some therapists recommend macrobiotics as a cure-all. Its forte, however, since macrobiotics represents a balanced and healthy way of eating (see page 2), lies in disease prevention.

Proof it works

Controlled trials (*see* page xix) have generally underscored the benefits to be derived from eating organic foods, in terms of prevention and the part they play in reducing the risk factors for various lifestyle diseases. But there is no scientific evidence to substantiate claims that a macrobiotic way of eating is a cure-all. The case reports and outcome studies (*see* page xx) that are available are of dubious worth.

Risks, cautions, and contraindications

Not very many patients will be able to tolerate all types of organic foods, so patients following a macrobiotic diet should be individually assessed. In children, macrobiotics should only be attempted, if at all, under the supervision of an experienced pediatrician or nutritionist. A macrobiotic diet could be life-threatening for infants and young children. Where a condition is persistent or recurrent, patients should consult their doctor for an examination and for conventional treatment where this is called for.

Patients should avoid rigid adherence to Oshawa's original dietary philosophy, which can cause severe deficiency symptoms and has in the past produced a number of fatalities.

Eating moldy grain can poison the liver with aflatoxins, which are also known to be carcinogenic.

Duration of treatment

Depending on the condition with which the patient presents and his or her individual needs, this form of nutritional therapy may be practiced in the short or medium term, possibly also becoming a permanent element of a new lifestyle.

Finding the right therapist

A reputable dietary therapist will generally not start treatment without the patient having obtained a conventional diagnosis. With the patient, he or she will define a treatment goal and propose an initially limited treatment plan (*see* page xxiii), to be used as a basis for checking that the diet is having the desired positive effect. No credence should be given to any therapist promising an instantaneous or complete cure (*see* Practitioner checklist, page xxv).

Therapeutic fasting

Rating
Useful as a short-term measure to improve mental outlook or as a prelude to an organic diet.
Not advised as the sole treatment for persistent complaints unless a conventional physician has diagnosed the patient's condition and made a proper risk–benefit assessment.

Method

A voluntary reduction in food intake is claimed to improve a person's mental outlook, speed up the elimination of waste products, and underpin the resolve to bring about a change of lifestyle.

Rationale and historical perspective

Various religions have practiced fasting for thousands of years. It was, and is, viewed as a way of drawing nearer to one's creator or to oneself. Therapeutic fasting has nothing at all to do with crash dieting (*see* page 6), in which the aim is to lose as much weight in as short a time as possible. The key elements of therapeutic fasting are the—frequently spiritual—ideals of purification, improved mental state, and mental or physical reorientation. Fasting is also said to be an excellent way of beating disease. After a few days of fasting, the body can become accustomed to a daily of intake of just 500–600 calories. This low figure can be achieved and sustained through water, tea, juice, whey, or Buchinger fasts (juice, vegetable broth, and herbal teas with a little honey).

For many doctors who recommend therapeutic fasting, the notion of detoxification and removal of waste materials is the central theme. They see the gut and connective tissues as storing up an excess of harmful waste that, among other things, weakens the immune system, ultimately leading to chronic disease. Mainstream doctors retort that even with the most sophisticated test equipment it has hitherto not been possible to detect any such "waste products" in the human body. For pragmatists, the idea of detoxification is a metaphor for a comforting and stimulating feeling of physical and emotional purification and wholeness.

Various forms of physical therapy (*see* pages 867–78) are recommended for typical fast-related complaints such as stomach cramps, sleeplessness, low blood pressure, or feeling cold. Enemas (*see* page 819) and increased intake of fluids are said to alleviate symptoms in what are termed "fasting crises," which may present as melancholia, irritability, or general malaise. Chewing a slice of lemon can remove an unpleasant taste from the mouth.

How it works

Therapeutic fasting can elicit various favorable effects. After a few days, energy requirements will be covered almost entirely from the body's fat reserves, so that, as a rule, a daily weight loss of about 1lb can be anticipated. This takes some of the mechanical load off the spine and joints. Cholesterol, triglycerides, and blood glucose values can be lowered; impaired liver function can be normalized. Occasionally, acute, or chronic inflammatory diseases can be made less active. The spiritual aspects of therapeutic fasting can have numerous positive effects on the mind and emotions, which may in turn underpin attempts by the patient to bring about a change in his or her lifestyle.

Indications

Some therapists see therapeutic fasting as a panacea. Typically, it is employed for detoxification, elimination of waste products, improving mental outlook, and bringing about a desired change of lifestyle.

Proof it works

Outcome studies and case reports (*see* page xx) have shown therapeutic fasting to be of some benefit in encouraging a changeover to an organic diet. Reports that therapeutic fasting has helped alleviate symptoms of neurodermatitis, rheumatic disorders, and chronic polyarthritis are common.

Risks, cautions, and contraindications

Not all patients can tolerate every form of fasting. Each fasting regimen should be checked for individual suitability. Study findings have not substantiated the claims occasionally made that therapeutic fasting is a cure-all. Where a condition is recurrent or persistent, the patient should consult his or her doctor for a conventional examination and to receive orthodox treatment where this is called for.

Therapeutic fasting should not be undertaken by pregnant or lactating women, by children, or by persons with diabetes, cancer, tuberculosis, a psychotic disorder, severe depression, liver cirrhosis, emaciation, or a gastric or duodenal ulcer. Persons fasting for longer than about five days must be kept under medical review.

Duration of treatment

Short therapeutic fasts last for about three to five days and can be carried out without medical supervision. It is usual for fasts to be preceded by two or three days of gentle, reduced-calorie food intake, generally supported by a laxative such as Epsom or Glauber's salt. Then follow the fast proper and the post-fast period. The subsequent transition phase, a time during which a changeover to an organic diet can be accomplished, should be equal to roughly a third of the total time spent fasting.

Finding the right therapist

A reputable fasting therapist or nutritionist will generally not start any treatment without the patient having obtained a conventional diagnosis. With the patient, he or she will define a treatment goal and propose an initially limited treatment plan (*see* page xxiii), to be used as a basis for checking that the fast is having the desired positive effect.

No credence should be given to any therapist promising an instantaneous or complete cure irrespective of disease and symptoms (*see* Practitioner checklist, page xxv).

Physical therapies

A physical therapy is one that is used to work the body in order to prevent or treat disease and illness. As well as the usual bodywork and physical manipulation techniques (osteopathy, chiropractic) the term is also taken as including therapies such as hydro- and hydrothermic therapy, exercise therapies, various forms of massage (*see* page 847), relaxation techniques (*see* page 888), and electroneural therapy (*see* TENS, page 886).

Exercise therapy

> **Rating**
> **Useful** as a preventive measure, for risk reduction following myocardial infarction or a stroke, and as a contribution to rehabilitation.
> **Not advised** as the sole treatment for persistent complaints unless a conventional physician has diagnosed the patient's condition and made a proper risk–benefit assessment.

Method

Specially devised exercise programs may be instrumental in preventing disease, alleviating symptoms, reducing the risk of heart attack and stroke, and helping patients recuperate from illness or injury.

Rationale and historical perspective

Up until just a couple of decades ago, many diseases were caused by sheer physical exhaustion; and the right way of taking the road to recovery was thought to be to cocoon oneself from the rigors of everyday life. The situation now, however, is that many modern lifestyle diseases are actually caused by a lack of exercise. There is no doubt that a measured dose of regular, sustained exercise and power training is effective in *preventing* disease (*see* Sport and exercise, page 8). However, conventional medicine has been slow to accept the *therapeutic* benefits of exercise for the treatment of various ailments. Even just a short while ago, the treatment of choice after a heart attack, stroke, or orthopedic surgery, for instance, was to confine the patient to bed for weeks on end. It is now recognized that a properly devised training program (e.g. under the supervision of a physiotherapist) can be a mainstay of treatment. Physiotherapy is nowadays also a cornerstone of conventional treatment for many other diseases and conditions.

How it works

Regular sustained and power exercise can be used to improve fitness and lessen a wide range of risk factors. Physiotherapy can be useful as a way of rehabilitation, alleviating symptoms, as a means of preventing embolism and muscle wastage in bedridden patients, and as a method of re-learning skills or speeding recovery from a number of diseases.

Indications

Various forms of exercise therapy are used to reduce risk factors. Physiotherapy is widely used for treating circulation disorders, problems with the musculoskeletal system, certain psychosomatic illnesses, nervous problems, cerebral dyskinesia in children, chronic constipation, and urinary incontinence. Following myocardial infarction and a stroke, exercise is used for rehabilitation and for reducing the risk of recidivation.

Proof it works

Numerous controlled clinical studies (*see* page xix) show various forms of exercise to be useful for preventing disease, for rehabilitation and as a means of reducing the risk of recidivation following a heart attack or stroke. Modern exercise therapies include many forms of physical activity, including walking, swimming, physiotherapy, and sports. Therapeutic exercises may also be helpful in a large variety of musculoskeletal, rheumatic, and neural disorders, as well as following operations and in intensive care.

Risks, cautions, and contraindications

Too much sporting activity, or sports carried out wrongly, can actually be harmful (*see* Sport and exercise, page 8). Persons engaging in sports, especially of advancing years taking up a sport, should be kept under medical review. There is presently no consensus as to what constitutes the optimum level of exercise.

Measures aimed at rehabilitating a patient should be instituted as early as possible.

Duration of treatment

The duration of exercise therapy will depend on the individual effects achieved and the condition for which treatment is being provided.

Finding the right therapist

A therapist should be properly qualified and registered with a professional organization. Physiotherapists are usually best qualified. Although in most cases this will give some assurance as to the quality of the training that the therapist will have received and the standard of treatment that the patient can expect, it does not automatically follow that exercise therapy will be the most appropriate treatment for the patient's condition.

A reputable therapist will generally not treat a persistent condition without a conventional diagnosis having been obtained. With the patient, he or she will define a treatment goal and propose an initially limited plan of treatment (*see* page xxiii) to be used as a basis for checking that the treatment is having the desired effect. No credence should be given to any therapist promising a complete or instantaneous cure (*see* Practitioner checklist, page xxv).

Hydrotherapy and hydrothermal therapy

> **Rating**
> **Useful** as an attempted treatment for the stated diseases and conditions and as a preventive measure. Anyone with a persistent or recurrent complaint must always obtain a conventional diagnosis before receiving this type of treatment. **Not advised** as the sole treatment for persistent complaints unless a conventional physician has diagnosed the patient's condition and made a proper risk–benefit assessment.

Method

Hydrotherapy is the use of water in the treatment of disease. Hydrothermal therapy additionally uses its temperature effects, as in hot baths, saunas, wraps, etc.

Rationale and historical perspective

Hydro- and hydrothermal therapy are traditional methods of treatment that have been used for the treatment of disease and injury by many cultures, including those of ancient Rome, China, and Japan. The practice of utilizing the beneficial effects of water slipped into oblivion in Europe during the Middle Ages, but was rediscovered in the 17th century when it became fashionable to "take the waters" at hot water spas such as Bath in England, Baden-Baden in Germany, and Spa in Belgium.

A Bavarian monk, Father Sebastian Kneipp (1821–97) also helped repopularize the therapeutic use of water in the 19th century. There are now many dozens of methods of applying hydrotherapy, including baths, saunas, douches, wraps, and packs, so there will almost invariably be a method ideally suited to a patient's specific needs.

How it works

The recuperative and healing properties of hydrotherapy are based on its mechanical and/or thermal effects. It exploits the body's reaction to hot and cold stimuli, to the protracted application of heat, to pressure exerted by the water and to the sensation it gives. The nerves carry impulses felt at the skin deeper into the body, where they are instrumental in stimulating the immune system, influencing the production of stress hormones, invigorating the circulation and digestion, encouraging blood flow, and lessening pain sensitivity.

Indications

Hydrotherapy and hydrothermal therapy are chiefly used to tone up the body, to stimulate digestion, the circulation, and the immune system, and to bring relief from pain.

Proof it works

Various case reports, observational studies (*see* page xx), and a number of controlled studies (*see* page xix) provide some evidence of success in the treatment of the particular conditions quoted, although there is probably wide variation in the degree of efficacy attained.

Risks, cautions, and contraindications

Persons with impaired temperature sensation (*see* Neuropathy, page 140) run the risk of scalding or frostbite at temperature extremes.

When a condition is recurrent or persistent, the patient's doctor should decide whether a physical therapy of this type is a suitable addition to the arsenal of conventional medical methods.

Duration of treatment

The length of treatment will depend on the efficacy of the particular treatment method in the individual and on the ailment being treated.

Finding the right therapist

Hydrotherapy and hydrothermal therapy lend themselves well to self-treatment. Qualified instruction is recommended though not absolutely essential.

Common techniques

Full and partial immersion baths

Various substances can be added to warm and rising temperature baths (*see* Medical herbalism, page 853 and Aromatherapy, page 786). The following are the different kinds of bath used:

- **Rising temperature hip bath**. This is taken in a tub filled with a hand's breadth of tepid water. Hot water is then gradually added until the level reaches the navel. The final temperature should be 103–104°C. Following this procedure, the patient is wrapped warm and proceeds to bed. It should last 15–30 minutes, not more than three times per week. *Indications*: incipient and abating common colds, back pain (sciatica). *Warning*: to be used with caution by persons with heart or circulation problems, hemorrhoids, or varicose veins.
- **Cold foot bath**. The feet are placed into a foot bath filled to calf depth with cold water. Stop when a cold stimulus is felt or when the water is no longer perceived as being particularly cold. Stroke off excess water, dress, and walk or run until dry. A special form of this treatment is "walking in water," which involves walking stork-like on a non-slip mat placed under the water. *Indications*: Varicose veins, susceptibility to edemas, headaches, low blood pressure, circulatory problems, sleeplessness, proneness to the

common cold, sweaty feet, or a contused ankle. *Warning*: This type of treatment is best avoided by people who suffer from cold feet, very high blood pressure, an irritable bladder, urinary tract infection, diabetes, or vascular occlusion.

- **Rising temperature foot bath, warm foot bath**. The feet are immersed in a foot bath filled with water at body temperature. Hot water is gradually added to give a final temperature of 103–104°C. In warm foot baths water of this temperature is added straight away. Keep warm afterwards. The procedure should last 10–15 minutes and can be done daily. *Indications*: Cold feet, start of a common cold, for relaxation. *Warning*: Best avoided by people with varicose veins, lymphostasis, or edema.

- **Cold arm bath**. A basin is filled with cold water until it reaches a depth several inches above the immersed elbow. If the treatment becomes intolerable, stop and repeat as desired. *Indications*: Headaches, sleeplessness. *Warning*: Best avoided by people with heart or circulatory problems.

- **Rising temperature arm bath**. In principle, this is the same as the rising temperature foot bath. It should be followed by a cold arm douche, then by half an hour's rest. *Indications*: Bronchitis, asthma, incipient respiratory infection, circulatory problems, angina pectoris.

- **Sitz bath**. This is generally taken in a hip bath as a cold, rising temperature, or warm sitz bath. Prior to a sitz bath, warm the feet, e.g. through a warm foot bath. Parts of the body not immersed in water should be covered. *Indications*: Cold sitz bath for hemorrhoids or inflammation of the anus; warm or rising temperature sitz bath for difficulty in voiding the bladder, an irritable bladder, inflammation or infection of the prostate, preparation for pregnancy. *Warning*: Do not use warm or rising temperature sitz baths for hemorrhoids.

Cold rubbings

Soak a linen cloth in cold water, wring out and briskly rub the upper and lower trunk, or the entire body. Go to bed until warm and dry. Indications: For invigoration, to tone up the body, to promote blood flow, for use in problems of circulation, or infections of the respiratory system.

Douches

Gentle douches can be carried out with a watering can or hose. The water should not splash, but gently envelop the skin. The water stream should always be directed from the periphery toward the heart. After douching, stroke off excess water, dress, and exercise. There are various types of douche:

- **Knee douche**. The water stream is directed from the right small toe, along the outside of the lower leg to the hollow of the knee, then back along the inside and over the sole of the foot. The process is then repeated for the left leg. *Indications*: Headaches and migraines, low blood pressure, sleeplessness, contusions, and varicose veins. This treatment influences the digestive and reproductive organs and can help ward off vascular damage. *Warning*: Not to be used for urinary tract infections, an irritable bladder, sciatica, or during menstruation.
- **Thigh douche**. The procedure is as for a knee douche, but includes the upper thigh. It can stimulate blood flow and help improve poor circulation. *Indications*: Varicose veins, muscular rheumatism, crural paralysis, coxarthritis. *Warning*: Not to be used for urinary tract infection, an irritable bladder, sciatica, or during menstruation.
- **Lower trunk douche**. The procedure is as for the thigh douche, but including the lower trunk. *Indications*: Diabetes mellitus, meteorism, enlargement of the liver, enlargement of the gallbladder, stone formation. *Warning*: Not to be used for urinary tract infections, an irritable bladder, sciatica, or during menstruation.
- **Arm douche**. Direct the water stream from the outside of the right hand to the shoulder, then back on the inside of the arm. Repeat the process for the left arm. *Indications*: Cold hands, nervous disorders, neuralgia and paralysis, rheumatism of the arms, heart problems, vertigo, headaches, catarrh in the nose and throat.
- **Chest douche**. Douche the arms first. *Indications*: Chronic bronchitis and bronchial asthma, angina pectoris. *Warning*: Moderate the temperature if there is risk of angiospasm.
- **Upper trunk douche**. This involves the upper torso and arms. It can be used to improve blood flow to the lungs, heart, and pleura. *Indications*: Bronchitis, bronchial asthma,

disease of the larynx and vocal cords, headaches, nervous excitability, varicose veins of the legs, for toning-up, and for stimulating cardiac and respiratory activity. *Warning*: Not to be used if there is blood stasis in the pulmonary circulation.

- **Back douche.** *Indications*: Weakened back muscles, back pain, spinal disease, multiple sclerosis, bronchial asthma, nearly all diseases of the lung. *Warning*: Not to be used in debilitated patients or those with neurasthenia.

- **Neck douche.** *Indications*: Headaches, migraines, tenseness in the shoulder and neck, hypersensitivity to changes in the weather, mild depression, tinnitus, vertigo, arthrosis of the hand and finger joints. *Warning*: Not to be used in persons with high blood pressure, enlargement of the thyroid, or raised intraocular pressure.

- **Face douche.** Proceed from the right temple downward to the chin, upward to the left temple, from right to left over the forehead, and repeatedly from the forehead to the chin, then in circles over the face. *Indications*: Headaches and migraines, trigeminal neuralgia, toothaches, for relaxing tired eyes. *Warning*: Keep the eyes closed.

Sauna

Various cultures have adopted the idea of purifying or therapeutic steam baths. The sauna was brought to Europe by the Finns from their original home in Asia Minor some 2,000 years ago. The "Turkish" bath originated not in Turkey but in Russia. Saunas and steambaths are similar in effect; the decision to take one rather than the other will be guided by personal preference. In a sauna the heat acts more quickly to eliminate toxins through the skin, though some consider the moist air of a steambath to have a more satisfying effect on the respiratory system.

A sauna is an eliminative procedure; it stimulates bloodflow, increases the heartrate, has an immune-modulating effect (*see* page 10), promotes hormone production, encourages mucosal secretions in the respiratory system, opens the airways, reduces resistance to respiration, regulates the vegetative system, relaxes, and can improve mental outlook. Children can start to take saunas at two or three years of age.

Indications: e.g. for "toning-up," for health promotion, as a way of treating pain caused by pulled back muscles, chronic rheumatoid arthritis, bronchial asthma, unstable hypertension (stages I and II), severely disturbed peripheral blood circulation. *Warnings*: Saunas should not be taken by persons with acute rheumatoid arthritis, acute infection, active tuberculosis, sexually transmitted diseases, acute mental disorder, inflammation of an inner organ or blood vessels, significant vascular changes in the brain or heart, circulatory problems or acute cancer.

Wraps

A wrap is primarily used as a supportive measure for treating fever and local inflammation. The person receiving treatment should first adopt a relaxed position. Then a linen cloth is moistened with cold water (warm water for respiratory diseases), well wrung out, and then wrapped tightly around the appropriate part of the body, but not so tightly as to cause constriction. The moist linen cloth is in turn wrapped with a dry cotton or linen cloth. The patient is then usually wrapped in a blanket or another cloth, and should rest for 45–60 minutes or, if the intention is to induce sweating, for up to three hours.

If the wrap is not felt to be warm after a quarter of an hour, heat should be applied in the form of a hot water bottle or by giving warm tea. The wrap should be removed immediately if the person complains of feeling unwell.

Wraps are used for the following indications:

- neck wrap: sore throat
- chest wrap: bronchitis, lung disease, neuralgia
- body wrap (between costal arch and pubic bone): inflammatory disease of the upper abdomen, gastric and duodenal ulcers, cramps, sleeplessness, fever
- trunk wrap (between pubic bone and armpits): high fever
- hip wrap (with gap between the legs): prostatitis, vaginitis, hemorrhoids, anal eczema, inflammation in the pelvic cavity
- calf wrap (between foot and knee): lymphostasis, edema, for withdrawing heat in fever and phlebitis; in varicose veins the effect can sometimes be amplified through the use of healing earth or loam poultices
- joint wraps: rheumatoid arthritis, arthrosis

Packs

- **Cold packs**. Cooled cataplasm is spread onto the wrapping cloth and placed on the patient. Crushed ice in a plastic bag may also be repeatedly applied for one minute, then removed for four. Indications: Various inflammatory arthropathies, sprains and strains, pleurisy. Ice packs can also be used for headaches. Warning: When using ice packs, place a thin cloth between the pack and the skin to prevent frostbite.
- **Warm packs**. A wrapping cloth is soaked in a hot infusion or decoction of herbs, then wrung out and applied to the patient's body. Alternatively, the wrap may receive a coating of hot mud, mustard flour, or fango. As a further alternative, hayseed may be placed in a sack and steamed. *Indications*: painful chronic diseases such as arthrosis, renal disease, or cystitis, and for stimulating bloodflow. *Warning*: Always check that the temperature is tolerable before applying a wrap.

Probiotics

Rating

May be of some use as a short-term attempt to treat chronic, recurrent infections and immune-system impairment. An individual risk–benefit assessment must be obtained when the symptoms are persistent.

Of little use for other diseases and associated symptoms for which the treatment is advocated by some of its proponents.

Not advised as the sole treatment for persistent complaints unless a conventional physician has diagnosed the patient's condition and made a proper risk–benefit assessment.

Method

Humans and bacteria live in a symbiotic relationship. Introducing certain bacteria into the gut is held to be a way of correcting deficiencies of the intestinal flora and thus of removing the cause of a number of ailments.

Rationale and historical perspective

Once the German bacteriologist Robert Koch had established the fundaments of modern bacteriology, people began to appreciate the significance of normal gut bacteria for the maintenance of good health. Following the discovery of penicillin, it also became clear that antibiotics can destroy friendly bacteria in the gut, upsetting the delicately balanced intestinal flora and weakening the person's immune status.

As a logical development of this concept, probiotics (or microbiological therapy) combines elements of immunization theory. Those therapists who have been instrumental in its evolution as a distinct healthcare practice proceeded from the premise that the bacterial population of the gastrointestinal tract, which is so vital in the proper functioning of the body's defence systems, can be damaged by unhealthy eating, by taking drugs, and by environmental factors. This bacterial imbalance (dysbacteria or dysbiosis) is characterized by the intestine not being populated with the "right" bacteria, or by their ratios of one to another being incorrect. An incorrect bacterial population can be a cause, as well as an effect, of disease.

Proponents of probiotics believe that the gut plays a central role in the human immune system. If its flora is held to be "non-physiological," it can, suggest many proponents of constructive symbiosis, lead to a number of conditions such as asthma, allergies, eczema, neurodermatitis, liver and gallbladder disease, rheumatic disorders, and even cancer.

The treatment of alleged or actual symbiotic disturbances aims, in the first phase of treatment, to reduce the number of incorrect bacteria and then to restore the flora to a normal balance through the use of physiological cultures of bacteria, which are swallowed or injected. Most products on the market contain either human gut bacteria (sometimes supplemented with other materials), lactic acid-forming bacteria or organisms that normally occur chiefly in the respiratory and urinary systems. Occasionally, so-called "autovaccines" are used to steer symbiosis. These are individually prepared formulations for injection containing inactivated bacteria derived from the patient's own feces, urine, nasal secretion, saliva, or pharyngeal smears.

How it works

Certain suitable bacteria are said to normalize an incorrect intestinal flora and improve the body's immune system. There is a lack of scientific proof, however, to validate claims that this treatment can also be used in diseases other than those affecting the respiratory tract, or following antibiotic therapy. Auto-intoxication through dysbiosis is a hitherto unproven hypothesis.

Indications

Constructive symbiosis, some of its proponents claim, is beneficial in a number of conditions including asthma, allergies, eczema, neurodermatitis, liver and gallbladder disease, rheumatic disorders, and even cancer. It is most commonly used to treat recurrent coughs and colds and for restoring the normal balance of an intestinal flora upset by treatment with antibiotics.

Proof it works

There is some evidence that probiotics is capable of normalizing damaged intestinal flora, e.g. following treatment with antibiotics, and of dealing with recurrent coughs and colds. For all other proposed indications, however, research into whether the treatment works has been patchy. Few controlled studies (*see* page xix) have been undertaken. The successes that case reports and other studies (*see* page xx) claim as having been achieved probably only hold true for a proportion of patients receiving treatment (*see* Placebo, page xxi).

Risks, cautions, and contraindications

Injection of auto–vaccines can trigger allergic reactions and (occasionally) shock.

Duration of treatment

A course of treatment generally lasts between eight and 17 weeks. There are various abbreviated forms of follow-up treatment.

Finding the right therapist

No credence should be given to therapists promising an instantaneous or total cure (*see* Practitioner checklist, page xxv). Any training that a therapist has received in this healthcare practice will usually give some assurance as to the standard of treatment the patient can expect, though it will not necessarily follow that the treatment will be that most appropriate for dealing with his or her condition.

A reputable therapist will generally not start treatment until the patient has consulted a physician for a conventional diagnosis. With the patient, he or she will define a treatment goal and propose a short-term treatment plan (*see* page xxiii) to be used as a basis for checking that the therapy is having the desired effect. Prescription-free products are suitable for self-treatment.

Reflex therapies

Reflex therapies are based on the idea that there are a number of lines or zones running the length of the body, and that the organs and structures within each zone are connected by a flow of energy, so that pain felt in one region, for instance, "reflects" a condition in a remote part of the body. The reflex zones can be treated through pressure, ice massage, cold sprays, or electrical stimulation.

For thousands of years numerous cultures have used a variety of therapeutic techniques (chiefly for pain relief) that are based on the belief that there are lines or channels connecting certain areas on the surface of the skin with the inner organs and structures.

At the end of the last century the British physician Henry Head discovered that when an organ becomes diseased, it can elicit particularly painful changes at certain areas on the skin with which it is associated. It was thought for a long time that the nerves connecting Head's zones with their respective organs must originate from the same segment of the spine (segment theory). By stimulating the nerve endings at the skin surface, it was conjectured, it must be possible to elicit a reflex response in the diseased organ, helping it to return to health. Meanwhile, new research seems to indicate that various parts of the brain, acting via reflex channels, are also implicated. One current research project into pain surmises that there is so-called "pain homunculus" located in or near the fourth ventricle of the brain: a miniature version of the nervous system. This novel approach is tending to supersede the original segment theory.

Reflex channels are exploited, too, in acupressure (*see* page 769), various forms of acupuncture (*see* page 772), and certain hydrothermic therapies (*see* page 871). Reflex therapies can be administered through the activation of reflex zones and trigger points, e.g. through massage techniques (*see* Reflexology, page 883), electrical impulses (*see* TENS, page 886), application of ice or heat (*see* Physical therapies, pages 871–8), or embrocation (*see* Aromatherapy, page 786).

Reflexology

Method

Massaging parts of the body thought to be linked to the principal organs via the bloodstream and neural pathways is said to have a curative effect on these organs.

Rationale and historical perspective

For thousands of years numerous cultures have used a variety of therpeutic techniques based on the belief that there are lines or channels connecting certain areas on the surface of the skin with the inner organs and structures. The most widespread application of these techniques has been in pain relief. Theories abound with regard to the mechanisms by which these techniques work. Belief in the existence of reflex channels is at the heart, too, of acupressure (*see* page 769), various forms of acupuncture (*see* page 772), TENS (*see* page 886), and certain hydrothermal therapies (*see* pages 871–8).

Many variations on the theme of reflex massage have evolved over the years, including massage of the connective tissue, colonic massage, and massage of the periosteum at various points (periosteal massage). In 1913, the American ENT specialist William Fitzgerald laid the foundations of what became known as "reflex zone massage;" he proposed that the body is divided into ten zones running the length of the body from head to toe, and that stimulating an area in one zone affects other parts of the body that are in the same zone. The work on reflex zone massage was continued by Eunice Ingham, who developed the concept of "reflex zone massage of the feet," now simply referred to as "reflexology." She claimed to be able to show that the entire body is reflected in the sides and soles of the feet and that any vital organ can be treated by massaging the appropriate part of the foot. Though normally carried out on the feet, reflexology is also said to work when points on the ear, hands, etc., are massaged.

Reflexology may at times be very painful.

How it works

There are many beliefs, theories, and systems for selecting the zone that is to receive reflex treatment as a proxy for the diseased organ. There is a broadly held view, based in part on experimental and clinical observations, that certain parts of the brain have an important role in linking areas of the skin with the internal organs.

An important concept in reflexology is that of referred pain, which can be initiated from so-called trigger points (*see* page 929). Treatment given at the trigger points helps alleviate referred pain and other conditions. In theory at least, painful treatment techniques are capable of providing powerful counter-stimuli that temporarily mask pain. Whether and to what extent reflexology can be used to treat individual organs are questions that have not been adequately researched.

Indications

Some of the proponents of reflexology see it as a holistic (*see* page 928) treatment, and apply it to a whole range of problems and disorders. Its chief uses are for providing relaxation, increasing the patient's general sense of well-being, and alleviating pain. Some reflexologists also claim to be able to use reflex zone massage for diagnosis. For example, an area of the foot found to be particularly painful is said to point to disease in its associated organ.

Proof it works

Numerous testimonials and case studies (*see* page xx), and a few controlled clinical studies (*see* page xix) do suggest that reflexology may be efficacious to a degree in the provision of relaxation and pain relief and in enabling the amounts of painkilling medications to be reduced. There is no clinical evidence, however, to corroborate frequently made claims that reflexology can be used as a diagnostic technique.

Risks, cautions, and contraindications

In patients with tumors or osteoporosis, reflexology should not be applied to parts of the body affected by disease. It should also not be attempted for persons with acute inflammation of the venous or lymphatic system, infectious or highly febrile diseases, psychosis, high-risk pregnancy, or certain conditions of the feet. Massage of the connective tissue is contraindicated by patients with acute inflammation, a tumor, or psychosis; also by patients who have recently suffered a heart attack.

Colonic massage should not be attempted for persons with inflammation of the bowel or abdominal cavity, nor for pregnant women or anyone with a tumor.

Some patients are unduly sensitive to manual stimuli; others find it hard to tolerate the close physical contact that is a crucial element of reflexology.

Duration of treatment

Reflexology is a form of stimulation therapy (*see* page 929) in which a single treatment will often not have any lasting effect. Generally, a series of at least six treatments will be required.

Finding the right therapist

Reflexology should be performed by a qualified reflexologist. Although in most cases this will give some assurance as to the quality of training the practitioner will have received and the standard of treatment the patient can expect, it does not automatically follow that reflexology will be the most appropriate form of treatment.

A reputable reflexologist will generally not treat a persistent or recurrent condition without the patient having obtained a conventional diagnosis. With the client, he or she will define a treatment goal and propose an initially limited treatment plan (*see* page xxiii) to be used as a basis for checking that reflexology is having the desired beneficial effect. No credence should be given to any reflexologist promising an instantaneous or total cure for a persistent or recurrent problem or a serious disease (*see* Practitioner checklist, page xxv).

Transcutaneous Electrical Nerve Stimulation (TENS)

> **Rating**
> **Useful** as a short-term attempt to provide relief from chronic pain.
> **Not advised** as the sole treatment for persistent complaints unless a conventional physician has diagnosed the patient's condition and made a proper risk–benefit assessment.

Method

A small battery-powered device is used to deliver a low voltage pulsating electrical current that is claimed to provide relief from pain.

Rationale and historical perspective

The use of electrical stimuli in pain relief came to the fore in the 19th century when devices for generating and applying electrical currents gradually became available. At the time, electrical energy was often equated with vital energy and seen as some sort of sovereign remedy.

The use of electrical stimuli for pain relief became widespread in the 1960s and 1970s, following the development of portable, battery-driven devices suitable for self-treatment. The devices deliver a low current electrical impulse (generally 0–60 milliamperes) directly to the skin through a system of electrodes and contact materials, the electrodes being applied either to the site of the pain, above the main nerve stem, at trigger (*see* page 929) and acupuncture (*see* page 772) points, in the appropriate neural segment or to the temples. The current can be regulated during treatment to suit the individual patient's requirements.

There are also various procedures that are similar in effect to TENS, e.g. the "electrical pill." This is a small disc-shaped device that is attached to the site of pain or to reflex zones and is claimed to alleviate pain.

How it works

How TENS works is not fully understood. It is thought to stimulate the release of endorphins and encephalins, the body's natural painkillers. These modulate the way pain is perceived and transmitted. TENS may also improve the circulation locally.

Indications

TENS is used to provide pain relief in virtually all types of medical condition.

Proof it works

Various controlled clinical studies (*see* page xix) suggest that TENS is more effective than a placebo (*see* page xxi) treatment for dealing with chronic pain.

Risks, cautions, and contraindications

TENS is a system of pain relief which, though it can alleviate symptoms, cannot cure the disease causing them. It should not be employed in patients wearing cardiac pacemakers, as the current generated may upset the pacemaker's electronic control system. As many as 10 percent of patients may suffer from allergic reactions as a result of electrodes being attached to the skin. Some patients are also allergic to contact gel or silicone electrodes. Since any form of electrical stimulation can burn the skin, persons with reduced temperature sensation (e.g. the elderly, diabetics and patients with polyneuropathy) may suffer some skin damage.

Duration of treatment

Depending on when pain relief actually starts, treatment may range in duration from 15 minutes to several hours. It is mostly given several times daily.

Finding the right therapist

With professional guidance (e.g. from a therapist or a doctor experienced in this treatment), TENS is suitable for do-it-yourself therapy.

Relaxation techniques

Autogenic training (basic level)

Rating
Useful for inducing relaxation and as an attempt to treat psychosomatic disorders and alleviate pain (usually supportively).
Not advised as the sole treatment for persistent complaints unless a conventional physician has diagnosed the patient's condition and made a proper risk–benefit assessment.

Method

Autogenic training (AT) is a relaxation technique that can help relieve overworked muscles, dispel inner tenseness, and treat psychosomatic disorders.

Rationale and historical perspective

Psychiatrist Johannes Schultz devised a relaxation technique based on autosuggestion to help him overcome his fear as he lay in the trenches in the First World War. Gradually and systematically, he fashioned the technique into a method in which the body and mind work together to develop a feeling of restfulness, relaxation, warmth, well-being, and calm. A state of near-hypnosis is induced through a series of phrases ("My right/left arm is very heavy," "I now feel quite at ease," "My heartbeat is calm and regular," "My breathing is easy and natural," "I feel a warmth in my stomach," "My forehead is pleasantly cool," and the like), which are visualized and repeated. Once these basic exercises, which can be carried out sitting or lying comfortably, have been mastered, the vegetative system, i.e. that which includes the heartbeat and breathing, can be effectively controlled.

From this basic stage you can move on to autogenic modification, which focuses on specific areas, to behavior control, and to autogenic meditation.

AT techniques are generally learned in groups and the exercises are carried out in a way that suits you.

How it works

AT is based on autosuggestion.

Indications

AT is useful for any stress-induced condition and is often used in support of psychotherapy to treat psychosomatic illness.

Proof it works

Case reports, case studies (*see* page xx), and a number of controlled trials (*see* page xix) have shown AT to be instrumental in inducing relaxation and relief from pain. In many cases it was noticed that AT helps patients suffering from pain or high blood pressure to manage with less medication.

Risks, cautions, and contraindications

AT is not recommended for persons with severe psychosis, depression, or obsessional neurosis, nor for debilitated patients or those with psychopathic personalities. Anyone suffering from a persistent illness should check first with his or her doctor, so as not to forgo the opportunity of receiving perhaps more appropriate treatment. Some organizations arranging teaching sessions are mystical or sect-like.

Duration of training

Training sessions generally take place once a week for seven to eight weeks. After this initial phase it is probably best to work on your own and then attend one or more general sessions some weeks after initial training to exchange experiences and discuss any points that have arisen.

Finding the right therapist

An AT trainer should be a member of a professional organization. Although in most cases this will give some assurance as to the quality of instruction that the trainer will have received and the standard of service that the patient can expect, it does not automatically follow that this treatment will be appropriate to the condition for which the patient is seeking treatment.

No credence should be given to trainers promising an instantaneous or total cure (*see* Practitioner checklist, page xxv).

Biofeedback

<table>
<tr><td>

Rating

Useful for inducing relaxation and as a (mostly supportive) attempt to treat psychosomatic disorders and alleviate pain when simpler relaxation techniques have not produced the desired results.

Not advised as the sole treatment for persistent complaints unless a conventional physician has diagnosed the patient's condition and made a proper risk–benefit assessment.

</td></tr>
</table>

Method

Biofeedback is a form of technologically supported relaxation therapy that can help release physical tenseness and inner unrest.

Rationale and historical perspective

Heart rate, skin conductivity, and muscle tension, which are normally not consciously perceived, are recorded and displayed on a computer screen or used to activate certain signals, melodies, or synthesizer instruments. Through this audio-visual feedback, patients learn how to read their body's functions and, in a second step, how to control them; they are ultimately able to achieve this aim without the need for technological aids.

Unlike traditional relaxation techniques, biofeedback is a relatively complex procedure. It also has a legitimate role in conventional medicine.

How it works

As with traditional relaxation techniques, biofeedback enables the patient to take effective control of certain body functions and to experience a feeling of profound relaxation.

Indications

Biofeedback is used to relax, alleviate anxiety and pain, and (as an adjunct to psychotherapy) to help overcome psychosomatic ailments.

Proof it works

Various field studies (*see* page xx) and a number of controlled trials (*see* page xix) have shown biofeedback therapy to be a valid means of inducing relaxation, of treating certain functional disorders, such as irritable bowel syndrome, constipation, and tension headaches, and of speeding recovery following a stroke.

Risks, cautions, and contraindications

Biofeedback therapy is not recommended for persons with severe psychosis, depression, or obsessional neurosis, nor for debilitated patients or those with psychopathic personalities.

Anyone suffering from a persistent illness should check first with his or her doctor, so as not to forgo the opportunity of receiving perhaps more appropriate treatment.

Duration of training

The patient should be able, after not more than 15 sessions, to control his or her physiological functions without any technological aids.

Finding the right therapist

A biofeedback trainer should have an appropriate qualification. Although in most cases this will give some assurance as to the quality of instruction that the trainer will have received and the standard of service that the patient can expect, it does not automatically follow that this treatment will be appropriate to the condition for which the patient is seeking treatment.

No credence should be given to trainers promising an instantaneous or total cure (*see* Practitioner checklist, page xxv).

Muscle relaxation according to Jacobson

Rating
Useful for rest and relaxation and as an attempt to treat psychosomatic disorders and relieve pain (usually supportively).
Not advised as the sole treatment for persistent complaints unless a conventional physician has diagnosed the patient's condition and made a proper risk–benefit assessment.

Method

Progressive muscle relaxation according to Jacobson can help ease physical tension, dispel inner unrest, overcome psychosomatic disorders, and relieve pain.

Rationale and historical perspective

Progressive muscle relaxation training was developed by Jacobson in the USA at about the same time that autogenic training (*see* page 888) appeared in Europe. At the start of each training program, which usually involves group sessions, participants learn how to flex and relax individual groups of muscles. In a defined sequence, they follow the therapist's instructions to clench a fist, frown, flex the stomach, or tighten the foot muscles for five to seven seconds at a time. Alternately flexing and relaxing the muscles is supposed to induce a state of relaxation and well-being.

Once training has been completed, progressive muscle relaxation according to Jacobson can be carried out independently, either on a daily basis or when there is an acute need. Most people find they can learn this technique more quickly than autogenic training, for instance.

How it works

At the heart of this technique is the "body over mind" principle. Alternately flexing and relaxing groups of muscles is said to provide a profound feeling of physical and mental relaxation.

Indications

The Jacobson technique is used to provide relaxation and to relieve anxiety. It is also used, often in support of other measures, for treating psychosomatic disorders.

Proof it works

Case reports and studies (*see* page xx) as well as various controlled clinical studies (*see* page xix) have shown this technique to be effective in inducing relaxation and pain relief.

Risks, cautions, and contraindications

Progressive muscle relaxation according to Jacobson is not suitable for persons with psychosis, depression, or obsessional neurosis, nor for debilitated persons or those with a psychopathic personality.

Duration of training

Profound relaxation, it has been found, can be achieved after three or four sessions per week over four to six weeks.

Finding the right trainer

Once the basic skills have been acquired from a trainer, muscle relaxation according to Jacobson is suitable for self-treatment. Information on how trainers can be contacted is generally available from adult education centers, doctors' practices, counselling centers, and hospital outpatient clinics.

Traditional Chinese medicine

Rating

May be of some use as a treatment attempt for psychosomatic illness and for alleviating symptoms of chronic disease. If symptoms persist, the patient must consult a physician for a conventional diagnosis.

Not advised as the sole treatment for persistent complaints unless a conventional physician has diagnosed the patient's condition and made a proper risk–benefit assessment.

Method

Traditional Chinese medicine (TCM) is a system of diagnosis and treatment that has its roots in ancient Chinese philosophy and utilizes therapeutic techniques such as acupuncture (*see* page 772), auricular therapy, acupressure (*see* page 769), moxibustion (*see* page 775), and Chinese herbalism.

The limited amount of documentation on TCM that is available in the West precludes a definitive assessment of how it works and of its efficacy in individual diseases and illnesses.

Rationale and historical perspective

TCM, which blends elements of Confucianism, Buddhism, and Taoism, has traditionally utilized various therapeutic procedures allied to acupuncture in association with herbal remedies and medicinal preparations of animal and mineral origin. However, such treatment methods have always been considered secondary to the tenet of not allowing the patient to become ill in the first place. Chinese doctors were, in fact, paid for keeping a person healthy—a principle that differs markedly from the modern Western system of doctors' remuneration, which is based on the restoration of sick people to health. The main aim of TCM has thus always been prevention.

Ancient Chinese practitioners had no knowledge of anatomy, physiology, and pathology in the modern sense; autopsies were forbidden, as were surgical operations. So any reference to an organ automatically implies its function within a system and not its anatomical structure. It is understandable, therefore, how TCM gradually lost ground to emerging modern Western medicine in the course of the last century, only enjoying a brief revival this century, initiated by Chairman Mao.

The origins of TCM can be found in ancient Chinese philosophical beliefs that were handed down verbally through the mists of time and, in the 2nd century BC, recorded in the *Huang-ti Nei-ching* (*The Yellow Emperor's Classic Textbook of Internal Medicine*) as a dialog between Huang-ti, the Yellow Emperor, and his personal physician, Chi Po. The principles enshrined in the book are still applied today.

TCM is based on the notion of yin and yang and a belief in "phases of change." The ancient Chinese ascribed development and change not to divine will, as in Western religions, but to Tao, the way of the universe. Tao is seen as the interaction of yin and yang, the opposing forces of nature, which in turn gives rise to the life force, chi. Traditional Chinese medicine upholds this principle of opposing forces, classifying disease symptoms according to a system of eight diagnostic criteria in four interacting pairs: yin and yang, internal and external, fullness and emptiness, hot and cold. The TCM doctrine has passed down through the millennia in a metaphorical language that is alien to the Western way of thinking. One Chinese concept, is for example, "liver wind," which covers such symptoms as headaches, migraines, and dizziness. Many Western critics of acupuncture (and indeed many of its proponents) are focusing on the question of how the imagery and terminology of TCM can be viewed against a modern scientific backdrop.

The link between diagnosis and therapy in TCM is also

thoroughly at odds with the teachings of Western academic medicine. Whereas practitioners of conventional Western medicine search for the cause of an illness (etiology, pathogenesis, diagnosis, therapy) in order to eliminate it, TCM defines illness not as the end product of a chain of circumstances and events but as a process in itself that can be influenced by encouraging the body's self-regulating powers—e.g. by restoring the chi energy balance. Chinese diagnosis, which is partly based on special techniques such as tongue diagnosis and pulse palpation, is followed by differentiated therapies that are carefully attuned to the individual and that can change from one treatment session to the next.

In modern China the importance of TCM is waning as mainstream medicine becomes more widespread. Those who bring these thoroughly disparate systems together find it difficult to reconcile their underlying concepts of disease and therapy.

Tibetan medicine

Tibetan medicine dates back to the 7th century AD, when various TCM and ayurvedic texts (*see* ayurveda, page 789) were translated into Tibetan. In a departure from the yin–yang principle of TCM, however, Tibetan medicine considers disease to be the result of an imbalance between three humors that exist in all living organisms. They are: chi, with the symbol for "wind;" shara, with the symbol for "bile;" and badgan, with the symbol for "phlegm." "Wind" relates to the spirit, thought, respiration, and movement, "bile" to the temperament and to the energetic and dynamic elements of life processes, and "phlegm" to sensory perception and material being. In Tibetan medicine all three humors are intimately interrelated. Only their full harmony assures the proper functioning of the seven "tissues" that make up the human body (lymph, blood, sperm, muscle, fat, bone, and bone marrow); without it, life and health are impossible.

Since the 1970s, Western medical science has shown increasing interest in the systematic study of the various herbal remedies that are used in Tibetan medicine.

Traditional Japanese medicine (kanpo)

TCM was introduced to Japan from Korea. Elements of other Asiatic medical traditions such as ayurveda (*see* page 789) were assimilated and, in time, Japan developed its own unique style of medicine known as *kanpo*. During the 17th century other systems started to evolve, including the Todo Yoshimasu school, which took a homeopathic approach, and the Toyo Yamawaki school which, because of doubts surrounding the traditional Chinese concepts of anatomy and physiology, concentrated on research into body structure through dissection. Unlike TCM, *kanpo* assimilated various surgical practices.

As Western medicine advanced into Japan, *kanpo* gradually began to decline in popularity, although after the end of the Second World War various Japanese universities started to teach it and to use modern methods to research its traditional drugs and healing techniques.

How it works

In TCM, the aim of treatment is to bring chi back into balance, thus removing the basis for the continued existence of the symptoms. These are notions that run counter to modern Western thinking and are difficult to transpose to a different cultural context. The traditional Chinese understanding of disease causation is in many respects incompatible with the teachings of modern scientific medicine.

Clinical proof of TCM's alleged ability to deal with acute conditions, as required by modern orthodox medicine, is absent. Many of the remedies that are used in TCM have not yet been the subject of scientific research.

Indications

In present-day China TCM is largely used for psychosomatic illnesses and as a supportive treatment for chronic disease and severe organ dysfunction. Though mostly used for pain relief and for treating psychosomatic and chronic illness, Western-style TCM is claimed to be effective against virtually any disease or condition, and even to be useful in medical emergencies.

Proof it works

Pharmacological research has only just been started into drugs used in TCM, Tibetan medicine, and *kanpo*. There have already been positive results with various drugs and drug combinations (phytopharmaceuticals) in patients with defined conditions.

Risks, cautions, and contraindications

Being of unproven efficacy, TCM should not be used to treat serious conditions. Anyone relying entirely on diagnosis by TCM is open to the risk of a diseased organ or cancer being overlooked and the chance of receiving an appropriate modern conventional therapy being missed. With oriental herbal medicines quality assurance is a problem. There have been isolated but persistent reports of remedies being adulterated with toxic plants or contaminated with heavy metals and other poisonous substances. Numerous deaths are on record.

Duration of treatment

Depending on the condition with which the patient presents, therapy may occasionally last for years or even call for lifelong treatment.

Finding the right therapist

A TCM therapist should be properly qualified and accredited with a professional foundation (*see* pages 930–7). In most cases accreditation will give some assurance as to the quality of training the therapist will have received and the standard of treatment that the patient can expect, but will not necessarily ensure that the therapy given will be appropriate to the patient's condition.

A reputable therapist will generally not offer treatment until the patient has consulted a medically qualified doctor for a conventional diagnosis. With the patient, he or she will define a treatment goal and propose a treatment plan (*see* page xxiii) to be used to monitor the patient's progress. No credence should be given to therapists promising an immediate or complete cure (*see* Practitioner checklist, page xxv).

Vitamins

> **Rating**
>
> Taking vitamins is **useful** when the patient has signs of vitamin deficiency or an increased vitamin requirement. However, maintaining a balanced diet remains the best way of ensuring a normal, adequate supply of vitamins.
>
> **May be of some use** when used preventively to lessen certain disease risks, e.g. arteriosclerosis, cardiovascular disease, neurological conditions. and various forms of cancer, and as an adjunct to other treatments.
>
> **Not advised** as the sole treatment for persistent complaints unless a conventional physician has diagnosed the patient's condition and made a proper risk–benefit assessment.

Method

Taking higher than normal doses of vitamins is believed to prevent diseases of modern living such as cancer (*see* page 701) and cardiovascular disease (*see* pages 409–511).

Rationale and historical perspective

Vitamins are substances that are essential to life and must form part of our regular intake of nutrients, as the body is unable to synthesize them for itself. For a long time the vitamin debate focused on avoidance of certain deficiency diseases, such as rickets, scurvy, and beriberi, which rarely occur nowadays, given a balanced diet. However, since the mid-1980s nutritional science and preventive medicine have turned their attention to the question of whether normal or raised doses of vitamins can act to prevent disease. One of the main proponents of this novel hypothesis was the American chemist and double Nobel prize-winner Linus Pauling, who died in 1994. He maintained that daily doses of vitamins C and E that far exceed the normal recommended doses can provide protection against infectious diseases and cancer, and even arrest the ageing process. This approach is also sometimes termed "orthomolecular medicine." It is a style of treatment that has its origins in the USA and employs a strategy of health maintenance and disease prevention based on high doses of vitamins, trace elements, and other important nutrients.

Considerable attention has been focused on the so-called antioxidative effect of vitamins C and E, of beta-carotene (provitamin A) and of the trace element selenium. No definitive suggestions can be given with regard to the recommended daily intake of these vitamins and antioxidants. Also unclarified is the question of whether the normal nutritional intake of vitamins is sufficient or whether it might not be better to take extra vitamins in the form of tablets to achieve a potentially preventive effect. Much of the evidence from recent years supports the latter notion.

Current recommendations vary considerably. While some organizations recommend a daily intake of 75mg of vitamin C, Pauling considered 10,000–18,000mg to be more appropriate. While some hold 12mg of vitamin E to be adequate, Pauling recommended 800. Beta-carotene recommendations are currently in the order of 2–6mg; Pauling made no recommendation. In the case of selenium, the daily dosage recommendations are sometimes vague; it should be borne in mind, however, that selenium taken in the long-term can lead to intoxication (warning signal: a metallic taste in the mouth).

Even within orthomolecular medicine, the recommended vitamin dosages vary widely, with some nutritional therapists, for example, recommending just 1.5g a day instead of Pauling's megadoses. Many doctors and nutritionists recommend exceeding today's daily vitamin recommendations by about 20 percent. There is little doubt, however, that certain conditions increase the need for vitamins and other nutrients. For example, mothers-to-be and breastfeeding mothers, women taking the pill, the elderly, people with stomach or intestinal disorders, alcoholics, and smokers all have increased vitamin requirements.

How it works

Modern research into vitamins proceeds from the premise that diseases of modern living, e.g. certain forms of cancer, atherosclerosis, coronary heart disease, various rheumatic disorders, and cataracts, are caused, *inter alia*, by so-called free radicals. Conversely, free radicals may also be formed in the course of a disease, exacerbating the ailment or producing complications.

A molecule becomes a free radical when it loses an electron through metabolic reactions or as a direct cause of pollutants entering the body. Each cell in the human body has to ward off such attacks thousands of times daily. Smog, cigarette smoke, stress, and exposure to harsh sunlight and ozone can make these attacks even more frequent. Having been attacked by a radical, the damaged molecule itself hunts for another molecule from which it can capture an electron to make up for the one it has lost. This sets up a chain of oxidative events that alters protein structures and damages the cell wall, leading ultimately to various diseases such as cancer, rheumatic disorders, and vascular disease. Free radicals are also suspected of being implicated in arteriosclerosis, an important risk factor for heart attacks and strokes. They are thought to be drawn especially to the harmful LDL cholesterol fraction and to be responsible for oxidizing these fatty acids. The rancid LDL cholesterol goes on to form a sort of fatty debris that is deposited on the inner walls of blood vessels and can lead via a number of complex metabolic reactions to arteriosclerosis. It is concluded from research to date that substances with an antioxidant effect are able to neutralize free radicals and thus nullify their effect. Despite the fact that there are still some gaps in our knowledge, it would seem appropriate to ensure that high doses of antioxidative vitamins and trace elements are taken as part of a balanced diet (fresh yellow and green vegetables, and fruit).

Indications

Advocates of high daily doses of vitamins commend this approach as a means of encouraging metabolism, invigorating the immune system, and preventing such conditions as cancer, arteriosclerosis, coughs and colds, rheumatic disease, and cataracts. Orthomolecular psychiatrists employ similar principles to treat psychiatric disorders.

Proof it works

Various controlled clinical studies (*see* page xix) have suggested that test subjects taking high daily doses of vitamins are less susceptible to cardiovascular disease and various types of cancer than a control group that received a placebo (*see* page xxi). However, in an extensive Finnish study in which test subjects were treated over several years with vitamin supplements, it was not possible to demonstrate any positive effect of beta-carotene or vitamin E in reducing the risk of lung cancer. The results recorded regarding the usefulness of antioxidants remain contradictory.

Risks, cautions, and contraindications

When taken in excessive doses, vitamin C can cause urinary calculi and diarrhea, while vitamin E may be implicated in muscle weakness and disturbed blood clotting. Excessive intake of vitamins A and D can induce various toxic symptoms. Selenium overdosage on a massive scale can cause serious intoxication. No definitive maximum limits can be stated based on the body of knowledge available today; it is known, however, that tolerance may differ from person to person.

   The promises made by some researchers and manufacturers can lead to the erroneous conclusion that taking large doses of vitamins will enable a person to perpetuate his or her unhealthy lifestyle.

Duration of treatment

As far as prevention is concerned, it may require years of taking vitamins to achieve the desired favorable effect.

Finding the right therapist

A reputable orthomolecular specialist will generally not start treatment until the patient has consulted a physician for a conventional diagnosis. With the patient, he or she will define a treatment goal and propose a short-term treatment plan (*see* page xxiii) to be used as a basis for checking that the treatment is having the desired effect.

No credence should be given to any therapist promising a total cure or maintaining that vitamin megadoses are able to offer general protection from disease (*see* Practitioner checklist, page xxv).

PART 3

The diagnostic techniques used in complementary medicine

Applied kinesiology (AK)

Rating
Not advised as the sole method of diagnosis.

Rationale and historical perspective

Applied kinesiology (Greek *kinesis*: "motion") is based on the idea that specific groups of muscles are related to the principal organs of the body. A diseased organ, or an organ dysfunction, is believed to upset the flow of vital energy through the body, manifesting itself as a weakening of the muscles associated with that organ. If the flow of energy is in balance and the organ in question is healthy, the muscle will be firm and responsive. The kinesiologist will tell the patient to raise an arm or a leg, then place one hand on the body above the organ being examined and, with the other, will apply light pressure to the associated arm or leg muscles. If the patient is able to exert an opposite pressure, the organ is healthy. Sagging of the limb when pressure is applied indicates that the organ is diseased.

Applied kinesiology can also be employed to test foods, drugs, and potential allergens. If drugs are being tested, the kinesiologist will hold them in turn against the body at a point above the organ thought to be diseased. A firm muscle allegedly shows that drug to be effective, while a sagging muscle shows it to be unsuitable. If the therapist is testing foods or trying to identify potential allergens, he or she will hold a series of foods or miscellaneous substances in one hand, while applying pressure to the relevant muscle group with the other. If the limb feels spongy, the food is not suitable for the patient or the substance is an allergen.

One variant of AK, edukinesthesia, is claimed to be able to detect a lack of cooperation between the two hemispheres of the brain said to be responsible for learning difficulties and poor concentration.

Any problems found will be treated with a drug that tests positively, or by massaging to unblock the energy flow. The "touch for health" variant of AK aims to ease stress-induced tension through physical contact, exercise therapy, and massage. Edukinesthesia uses physical and mental exercises to promote cooperation between the two brain hemispheres.

Indications

Kinesiologists use AK to diagnose organ dysfunction and energy blockage. More controversial, however, is its use for allergy testing and testing for drug response.

Proof it works

The beliefs on which AK is based are inconsistent with the principles of modern anatomy. There has not been any formal clinical research into specific links between muscle response and organ disease, nor have there been any controlled clinical studies (*see* page xix) showing the method to be accurate enough to be used as a diagnostic tool. Several controlled clinical studies have been unable to corroborate kinesiologists' claims.

Risks, cautions, and contraindications

There is a very high risk of a disease remaining undetected, of a condition being wrongly diagnosed, or of an unsuitable medication being given unnecessarily.

Bioelectronics according to Vincent

Rating
Not advised as the sole method of diagnosis.

Rationale and historical perspective

This diagnostic technique is founded on the belief that the acidity (pH), resistance, and electrical potential of the blood, saliva, and urine of test subjects can give an insight into their resistance or otherwise to disease.

The theory originates from the discovery by the French scientist Louis-Claude Vincent that these three parameters are useful in the assessment of drinking water quality. Vincent concluded from his work that these parameters must also be instrumental in deciding a person's state of health.

Some bioelectronics therapists advise people found to have an alleged susceptibility to a disease to undergo an (often expensive) course of preventive treatment.

Indications

Proponents claim to be able to utilize Vincent's principle to determine a person's resistance to disease, "biological age" (which can, it is claimed, be different from the person's actual age), any metabolic disorders from which they may be suffering, and their susceptibility to certain diseases.

Proof it works

The theory on which bioelectronics according to Vincent is based does not accord well with the principles of modern science. There has not been any formal clinical research into the diagnostic capabilities of this method (*see* page xix).

Risks, cautions, and contraindications

There is a high risk of a real disease remaining undetected or of a condition being wrongly diagnosed.

Dowsing

Rating
Not advised as the sole method of diagnosis.

Rationale and historical perspective

Dowsing is believed to be useful for locating water courses, minerals, and other materials underground. Medical dowsers believe that geological faults and water courses produce geopathic energies or forces. Where these forces are particularly concentrated (along ley lines, for instance), they are believed to be (co-)responsible for a whole raft of complaints ranging from sleeplessness to cancer.

The divining rods that dowsers use may consist of a number of materials, including wood, plastic, and metal. More recently, computer-assisted devices have been used to trace geopathic energies. Using their divining rods, dowsers will scan homes and offices in an attempt to sense negative geopathic energies. A positive response by the rods shows such energies to be present.

Some dowers claim they can sense energies simply by

examining charts or maps. Having located a bad radiation, they will generally advise moving a bed or office chair away from the area, or recommend that it be specially "decontaminated."

When used for diagnosing disease, the divining rods may well be passed along the client's body. Those parts of the body above which the rods respond are allegedly diseased. Many dowsers claim to be able to sense disease by testing a polaroid image or a drop of blood.

Indications

Most dowsers claim not only to be able to identify virtually any disease but also to be able to prevent illness by locating bad ley lines.

Proof it works

There is no scientific proof that there is any such thing as bad radiations or energies. The principle on which diagnosis by dowsing is based is unproven. There has not been any controlled clinical research (*see* page xix) into the question of whether the technique can furnish an accurate diagnosis. Older studies have shown that the diagnostic "hits" obtained by dowsing are due to nothing more than chance. Such studies are not negated by the sometimes extraordinary successes achieved by dowsers in their search for water.

Examination of "decontamination devices" has failed to reveal any element that would be capable of locating alleged natural energies; indeed, some contained only such materials as pebbles, putty, or wool.

Risks, cautions, and contraindications

There is a high risk of a real disease being overlooked.

Electroacupuncture according to Voll (EAV)

Rating
Not advised as the sole method of diagnosis.

Rationale and historical perspective

Several decades ago the German physician Reinhold Voll developed a diagnostic principle to serve as a basis for his treatment methods. He used an ohmmeter to measure the electrical resistance of the skin at various acupuncture points and other defined sites, claiming that the electrical conductivity of the skin reflects the reactive properties of that part of the body associated with the point in question.

Assuming the normal state (test subject in good health) to be when the needle is deflected halfway along an ohmmeter scale, values that are higher than the norm are believed to indicate an inflammation, while those that are lower suggest that the person is run-down or suffering from "degenerative processes." A gradual falling back of the needle from its initial position allegedly indicates the presence of toxins (*see* page 929), remains of an earlier disease, or foci (*see* page 928). The reading halfway along the scale is said to prove that the remedy in question is efficacious.

Indications

Proponents of EAV believe it to be capable not only of discovering foci or toxins said to be responsible for a wide variety of illnesses but also of detecting immune system disorders and diseases even before they have manifested themselves.

Proof it works

The theory underlying EAV is inconsistent with the principles of modern science. There have not been any reports of formal clinical research adequately proving a link between electrical resistance of the skin, foci or toxins, and disease. Experiments have shown, however, that the results obtained are affected by artifacts such as the pressure with which the probes are applied to the skin, moisture, and the thickness of subcutaneous fatty tissues.

While there have so far not been any rigorous tests into the diagnostic accuracy of this technique, experiments have shown, conversely, that multiple attempts at EAV diagnosis in one and the same person have often produced different results.

Risks, cautions, and contraindications

There is a high risk of a disease remaining undetected, of a condition being misdiagnosed, or of an unsuitable medication testing positive. Persons should be very wary in particular of EAV therapists' frequent tendency to recommend the elimination of pathogenic foci. Patients should at all events consult a physician for a second opinion before agreeing to surgical removal of their tonsils, appendix, teeth, ovaries, or prostate, or to any other expensive surgical measures or interventions.

Electroneural diagnosis according to Croon

Rating
Not advised as the sole method of diagnosis.

Rationale and historical perspective

At about the same time as his work on electroneural therapy in the 1950s (*see* page 807), the German physician Richard Croon also developed a diagnostic system based on the same technology. His method exploits more than 200 so-called reactive sites on a person's skin, located chiefly in the head and back region, each having a diameter of $3/4$–$1^1/4$ inches. These points, which Croon matched to specific organs, allegedly exhibit lower electrical resistance and thus higher conductivity than the areas surrounding them. Key values that are found to be outside Croon's defined "normal range" are plotted on an electroneural somatogram and are claimed to give a diagnostic insight into the person's overall state of health, to be able to detect possible organ disease, to locate pathogenic foci, and to identify causes of disease. Patients subsequently receive a course of electroneural stimulation.

Indications

Proponents claim that electroneural diagnosis according to Croon can be used to diagnose a multitude of diseases, including serious ailments such as diabetes and cancer.

Proof it works

The concept at the heart of electroneural diagnosis is inconsistent with modern medical science. There are no reports of there having been any rigorous tests into a possible relationship between raised conductivity readings and disease. Nor have there been any tests showing the method to be accurate enough to be used as a diagnostic tool.

Risks, cautions, and contraindications

There is a high risk of a disease remaining undetected, or of a patient's condition being misdiagnosed.

Hair mineral analysis

Rating
Not advised as the sole method of diagnosis.

Rationale and historical perspective

Hair mineral analysis is based on the belief that the mineral make-up of human hair, its toxic metal content, and the amounts of trace elements it contains can provide an insight into a person's general state of health and highlight possible mineral deficiencies. While conventional practitioners might use chemical analysis of hair to detect possible long-term exposure to heavy metals or other environmental pollutants and poisons, complementary hair mineral analysis is used as a diagnostic tool that purportedly can even show a person's tendency to acquire serious disease.

Mail order hair mineral analysis is also available to would-be patients. Prospective clients are instructed to cut off a lock of hair weighing approximately .03oz from the back of the head as close to the scalp as possible and to send it in to a laboratory. There the hair is cleaned, dissolved in acid, and subjected to chemical analysis. Clients are then informed in writing of the alleged deficiencies that the analysis has revealed, the recommended remedy, and sometimes even a detailed diagnosis of possible illnesses or disease susceptibilities. A complementary therapy may also be proposed. Any trace elements and minerals that are recommended will possibly be manufactured and sold by the same company as has performed the hair mineral analysis.

Indications

Proponents of hair mineral analysis hold the view that it can determine whether a person has been exposed to toxic heavy metals or other substances, detect a lack of trace elements and minerals, and even identify illnesses and susceptibility to disease.

Proof it works

The principles of complementary hair mineral analysis are inconsistent with modern medical science. There is no proven relationship between the mineral content of hair and physiological deficiencies. A deficit (or excess) of minerals in the hair can have a variety of causes. That one is able to deduce the presence of an illness or a proneness to disease based on hair composition is an unproven hypothesis.

Results differ from one laboratory to another. Hair samples, for instance, from two persons that were submitted for analysis to 13 different laboratories gave contradictory results, even for two hair samples from the one person sent in to the same laboratory. Altogether, the results failed to show any consistency.

Risks, cautions, and contraindications

Present findings show there to be a high risk of a real disease remaining undetected, or of a person's condition being mis-diagnosed. There is also a tendency for inappropriate and/or expensive preparations to be prescribed.

Iridology

Rating
Not advised as the sole method of diagnosis.

Rationale and historical perspective

Iridologists believe that the iris of the eye reflects a person's state of health and the condition of his/her internal organs. The iris, they say, represents a body map with the left eye corresponding to the lefthand side of the body, the right eye to the righthand side. The map divides the iris into segments, with each segment allegedly representing a part of the body. Possible diseases show up as pigmentation irregularities or as white or dark streaks, spots, or flecks. According to iridologists, this shows how the whole body is linked to the eyes through a neural network. Some modern iridologists take color photographs or transparencies that they magnify and read.

Iridology actually dates back to the 17th century, though it is probably fair to say that modern iridology developed when the Hungarian homeopath Ignaz von Péczely, as a boy, tended an owl with a broken leg and noticed changes in the eye of the bird as it recovered.

Iridology is now a popular tool in complementary medicine. A number of variants have developed, including pupil diagnosis.

Indications

Iridology, it is claimed, is capable not only of diagnosing various complaints but also of providing an insight into hereditary disease factors or proneness to certain diseases such as cancer.

Proof it works

The ideas on which iridology is based are inconsistent with modern anatomical science. There are no neural pathways directly linking the principal organs of the body with the iris. Comparison of the available eye maps also reveals some notable inconsistencies. In trials that were designed to test the accuracy of iridology as a diagnostic tool, its practitioners were unable to substantiate their claimed ability to pinpoint certain diseases. When, for example, they were shown iris photographs of patients suffering from gallbladder disease and of persons from a healthy control group, the proportion of diagnostic "hits" was just 50 percent—no better than chance. The figures were similar in studies with kidney patients.

Risks, cautions, and contraindications

There is a high risk of a real disease being overlooked, or of a person's condition being misdiagnosed. An iridologist's claim to have discovered a proneness to a certain disease (cancer, for instance) in a patient is likely to cause considerable anguish.

Kirlian photography

Rating
Not advised as the sole method of diagnosis.

Rationale and historical perspective

Inspired by the theories of Rudolf Steiner, the founding father of anthroposophy (*see* page 781), concerning the physical and the etheric body, the Russian husband and wife team Semyon and Valentina Kirlian developed a photographic technique that is said to be able to detect a patient's aura or energy flow. A high voltage, high frequency electrical charge is passed through a sensitive photographic plate to make an image of the patient's hand, following which the photograph is developed to reveal what appear to be flares of emitted electrical energy.

Modern Kirlian diagnosticians use an updated version of the technique originally devised by the Kirlians. Nowadays a hand, foot, or individual finger is placed on a discharge plate above a photosensitive film and the emissions are recorded. The film is developed to produce a colored image of the person's so-called bio-aura, which the therapist then interprets to discover any possible physical or psychological problems in need of treatment. Patients are sometimes recalled for further imaging to enable the success of a treatment that has been prescribed for an allegedly disturbed bio-aura to be checked.

Indications

Kirlian photography, its proponents claim, can be used to diagnose various diseases including serious ones such as cancer.

Proof it works

The theories on which Kirlian photography is based are inconsistent with modern science. There is no verifiable proof that the results obtained by this diagnostic procedure are anything more than hit and miss. There have not so far been any tests into the alleged diagnostic capabilities of the method. The energy emission patterns depend very much on the conditions under which the technique is applied.

Risks, cautions and contraindications

There is a high risk of a real disease being overlooked or of the patient's condition being misdiagnosed.

Optical blood testing

Rating
Not advised as the sole method of diagnosis.

Rationale and historical perspective

This diagnostic procedure is based on the notion that the appearance and behavior of human blood, after it has been prepared in a special way, can help pinpoint various ailments. Doctors with an anthroposophical leaning (*see* Anthroposophical medicine, page 781), occasionally employ the Pfeiffer crystallization test, in which, under controlled climatic conditions, a patient's blood is trickled into copper chloride. The shape of the crystals that form, they say, enables them to diagnose an existing disease or a risk to the person's health.

In the Kaelin capillary dynamic blood test, filter paper is immersed in the patient's blood. The blood is drawn into the paper and migrates upward forming shapes, the edge patterns of which are used as the basis for "diagnosing" the patient's condition. Mushroom-shaped images, for example, are said to signify cancer.

In holistic blood diagnosis or auroscopy, blood is spread on a flat surface. If the blood exhibits irregular coloration, the darker regions, it is claimed, assume the shape of the organ that is diseased.

Indications

Complementary therapists who practice optical blood testing claim it to be useful for diagnosing a variety of diseases including serious ones such as cancer; and additionally for detecting disease precursors, incipient illness, and proneness to certain medical conditions.

Proof it works

There is no verifiable indication of how the technique works, if indeed it does; nor a scrap of proof that optical blood testing has any diagnostic value whatsoever.

Risks, cautions, and contraindications

There is a high risk of a real disease being overlooked, or of a fictitious disease being "discovered."

Pendulum diagnosis

Rating
Not advised as the sole method of diagnosis.

Rationale and historical perspective

Pendulums exist in a variety of shapes and materials, and often resemble a plumb bob. Diagnosticians generally hold the pendulum on a chain or thread in one hand and gently swing it to and fro a short distance from the patient's body, starting with the head and finishing with the feet. The motion of the pendulum is said to show up any part of the body that is affected by disease. A serious disease is allegedly present if the pendulum stops moving; if it moves obliquely, it is said to forewarn of cancer.

During examination, the diagnostician may interrogate the pendulum about the patient's state of health or may hold a series of foods in one hand and ask whether the patient tolerates them. Some pendulum diagnosticians even claim to be able to perform long-range diagnoses by swinging the pendulum over an item of clothing or a letter sent in by the client.

Indications

Proponents suggest that the pendulum can pinpoint parts of the body that are diseased and even be used to select suitable remedies, which are frequently homeopathic preparations (*see* page 831) or flower remedies (*see* page 828).

Proof it works

There is nothing to substantiate the claimed diagnostic principle at the heart of pendulum diagnosis. The motion of the pendulum is determined above all by muscle tension in the diagnostician's arm and by his or her subconscious expectations. There have not so far been any tests (*see* page xix) into the ability of this method to identify disease.

Risks, cautions, and contraindications

There is a high risk of a real disease being overlooked or of unsuitable medications being recommended.

Thermoregulation diagnosis (TRD)

Rating
Not advised as the sole method of diagnosis.

Rationale and historical perspective

The German physician Ernst Schwamm initially devised his technique of thermoregulation diagnosis in the 1950s; a colleague of his, Arno Rost, developed the method further in the 1970s.

TRD, also called regulation thermography, starts with measurement of the "normal" skin temperature of a patient, this reading was then compared with temperature changes induced by exposing the person to a low temperature stimulus. Temperature changes form the basis on which a diagnosis can be formulated, either covering the entire body or concentrating on individual organs. They provide, it is claimed, an indication of the person's general state of health or of any illness present.

Rost's theory is that various diseases in the body are characterized by local temperature change that occurs without there being any sign of feverishness. However, disease *is* signalled by a change in temperature at points connected through so-called energy links (*see* page 928) to the diseased organ in question.

The patient, who preferably will not have taken any medication in the preceding 24 hours, will remain for half an hour in a room maintained at 70–73°F, and then have his or her skin temperature measured at various points with a thermal probe. He or she will subsequently be exposed to a low temperature stimulus (being asked to sit unclothed for ten minutes), following which the skin temperature will be remeasured. If the temperature remains virtually constant, the TRD therapist concludes there is an energy blockage (*see* page 927) that is due, possibly, to a pathogenic focus (*see* page 928). If there is a temperature difference of more than two degrees, the regulatory mechanism is said to have "overshot"—an indication of a possibly serious disease. A difference of between 1 and 2°F is normal.

Nowadays the temperature differences are even computer evaluated, a fact which allegedly makes the diagnosis more precise.

Indications

TRD, its proponents claim, can detect factors conducive to illness and diagnose early stages of various diseases (such as cancer). TRD is also allegedly useful for discovering causes of disease such as pathogenic foci, for measuring to what extent a disease has taken hold, for deciding on the optimum form of treatment, and for ruling out less appropriate therapies. Proponents of TRD also believe it to be useful for monitoring the patient's progress and for providing documentary evidence of a successful outcome.

Proof it works

The ideas on which thermoregulation diagnosis is founded are only partially consistent with the principles of modern medicine. There is at present nothing to prove the claimed link between thermoregulation and the occurrence of individual physical conditions. Nor have there been any controlled clinical studies (*see* page xix) into this technique as a means of providing accurate diagnoses. Although there are indications that TRD could provide certain information, the suggestion that it is a precise diagnostic method have not been borne out scientifically.

Risks, cautions, and contraindications

There is a high risk of a real disease being overlooked, or of fictitious diseases or factors purportedly conducive to disease being "discovered." A medically qualified practitioner must always be consulted for a second opinion before any surgical intervention is undertaken to "eliminate foci."

Tongue diagnosis

Rating
Not advised as the sole method of diagnosis.

Rationale and historical perspective

Practitioners who use tongue diagnosis believe that each part of the tongue reflects a different internal organ: the heart and lung at the tip, liver on the right side, stomach on the left. The appearance, color, and quality of the tongue at various points give an insight into the state of health of each organ. Practitioners for whom tongue diagnosis is part of the standard repertoire believe the tongue and principal organs to be linked via the sympathetic nervous system.

Tongue diagnosis has its origins in traditional Chinese medicine and, in recent years, has become popular among certain complementary practitioners and medical doctors with a leaning toward TCM. Tongue diagnosis, without the clutter of claims made about it in the complementary sphere, is a legitimate and valuable part of conventional medical diagnosis.

Indications

Practitioners believe tongue diagnosis to be a useful way of discovering whether internal organs such as the liver, stomach, heart, or lungs are affected by disease.

Proof it works

The ideas on which complementary tongue diagnosis is based are inconsistent with modern medical science. There has so far not been any controlled clinical research into whether the method is capable of providing a reliable diagnosis.

Risks, cautions, and contraindications

There is a high risk of a real disease being overlooked.

Glossary

Constitution. Describes the sum of all inherited and socially acquired physical and mental characteristics that are believed to sustain and perpetuate a predisposition to certain diseases. Many complementary treatments pay more attention to a person's constitution than to his or her particular disease.

Energize. To impart vital energy or amplify its effect, usually through complementary healthcare procedures.

Energy, energetic. In complementary medicine, "energy" has a number of meanings. Sometimes the term is used to denote intangible links—for example, the communication links within the human body, between a patient and the therapist, or between the patient and the environment. Also, there may be energy links between the body and soul. "Energy" is often a synonym for "life force" (qv) or "healing power," i.e. for the driving force deep within us.

Energy blockage. Denotes a situation in which the body's energies are blocked or become stagnant (*see* Foci), so lessening its self-healing power and limiting the therapeutic possibilities. Clearing energy blockages is thus a central theme in many complementary practices.

Energy imbalance. Much of nonorthodox medicine sees health as a delicate balance between certain energies, forces, etc., and disease as an imbalance between them or as a preponderance of one or other of them. Various therapeutic measures are taken in an attempt to restore balance.

Energy links. In reflexology, these are interactive channels between the surface of the body and its inner tissues and organs. An imbalance or disease in one zone of the body is believed to have an effect on other zones or organs. Reflexologists exploit these links.

Foci. Phenomena that trigger and perpetuate disease and that also affect a person's well-being and normal body function (*see also* Energy blockage). Depending on the rationale underlying the particular therapeutic approach, foci may be seen as structural (e.g. scars, diseased organs, localized or general buildup of toxins, chronic inflammation, remains of an earlier disease, etc.), or as events in the patient's life. Foci sometimes are defined in terms of a lack or deficit of life force (qv) or as blockage or imbalance of energies coursing through the body. These notions are only plausible as long as they appear to have a therapeutic effect.

Holistic. Holistic medical philosophies are those which see disease as the manifestation of physical, mental, and emotional disturbance and consider the body and soul to be a single entity. In what is essentially a cosmic approach, all aspects of the patient's personal and social lifestyle are duly considered, as well as his or her links with nature and the environment. Treatment must take all of these important factors into account and has, as one of its foremost principles, the notion that the individual carries exclusive responsibility for his or her own well-being.

Immunomodulation. Immunomodulation is based on the supposition that various immunostimulant and immuno-suppressive influences co-exist, and indeed are interlinked, in the human body. Certain complementary therapies aim to control or modulate immune processes in the body to stop a disease from progressing or, in some cases, to eradicate it altogether.

Life force. A frequently used synonym for "vital energy," "self-healing power," "the will to get well," or "healing potential."

Randomized. Randomized double blind trials are studies in which patients are split up randomly into subgroups and assigned to a doctor, with neither the doctor nor the patient knowing whether the treatment is the real one or the control treatment; both the doctor and patient are "blind."

Referred pain. Pain that is felt at a site other than that at which it originates (*see* Energy links). Treatment should therefore be aimed not at the site where pain is experienced but at the trigger points (qv).

Self-healing power. *See* Life force.

Stagnation. *See* Energy blockage.

Stimulation therapy. Individually dosed stimuli are applied to the body in an attempt to clear energy blockages (*see* Foci, Energy blockage), to invigorate the body's self-healing power, or to make a disease amenable to treatment.

Toxins. Include environmental poisons, waste products in the body, bacterial poisons, drugs, etc. Together they may be considered as a sort of generalized focus (*see* Foci).

Trigger points. Points or zones which can produce and sustain energy imbalance, organ dysfunction and, above all, pain. Trigger points are believed to exist throughout the body, are often pressure-sensitive, and can be the origin of referred pain (qv).

Vital energy. *See* Life force.

Useful addresses

Australia

Australian Federation for
Homoeopathy
PO Box 806
Spit Junction
New South Wales
2088

Australian Society of Teachers of
the Alexander Technique
(AUSTAT)
PO Box 716
Darlinghurst
New South Wales
2010

Australian Traditional Medicine
Society Limited
ATMS
PO Box 1027
Meadowbank
New South Wales
2114

Martin & Pleasance
(Bach Flower Remedies)
137 Swan Street
Richmond
Victoria
3121

National Herbalists Association
of Australia
Suite 305
BST House
3 Smail Street
Broadway
New South Wales
2007

Reflexology Association of
Australia
15 Kedumba Crescent
Turramurra
New South Wales
2074

Society of Clinical Masseurs
PO Box 483
9 Delhi Street
Mitchum
Victoria
3131

UK

Anglo-European College of
Chiropractic
13–15 Parkwood Road
Boscombe
Bournemouth
Dorset
BH5 2DF

Aromatherapy Organizations
Council
3 Latymer Close
Braybrooke
Market Harborough
Leicestershire
LE16 8LN

Association of Holistic Therapists
39 Prestbury Road
Cheltenham
Gloucestershire
GL25 2PT

Association of Massage
Practitioners
Flat 3
52 Redcliffe Square
London
SW10 9HQ

Association of Medical
Aromatherapists
Abergare
Rhu Point
Helensburgh
G84 8NF

Association of Natural Medicine
27 Braintree Road
Witham
Essex
CM8 2DD

Association of Physical and
Natural Therapists
68a The Avenue
Worcester Park
Surrey
KT4 7HJ

British Acupuncture Association
& Register (BAAR)
34 Alderney Street
London
SE1 4EU

British College of Acupuncture
8 Hunter Street
London
WC1N 1BN

British College of Naturopathy
and Osteopathy
6 Netherhall Gardens
London
N3 5RR

British Complementary Medicine
Association
Mental Health Unit
St Charles' Hospital
Exmoor Street
London
W10 6DZ

British Herbal Medicine
Association
Sun House
Church Street
Stroud
Gloucestershire
GL5 1JL

British Holistic Medical
Association
179 Gloucester Place
London
NW1 6DX

British Homoeopathic Research
Group
1 Upper Wimpole Street
London
W1M 7TD

British Reflexology Association
Monk's Orchard
Whitbourne
Worcester
WR6 5RB

British Register of
Complementary Practitioners
Institute of Complementary
Medicine
PO Box 194
London
SE16 1QZ

British School—Reflex Zone
Therapy of the Feet
Oakington Avenue
Wembley Park
London
HA9 8HY

Centre for the Study of
Complementary Medicine
51 Bedford Place
Southampton
SO15 2DT

College of Homoeopathy
26 Clarendon Rise
London
SE13 5EJ

College of Osteopaths
Practitioners' Association
13 Furzhill Road
Borehamwood
Herts
WD6 2DG

Community Health Foundation
188–194 Old Street
London
EC1V 9BP

Consumers' Association
2 Marylebone Road
London
NW1 4DF

Council for Complementary and
Alternative Medicine
179 Gloucester Place
London
NW1 6DX

Dept of Homoeopathic Medicine
United Bristol Healthcare NHS
Trust
Cotham Hill
Cotham
Bristol
BS6 6JU

European School of Osteopathy
104 Tonbridge Road
Maidstone
Kent
ME16 8SL

European Shiatsu School
Central Administration
High Banks
Lockeridge
Nr Marlborough
Wiltshire
SN8 4EQ

Foundation of Traditional
Chinese Medicine
122A Acomb Road
York
YO2 4EY

General Council and Register of
Naturopaths
Frazer House
6 Netherhall Street
London
NW3 5RR

General Council and Register of
Osteopaths
56 London Street
Reading
RG1 4SQ

Glasgow Homoeopathic Hospital
1000 Great Western Road
Glasgow
G12 QAA

Hearing Voices Network
Creative Support
67 Abbot's Court
Gateshead
Tyne and Wear
NE8 3JY

Hahnemann Society
Humane Education Centre
Bounds Green Road
London
N22 4EV

Healing Herbs of Dr Bach
PO Box 65
Hereford
HR2 0UW

Homoeopathic Development
Foundation
19a Cavendish Square
London
W1M 9AD

Homoeopathic Medical Research
Council
Royal London Homoeopathic
Hospital
Great Ormond Street
London
WC1N 3HR

Incorporated Society of
Registered Naturopaths
1 Albemarle Road
The Mount
York
YO2 1EN

Institute of Complementary
Medicine
PO Box 194
London
SE16 1QZ

Institute of Dream Analysis
8 Willow Road
London
NW3 1TJ

Institute of Family Therapy
43 New Cavendish Street
London
W1M 7RG

Institute of Optimum Nutrition
Blades Court
Deodar Rd
London
SW15 2NU

International Federation of
Aromatherapists
Department of Continuing
Education
Royal Masonic Hospital
Ravenscourt Park
London
W6 0TN

International Federation of
Iridologists
c/o Vicki Pitman
Hayes Corner
South Cheriton
Templecombe
Somerset
BA8 0BR

International Institute of
Reflexology
Francis Wagg, UK Director
15 Hatfield Close
Tonbridge
TN10 4JP

International Register of Oriental
Medicine (UK)
4 The Manor House
Colley Lane
Reigate
Surrey
RH2 9JW

International Society of
Professional Aromatherapists
Hinckley and District Hospital
The Annex
Mount Road
Hinckley
Leicestershire
LE10 1AG

Michio Kushi Institute
188 Old Street
London
EC1V 9FR

National College of Hypnosis
and Psychotherapy
12 Cross Street
Nelson
Lancashire
BB9 7EN

Pain Relief Foundation
Rice Lane
Liverpool
L9 1AE

Register of Traditional Chinese
Medicine (RTCM)
19 Trinity Road
London
N2 8JJ

Research Council for
Complementary Medicine
60 Great Ormond Street
London
WC1N 3JF

School of Phytotherapy
Bucksteep Manor
Bodle Street Green
Near Hailsham
East Sussex
BN27 4RJ

Scientific & Medical Network
Lesser Halings
Tilehouse Lane
Denham
Uxbridge
UB9 5DG

Scottish Homoeopathic Research
and Education Trust
c/o Royal Bank of Scotland PLC
98 Buchanan Street
Glasgow
G1 3BA

Shiatsu Society
14 Oakdene Road
Redhill
RH1 6BT

Society of Homoeopaths
2 Artizan Road
Northampton
NN1 4HU

Society of Teachers of the
Alexander Technique (STAT)
20 London House
266 Fulham Road
London
SW10 9EL

Traditional Acupuncture Society
1 The Ridgeway
Stratford-upon-Avon
Warwickshire
CV37 9JL

UK Homoeopathic Medical
Association
6 Livingstone Road
Gravesend
Kent
DA12 5DZ

Yoga Biomedical Trust
PO Box 140
Cambridge
CB4 3SY

USA

American Association of Oriental
Medicine (AAOM)
433 Front Street
Catasauqua, PA 18032

American Board of
Homeotherapeutics/National
  Center for Homeopathy
801 North Fairfax Street,
Suite 306
Alexandria, VA 22314

American Chiropractic
Association
1701 Clarendon Blvd
Arlington, VA 24203

American College of
Advancement in Medicine
P.O. Box 3427
Laguna Hills, CA 92654

American Foundation
for Homeopathy
1508 Glencoe Street, Suite 44
Denver, CO 80220-1338

American Herb Association
P.O. Box 1673
Nevada City, CA 95959

American Holistic
Medical Association
6728 Old McLean Village Drive
McLean, VA 22101

American Institute of Massage
Therapy
2156 Newport Blvd
Costa Mesa
CA 92627

American Massage Therapy
Association
820 Davis, Suite 100
Evanston, IL 60201–4444

The Aromatherapy
Institute and Research
P.O. Box 1222
Fair Oaks, CA 95628

The Ayurveda Institute
P.O. Box 282
Fairfield, IA 52556

Behavioral Science Association
Association for Applied
Psychophysiology
and Biofeedback
Johns Hopkins University
Baltimore, MD 21203

California School of Herbal
Studies
PO Box 39
Forestville, CA 95436

Citizens for Health Education
2233 S Huron Pkwy
Ann Arbor, MI 48104

Dr Edward Bach Healing Society
644 Merrick Road
Lynbrook , NY 11563

Ellon (Bach U.S.A.), Inc.
P.O. Box 32
Woodmere, NY 11598

Fetzer Institute
9292 West KL Avenue
Kalamazoo, MI 49009

Flower Essence Society
PO Box 1769
Nevade City, CA 95959

Healthinform
PO Box 306
Montrose, NY 10548

International Council of
Reflexologists
PO Box 621963
Littleton, CO 80162

International Foundation for
Homeopathy
2366 Eastlake Avenue E, Suite 301
Seattle, WA 98102

National Holistic Institute
5900 Hollis st
Suite J
Emeryville
CA 94608-2008

NIH Office of Alternative
Medicine
6120 Executive Blvd, Suite 450
Executive Plaza South Building
Rockville , MD 20892

New York State Licensed
Acupuncturist's Association
350 Central Park West
New York, NY 10025

Older People in Society
National Institute on Aging
Gateway Building, Suite 533
7201 Wisconsin Avenue MSC
9205
Bethesda, MD 20892-9205

Society for Acupuncture
Research
Suite 804
4733 Bethesda Avenue
Bethesda, MD 20814

Traditional Acupuncture Institute
American City Building
10227 Wincopin Circle, Suite 100
Columbia, MD 21044-3422

Authors and advisers

Roland Bettschart, M Phil, born 1955 in Trieste, studied Social Sciences and International Relations in Vienna and Bologna. From 1989 to 1993 he was editor of the Austrian weekly magazine *profil*. Both before and after this he was a freelance writer and journalist: for German and English TV, Austrian Radio, the Hamburg weekly *Die Woche*, the Swiss weekly *Weltwoche*, the *Neue Zürcher Zeitung*, and *profil*. He is the co-author of *Reportagen aus der Zukunft* ("Reports from the Future"), 1991, and *Kursbuch Kinder* ("Childhood—a Handbook"), 1993.

Edzard Ernst, medical doctor and university professor, born 1948 in Wiesbaden, studied medicine in Munich, and held professorships in Hannover and Vienna. Since 1993 he has been Professor of Complementary Medicine and Director of the Department of Complementary Medicine at the University of Exeter. His special fields are: complementary medicine, physical medicine, hemorrhology and sports medicine. He has published several hundred papers and is the author or editor of 23 books. He had founded and edits three journals, and is an editor or adviser on many other journals. He has received 8 scientific awards for his work.

Gerd Glaeske, Doctor of Natural Sciences, born 1945 in Quedlinburg, studied physics and pharmacy in Aachen and Hamburg. Since 1987 he has directed the pharmacological advisory services for health insurance organizations. He is presently director of the department of Health Studies and Principal of Medical Care at the Health Insurers Association (VdAK). He is a member of the Standards Commission at the government Institute for Medicines, and of the Drug Utilization group of the World Health Organization (WHO). He is a lecturer on Medicine Epidemiology at Bremen University. He has published numerous articles in specialist fields, and the following books: *Positivliste für Arzneimittel* ("Choosing Your Medicine"), co-author, 1988; *Altern ist keine Krankheit* ("Aging isn't an Illness"), co-author, 1989; *Lieber Handeln als Schlucken* ("Better to act than Swallow"), co-author, 1990; *Arzneimittelsicherheit und Länderüberwachung* ("Medicine Safety and International Monitoring"), co-author, 1993; *Was hilft—ein Medikamentenratgeber für Frauen* ("Something to Help—a Medicine Handbook for Women"), co-author, 1994. He has contributed in an advisory capacity to *Bittere Pillen* ("Bitter Pills"), 1983 onwards; *Krankheit auf Rezept* ("Illness on Prescription"), 1984; and *Kursbuch Gesundheit* ("Health—a Handbook"), 1990.

Kurt Langbein, born 1953 in Budapest, studied Sociology in Vienna. From 1979 to 1989 he was a documentary filmmaker, and a journalist for Austrian Radio; from 1989 to 1992 head of the national news department of the Austrian news magazine *profil*. Since then he has been a freelance author and journalist for, among others, the Hamburg weekly *Die Woche*, for *profil*, for SAT 1, RTL and Austrian Radio. He is co-author of the following books: *Gesunde Geschäfte* ("Healthy Shopping"), 1981; *Bittere Pillen* ("Bitter Pills"), 1983, revised edition 1993; *Gift-Grün Chemie in der Landwirtschaft* ("Toxic Green: chemical agriculture"), 1986; *Sozialstaat Österreich* ("Austria's Welfare State"), 1987; *Kursbuch Gesundheit* ("Health—a Handbook"), 1990; *Land der Sinne—Liebe, Sex und Partnerschaft in Österreich* ("Land of the Senses—Love, Sex and Partnership in Austria"), 1991; *Kursbuch Kinder* ("Childhood—a Handbook"), 1993; *Kursbuch Küche* ("Cookery—a Handbook"), 1995; and *Kursbuch Lebensqualität* ("Quality of Life—a Handbook"), 1995.

Reinhard Saller, medical doctor, university professor, born 1947 in Lower Bavaria, studied medicine in Frankfurt and Würzburg. Worked as internist, in naturopathic medicine listing, and physical therapy. Until 1994 he was director of the department of "New Research and Treatment Methods—Unconventional Medicine" of the Hessen health insurance medical service. Since then he has been Professor of Naturopathy in the department of internal medicine at the University Hospital, Zurich. His special fields are: complementary medicine, internal medicine, medicinal therapy, physical medicine, medicine consultation for both conventional and unconventional treatments. He has published roughly 150 specialist papers, and is the author or editor of 16 books, the editor of two magazines, and the editor or adviser to several other specialist periodicals.

Christian Skalnik, born 1963 in Vienna, where he studied journalism. From 1987 to 1992 he was editor in the national news section of the Austrian news magazine *profil*. Since then he has been a freelance author and journalist for, among others, the Hamburg weekly *Die Woche*, for *profil*, for SAT 1, RTL, and Austrian Radio. He is the co-author of *Kursbuch Kinder* ("Childhood—a Handbook"), 1993; *Kursbuch Küche* ("Cookery—a Handbook"), 1995; *Kursbuch Lebensqualität* ("Quality of Life—a Handbook"), 1995.

Index

Abies sibirica 34, 46, 192
ACE (angiotensin-converting enzyme) inhibitors 431, 475
acetylcholine 149
acetylsalicylic acid (aspirin) 24, 36, 49, 464
Achillea millefolium 563, 583, 598, 691, 764
acid-forming foods 859
acne 314–22
acupressure 769–71
acupuncture 772–80
addiction 24, 57–66
Adonis vernalis 487
aerobic exercise 9
Aesculus hippocastanum 221, 509, 756
aflatoxins 864
agnus-castus fruit 321, 655, 663, 681, 689
Agrimonia eupatoria 533
agrimony 533
Agropyron repens 387
AIDS (Acquired Immune Deficiency Syndrome) 715–25
Alchemilla vulgaris 534
alcohol 3
    dependence 66
    withdrawal 66–75
alder buckthorn 521
alkali-forming foods 859
allergies 304–13
Allium cepa 596
Allium sativum 429, 441, 473, 497, 640, 739
allopurinol 180

Aloe barbadensis 522
Aloe ferox 522
aloe sap 522
Alpinia officinarum 560, 595
alternative medicine xx–xxi
Althaea officinalis 253, 275, 759
Alzheimer's disease 75–83
ama 790
amalgam fillings 48
amaroids 584
Ananas comosus 221, 296
analphylactic shock 304, 305
Angelica archangelica 557, 592
angelica root 557, 592
angina pectoris 409–19
anthelmintics 624
anthroposophical medicine (AM) 781–6
antibiotics 239, 261, 277, 287, 298, 359, 364, 401, 715, 879
antidepressants 94, 101
antihistamines 287, 304, 364
antioxidants 901, 902
antipsychotic drugs 157
anus 564
anxiety and worry 84–93
anxiolytic drugs 84
appetite, lack of 583–98
appetite stimulants 584
appeite suppressants 57
applied kinesiology (AK) 907–8
Arctosaphylos uva-ursi 390, 763
arm baths 874
arm douche 875
Armoracia rusticana 178, 193, 387

arnica flowers 220, 509
Arnica montana 220, 509
aromatherapy 786–8
arsenic 836
Artemisia absinthium 547, 563, 597
arteriosclerosis 464, 635, 902
arthritis 202–3
arthrosis 202
Aschner, Bernard 809
Asiatic ginseng 139, 740
Asparagus officinalis 386
asparagus root 386
aspirin (acetylsalicyclic acid) 24, 36, 49, 464
asthma 229–39
astral body 782
atherosclerosis 420–30
Atropa belladonna 156
aura 919
auroscopy 920
autogenic training 839, 888–90
autovaccines 880, 881
Avena sativa 119, 337
ayurveda 789–93

Bach, Edward 828–9
Bach Rescue Remedy 829, 830
back douche 876
back pain 167–80
bacteria 3, 548, 664, 879–80
bacterial prostatitis 400
bad humors 809, 810, 811, 812, 813
badgan 897
balm extract 362
balsam of Tolú 571
barberry bark 361
basal metabolic rate 8
baths 873–4
bean pod tea 634
Beard, John 825
Beatles 790
bedwetting (enuresis) 93–100
benzodiazepine 58, 84
Berberis vulgaris 361
beta-blockers 409, 431, 464, 641
beta-carotene 5, 901
beta-sympathomimetics 229
Betula pendual 390

bilberries 533, 754
bile 3
bile ducts 536
bio-aura 919
biocommunication 794
bioelectronics according to Vincent 909–10
biofeedback 891–2
bioresonance therapy (BRT) 794–6
black cohosh root 202, 664, 681, 690
blessed thistle 557, 592
blood glucose levels 5, 627, 628, 866
bloodletting 810–12
blood pressure *see* high blood pressure; low blood pressure
blood testing *see* optimal blood testing
body lice 338
bone density 195
bones, muscle, and joints 167–228
boneset 19
borage oil 349
Borago officinalis 349
brain hemispheres 908
brain meninges 322, 363
brain nerve cells 149
breast disorders 648–55
brewer's yeast 322
brittle bones (osteoporosis) 195–202
bronchitis (herbal remedies) 249–50
BSE 799
Buchinger fasts 865
buck bean leaves 557, 592
Buddhism 895
bugleweed 647, 655
bursitis 222
butterbur root 386

caffeine 23, 24, 33, 452
cajeput oil 33, 45, 177, 190, 213
calcium 7, 195, 801
   with echinacea 313
calcium antagonists 409–10, 431
calcium-retaining hormone 195
Calendula officinalis 313, 349, 759
California poppy 118
calorie intake 8
camomile

baths 362
  tincture combinations 274
  see also German camomile
camphor 177, 191, 213, 227, 453, 812
camphor oil 787
cancer 701–14
cantharidin 699, 812
cantharide poultices 812–14
capillary dynamic blood tests 784,
  920
Capsella bursa-pastoris 691
Capsicum frutescens 179, 193
caraway
  oil 620, 788
  seeds 621
carbamazepine 36
carbo coffeae 533, 754
carbohydrates 4, 7, 636, 859
carbon monoxide poisoning 149, 373
cardiac arrhythmia 454–63
cardiac insufficiency (heart failure)
  474–88
cardiospermum ointment 313
Carica papaya 626, 825
Carmelite water (spirit of melissa)
  118, 191
Carum carvi 620, 621
Caryophylli atheroleum 56, 760
cascara sagrada 522
case reports xx
case studies xx
Cassia angustifolia 525
cassia oil 787
Cassia senna 525
celandine, greater 546
cell therapy 796–800
Centaurium minus 558, 593
centaury 558, 593
Cetraria islandica 252, 561, 596, 757
Chamomilla recutita 257, 560, 571, 581,
  671, 756
chelation therapy 800–2
Chelidonium majus 358, 546
chemoprevention 5
chest douche 875
chi (Chinese) 773, 896
chi (Tibetan) 897
Chi Po 896

chicken pox 322
chicory leaves and root 558, 593
children's ailments 742–65
Chinese cinnamon bark 558
Chinese wormwood 775
chiropractic 844–7
cholesterol 2, 5, 409, 866, 902
  high 635–40
chronic arthritis 202
chronic fatigue 130–40
chronic venous insufficiency 499–511
Chrysanthemum cineraria 341
chylomicrons 635
Cichorium intybus var. *intybus* 558,
  593
Cimicifuga racemosa 202, 664, 681,
  690
cinchona bark 559, 593, 621
Cinchona pubescens 559, 593, 621
Cinchona succirubra 559, 593, 621
cineol 295
Cinnamomum aromaticum 558
Cinnamomum camphora 177, 191, 213,
  227, 453
Cinnamomum verum 559, 594, 621
cinnamon
  bark 559, 594, 621
  oil 787
cirrhosis 599
Citrus aurantium ssp. *aurantium* 562,
  592
Citrus sinensis 561, 596
classical massage 847–50
clove oil 56, 760
Cnicus benedictus 557, 592
cocaine 57
codeine 49, 57
Coffea arabica 533, 754
coffee 23, 35
coffee-withdrawal headache 23
Cola nitida 139
colchicine 181
Colchicum autumnale 181
cold arm baths 874
cold foot baths 873–4
cold packs 878
cold rubbings 874
colds 239–61

coli bacteria 664
colonic hydrotherapy (colonic
    irrigation) 820
coltsfoot
    flowers, aerial parts and roots 250
    leaves 250, 266, 274
comfrey leaves and root 221
Commiphora molmol 275
complementary medicine xxi
compositions 783
condoms 664
condurango bark 594
Confucianism 895
conjunctivitis 359–62
constipation 512–25
constitution 927
contraceptive pill 648
controlled clinical studies xix
Convallaria majalis 486
copper 800
coriander
    oil 787
    seeds 559, 594
Coriandrum sativum var. *vulgare* 559,
    594
cortisone 203, 222
Corydalis cava 118
Cornanthe yohimbe 700
couch grass root 387
coughs (herbal remedies) 250–5
cowslip root 251, 754
crab lice 338
crack 57
crash diets 6–8
Crataegus laevigata 419, 441, 453, 485,
    741
Crataegus monogyna 419, 441, 453,
    485, 741
creeping juniper leaves/tincture 357
Croon, Richard 807, 914
Cucurbita pepo 399, 761
cupping, bloody 815–17
cupping, unbloody 817–18
Cyamopsis tetragonolobus 634
Cynara scolymus 545, 640
cystic mastopathy 648
cystitis 391, 664
cytostatics 350

dairy products 3
dandelion 560, 595, 622
    root and leaves 545
deadly nightshade 156
decoctions 853, 854
Delphinium consolida 625
dementia 75
depression 100–9
detoxification 865
devil's claw 177, 191
diabetes 627–35
diarrhea 525–36
diet 2–8 *see also* nutritional therapies
dietary fiber 3, 5
dietary pharmacology 5
dieting 6–8
digestive system 512–626
digoxin 475
diphenhydramine 119
diuretics 431, 475
diverticulitis 512
dopamine 149
doshas 790–1
douches 875–6
dowager's hump 195
dowsing 910–11
drinking (alcohol) 66
Drosera rotundifolia 255, 762
drug addiction 57–66
Dryopteris filix-mas 626
duodenal ulcer 548–56
    herbal remedies 564
dysbacteria 879
dysbiosis 879

ear acupuncture 776
earache 363–71
ears 363–79
echinacea 313
    combination preparations 20
    coneflowers 19, 389, 713, 724, 755
    root 19, 713, 724, 755
    with calcium 313
Echinacea angustifolia 19
Echinacea pallida 19, 713, 724, 755
Echinacea purpurea 19, 313, 389, 713,
    724, 755
echinacin ointment 313, 755

edukinesthesia 908
ego 782
elderflowers 256, 260
elderly people's ailments 726–41
electrical pills 887
electroacupuncture 776
electroacupuncture according to Voll
   (EAV) 776
  diagnosis 912–13
  treatment 802–6
electroneural somatogram 807
electroneural therapy according to
   Croon (ENT)
  diagnosis 914–15
  treatment 806–7
Eleutherococcus senticosus 138, 740
eliminative methods 809–24
endorphins 777
enemas 819–21
energize 927
energy, energetic 927
energy blockage 927
energy imbalance 927
energy links 928
enuresis (bedwetting) 93–100
enzyme therapy 824–8
enzymes 825
ephedra 239, 251, 453
Ephedra sinica 239, 251, 453
Epsom salt 867
Equisetum arvense 387, 756
Eschscholzia californica 118
Eskimo diet 3
esterase 825
estrogen 672–3
etheric body 782
ethylenediamine tetraacetic acid
   (EDTA) 800, 801
Eucalyptus globulus 178, 192, 214, 256,
   257, 295, 296
eucalyptus
  leaves 256, 296
  oil 178, 192, 214, 257, 295
Eupatorium perfoliatum 19
Euphrasia officinalis 362
evening primrose oil 130, 349, 690
exercise 8–10
exercise therapy 868–70

extensor tendons 217, 222
eyebright 362
eyes 359–62

face douche 876
fasting, therapeutic 864–7
fat-related disorders 635
fatigue, chronic 130–40
fats 2, 3, 4, 636
  high-fat diets 6–7
femidoms 664
fennel
  honey 755
  oil 622
  seeds 622
  water 362
fenugreek seeds 595
fertility problems 656–64
fiber *see* dietary fiber
fibrocystic disease 648
Filipendula ulmaria 258, 260, 759
fir needle oil 34, 46, 192
fitness 8–10
Fitzgerald, William 883
flatulence 613–23
fleawort seeds (dark psyllium) 523, 756
flexor tendons 217, 222
flower remedies 828–30
foci 928
focus theory 804
Foeniculum vulgare 622, 755
foot baths 873–4
Fraxinus ornus 523
free radicals 902
fresh cell cure 797, 798
Freud, Sigmund 838
Freund, Ernst 825
Fumaria officinalis 545
fumitory 545
functiotropic homeopathy 833

galangal root 560, 595
gall bladder disease 536–47
garlic
  combination preparations 474, 498
  corms 429, 441, 473, 497, 640, 739
  oil maceration products 430, 474,
   498, 640, 739

gastric ulcer 548–56
herbal remedies 564
gastritis 548–63
genital herpes 322
gentian root 595, 623
Gentiana lutea 595, 623
German camomile
flowers 560, 571, 581, 671, 756
leaves 257
ginger
root 613
with moxa cones 775
gingko
extract 378, 430, 498, 739
leaves 379, 430, 498
Ginkgo biloba 83, 378, 379, 430, 498,
739
ginseng, Asiatic 139, 740
ginseng, Siberian 138, 740
Glauber's salt 867
globe artichoke leaves 545
extract 640
Glycine max 430, 597, 640, 741
Glycyrrhiza glabra 253, 564, 758
goiter *see* thyroid disorders
gold injections 203
goldenrod 387
golden seal 856
gout 180–7
Graminis flos 178, 192, 214
grapevine 784
greater celandine sap 358
green beans, seedless 400
pods 635
grindelia 251
Grindelia robusta 251
guar meal 634

H₂ antagonists 548
Hahnemann, Samuel 831–2
hair mineral analysis 915–16
Hamamelis virginiana 277, 511, 573, 672
Harpagophytum procumbens 177, 191
hashish 57
hawthorn
combination preparations 485
leaves and blossom 419, 441, 453,
485, 741

Hay, Howard 858–9
hayfever 304
herbal remedies 313
Hay's diet 858–61
hayseeds 178, 192, 214, 878
Head, Henry 882
head lice 338
headache 23–35
healing-earth poultices 371
healthy eating 2–4
heart and circulation 409–511
heart attack 464–74
heart failure (cardiac insufficiency)
474–88
heartburn 548–64
Hedera helix 249, 252, 757
Helicobacter pylori 548
hemorrhoids 564–73
heparin 464
hepatitis 598, 599
hepatodoron 784
herbal teas 853–4
herbalism, medical 853–7
Hering, Constantin 833
heroin 57
herpes 322–30
Herpes simplex 322
Herpes zoster 36, 322
hibiscus flowers 258
Hibiscus sabdarifla 258
high blood pressure (hypertension)
431–42
hip baths 873
Hippocrates 789–90, 809, 841
hirudin 822
Hirudo medicinalis officinalis 822
HIV (human immunodeficiency
virus) 715
hoarseness 261–7
holewort root 118
holistic 928
holistic blood diagnosis (auroscopy)
920
homeopathy 831–7
homotoxicology 834
hops 91, 118
hormone replacement therapy (HRT)
672–3

horse chestnut 221
  combination preparations 510
  extract 509, 756
horseradish root 178, 193, 387
horsetail 387, 756
Huang Ti 896
Humulus lupulus 91, 118
hydrotherapy 871–8
hydrothermal therapy 871–8
hyperglycemia 627
Hypericum perforatum 100, 109, 166,
  725, 762
hypertension (high blood pressure)
  431–42
hyperthyroidism *see* thyroid
  disorders
hypnosis 837–40
hypothyroidism *see* thyroid disorders

ibuprofen 24, 36, 49
ice packs 878
Iceland moss 252, 561, 596, 757
Ilex paraguariensis 140
immune complexes 826
immune system modulation
    (immunomodulation) 10–20,
    121, 928
immunosuppression 11
infertility *see* fertility problems
infusions 853, 854
Ingham, Eunice 884
injection acupuncture 776
insomnia (sleeplessness) 109–20
insulin 627, 628
intercostal neuralgia 36
interferons 121, 598
intestinal flora 820, 878–81
iridology 917–18
irritable bowel syndrome (IBS)
    574–83
itch mites 338
itching 331–8
ivy leaves 249, 252, 757
  extract 757

Jacobson 893
Jamaica dogwood 118
jambul 533

joints, muscle and bone 167–228
Juglans regia 573
juniper 856
Juniperus sabina 357

Kaelin capillary dynamic blood test
    920
kanpo 898
kapha 790
kava
  root 92, 166, 757
  with St. John's wort 109
kidney disease 380–90
kidney stones 380
Kirlian, Semyon and Valentina and
    919
Kirlian photography 918–20
knee douche 875
Kneipp, Sebastian 871
Koch, Robert 879
kola seeds 139
Krameria triandra 275
Kushi, Michio 862

lactic acid 187
lactic acid bacteria 3
lady's mantle 534
Lamium album 277
larkspur flowers 625
laryngitis 261–7
Lavandula angustifolia 92, 119, 454, 690
lavender flowers 92, 119, 454, 690
laxatives 57, 513, 564, 867
LDL cholesterol 635, 902
lead 372, 785, 800, 836
lecithin with vitamins 140 *see also* soy
    lecithin
leeches 822–4
lemon 865
  juice with coffee 25
  oil 787
lemon balm leaves 93, 119, 330, 561,
    623, 691, 758
Leonurus cardiaca 647
Levisticum officinale 388
lice 338–41
Lichen islandicus 561, 596, 757
licorice root 253, 564, 758

life force 928
ligamental sprains 216
ligaments 222–8
lily of the valley 486
    combination preparations 486
limeflowers 252, 258, 260
limited period trials xxiii-xiv
linseed 523, 582, 758
Linum usitatissimum 523, 582, 758
lipoprotein lipase (LPL) 7–8
lipoproteins 635
liver disease 598–608
lovage root 388
low blood pressure (hypotension)
    443–54
lower pole of body 782
lower trunk douche 875
Lycopus europaeus 647, 655
lymphatic drainage 850–2

macrobiotics 861–4
magnesium 195
magnetic field therapy 841–3
Maharishi-Ayur-Veda 790, 792
Maharishi Mahesh Yogi 790
malaria 831
male fern leaves and root 626
mallow leaves and flowers 253,
    758
Malva neglecta 253, 758
Malva sylvestris 253, 758
manganese 800
manic depression 157
manna 523
manual therapies 844–7
Mao Zedong 896
marigold
    flowers 349, 759
    ointment 313
marijuana 57
marjoram 856
Marrubium vulgare 562, 597, 623
Marsdenia cundurango 594
marsh mallow root and leaves 253,
    275, 759
massage 847–52
mastodynia *see* breast disorders
mastopathy *see* breast disorders

maté leaves 140
meadowsweet flowers and leaves
    258, 260, 759
meat eating 2, 3–4
medical herbalism 853–7
Melaleuca alternifolia 322
Melaleuca leucadendron 33, 45, 177,
    190, 213
Melilotus officinalis 222, 338, 510, 573
Melissa officinalis 93, 119, 330, 561,
    623, 691, 758
melon tree
    fruit 825
    leaves 626, 825
meninges 322, 363
menopause 672–81
Mentha arvensis 34, 46, 228, 760
    var. *piperascens* 259, 275
Mentha piperita 34, 215, 228, 259, 296,
    546, 547, 561, 562, 583, 761
menthol 228, 337
Menyanthes trifoliata 557, 592
mercury 48, 372, 785, 793, 800, 836
meridians 773
metabolism 627–47
meteorism 613–23
methadone 58
methotrexate 203
microbiological therapy 879
middle ear infection (otitis media)
    363–71
middle region of body 782
migraine 23–35
milk thistle seeds 608
mint oil 34, 46, 228, 259, 275, 760, 788
mistletoe 179, 784, 785
    injections 20, 714, 725
    stem and leaves 442
mites 338–41
moratherapy 794
Morell, Franz 794
mother tincture 832
motherwort 647
motor-digestive system 783
mouth ulcers 267–77
moxa 775
    cigars 775
    cones 775

moxibustion 775–6
mugwort 856
mullein 254, 760
Multicom 795
multiple sclerosis (MS) 120–30
muscle, bones, and joints 167–228
muscle relaxation according to
    Jacobson 893–4
muscle-relaxing tranquilizers 168
muscle soreness 187–94
muscle strain 216
muscular rheumatism 202
mustard oil 812
mustard seeds for compresses 179,
    193, 214
myalgic encephalomyelitis (ME)
    130–40
myocardial infarction (MI) 464
Myroxylon balsamum var. *pereira* 571
myrrh 275

Naegeli, Otto 844
nasal polyps 286, 287, 363
neck douche 876
nerve-sense system 783
nerve transmitters 149
nervous system and psyche 57–166
nettle 388
    root 399
neuralgia 36–47
neurodermatitis 341–9
neuroleptin 149
neuropathy 140–8
nicotine withdrawal 66–75
Niehans, Paul 797
nifedipine 409
nitroglycerin 409
nits 338
nonbacterial prostatitis 400
nosodes 833–4
nutmeg oil 787
nutritional therapies 858–67

oak bark 534, 572
oat straw 337
oats 119
obesity 2, 6–8
Oenothera biennis 130, 349, 690

onion 596
    rings 371
Ononis spinosa 389
opium tincture 534
optimal blood testing 920–1
orange peel 561, 596 *see also* Seville
    orange peel
organic diets 4–5
organic nitrate preparations 409
organotropic homoeopathy 833
orthomolecular medicine 901
orthosiphon leaves 388
Orthosiphon spicatus 388
Oshawa, Georges 862
osteoarthritis 202–3
osteopathy 844–7
osteoporosis (brittle bone disease)
    195–202
otitis media (middle ear infection)
    363–71

pacemakers 455, 843, 887
packs 878
pain 23–56
pain homonculus 882
painkillers 24, 36, 49, 57, 58, 168, 187,
    222
pale psyllium 524, 582, 761
Palmer, David Daniel 844
Panax ginseng 139, 740
pancreas 627, 825
pansy 761
Papaver somniferum 534
paprika-containing poultices or
    ointments 179, 193
paracetamol 24, 36, 49
Parkinson's disease 149–56
parsley herb and root 389
Passiflora incarnata 93, 119
passionflower 93, 119
Pauling, Linus 901
pectin 534
Péczely, Ignaz von 917
pendulum diagnosis 921–2
pennyroyal 856
    oil 788
peppermint
    leaves 546, 561

peppermint (*continued*)
  oil 34, 215, 228, 259, 296, 547, 562,
    583, 761
periodontosis 47, 48
peripheral nervous system 141
Petasites hybridus 386
Petroselinum crispum 389
Pfeifer crystallization test 920
Phaseolus vulgaris 400, 634, 635
phlebitis 499–511
physical body 782
physical therapies 867–78
physiotherapy 869
phytochemicals 5–6
phytotherapeutic/sedative
    combinations 119
phytotherapy 853–7
pine needle oil 35, 46, 180, 194, 215,
    787
pineapple 825
pineapple enzyme 221, 296
Pinus australis 250
Pinus pinaster 35, 46, 180, 194, 215, 250
Piper methysticum 92, 166, 757
Piscidia erythrina 118
pitta 790
placebos xxi–xxii
Plantago indica 523, 756
Plantago isphaghula 524, 582, 761
Plantago lanceolata 254, 276
Plantago ovata 524, 582, 761
Plantago psyllium 523, 756
plaque 47–8
pneumonia 277–86
pokeroot 856
pollen 140, 596
Polygala senega 254
poplar buds 572
Populi gema 572
Populus tremuloides 400
post-marketing surveillance
    studies xx
Potentilla anserina 535, 691
Potentilla erecta 276, 535
potentization 832
practitioner checklist xxv–xxvi
prakriti 791
premenstrual syndrome (PMS)
    682–91
Primula veris 251, 754
probiotics 878–81
prostate enlargement 391–400
prostratitis 400–8
proteins 2, 636, 859
  high-protein diets 6–7
proteolytic enzymes (proteases) 826
psyche and nervous system 57–166
psychoneuroimmunology xxi–xxii
psychotic disorders 157–66
pulse 8–9
pumpkin seeds 399, 761
purines 3
pyrethrins 341

Quercus petraea 534
Quercus robur 534, 572
Quillaja saponaria 255
quinine 831

radish root 547
randomized 928–9
Raphanus sativus var. *niger* 547
Rasche, Erich 794
rating system xviii–xx
rauwolfia
  root 442
  with St John's wort 109
Rauwolfia serpentina 442
reactive sites 807, 914
Reckeweg, Hans-Heinrich 834
referred pain 884, 929
reflex therapies 881–8
reflex zone massage 883–4
reflexology 883–6
regulation thermography *see*
    thermoregulation diagnosis (TRD)
relaxation techniques 888–94
renal colic 380
Rescue Remedy 829, 830
respiratory ailments 229–303
restharrow root 389
Rhamnus frangula 521
Rhamnus purshiana 522
rhatany root 266, 275
Rheum officinale 524
Rheum palmatum 524

rheumatic fever 202
rheumatism 202–16
rheumatoid arthritis 202, 203
Rhododendri folium 442
rhododendron leaves 442
rhubarb root 524
ribwort 254, 276
rising temperature arm baths 874
rising temperature foot baths 874
rising temperature hip baths 873
risk/benefit evaluation xxii–xxiii
Rosae pseudofructus 259
rose hips 259
rosemary
    leaves 180, 194, 215, 454
    oil 180, 194, 215, 787
    wine 741
Rosmarinus officinalis 180, 194, 215,
    454, 741
Rost, Arno 923
roughage *see* dietary fiber
roundworms 624
Ruscus aculeatus 221, 337, 510, 572

Saccharomyces cerevisiae 322, 535, 765
sage 856
    leaves 267
    oil 788
    oil combination preparations 276
salicylic acid preparations 350
Salix fragilis 35, 194, 202, 216, 261,
    764
Salvia officinalis 276
Sambucus nigra 256, 260
Sandberg 797
Santalum album 390
Saponaria officinalis 254
saunas 876–7
saw palmetto berries 400
scabies 338
schizophrenia 157
Schultz, Johannes 889
Schwamm, Ernst 923
sebum 314
secondary elements of plants 855
selenium 5, 901, 903
self-healing power *see* life force
self-hypnosis 837–40

senna fruits and leaves 525
separation diets 859
Serenoa repens 400
serous otitis 363
Seville orange peel 562, 597
sexual organs, infection and
    discharge 664–72
sexual problems 692–700
shara 897
shepherd's myrtle root 221, 337, 510,
    572
shepherd's purse 691
shiatsu 769–71
shingles 322
Siberian ginseng 138, 740
silver birch leaves 390
silverweed 535, 691
Silybum marianum 608
Sinapsis alba 179, 193, 214
sinusitis 286–96
sitz baths 874
skin 314–58
sleeping tablets 57, 110
sleeplessness (insomnia) 109–20
smoking 66
snake root 254
sniffles and sneezes (herbal
    remedies) 256–9
soapbark 255
soapwort root 254
Solidago virgaurea 387
sore throat 297–303
sour (Seville) orange peel 562, 597
soy lecithin 430, 640, 741
soybean phospholipids 597
spagyric 834–5
Spanish fly ("blister beetle") 699, 812
Spiritus melissae 118, 191
sport 8–10
sprains and strains 216–22
spring adonis 487
    fluid extract in combination 487
spurge 825
squill 488
    combination preparations 488
St. John's wort 100, 109, 166, 725, 762
    oil 762
    with kava 109

with rauwolfia 109
with valerian 120
stagnation *see* energy blockage
steam baths 876–7
Steiner, Rudolf 781–2, 919
Still, Andrew Taylor 844
stimulation therapy 929
Stomach, intestine and digestive
    system 512–626
strawberry, wild 784
stroke 488–98
sundew 255, 762
sweet clover 222, 338, 510, 573
Symphytum officinale 221
synergism 855
synovial bursae 222
Syzygium cumini 533

Tao 896
Taoism 895
tapeworms 624
Taraxacum officinale 545, 560, 595, 622
TCM-style acupuncture 774
tea tree oil 322
tendons 222–8
tenosynovitis 222
Terebinthina laricina 35, 47, 216
testimonials xx
therapeutic fasting 864–7
therapists xxiv–xxvi
thermoregulation diagnosis (TRD)
    923–5
thigh douche 875
threadworms 624
throat *see* laryngitis; sore throat
thuja 20, 763
    drops 714, 725
    oil 787
    tincture 358
Thuja occidentalis 20, 358, 714, 725,
    763
thyme
    common 249, 255, 763
    oil 788
    wild 249
Thymus serpyllum 249
thymus therapy 797, 798, 799
Thymus vulgaris 249, 255, 763

thyroid disorders 641–7
Tibetan medicine 897
Tilia cordata 252, 258, 260
tinnitus 372–9
    maskers 372
tobacco 66
Todo Yoshimasu school 898
tongue diagnosis 925–6
tooth decay 47–8
toothache 47–56
tormentil root 267, 276, 535
touch for health 908
toxins 929
Toyo Yamawaki school 898
traditional Chinese medicine (TCM)
    895–9
traditional Japanese medicine (*kanpo*)
    898
tranquilizers 57
transcutaneous electrical nerve
    stimulation (TENS) 776, 886–8
treatment plans xxiii–xiv
tridosha principle 790
trigeminal neuralgia 36
trigger points 929
triglycerides 866
Trigonella foenum-graecum 595
tumor cells 825–6
turpentine 812
    oil 35, 47, 216, 250
Tussilago farfara 250, 274
Type I (insulin-dependent) diabetes
    627
Type II (non-insulin-dependent)
    diabetes 627

upper pole of body 782
upper trunk douche 875–6
Urginea maritima 488
uric acid 6, 180, 409
urinary system 380–408
urinary tract disease 380–90
Urtica dioica 388, 399
uva-ursi leaves 390, 763
uzara root 536, 764

Vaccinium myrtillus 533, 754
vagina 664

valerian
  root 93, 120, 764
  with St John's wort 120
Valeriana officinalis 93, 120, 764
varicose veins 499–511
vata 790
veganism 3
vegetarianism 3
venous insufficiency, chronic 499–511
Verbascum densiflorum 254, 760
Verbena officinalis 255
vervain 255
vesicants 812
Vincent, Louis-Claude 909
Viola tricolor 761
viruses 322, 350, 664, 715
Viscum album 179, 442, 714, 725
vital energy *see* life force
vitamins 900–4
  A 903
  C 5, 901, 903
  D 195, 903
  E 5, 140, 901, 903
Vitex agnus-castus 321, 655, 663, 681, 689
Vodder 851
Voll, Reinhold 803, 912
vomiting 608–13

walnut leaves 573
warm foot baths 874
warm packs 878
warts 350–8
Wegman, Ita 781–2

weight 6–8
Western acupuncture 774–5
white dead nettle flowers 277
white horehound 562, 597, 623
white poplar extract 400
white sandalwood 390
willow bark 194, 202, 216, 261, 764
  extract 35, 764
wind 613–23
witch hazel 362
  bark 511, 672
  leaves 277, 511, 573, 672
Wolf, Max 825–6
World Health Organization (WHO) 1, 777
worms 624–6
wormwood 547, 563, 597
  Chinese 775
worry *see* anxiety and worry
wraps 877

Xysmalobium undulatum 536, 764

yarrow
  flowers and leaves 691, 764
  shoot and flowers 563, 583, 598
yeast, dried 535, 765
yin and yang 773, 862, 896
yohimbé bark 700

Zen Buddhism 862
zinc 800
Zingiber officinale 613